Methods in Molecular Biology

Series Editor
John M. Walker
School of Life and Medical Sciences
University of Hertfordshire
Hatfield, Hertfordshire, UK

For further volumes:
http://www.springer.com/series/7651

For over 35 years, biological scientists have come to rely on the research protocols and methodologies in the critically acclaimed *Methods in Molecular Biology* series. The series was the first to introduce the step-by-step protocols approach that has become the standard in all biomedical protocol publishing. Each protocol is provided in readily-reproducible step-by-step fashion, opening with an introductory overview, a list of the materials and reagents needed to complete the experiment, and followed by a detailed procedure that is supported with a helpful notes section offering tips and tricks of the trade as well as troubleshooting advice. These hallmark features were introduced by series editor Dr. John Walker and constitute the key ingredient in each and every volume of the *Methods in Molecular Biology* series. Tested and trusted, comprehensive and reliable, all protocols from the series are indexed in PubMed.

Regulatory B Cells

Methods and Protocols

Second Edition

Edited by

Francesca Mion and Silvia Tonon

Department of Medicine, University of Udine, Udine, Italy

Humana Press

Editors
Francesca Mion
Department of Medicine
University of Udine
Udine, Italy

Silvia Tonon
Department of Medicine
University of Udine
Udine, Italy

ISSN 1064-3745 ISSN 1940-6029 (electronic)
Methods in Molecular Biology
ISBN 978-1-0716-1236-1 ISBN 978-1-0716-1237-8 (eBook)
https://doi.org/10.1007/978-1-0716-1237-8

Illustration of the cover page by Paola Tonon

This Humana imprint is published by the registered company Springer Science+Business Media, LLC, part of Springer Nature.
The registered company address is: 1 New York Plaza, New York, NY 10004, U.S.A.

Preface

The immune system is constantly working to ensure what has been appropriately defined as a "dynamic balance." Different immune cell types cooperate one with each other and with the specific environment to restore homeostasis following an insult (e.g., infectious agents, stress, injury, and xenobiotic substance). In this context, regulatory cells constitute a double-edged sword since their suppressive function is beneficial for preventing autoimmunity and chronic inflammation but results detrimental in other contexts, such as in the fight against cancer. In this light, it is easy to understand the interest unleashed in the scientific community when it was understood that even the B cell, mainly known for antibody production, could have a suppressive role on the immune response. The very first reports showed the role of these cells in regulating autoimmunity and chronic inflammation, and, within 20 years, regulatory B cells (Bregs) were described as active actors in different scenarios such as cancer, transplantation, and pregnancy. The interest in this functional B-cell subset emerged also through the relentless search for a unique marker that could univocally identify Bregs. However, despite the great effort devolved to this aim, several intracellular and extracellular markers have been associated to the regulatory phenotype of B cells, rendering somehow confusing the analysis of this population. In order to try to overcome these problematics, in the last few years several groups have started to apply cutting-edge molecular biology technologies for the study of Bregs, both in the murine and human context.

This second edition of the "Regulatory B Cells—Methods and Protocols" book reflects all these aspects. Following a first part that collects the protocols for the purification and characterization of B-cell subsets linked to the regulatory phenotype, the methods for characterizing the Breg suppressive mechanisms are presented. This second part of the book has significantly strengthened since the first edition, precisely as a consequence of the identification of new cellular markers associated with Bregs. The third part of the book is perhaps the most innovative because it collects those cutting-edge molecular methodologies helpful for the study of the intracellular pathways involved in the development and/or differentiation of Bregs. In this context, there is still much to do and to discover, and we think that, in the coming years, there will be a significant increase in studies exploiting these methodologies. The last part is focused on the analysis of Bregs in pathological settings, but, this time, our choice fell on different diseases as a demonstration of the very different conditions in which these Bregs play a role.

The use of reliable and highly reproducible methods is always the best starting point when looking for the answer to a scientific question. We hope that the protocols presented in this book will be useful to the scientific community and that they can serve to clarify some still unsolved aspects of Bregs research.

Udine, Italy

Francesca Mion
Silvia Tonon

Contents

Contributors

RITA AGAYBY • *Department of Medicine, Division of Respirology, McMaster University, Hamilton, ON, Canada*
ROWA Y. ALHABBAB • *Facility of Applied Medical Sciences, Medical Laboratory Technology Department, Immunology Group, King Abdulaziz University, Jeddah, Saudi Arabia*
ALAITZ ARANBURU • *Department of Rheumatology and Inflammation Research, University of Gothenburg, Gothenburg, Sweden*
UTTIYA BASU • *Department of Microbiology and Immunology, Vagelos College of Physicians and Surgeons, Columbia University, New York, NY, USA*
NICOLE BAUMGARTH • *Center for Immunology & Infectious Diseases, Schools of Medicine and Veterinary Medicine, University of California, Davis, CA, USA; Dept. Pathology, Microbiology and Immunology, Schools of Medicine and Veterinary Medicine, University of California, Davis, CA, USA*
JOANNE BOLDISON • *Division of Infection and Immunity, Cardiff University School of Medicine, Cardiff, UK*
HANNAH F. BRADFORD • *Centre for Rheumatology, Division of Medicine, University College London, London, UK*
SOPHIE BROUARD • *CHU Nantes, Université de Nantes, Inserm, Centre de Recherche en Transplantation et Immunologie, UMR 1064, ITUN, Nantes, France; Labex IGO, Nantes, France; Centre d'Investigation Clinique en Biothérapie, Centre de ressources biologiques (CRB), Nantes, France*
SEBASTIEN CALBO • *INSERM U1234, Normandy University, Rouen, France*
RITA CARSETTI • *B Cell Physiopathology Unit, Immunology Research Area, Bambino Gesù Children Hospital, Rome, Italy*
SIMONA CASCIOLI • *B Cell Physiopathology Unit, Immunology Research Area, Bambino Gesù Children Hospital, Rome, Italy*
MATHILDE A. M. CHAYÉ • *Department of Parasitology, Leiden University Medical Center, Leiden, The Netherlands*
MÉLANIE CHESNEAU • *CHU Nantes, Université de Nantes, Inserm, Centre de Recherche en Transplantation et Immunologie, UMR 1064, ITUN, Nantes, France; Labex IGO, Nantes, France*
JIN KYEONG CHOI • *Molecular Immunology Section, Laboratory of Immunology, National Eye Institute (NEI), National Institutes of Health, Bethesda, MD, USA; Department of Immunology, Jeonbuk National University Medical School, Jeonju, Jeonbuk, Republic of Korea*
VAN DUC DANG • *Deutsches Rheuma-Forschungszentrum, a Leibniz Institute, Berlin, Germany; Department of Cell Biology, Faculty of Biology, University of Science, Vietnam National University, Hanoi, Vietnam; Vinmec Institute of Stem Cell and Gene Technology, Vinmec Healthcare System, Hanoi, Vietnam*
LARISSA CAMARGO DA ROSA • *Division of Infection and Immunity, Cardiff University School of Medicine, Cardiff, UK*
QING DING • *Department of Surgery, Thomas E. Starzl Transplantation Institute, University of Pittsburgh School of Medicine, Pittsburgh, PA, USA*
BONNIE N. DITTEL • *Versiti Blood Research Institute, Milwaukee, WI, USA*

Charles E. Egwuagu • *Molecular Immunology Section, Laboratory of Immunology, National Eye Institute (NEI), National Institutes of Health, Bethesda, MD, USA*
Simon Fillatreau • *Institut Necker-Enfants Malades, INSERM U1151-CNRS UMR 8253, Paris, France; Faculté de Médecine, Université de Paris, Paris, France; AP-HP, Hôpital Necker Enfants Malades, Paris, France*
Gail M. Gauvreau • *Department of Medicine, Division of Respirology, McMaster University, Hamilton, ON, Canada*
Ezio Giorda • *B Cell Physiopathology Unit, Immunology Research Area, Bambino Gesù Children Hospital, Rome, Italy*
Jeremy W. Herzog • *Center for Gastrointestinal Biology and Disease, Department of Medicine, Division of Gastroenterology and Hepatology, University of North Carolina at Chapel Hill, Chapel Hill, NC, USA*
Shunji Ishihara • *Department of Internal Medicine II, Shimane University Faculty of Medicine, Izumo, Japan*
Mohamed Khalil • *Versiti Blood Research Institute, Milwaukee, WI, USA; Molecular Biology Department, National Research Centre, Cairo, Egypt*
Hoa Le Mai • *CHU Nantes, Université de Nantes, Inserm, Centre de Recherche en Transplantation et Immunologie, UMR 1064, ITUN, Nantes, France; Labex IGO, Nantes, France*
Xiang Lin • *School of Chinese Medicine and Shenzhen Institute of Research and Innovation, The University of Hong Kong, Hong Kong, China*
Andreia C. Lino • *Deutsches Rheuma-Forschungszentrum, a Leibniz Institute, Berlin, Germany*
Bo Liu • *Center for Gastrointestinal Biology and Disease, Department of Medicine, Division of Gastroenterology and Hepatology, University of North Carolina at Chapel Hill, Chapel Hill, NC, USA*
Giovanna Lombardi • *MRC Centre for Transplantation, School of Immunology & Mucosal Biology, King's College London, London, UK*
Liwei Lu • *Department of Pathology and Shenzhen Institute of Research and Innovation, The University of Hong Kong, Hong Kong, China*
Steven K. Lundy • *Graduate Program in Immunology, Program in Biomedical Sciences and Division of Rheumatology, Department of Internal Medicine, University of Michigan Medical School, Ann Arbor, MI, USA*
Maik Luu • *Institute for Medical Microbiology and Hygiene, Philipps-University Marburg, Marburg, Germany*
Maud Maho-Vaillant • *INSERM U1234, Normandy University, Rouen, France; Dermatology Department, Rouen University Hospital, Rouen, France*
Eleonora Martinis • *Department of Medicine (DAME), University of Udine, Udine, Italy*
Diana E. Matei • *Centre for Rheumatology, Division of Medicine, University College London, London, UK*
Claudia Mauri • *Centre for Rheumatology, Division of Medicine, University College London, London, UK*
Daniel Michaud • *Department of Cell Biology and Physiology, The University of North Carolina at Chapel Hill School of Medicine, Chapel Hill, NC, USA*
Francesca Mion • *Department of Medicine (DAME), University of Udine, Udine, Italy*
Bhalchandra Mirlekar • *Lineberger Comprehensive Cancer Center, The University of North Carolina at Chapel Hill School of Medicine, Chapel Hill, NC, USA*

YOSHIYUKI MISHIMA • *Department of Internal Medicine II, Shimane University Faculty of Medicine, Izumo, Japan*

KANISHKA MOHIB • *Department of Surgery, Thomas E. Starzl Transplantation Institute, University of Pittsburgh School of Medicine, Pittsburgh, PA, USA*

AKIHIKO OKA • *Center for Gastrointestinal Biology and Disease, Department of Medicine, Division of Gastroenterology and Hepatology, University of North Carolina at Chapel Hill, Chapel Hill, NC, USA; Department of Internal Medicine II, Shimane University Faculty of Medicine, Izumo, Shimane, Japan*

JOHN PAUL OLIVERIA • *School of Medicine, Department of Pathology, Stanford University, Stanford, CA, USA; Department of Medicine, Division of Respirology, McMaster University, Hamilton, ON, Canada*

ARIFA OZIR-FAZALALIKHAN • *Department of Parasitology, Leiden University Medical Center, Leiden, The Netherlands*

GIADA PACE • *Department of Medicine (DAME), University of Udine, Udine, Italy*

CARLO E. M. PUCILLO • *Department of Medicine (DAME), University of Udine, Udine, Italy*

YULIYA PYLAYEVA-GUPTA • *Lineberger Comprehensive Cancer Center, The University of North Carolina at Chapel Hill School of Medicine, Chapel Hill, NC, USA; Department of Genetics, The University of North Carolina at Chapel Hill School of Medicine, Chapel Hill, NC, USA*

AVIJIT RAY • *Versiti Blood Research Institute, Milwaukee, WI, USA*

M. MANUELA ROSADO • *B Cell Physiopathology Unit, Immunology Research Area, Bambino Gesù Children Hospital, Rome, Italy*

ELIZABETH C. ROSSER • *Centre for Rheumatology, Division of Medicine, University College London, London, UK*

DAVID M. ROTHSTEIN • *Department of Surgery, Thomas E. Starzl Transplantation Institute, University of Pittsburgh School of Medicine, Pittsburgh, PA, USA; Department of Immunology, University of Pittsburgh, Pittsburgh, PA, USA*

R. BALFOUR SARTOR • *Center for Gastrointestinal Biology and Disease, Department of Medicine, Division of Gastroenterology and Hepatology, University of North Carolina at Chapel Hill, Chapel Hill, NC, USA; Department of Microbiology and Immunology, University of North Carolina at Chapel Hill, Chapel Hill, NC, USA; National Gnotobiotic Rodent Resource Center, University of North Carolina at Chapel Hill, Chapel Hill, NC, USA*

MARCO SCARSELLA • *B Cell Physiopathology Unit, Immunology Research Area, Bambino Gesù Children Hospital, Rome, Italy*

HERMELIJN H. SMITS • *Department of Parasitology, Leiden University Medical Center, Leiden, The Netherlands*

JIANBO SUN • *Guanghua School of Stomatology, Hospital of Stomatology, Sun Yat-Sen University, Guangzhou, China*

SOPHINA H. TAITANO • *Graduate Program in Immunology, Program in Biomedical Sciences and Division of Rheumatology, Department of Internal Medicine, University of Michigan Medical School, Ann Arbor, MI, USA*

SILVIA TONON • *Department of Medicine (DAME), University of Udine, Udine, Italy*

CHIARA TONTINI • *Allergy Unit, Department of Internal Medicine, University Hospital of Ancona, Ancona, Italy*

Viviana Valeri • *Department of Medicine (DAME), University of Udine, Udine, Italy; Faculté de Médecine, Institut Necker-Enfants Malades (INEM), INSERM U1151-CNRS UMR8253, Université de Paris, Paris, France*

Luciën E. P. M. van der Vlugt • *Division of Rheumatology, Department of Internal Medicine, University of Michigan Medical School, Ann Arbor, MI, USA*

Alexander Visekruna • *Institute for Medical Microbiology and Hygiene, Philipps-University Marburg, Marburg, Germany*

Astrid L. Voskamp • *Department of Parasitology, Leiden University Medical Center, Leiden, The Netherlands*

Xiaohui Wang • *Department of Pathology and Shenzhen Institute of Research and Innovation, The University of Hong Kong, Hong Kong, China*

F. Susan Wong • *Division of Infection and Immunity, Cardiff University School of Medicine, Cardiff, UK*

Vanessa Yenson • *Center for Immunology & Infectious Diseases, Schools of Medicine and Veterinary Medicine, University of California, Davis, CA, USA; University of Technology Sydney, Sydney, NSW, Australia*

Part I

Purification and Phenotypic Characterization of B Cell Subsets with Breg Traits

Chapter 1

Purification and Characterization of Murine MZ and T2-MZP Cells

M. Manuela Rosado, Alaitz Aranburu, Marco Scarsella, Simona Cascioli, Ezio Giorda, and Rita Carsetti

Abstract

The spleen is the second major reservoir of B cells in the adult. In the spleen, cells, generated in the bone marrow, are selected, mature, and become part of the peripheral B-cell pool. Murine spleen comprises several B-cell subsets representing various maturation stages and/or cell functions. The spleen is a complex lymphoid organ organized into two main structures with different functions: the red and white pulp. The red pulp is flowed with blood while the white pulp is organized in primary follicles, with a B-cell area composed of follicular B cells and a T-cell area surrounding a periarterial lymphatic sheath. The frontier between the red and white pulp is defined as the marginal zone (MZ) and contains the MZ B cells. Because B cells, localized in different areas, are characterized by distinct expression levels of B-cell receptor (BCR) and of other surface markers, splenic B-cell subsets can be easily identified and purified by flow cytometry analyses and fluorescence-activated cell sorting (FACS).

Here, we will focus on MZ B cells and on their precursors, giving some experimental hints to identify, generate, and isolate these cells. We will combine the use of FACS analysis and confocal microscopy to visualize MZ B cells in cell suspensions and in tissue sections, respectively. We will also give some clues to analyze B-cell repertoire on isolated MZ-B cells.

Key words Flow cytometry, Transitional B cells, Marginal zone B cells, Spleen, Heavy chain sequencing, Heavy chain repertoire

1 Introduction

B lymphocytes can be classified into different subsets according to their origin, function, and localization. Each B-cell subset expresses a combination of cell surface markers that allow its identification/purification using flow cytometry analysis and cell sorting [1]. The primary B-cell marker, which also confers B-cell identity, is the B-cell antigen receptor (BCR), i.e., the membrane-bound antibody molecule [2]. BCRs possess two identical heavy and light chains that together form the antibody on the B-cell surface. BCRs are generated by highly controlled DNA rearrangements by a process

Francesca Mion and Silvia Tonon (eds.), *Regulatory B Cells: Methods and Protocols*, Methods in Molecular Biology, vol. 2270, https://doi.org/10.1007/978-1-0716-1237-8_1, © Springer Science+Business Media, LLC, part of Springer Nature 2021

known as V(D)J recombination where discrete germ line gene segments known as variable (V), diversity (D), and joining (J) are assembled during early B-cell differentiation [2]. In the mouse, the first BCR-expressing cells appear as early as at the embryonic day 16 (ED16) of gestation and are generated from fetal liver hematopoietic stem cells (HSCs) [3, 4]. Although HSCs start to colonize the embryonic spleen at ED12 and bone marrow at ED15–16, the fetal liver retains hematopoietic functions until birth [5]. After birth, the majority of B cells originate in the bone marrow with the exception of a minor B-cell population originating in the spleen [6]. B cells exit the bone marrow at immature/transitional developmental stage [7, 8] and migrate to the peripheral organs [7] where they differentiate into mature, memory, and antibody-secreting cells (ASC) (*see* Fig. 1a–c). Bone marrow-derived B cells preferentially replenish B-cell pools that will generate the acquired immune responses, mostly follicular B cells in the lymph nodes and in the spleen and B2 cells in the peritoneal cavity [7]. Although B-cell turnover at the periphery is low [9], the daily B-cell output from the bone marrow allows a continuous "refreshment" of the antigenic specificities of the follicular/B2 B-cell pools in lymph nodes, peritoneal cavity, and spleen. The fate of immature B cells, once they arrive into the periphery, is mostly determined by the BCR specificity and consequently on the signal strength (survival or cell death) delivered through the BCR [10, 11].

The spleen consists of three different interrelated areas: the red pulp, the white pulp, and the marginal zone, each of them performing different functions [12], whereas the red pulp is a sponge-like tissue filled with blood where damaged circulating cells and particulate antigen are removed, the white pulp is a lymphoid tissue, similar to a lymph node, made of defined T- and B-cell areas (*see* Fig. 2a, b). The most peculiar area of the spleen is the marginal zone (MZ) surrounding the white pulp and in contact with the blood flowing in the open circulation of the red pulp. The MZ is composed of a reticular network of metallophilic macrophages (MMM), located in the inner part of the MZ near the white pulp, marginal macrophages (MZM), which can be found in the outer MZ toward the red pulp, and the marginal zone B cells (*see* Fig. 2c, d), a layer of B cells ready to generate plasma cells and produce antibodies [13, 14].

Table 1 describes several mouse models in which the development of MZ B cells is impaired. In addition to mature B cells, the spleen contains B-cell precursors of fetal origin that can generate B cells "on demand." These precursors sustain the production of the so-called innate B cells, specifically B-1a B cells, in the body cavities and marginal zone B cells in the spleen [6]. In spite of the lack of consensus on the origin of certain B-cell subsets, such as the dichotomy of B-1 versus B-2 B cells, the characterization of the mouse B-cell compartments is well established. Indeed, through

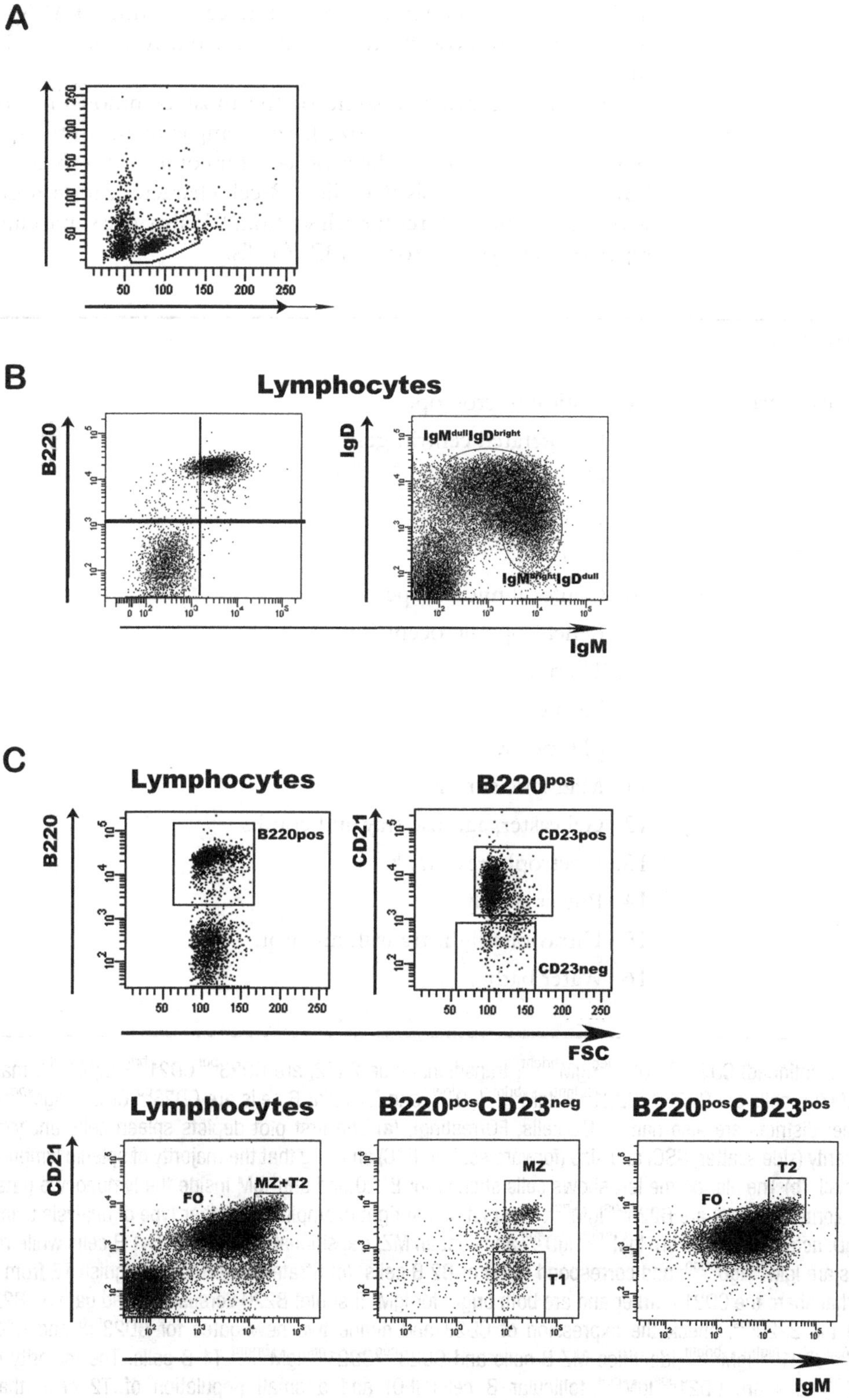

Fig. 1 Representative flow cytometry plots showing spleen cell suspensions analyzed for the expression of CD21, CD23, B220, IgM, and IgD molecules. Spleen B cells can be classified into various subsets according to the expression of CD21, CD23, IgD, and IgM. Briefly, transitional type 1 (T1) B cells are

multiparametric fluorescence-activated cell sorting (FACS) analyses, it is now possible to identify and purify almost all B-cell subsets.

Herein, we describe some of the most common procedures used to isolate and characterize B-cell compartments of the spleen. In particular, we present the protocols for confocal microscopy and flow cytometry analysis that allow B-cell characterization together with staining procedures for cell sorting. We also give some clues on repertoire analysis on sorted MZ B cells.

2 Materials

2.1 Equipment

1. Optical microscope.
2. Refrigerated centrifuge.
3. Flow cytometer.
4. Cell sorter.
5. Cryostat.
6. Confocal microscope.
7. Bench top microcentrifuge.
8. Thermal cycler.
9. Balance.
10. pH meter.
11. Magnetic stirrer.
12. Gel caster, agarose tray and combs.
13. Electrophoresis tank.
14. Power supply.
15. Ultraviolet light transilluminator.
16. Water bath.

Fig. 1 (continued) CD23^{neg}CD21^{neg}IgM^{bright}, transitional type 2 (T2) are CD23^{pos}CD21^{bright}IgM^{bright}, marginal zone (MZ) B cells are CD23^{neg}CD21^{bright}IgM^{bright}IgD^{low}, and follicular B cells are CD23^{pos}CD21^{pos}IgM^{pos}IgD^{pos} (in other districts are also named B2 cells, FO/resting). (**a**) The first plot depicts spleen cells analyzed for granularity (side scatter, SSC) and size (forward scatter, FSC) showing that the majority of splenic lymphocytes are small. (**b**) The plot on the left shows cells stained for B220 and anti-IgM inside the lymphocyte gate, and the majority of B cells are B220^{pos}IgM^{pos}. The plot on the right exemplifies another type of analysis using IgM and IgD: activated B cells are IgM^{bright}IgD^{dull} and contain MZ, transitional B cells, and B-1 B cells while resting B cells are IgM^{dull}IgD^{bright} and correspond to FO or B2 B cells. (**c**) Strategy used to distinguish T2 from MZ B cells that share the CD21 marker and are both bright for IgM: first plot B220 versus FSC and gate on B220^{pos}; inside the B220^{pos}, check the expression of CD23 and define two new gates for CD23^{neg} and CD23^{pos}. CD23^{neg}CD21^{high}IgM^{bright} identifies MZ B cells and CD23^{neg}CD21^{neg}IgM^{bright} T1 B cells. The majority of the CD23^{pos} cells are CD21^{pos}IgM^{pos} follicular B cells (FO) and a small population of T2 cells that are CD21^{high}IgM^{bright}

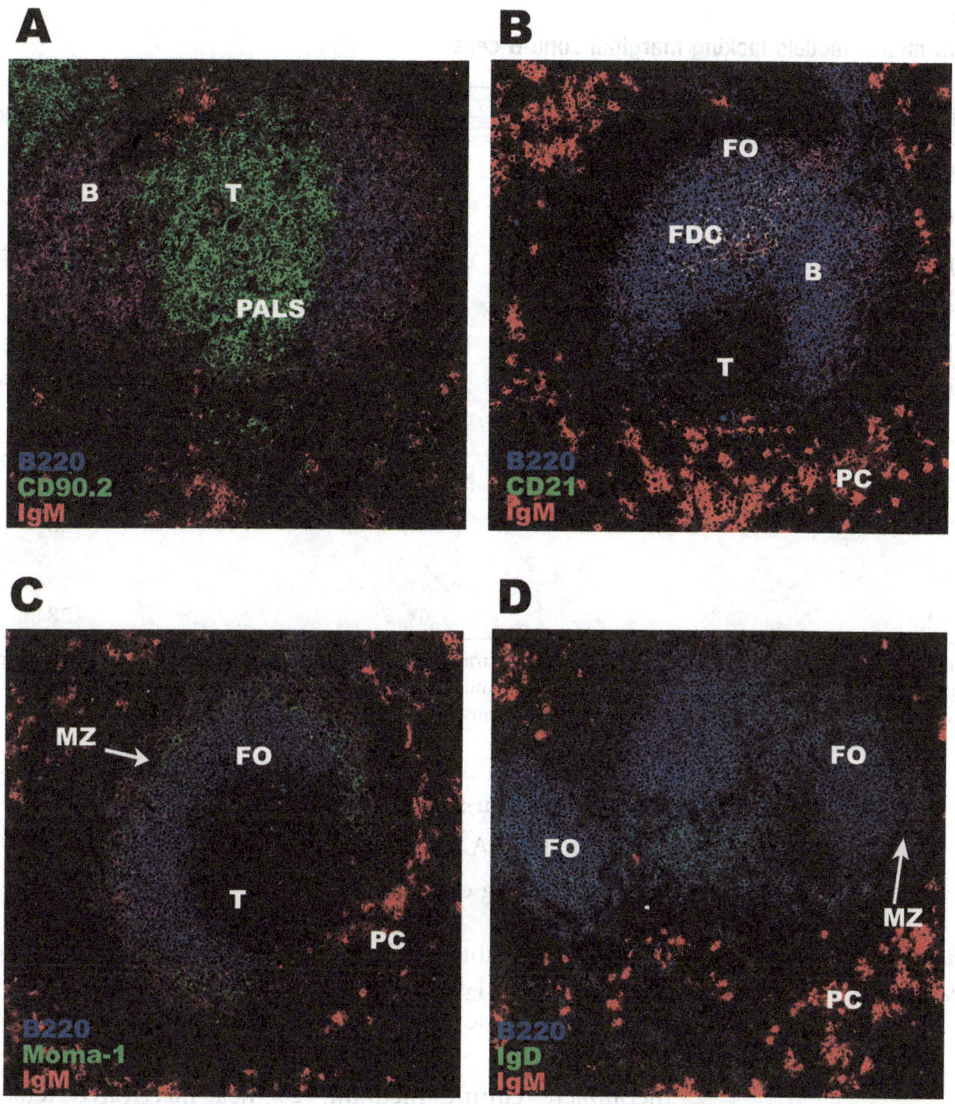

Fig. 2 Representative confocal images showing the expression of B220 (formally CD45R), CD21, CD90, Moma-1, IgD, and IgM in adult spleens. (**a**) Spleen sections from 8- to 10-week-old mice were stained for B220 (*blue*), IgM (*red*), and CD90.2 (*green*). Primary follicles (FO) are visible with the T-cell area (T) around the periarteriolar lymphoid sheath (PALS) and more externally the B-cell areas (B). (**b**) The panel shows a representative example of a spleen section stained for B220 (*blue*), IgM (*red*), and CD21 (*green*). CD21 stains follicular reticular dendritic cells that can be observed as a net inside the primary follicle (yellow staining inside the FO). Outside the follicle, a considerable proportion of cells is IgM^{bright} B220^{low} and most probably corresponds to IgM-producing cells (PC). (**c**) Sections were stained for B220 (*blue*), IgM (*red*), and Moma-1 (*green*). Moma-1^{pos} cells, surrounding the primary follicle (FO), correspond to the marginal zone (MZ, see *arrow*) with IgM^{bright} B220^{pos} MZ B cells lining externally to the ring of the Moma-1^{pos} cells. IgM^{bright} B220^{low} plasma cells (PC) are found outside the MZ. (**d**) The panel presents sections of the adult spleen stained for B220 (*blue*), IgM (*red*), and IgD (*green*). All B cells inside the primary follicle (FO) are IgD^{pos} IgM^{pos} B220^{pos} corresponding to mature follicular B cells. MZ B cells are found around the FO as IgD$^{dull/neg}$ IgM^{pos} B220^{pos} (MZ, *arrow*). All images were acquired at $\times 40$ objective amplification

Table 1
Mutant mouse models lacking marginal zone B cells

Deficient gene or molecule	References
LTα	[16]
LT-β	[17]
LT-β and TNF	[18]
LT-α, LT-β, and TNF	[19]
LT-βR	[20]
NIK	[21, 22]
NF-κB p50	[23, 24]
REL-B	[25]
PyK2	[26]
Aiolos	[27]
NKX2.3	[28]

LT lymphotoxin, *LT-βR* LT-β receptor, *NF-κB* nuclear factor-κB, *NIK* NF-κB-inducing kinase, *PYK2* protein tyrosine kinase 2, *Aiolos* zinc finger protein, also known as Ikaros family zinc finger protein 3, *NKX2.3* NK2-transcription factor-related locus 3. Note that the references cited in this table must be considered as a starting point since they are just a small part of the present literature on these topics

17. Shaking and non-shaking incubators at 37 °C.
18. Automated DNA plasmid purification robot (*see* **Note 1**).
19. Burker counting chamber.

2.2 Solutions for Cell Preparation

1. 10× phosphate-buffered saline (PBS), pH = 7.2: dissolve 43 g of $NaH_2PO_4{\cdot}2H_2O$, 258 g of $Na_2HPO_4{\cdot}12H_2O$, and 850 g of NaCl to a volume of 10 l of distilled H_2O, check the pH, and store at 4 °C.
2. Incomplete culture medium: 2% heat-inactivated fetal calf serum (FCS) in RPMI 1640 (*see* **Note 2**).
3. Gey's solution: it should be prepared fresh each time by mixing 14 mL sterile H_2O, 4 mL solution A (35 g NH_4Cl, 1.85 g KCl, 1.5 g $Na_2HPO_4{\cdot}12H_2O$, 0.119 g KH_2PO_4, 5 g glucose, 25 g gelatin, and 0.05 g phenol red in 1 l of distilled H_2O), 1 mL solution B (0.14 g $MgSO_4{\cdot}7H_2O$, 0.42 g $MgCl_2{\cdot}6H_2O$, and 0.34 g $CaCl_2{\cdot}2H_2O$ in 100 mL of distilled H_2O), and 1 mL solution C (2.25 g $NaHCO_3$ in 100 mL of distilled H_2O). Autoclave solutions A, B, and C at 120 °C and store in dark at 4 °C.
4. Trypan blue solution: dilute Trypan blue stock solution 1:1 in 1× PBS.
5. Cryostat embedding medium: optimum cutting temperature (OCT) compound.

Table 2
Monoclonal antibodies used to characterize mouse B-cell subsets

Anti-mouse	Clone
CD1b (Ly-38)	1B1
CD16 (FcγIII/IIR)	2.4G2
CD19	1D3
CD21	7G6
CD23	B3B4
CD43	S7
CD45R (B220)	RA3-6B2
CD80 (B7–1)	16-10A1
CD86 (B7–2)	GL1
CD90.2 (Thy1.2)	53–2.1
IgM	2911
IgD	11.26c
Moma-1	MCA947F

2.3 Flow Cytometry Analysis

1. FACS buffer: 2% FCS, 0.01% sodium azide, in 1× PBS (*see* **Note 3**).
2. FACS buffer for cell sorting: 2% FCS in 1× PBS.
3. Antibodies routinely used for mouse B cell population staining (*see* Table 2).

2.4 Immuno-fluorescence

1. Cold acetone (+4 °C).
2. Blocking solution: 5% bovine serum albumin (BSA) in 1× PBS.
3. Hoechst 33342 fluorescent stain.
4. Anti-fade reagent.

Mouse antibodies: anti-CD21, anti-CD90.2, anti-Moma-1, anti-IgM, and anti-IgD (*see* Table 2).

2.5 RNA Isolation and cDNA Synthesis for Repertoire Analysis

1. RNA extraction kit (*see* **Note 4**).
2. Ethanol (95–99% purity).
3. Nuclease-free water.
4. Kit for complementary DNA (cDNA) synthesis, usually made of random hexamers, dNTPs, buffers, and reverse transcriptase.

Table 3
PCR amplification oligonucleotides used for repertoire analysis

Oligo name	5′–3′ sequence	
5′ MsVHE	GGGAATTCGAGGTGCAGCTGCAGGAGTCTGG	Forward
3′ Cμ outer	AGGGGGCTCTCGCAGGAGACGAGG	Reverse

2.6 PCR Amplification, Product Purification, Subcloning, and Propagation in Bacteria

1. High-fidelity PCR amplification system including high-fidelity enzyme mix (a blend of thermostable DNA polymerases with proofreading activity), high-fidelity buffer, $MgCl_2$, dNTP mix, and nuclease-free water.
2. PCR amplification oligonucleotides used for repertoire analysis (*see* Table 3 and [15]).
3. Cloning kit containing vectors for sequencing (*see* **Note 5**).
4. Agarose powder.
5. 10× Tris-borate-EDTA (TBE) buffer: dissolve 108 g of Tris base, 55 g of boric acid, and 7.4 g of ethylenediaminetetraacetic acid (EDTA) to a volume of 1000 mL of distilled H_2O, and store at 15–20 °C (*see* **Note 6**).
6. 1× TBE buffer: dilute 100 mL of 10× TBE buffer to 1 L with deionized water.
7. Dye for nucleic acid detection in gel (*see* **Note** 7).
8. Orange G loading dye.
9. DNA ladder.
10. PCR cleanup and purification kit.
11. High-efficiency competent bacteria supplied/recommended by the choice of cloning kit.
12. Luria Bertani (LB) liquid and solid media.
13. Agar.
14. Kanamycin.
15. Sterile disposable loops.

3 Methods

3.1 Tissue Collection for Immunohistochemistry

1. Sacrifice mice by cervical dislocation (*see* **Note 8**). Collect the spleen and divide it in half with a longitudinal cut, using a sterile scalpel.
2. Prepare a small square of aluminum foil (*see* **Note 9**), roll it around the finger to make a small cylinder, close one side, put half of the spleen inside adding OCT, fold the paper to close in a pack, and drag it in liquid nitrogen (*see* **Note 10**).
3. Store tissues at −80 °C.

3.2 Cell Preparation

1. Prepare single-cell suspensions from the remaining half of the spleen by smashing the organ between two frosted slides in 5 mL of incomplete culture medium. Leave the splenocytes on ice for 5 min to allow debris to sediment and then transfer cells into clean 15 mL tubes. Wash the cells by centrifuging the tubes at 250 × *g* for 10 min at 4 °C.
2. Lyse red blood cells by resuspending the cell pellet in 5 mL of Gey's solution and incubating for 1 min at room temperature. Add 5 mL of incomplete culture medium and wash the cells by centrifuging the tubes at 250 × *g* for 10 min at 4 °C. Resuspend cells in 5 mL incomplete culture medium and keep the tubes on ice (*see* **Note 11**).
3. Count viable nucleated cells by trypan blue exclusion on a Burker counting chamber. Take 10 μL of the cell suspension and mix it with 90 μL of Trypan blue solution.

3.3 Staining Procedures for Flow cytometry Analysis

For each tissue, prepare a scheme with all the B-cell populations you want to analyze and choose the surface antibodies for the staining procedures accordingly. Table 4 shows a combination of useful markers that one should follow to characterize the main peripheral B-cell subsets, with some suggested bibliography. Carry out all procedures on ice and protect the samples from light.

1. For each staining condition, collect 1 × 10^6 cells in a round-bottom 96-well plate.
2. Centrifuge plate at 250 × *g* for 5 min at 4 °C and remove the supernatant by inverting the plate (*see* **Note 12**).

Table 4
B-cell subsets in peripheral lymphoid organs

	Main surface markers	Main localization	References
Recirculating B	B220^{bright}IgM^{pos}IgD^{pos}	Bone marrow blood	[29]
Transitional 1	B220^{pos}IgM^{bright}CD21^{neg}CD23^{neg} CD43^{neg}	Spleen	[7]
Transitional 2	B220^{pos}IgM^{bright}CD21^{bright}CD23^{pos}	Spleen	[7]
Follicular or B2	B220^{pos}IgD$^{pos/bright}$IgM^{pos}CD5^{neg} CD21^{pos}CD23^{pos}	Spleen/lymph node peritoneal cavity	[11]
Marginal zone	B220^{pos}IgM^{bright}CD1^{high}CD21^{bright} CD23^{neg} CD80^{pos} CD86^{pos}	Spleen	[12, 14]
B-1a	B220^{low}IgM^{bright}IgD^{dull}CD5^{pos} CD11b^{pos}	Peritoneal cavity	[30, 31]
B-1b	B220^{low}IgM^{bright}IgD^{dull}CD5^{neg} CD11b^{pos}	Peritoneal cavity	[32]

Note that because we still lack a unique phenotypic marker able to distinguish memory B cells from naïve B cells in the mouse, the memory B-cell subset was not included in the table

3. According to the specific experimental design, add 10 μL of each required antibody (*see* Table 2) diluted in FACS buffer to the cell pellet and shake gently (*see* **Note 13**). Make sure that the cell pellet is resuspended.
4. Incubate the cells on ice for 20 min and protect from light. At the end of the incubation, add 200 μL of FACS buffer and spin at 250 × *g* for 5 min at 4 °C.
5. Remove supernatant and resuspend the pellet in 200 μL of FACS buffer. Transfer the cells into FACS tubes. Wash the wells with an additional 200 μL of FACS buffer to recover all the cells and add to the tubes. Analyze using a flow cytometer (*see* **Note 14**).
6. Perform doublet exclusion by gating diagonal signals on forward height (H)/forward width (W) scatter plot. Dead cells can be excluded from the analysis by gating (*see* Fig. 3a and **Note 15**).

3.4 Staining Procedures for Cell Sorting

Follicular B cells are the most abundant B-cell subset in the spleen followed by MZ-B cells, and transitional B cells which are the rarest. In fact, because they represent 0.5–0.7% of the total number of spleen cells, the sorting procedure requires no less than 20×10^7 nucleated cells as starting material. Under these conditions, the final yields will be approximately 1×10^6 sorted cells. Consider that with this number of cells as starting point, this implies to use 4–5 mouse spleens for each experiment (*see* **Note 16**). After splenocytes isolation, carry out all procedures on ice and protect the samples from light.

1. Collect 1×10^7 spleen cells in a 5 mL FACS tube and adjust to 4 mL of the final volume by adding FACS buffer for cell sorting.
2. Centrifuge tubes at 250 × *g* for 8 min at 4 °C and remove the supernatant by aspiration with the help of a vacuum pump connected to a Pasteur pipette.
3. Add to the cell pellet the optimal amount of anti-mouse CD21 FITC, anti-mouse-CD23 PE-Cy5, and anti-mouse IgM PE antibodies (*see* **Note 17**), diluted in 100 μL of FACS buffer for cell sorting. Shake gently.
4. Incubate the cells on ice for 20 min and protect from light. At the end of the incubation, add 2 mL of FACS buffer for cell sorting and spin for 10 min at 250 × *g* at 4 °C.
5. Dilute cells at a final concentration of 5×10^6 cells/mL in 1× PBS and prepare the cell sorter.
6. Prepare sterile 5 mL polypropylene FACS tubes with 200 μL of FCS to collect cells during cell sorting. Clearly identify each tube with a label corresponding to the single-cell population you are purifying.

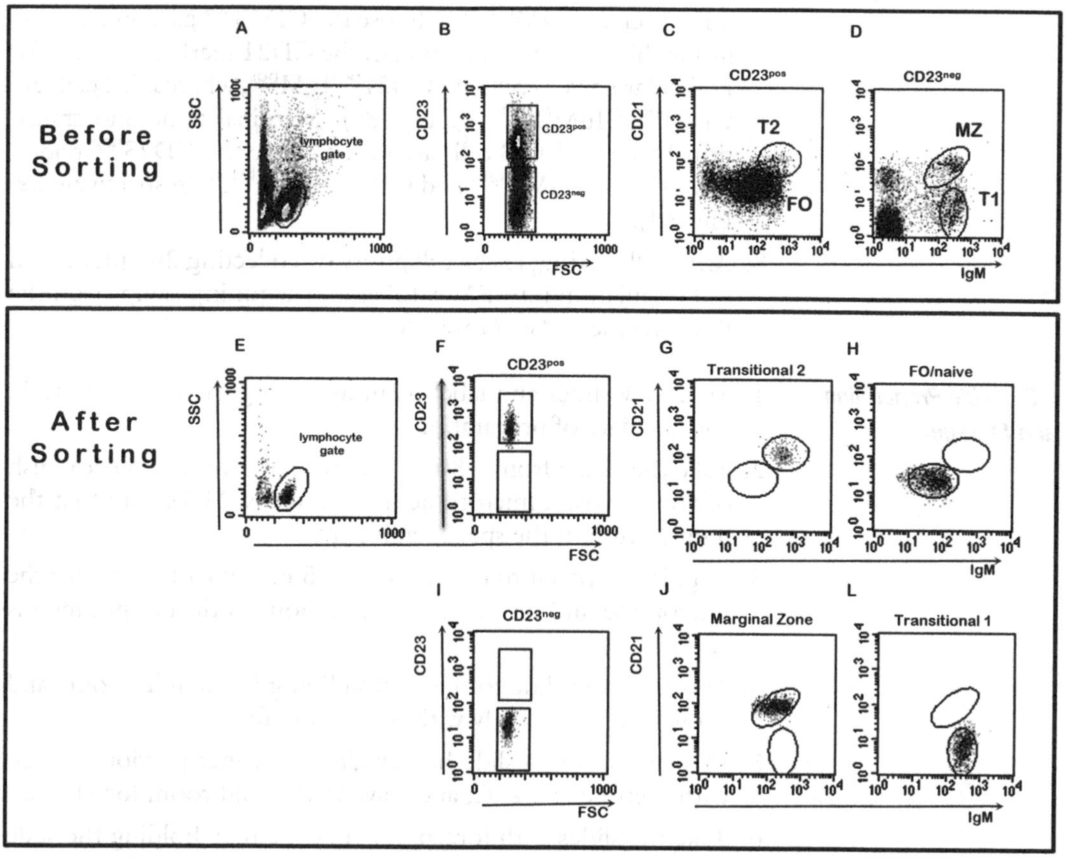

Fig. 3 Representative example of the cell sorting strategy used to purify transitional type 1 and type 2, marginal zone, and follicular naïve B cells from the spleen of adult mice. (**a–d**) B-cell subset analysis of spleen cells before cell sorting. (**a**) Dead cells, debris, doublets, granulocytes, and macrophages are excluded by defining a first gate on lymphocytes using the side/forward scatter (SSC/FSC) parameters. (**b**) Inside the lymphocyte gate, cells can be divided according to the expression of CD23 marker in two rectangular regions corresponding to $CD23^{pos}$ and $CD23^{neg}$ cells. (**c**) From the analysis of the $CD23^{pos}$ compartment for the expression of CD21 and IgM, follicular/naïve ($CD21^{pos}IgM^{pos}$) B cells can be discriminated from transitional type 2 (T2-$CD21^{bright}IgM^{bright}$) B cells. (**d**) Marginal zone (MZ) and transitional type 1 (T1) B cells can be identified inside the $CD23^{neg}$ region as $CD21^{bright}IgM^{bright}$ and $CD21^{neg}IgM^{bright}$, respectively. (**e–l**) Dot plot panels represent previously described B-cell populations analyzed after cell purification by cell sorting

7. Proceed with cell sorting. Figure 3 summarizes an example of a 4-way cell sorting strategy in which, combining different gates, the sorting machine selects and purifies four cell types simultaneously. Dead cells, debris, doublets, granulocytes, and macrophages can be excluded from the analysis by side/forward scatter gating by drawing a first region on lymphocytes (*see* Fig. 3a). Inside the lymphocyte gate, plot events according to the expression of the CD23 marker and forward scatter and depict two rectangular regions corresponding to $CD23^{pos}$ and $CD23^{neg}$ cells (*see* Fig. 3b). To discriminate follicular/naïve from transitional type 2 (T2) B cells (which already express

CD23 but are IgM^{bright}), choose the $CD23^{pos}$ gate and analyze inside this gate the expression of the CD21 marker and of IgM. Follicular naïve B cells are $CD21^{pos}IgM^{pos}$, whereas T2 cells are $CD21^{bright}IgM^{bright}$ (*see* Fig. 3c). Marginal zone and transitional type 1 (T1) B cells are found inside the $CD23^{neg}$ region as $CD21^{bright}IgM^{bright}$ and $CD21^{neg}IgM^{bright}$, respectively (*see* Fig. 3d).

8. After cell sorting, check cell purity by collecting 200 μL of each cell population into FACS tubes and acquiring samples on the flow cytometer (*see* **Note 18**).

3.5 Slide Preparation and Storage

1. Take new slides and label them indicating the tissue of origin and the date of preparation.
2. Take the tissue from −80 °C and mount it on the vertical dish of your cryostat microtome using forceps. Make sure that the temperature of the specimen is kept.
3. Regulate cryostat to cut sections of 5 μm. Start to cut with the microtome and discard the first sections until the specimen is visible.
4. Approach the slide to the section lining in the microtome and allow it to stick slowly without making folds.
5. Plunge slides in a slide-holder glass container previously filled with acetone at +4 °C, and leave in the cold room for 10 min.
6. Take the slides with forceps and dry them by holding the slide in vertical keeping one corner in contact with absorbent paper.
7. Keep the extra slides in a slide box at −20 °C.

3.6 Confocal Microscopy Staining

1. Take the slides from the −20 °C freezer, put them on towel paper, and leave on the bench for 1 h. Make sure slides reach room temperature.
2. Place the slide in a humid chamber and add 20 μL of blocking solution; incubate for 30 min and protect from the light.
3. Plunge slides in a slide-holder glass container with 1× PBS for 5 min.
4. Remove the slides from the slide holder and drain them by holding the slide in vertical, keeping one corner in contact with absorbent paper.
5. Place the slide in a humid chamber and add 20 μL of 1× PBS supplemented with the optimal amount of the required antibodies (*see* Table 2 and **Note 13**). Incubate for 45 min and protect from light.
6. Wash slides as in **Step 3** followed by **Step 4**.

7. Place the slide in a humid chamber and add 20 μL of Hoechst 33342 fluorescent stain diluted 1:10000 in 1× PBS. Incubate for 30 s protected from light (*see* **Note 19**).
8. Wash and drain slides as described in **Steps 3** and **4**.
9. Add 20 μL/section of an anti-fade reagent (*see* **Note 20**) and cover the slide with the coverslip. Leave overnight at room temperature protected from light.
10. Seal coverslips to the slides with polish and visualize them with confocal microscope (*see* **Note 21**).

3.7 RNA Isolation and cDNA Synthesis for Repertoire Analysis

1. Gently spin down sorted cells (*see* Subheading 3.4), carefully remove supernatants, and extract total RNA by lysing and homogenizing the sample (*see* **Note 22**). Continue by following the guidelines provided by the manufacturer of the specific RNA extraction kit employed (*see* **Note 23**).
2. Elute total RNA in a minimum volume of 20 μL of nuclease-free water and keep samples on ice until next step. Alternatively, freeze samples at −80 °C, until processing them further.
3. Proceed with cDNA synthesis. Transfer 8 μL of total RNA in 0.2 mL PCR tubes and add the reagents provided by the employed first-strand cDNA synthesis kit, specifically random hexamers, dNTPs, reverse transcriptase enzyme, and a suitable buffer up to a total volume of 20 μL/reaction (*see* **Note 24**).

3.8 PCR Amplification and Purification of Immunoglobulin Heavy Chains for Repertoire Analysis

1. To perform immunoglobulin heavy chain amplification, set every PCR sample with 1 μL of cDNA and using a high-fidelity PCR amplification system. Follow manufacturer's instructions to complete the reaction. Perform a 30-cycle amplification and use the oligonucleotides described in Table 3.
2. While the PCR is running, prepare an 1.8% agarose gel. Weigh 1.8 g of agarose into a relatively large bottle or flask (heat resistant) that will allow swirling, and dissolve the powder in 100 mL of 1× TBE solution. Heat the agarose/TBE solution in a microwave, stirring regularly until all agarose lumps have been completely dissolved. Add dye for detection of nucleic acid to the indicated concentration (*see* **Note 7**) and pour the gel onto the agarose tray with fitted combs previously assembled onto a gel caster.
3. Once the PCR reaction is complete, samples can either be stored at −20 °C until further processing or directly checked and purified (as described in **Step 5**) via agarose gel electrophoresis. In this second case, add 2.5 μL of the Orange G loading dye (1:10) to each PCR sample and load all the volume from each PCR product onto the 1.8% agarose gel. Load a DNA ladder to estimate the size of the main PCR products (*see* **Note 25**).

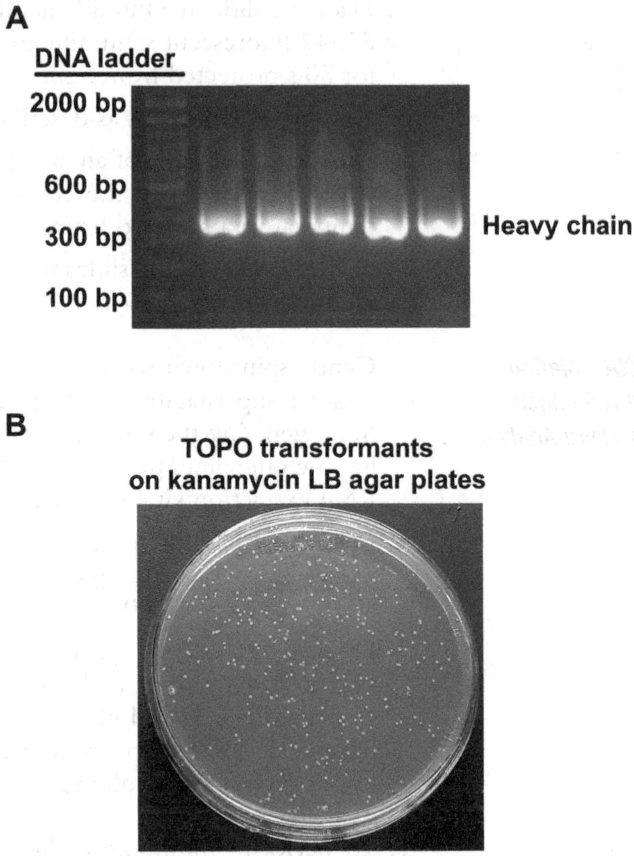

Fig. 4 PCR amplification of immunoglobulin heavy chains and subcloning into cloning/sequencing vectors. (**a**) Example of a typical result after agarose gel electrophoresis of PCR products containing amplified heavy chains from sorted B cells. The DNA ladder is the first line on the left. Samples were run long enough to separate the main product from non-incorporated primers. The gel was scanned in order to verify the right product size and to keep record of the experiment. Bp: base pair. (**b**) Example of bacterial colonies growth under antibiotic selection (kanamycin) as a result of the transformation of competent bacteria with the plasmid containing the antibiotic-resistance gene and the purified PCR product

4. Run the agarose gel in 1× TBE buffer for approximately 1 h at 110 mA electrical current in a medium-sized electrophoresis unit (*see* **Note 26**). As shown in Fig. 4a, as a result of the primer pair used in the PCR reaction (*see* Table 4), the PCR products of interest will be approximately 350 base pairs long.
5. Proceed with the purification of immunoglobulin heavy chains DNA. With the help of a clean scalpel, cut out the main PCR products from the agarose gel and place the sliced pieces of gel into pre-weighed empty 1.5 mL tubes. Add an appropriate volume of the membrane-binding solution (provided by the

PCR cleanup and purification kit) relative to the weight of agarose contained in each tube. Follow the instructions of the employed PCR cleanup and purification kit (*see* **Note 27**). Keep freshly purified PCR products on ice.

3.9 Subcloning into TOPO Cloning/Sequencing Vectors

1. The choice of the cloning vector should be made to allow cloning of blunt-end PCR products, preferably keeping short distance between sequencing primer and insert sites. It should include an antibiotic-resistance marker and conventional flanking restriction sites, e.g., EcoRI, for simplified excision of cloned PCR products, if needed. Take the purified PCR product, salt solution (if provided by manufacturer), sequencing vector, and water (if needed) to the recommended reaction volume (*see* **Note 28**).
2. Subclone blunt-end purified PCR products into the cloning vector of choice. Mix the reaction gently and incubate according to vector specifications, e.g., room temperature for 20–30 min.
3. After cloning, place the reactions on ice and proceed to transform competent bacteria by following the instructions provided in the user manual. A successful transformation will yield hundreds of bacterial colonies the day after (*see* Fig. 4b).

3.10 Bacterial Plasmid DNA Purification and Sequencing of Immunoglobulin Heavy Chains

1. Using a sterile disposable loop, pick a single bacterial colony from the transformation of competent bacteria (*see* Subheading 3.9) and gently re-streak an LB-agar plate supplemented with 50 μg/mL kanamycin and, using the same loop inoculate 2 mL of sterile LB liquid medium supplemented with 50 μg/mL kanamycin in a sterile 14 mL round-bottom loose-capped tube (*see* **Note 29**).
2. Set up the overnight bacterial culture in shaking incubators at 37 °C (*see* **Note 30**).
3. The day after, spin down overnight bacterial cultures at top speed in a benchtop microcentrifuge for 10 min. Discard the supernatants (*see* **Note 31**).
4. Isolate bacterial plasmid DNA. Since there are several different protocols for the isolation of plasmid DNA from bacteria, some of which do not require the use of a commercial kit, choose the system that best suits your needs (*see* **Note 32**).
5. Sequence the subcloned heavy chains using forward and reverse oligonucleotides nearby to the cloning site in the cloning/sequencing vector (*see* **Note 33**).

3.11 Analysis of the Immunoglobulin Heavy Chain Repertoire

Compare obtained sequences with germline sequences using the V-QUEST tool provided by the international ImMuno-GeneTics information system (http://www.imgt.org). IMGT/V-QUEST is the IMGT tool for nucleotide sequence alignment and analysis of immunoglobulin (IG) or antibody, T-cell receptor (TR), and major histocompatibility (MH) of human and other vertebrate species.

1. Select species (***Mus musculus*** or house mouse) and type of receptor (IGH) as indicated by the red arrow in Fig. 5a.
2. Then insert provided sequence containing the heavy chain sequence in FASTA format into the blank space provided at the IMGT/V-QUEST tool as indicated by the red arrow in Fig. 5b. Start the search.
3. After a while, a summary of the results will be displayed (*see* Fig. 5c).
4. Exclude from the analysis the first nine nucleotides of each heavy chain variable region because of the partial overlap with forward primer sequences (indicated with a red arrow and a red line in Fig. 5d).

4 Notes

1. Although the use of this technology is not fundamental and one could isolate DNA plasmids with conventional methods, the purpose of using the automated DNA plasmid purification robot is rather to speed up the process of plasmid DNA isolation because of the large number of clones to sequence.
2. Fetal calf serum should be heat inactivated by incubating for 30 min in a water bath at 56 °C.
3. Handle sodium azide with care, using protective clothing and gloves in order to avoid direct contact with skin, eyes, and/or accidental inhalation or ingestion.
4. Very reliable RNA extraction kits are commercially available and produce good-quality RNA. Alternatively, the classic single-step method of RNA isolation by acid guanidinium thiocyanate-phenol-chloroform extraction can be used. Although this method is widely used for isolating total RNA from biological samples of different sources, RNA extraction kits have the advantage of being quick to use and of giving a higher grade of purity.
5. There are different cloning kits commercially available. We used the TOPO cloning kit from Invitrogen.
6. Dissolve the indicated amounts of Tris, boric acid, and EDTA into 800 mL of distilled water. Undissolved white clumps may be made to dissolve by placing the bottle of solution in a hot water bath or hot plate/stirrer with the help of a magnetic stir bar to facilitate dissolution. Adjust the pH to 8.3 using a pH meter and dropwise addition of concentrated hydrochloric acid

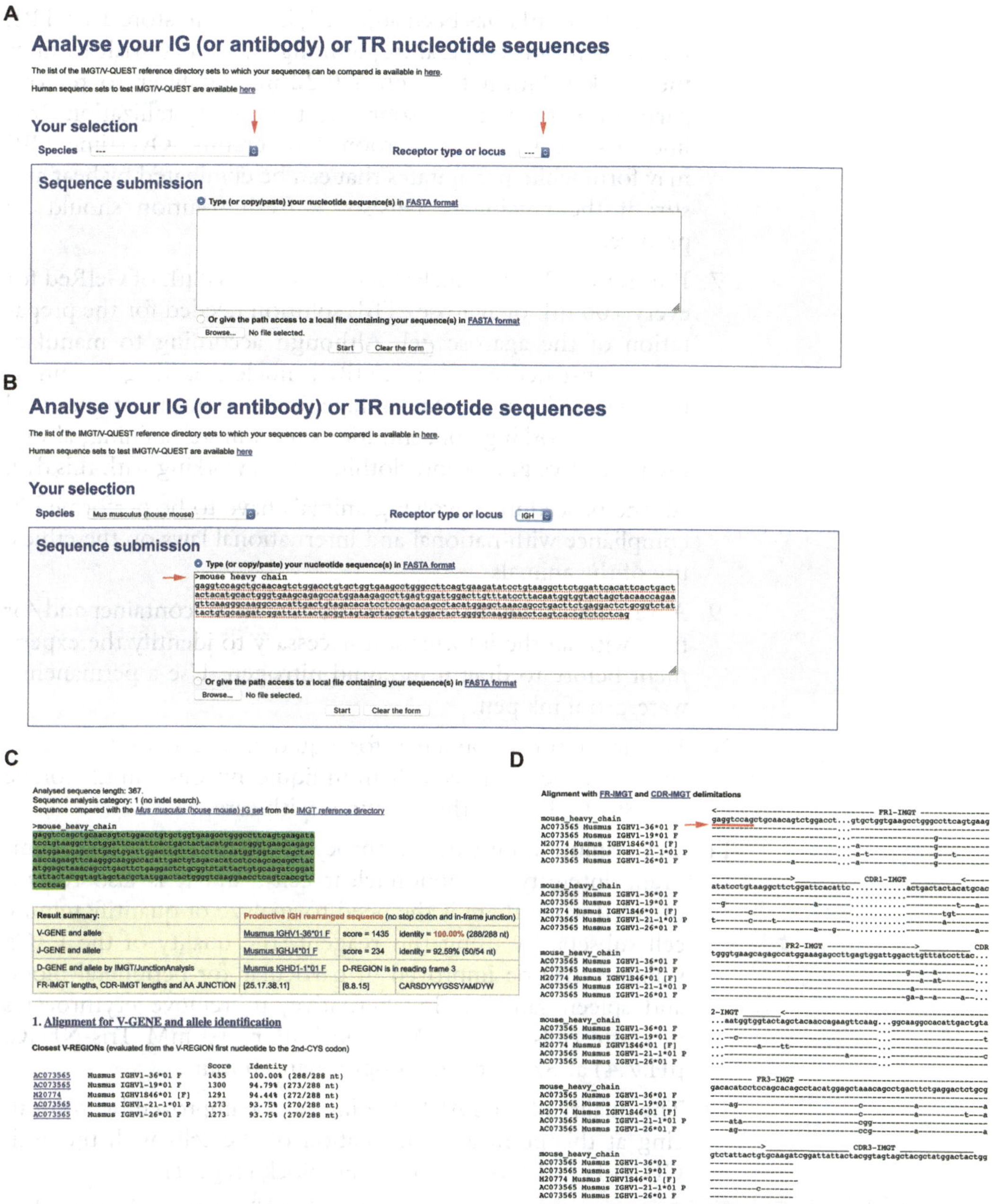

Fig. 5 Brief illustration of the IMGT sequence alignment software for immunoglobulins (IG) and T-cell receptor (TR) sequences. (**a**) Red arrows indicate where to select the species and receptor type or locus to study. (**b**) In this example "Mus musculus" and "IGH" have been selected because a mouse heavy chain sequence has been inserted in the sequence submission form. Note that the ">" or fasta symbol needs to be placed before the header of the sequence (red arrow). (**c**) Summary of the results retrieved by IMGT where IGHV (variable) 1–36*01, IGHD (diversity) 1–1*01, and IGHJ (joining gene) 4*01 are listed together with the H-CDR3 junction (CARSDYYYGSSYAMDYW). (**d**) Sequence alignment of the closest germline IGHV genes to the sequence of interest (=inserted in the sequence submission box). Underlined nucleotides indicated with an arrow should not be analyzed because these overlap with the forward oligonucleotide (5′ MsVHE in Table 3) used in the PCR amplification for repertoire analysis

(HCl). Once pH has been adjusted, it is fine to store 10× TBE buffer at room temperature, although you may wish to filter the stock solution through a 0.22-micron filter to remove particles that may act as source to foment crystallization. It is fine to store 10× TBE at room temperature. Overtime TBE may form white precipitates that can be eliminated by heat and stir; if the precipitate persists, a fresh solution should be prepared.

7. If using GelRed for nucleic acid stain, use 10 μL of GelRed for every 100 mL of agarose/TBE solution needed for the preparation of the agarose gel. Although according to manufacturer's instructions, the GelRed nucleic acid gel stain is non-cytotoxic and non-mutagenic at concentrations well above the working concentrations used in gel staining, always use protective gloves and clothing when working with this dye.

8. All the procedures involving animals have to be performed in compliance with national and international laws on the ethical use of the animals.

9. Always remember to pre-label the aluminum container and/or tube with all the information necessary to identify the experiment before to drag it in liquid nitrogen. Use a permanent/waterproof ink pen.

10. Prepare a small container for liquid nitrogen to fast freeze tissue samples and keep them in liquid nitrogen until storage at −80 °C. Handle the container with care.

11. Gey's solution destroys erythrocytes while maintaining membrane integrity of mononuclear cells, and it is also recommended when there is the need to analyze or quantify minute cell subsets. By using this reagent, the quality of the FACS staining may be improved in particular for peripheral blood and spleen samples. In alternative, to remove erythrocytes incubate cells with ACK lysing buffer (10 mM Tris-NH_4Cl pH 7.4) at 37 °C for no longer than 10 min.

12. The quality of the FACS staining can be improved by introducing at this point a preincubation of the cells with the anti-CD16-FcγIII/IIR antibody (Fc-block reagent).

13. Before using labeled or unlabeled antibodies, make sure they specifically bind to the receptor of interest and that the antibodies are appropriately diluted. Antibodies to be used in the FACS analysis should be diluted in FACS medium each time. To remove fluorescent precipitates, we recommend centrifuging the antibody dilution in a microfuge for 10 min at 1700 × *g* before use. This also applies to antibodies to be used in immunofluorescence staining for confocal microscopy analysis although, in this case, the antibodies are diluted in 1× PBS.

14. If cell acquisition is not possible shortly after the staining procedure, consider fixing the cells. After the surface staining and the last wash, add 200 μL of 1% paraformaldehyde in 1× PBS to the cells and incubate at 4 °C for 20 min in the dark. Transfer cells from the plate into FACS tubes and add 200 μL of FACS buffer.

15. If samples have been preserved at −80 °C, in N_2 or have to be analyzed after culture, consider using a specific dead cell reagent to exclude dead cells from your analysis. There are many live/dead cell stain reagents available from various companies, and in general they are to be added at the end of the cell surface staining procedure.

16. For the sorting procedures, consider using a pool of cells isolated from age- and sex-matched independent mice in order to reduce possible bias caused by individual variability.

17. The optimal antibody concentration must be determined experimentally for each assay, and it is usually obtained by a titration experiment. Consider that also FACS analyzers may be more or less sensitive depending on the producer and on the settings of the machine. Moreover, if you intend using the purified cells for in vitro culture assays, remember to remove azide from the antibodies by dialysis or to use azide-free antibody preparations before the staining for cell sorting. Cells should be manipulated under sterile conditions and washed with 1× PBS.

18. In spite of the excellent performance of most cell sorter machines, purity of minor populations is not always easy to obtain. Moreover, a certain degree of cell death is to be taken into account. Do not consider the use of cell populations that after sorting did not reach a purity of ≥99%.

19. Cell staining with the Hoechst 33342 fluorescent dye will allow the visualization of the nucleus, and this can be helpful to localize and identify nucleated cells inside the specimen. 4′,6-Diamidino-2-phenylindole, dilactate (DAPI) can also be used since it performs similar functions of nuclear counterstain. DAPI stains dsDNA in fluorescent blue. In alternative, cell contour and tissue structure can be pictured by using fluorescent phalloidin (bicyclic peptide belonging to a family of toxins isolated from *Amanita phalloides*) that specifically binds active F-actin.

20. The use of anti-fade reagents, which increase photostability of many common fluorophores, is critical when target molecules are of low abundance or when excitation light is of high intensity or long duration. Prolong®, one of the most commonly used anti-fade reagents, is a semirigid gel with anti-fade properties that protects slides from the loss of fluorescence through irreversible photo-bleaching.

21. Non-stained slides can be stored for a maximum time lapse of 6 months at −80 °C, whereas fluorescent-labeled slides can be stored for longer periods of time at +4 °C; make sure they remain free of contamination by fungi.
22. Before proceeding with RNA isolation, clean the bench with surface decontamination solutions commercially available to destroy RNases on contact. When working with RNA, always use gloves and change them as often as needed if suspected that a non-decontaminated surface has been touched.
23. We used the RNeasy Mini kit (Qiagen). As indicated by manufacturer's instructions, add the RLT cell lysis buffer, containing 2-mercaptoethanol, to the cells and proceed with the RNA isolation step. Since 2-mercaptoethanol is a hazardous chemical, work under appropriate fume hood when handling RNA lysis buffer. Handle this reagent with care and use protective clothing in order to avoid direct contact with skin, eyes, and/or accidental inhalation or ingestion. Some of the buffers included in this kit require ethanol for reconstitution.
24. When the amount of RNA is limiting, or when the same amount of RNA cannot be recovered from different cell populations, particularly if these are obtained from a sorting procedure, then it is advisable to use the maximum amount of RNA allowed by the capacity and reaction volume of the kit. For example, the volume of RNA used was of 8 μL in a reaction volume of 20 μL. This is valid when the purpose of the cloning experiment is to get a large number of transformants.
25. This step allows the detection of all products amplified through PCR. Indeed, occasionally other bands may appear beside the specific product. A 100 base pair DNA ladder is suitable to assess the right size of the fragment of interest.
26. Agarose gel electrophoresis allows the separation of the main PCR products from non-incorporated oligonucleotide primers and unfinished PCR products. At the end of electrophoretic run, make sure that the PCR products are well separated from non-incorporated primer pairs. Time given for the electrophoretic run is indicative and may depend on the equipment used in the laboratory.
27. Make sure to cut only the agarose gel containing the PCR product of interest, avoiding other closely migrating bands, if any. Also, make sure not to cut a great excess of agarose since it will prolong the time of melt down.
28. We used TOPO sequencing vectors with 0.5–4 μL of purified PCR product in a reaction volume of 6 μL containing salt, sequencing vector and water where necessary.

29. Re-streaking onto fresh LB-Agar kanamycin plates ensures each colony is preserved for the future. Repeat this procedure for all the selected transformants.
30. The number of colonies to pick, re-streak onto new LB-Agar plates and inoculate into LB liquid medium (supplemented with antibiotics) will depend on the nature of the experiment and whether there is an automated DNA plasmid purification robot on the premises. However, a minimum of 10 colonies per sample is recommended. If using a TOPO cloning kit One Shot®, TOP10 competent cells are a good choice of high-efficiency competent bacteria.
31. Make sure that the supernatants are clear, and the pellet is compact. Invert the tubes to discard supernatants and dry off excess draining from the walls by blotting onto tissue paper before tubes are placed again on the tube rack facing up.
32. Since we had many hundreds of colonies from which we had to purify plasmid DNA, we used an automated DNA plasmid purification robot in combination with a 96-well plate format NucleoSpinR©8/96 Plasmid Kit (Macherey-Nagel).
33. For sequencing of the plasmid DNA, carefully examine the backbone of the cloning/sequencing vector in order to select the appropriate forward and reverse oligonucleotide primers. Follow necessary instructions provided by the sequencing unit at your laboratory. We sequenced immunoglobulin heavy chains using BigDye™ chemistry (ThermoFisher), with help from a DNA analyzer.

Acknowledgments

We thank Dr. Claudio Pioli for his critical review of the manuscript.

References

1. Cossarizza A, Chang HD, Radbruch A, Acs A, Adam D, Adam-Klages S et al (2019) Guidelines for the use of flow cytometry and cell sorting in immunological studies (second edition). Eur J Immunol 49(10):1457–1973. https://doi.org/10.1002/eji.201970107
2. Cumano A, Berthault C, Ramond C, Petit M, Golub R, Bandeira A, Pereira P (2019) New molecular insights into immune cell development. Annu Rev Immunol 37:497–519. https://doi.org/10.1146/annurev-immunol-042718-041319
3. Godin I, Cumano A (2002) The hare and the tortoise: an embryonic haematopoietic race. Nature Reviews 2(8):593–604
4. Elsaid R, Yang J, Cumano A (2019) The influence of space and time on the establishment of B cell identity. Biom J 42(4):209–217. https://doi.org/10.1016/j.bj.2019.07.008
5. Ghosn EE, Sadate-Ngatchou P, Yang Y, Herzenberg LA, Herzenberg LA (2011) Distinct progenitors for B-1 and B-2 cells are present in adult mouse spleen. Proc Natl Acad Sci U S A 108(7):2879–2884
6. Rosado MM, Aranburu A, Capolunghi F, Giorda E, Cascioli S, Cenci F, Petrini S, Miller E, Leanderson T, Bottazzo GF, Natali PG, Carsetti R (2009) From the fetal liver to spleen and gut: the highway to natural antibody. Mucosal Immunol 2(4):351–361

7. Carsetti R, Kohler G, Lamers MC (1995) Transitional B cells are the target of negative selection in the B cell compartment. J Exp Med 181(6):2129–2140
8. Rolink AG, Andersson J, Melchers F (2004) Molecular mechanisms guiding late stages of B-cell development. Immunol Rev 197:41–50
9. Carsetti R, Rosado MM, Wardmann H (2004) Peripheral development of B cells in mouse and man. Immunol Rev 197:179–191
10. Freitas AA, Rosado MM, Viale AC, Grandien A (1995) The role of cellular competition in B cell survival and selection of B cell repertoires. Eur J Immunol 25(6):1729–1738
11. Casola S, Otipoby KL, Alimzhanov M, Humme S, Uyttersprot N, Kutok JL, Carroll MC, Rajewsky K (2004) B cell receptor signal strength determines B cell fate. Nat Immunol 5 (3):317–327
12. Chen X, Martin F, Forbush KA, Perlmutter RM, Kearney JF (1997) Evidence for selection of a population of multi-reactive B cells into the splenic marginal zone. Int Immunol 9 (1):27–41
13. Mebius RE, Kraal G (2005) Structure and function of the spleen. Nature Reviews 5 (8):606–616
14. Oliver AM, Martin F, Gartland GL, Carter RH, Kearney JF (1997) Marginal zone B cells exhibit unique activation, proliferative and immunoglobulin secretory responses. Eur J Immunol 27(9):2366–2374
15. Tiller T, Busse CE, Wardemann H (2009) Cloning and expression of murine Ig genes from single B cells. J Immunol Methods 350 (1–2):183–193. https://doi.org/10.1016/j.jim.2009.08.009
16. De Togni P, Goellner J, Ruddle NH, Streeter PR, Fick A, Mariathasan S, Smith SC, Carlson R, Shornick LP, Strauss-Schoenberger J et al (1994) Abnormal development of peripheral lymphoid organs in mice deficient in lymphotoxin. Science 264(5159):703–707
17. Alimzhanov MB, Kuprash DV, Kosco-Vilbois MH, Luz A, Turetskaya RL, Tarakhovsky A, Rajewsky K, Nedospasov SA, Pfeffer K (1997) Abnormal development of secondary lymphoid tissues in lymphotoxin beta-deficient mice. Proc Natl Acad Sci U S A 94(17):9302–9307
18. Kuprash DV, Alimzhanov MB, Tumanov AV, Anderson AO, Pfeffer K, Nedospasov SA (1999) TNF and lymphotoxin beta cooperate in the maintenance of secondary lymphoid tissue microarchitecture but not in the development of lymph nodes. J Immunol 163 (12):6575–6580
19. Kuprash DV, Alimzhanov MB, Tumanov AV, Grivennikov SI, Shakhov AN, Drutskaya LN, Marino MW, Turetskaya RL, Anderson AO, Rajewsky K, Pfeffer K, Nedospasov SA (2002) Redundancy in tumor necrosis factor (TNF) and lymphotoxin (LT) signaling in vivo: mice with inactivation of the entire TNF/LT locus versus single-knockout mice. Mol Cell Biol 22 (24):8626–8634
20. Futterer A, Mink K, Luz A, Kosco-Vilbois MH, Pfeffer K (1998) The lymphotoxin beta receptor controls organogenesis and affinity maturation in peripheral lymphoid tissues. Immunity 9(1):59–70
21. Koike R, Nishimura T, Yasumizu R, Tanaka H, Hataba Y, Watanabe T, Miyawaki S, Miyasaka M (1996) The splenic marginal zone is absent in alymphoplastic aly mutant mice. Eur J Immunol 26(3):669–675. https://doi.org/10.1002/eji.1830260324
22. Yamada T, Mitani T, Yorita K, Uchida D, Matsushima A, Iwamasa K, Fujita S, Matsumoto M (2000) Abnormal immune function of hemopoietic cells from alymphoplasia (aly) mice, a natural strain with mutant NF-kappa B-inducing kinase. J Immunol 165 (2):804–812
23. Weih F, Caamano J (2003) Regulation of secondary lymphoid organ development by the nuclear factor-kappaB signal transduction pathway. Immunol Rev 195:91–105
24. Cariappa A, Liou HC, Horwitz BH, Pillai S (2000) Nuclear factor kappa B is required for the development of marginal zone B lymphocytes. J Exp Med 192(8):1175–1182
25. Weih DS, Yilmaz ZB, Weih F (2001) Essential role of RelB in germinal center and marginal zone formation and proper expression of homing chemokines. J Immunol 167 (4):1909–1919
26. Guinamard R, Okigaki M, Schlessinger J, Ravetch JV (2000) Absence of marginal zone B cells in Pyk-2-deficient mice defines their role in the humoral response. Nat Immunol 1 (1):31–36. https://doi.org/10.1038/76882
27. Cariappa A, Tang M, Parng C, Nebelitskiy E, Carroll M, Georgopoulos K, Pillai S (2001) The follicular versus marginal zone B lymphocyte cell fate decision is regulated by Aiolos, Btk, and CD21. Immunity 14(5):603–615
28. Pabst O, Forster R, Lipp M, Engel H, Arnold HH (2000) NKX2.3 is required for MAdCAM-1 expression and homing of lymphocytes in spleen and mucosa-associated lymphoid tissue. EMBO J 19(9):2015–2023. https://doi.org/10.1093/emboj/19.9.2015

29. Kitamura D, Roes J, Kuhn R, Rajewsky K (1991) A B cell-deficient mouse by targeted disruption of the membrane exon of the immunoglobulin mu chain gene. Nature 350 (6317):423–426
30. Hayakawa K, Hardy RR, Honda M, Herzenberg LA, Steinberg AD, Herzenberg LA (1984) Ly-1 B cells: functionally distinct lymphocytes that secrete IgM autoantibodies. Proc Natl Acad Sci U S A 81(8):2494–2498
31. Wardemann H, Boehm T, Dear N, Carsetti R (2002) B-1a B cells that link the innate and adaptive immune responses are lacking in the absence of the spleen. J Exp Med 195 (6):771–780
32. Baumgarth N (2011) The double life of a B-1 cell: self-reactivity selects for protective effector functions. Nature Reviews 11(1):34–46

Chapter 2

Purification and Immune Phenotyping of B-1 Cells from Body Cavities of Mice

Vanessa Yenson and Nicole Baumgarth

Abstract

B-1 cells are fetal-origin B lymphocytes with unique developmental and functional characteristics that can generate natural, polyreactive antibodies with important functions in tissue homeostasis and immune defense. While B-1 cell frequencies in bone marrow and secondary lymphoid tissues are low, relative high frequencies exist within peritoneal and pleural cavities of mice, including both $CD5^+$ and $CD5^-$ B-1 cells. These cells represent B-1 reservoirs that, when activated, migrate to lymphoid tissues to secrete antibodies and/or cytokines. Here, we outline efficient methods for the extraction and magnetic isolation of $CD5^+$ B-1 cells from the peritoneal and pleural cavities as well as the separation and phenotypic characterization of $CD5^+$ and $CD5^-$ B-1 cells by flow cytometry.

Key words B-cell subsets, B-cell isolation, B-1 cell isolation, Innate-like B cells, Natural antibodies, Peritoneal cavity

1 Introduction

The B-cell compartment of mice contains two distinct B-cell lineages: B-1 and B-2. They arise from distinct progenitors during fetal and adult development, respectively, and differ in tissue distribution, phenotype, responsiveness to antigen and function [1, 2]. B-2 cells are also known as "conventional" B cells and contribute to the vast majority of B cells in lymphoid tissues. The fetal-derived B-1 cell compartment has been further differentiated into two subsets: B-1a and B-1b, based on their differential expression of CD5 [3]. However, recent evidence showed that the expression of CD5 can be lost upon TLR-mediated activation, suggesting that expression of CD5 may not differentiate discrete cell lineages, but rather distinct activation states of B-1 cells [4]. B-1 cells are the source of >80% of natural serum antibodies [5], which are produced in the absence of previous antigen exposure [6–8]. These

Francesca Mion and Silvia Tonon (eds.), *Regulatory B Cells: Methods and Protocols*, Methods in Molecular Biology, vol. 2270, https://doi.org/10.1007/978-1-0716-1237-8_2,

antibodies are germline encoded [9, 10, 18] and polyreactive [11, 18], recognizing both self and foreign antigens [12–14], making them more akin to innate immune effectors. Natural antibodies contribute to both tissue homeostasis and immune defense. They aid tissue homeostasis by binding to altered self-antigens expressed by dead and dying cells (phosphatidylcholine and annexin V), facilitating increased phagocytosis by immature dendritic cells [15], thereby suppressing tissue inflammation [16]. However, under certain circumstances (such as ischemia-reperfusion injury), self-reactive antibodies intended to aid apoptosis can cause tissue damage by activating the complement cascade [17, 18].

Recognition of self-antigens may influence the B-cell receptor (BCR) repertoire of B-1 cells by enriching for poly-specific receptors able to bind also to foreign antigens, i.e., pathogens [14]. Indeed, B-1 cell-derived IgM has been shown to contribute to immune protection from numerous infectious diseases, including influenza virus, *Streptococcus pneumonia*, *Borrelia hermsii* among others (reviewed in [19]). B-1 cells produce polyreactive IgM antibodies at the site of infection [20, 21], which can neutralize pathogens, in part via complement binding [22], thereby hindering early pathogenic expansion and increasing survival from infection [20, 23–26]. In addition, B-1 cells have also been identified as important sources of cytokines such as IL-10 [27] and GM-CSF [28]. Production of the latter may protect from LPS-induced sepsis.

B-1 cells are the predominant B-cell population found in the peritoneal and pleural cavities (35–70%). The ratio of $CD5^+$ (B-1a) to $CD5^-$ (B-1b) B-1 cells is about 3:1 to 4:1, depending on the mouse strain and the age of the mice [29–32]. Most studies on purified B-1 cells have therefore been conducted with body cavity B-1 cells. These cells do not spontaneously produce significant amounts of natural antibodies [31, 33, 34]. Instead, they respond to in vivo stimulation with rapid migration to secondary lymphoid tissues, such as spleen and lymph nodes, where they differentiate to IgM-secreting cells by mechanisms that are largely unexplored [32, 35, 36]. For example, systemic challenge with *Streptococcus pneumoniae* [35], LPS [32, 37, 38], or exogenous cytokines (IL-5 and IL-10) [39] induce migration of B-1 cells from the reservoirs in the body cavities to the spleen [32, 35, 36] and mucosal sites, such as the intestinal lamina propria [39, 40] depending on the type and delivery of the insult. This results in the differentiation of B-1 cells into IgM- or IgA-secreting cells with differing degrees of proliferation, depending on the stimuli [38]. As cytokines alone can initiate cell migration, antigen binding to the BCR does not appear to be required for B-1 cell activation [39]. Interestingly, B-1b cells have been proposed to clonally expand in response to antigen, thereby establishing a form of "memory" within the body cavities [41–43]. Thus, body cavity B-1 cells represent a pool of cells not actively secreting antibodies but poised to do so rapidly. Memory-like B-1 cells may also be present at those sites.

Smaller frequencies of B-1 cells are found in the spleen (1–2%) [30, 32, 34], lymph nodes (0.1–0.3%) [21, 29], bone marrow (0.1–0.2%), blood (0.3–0.5%), and mucosal sites [34]. B-1 cells within the lung parenchyma produce IgM and IgA (0.4–0.6%) [21] and those within the intestinal lamina propria produce IgA (up to 50% of all IgA generated) [44, 45]. B-1 cells in spleen and bone marrow spontaneously produce high levels of natural IgM and IgG3 [34, 46].

Studies of these intriguing fetal-derived B cells require their isolation, which is most easily achieved from the body cavities of mice because of their large frequencies [29–32]. Retrieval of cells from these sites requires thorough washes of the body cavities, which yields heterogeneous populations of single cells. Isolation of B-1 cells from this cell mix can be achieved by flow cytometry or by magnetic cell separation. The latter method is considerably faster and can be done in a way that leaves B-1 cells untouched for in vitro and in vivo investigations as outlined below. However, we have noted that even the physical stress of passing cells over a column can activate some to secrete antibodies (Savage, H.P and Baumgarth, N., unpublished). Isolation of subsets of $CD5^+$ and $CD5^-$ B-1 cells, or of B-1 cells from other tissue sources such as spleen and bone marrow, requires flow cytometry to obtain sufficiently high purities.

B-1 cells, while distinct in phenotype from conventional B cells, can be difficult to identify, as no single marker distinguishes this cell population. Instead, combinations of surface markers must be used, including CD19, CD23 (or CD24 in bone marrow), CD43, IgM, IgD, and CD5 [20, 47]. The presence of CD5 differentiates B-1a ($CD5^+$) from B-1b cells ($CD5^-$). The majority of B-1 cells in the body cavities are $CD43^+$ (as detected using the monoclonal antibody clone S7); however, about 20–30% of B-1 cells are $CD43^-$ [48]. In other tissues, CD43 expression is uniformly high. It is important to note also that body cavity B-1 cells, but not B-1 cells in other tissues, are $CD11b^+$ [3, 49], a marker that these cells share with NK cells and cells of the myeloid lineage.

In summary, B-1 cells are key effectors of tissue homeostasis and immune defense. Like many effectors of the immune system, their presence and function can be both advantageous and detrimental, depending on the circumstances and stimuli leading to their activation. There are many unanswered questions regarding their regulation, migration, and activation. In this chapter, we describe how to collect, sort, and immune-phenotype B-1 cells from various tissues.

2 Materials

2.1 Mice

Female inbred mice (BALB/c or C57BL/6), 8–15 weeks of age, as source of peritoneal cavity and/or pleural cavity lavage (*see* **Note 1**) as well as splenocytes as source of cells for flow cytometry compensation samples (*see* Subheading 3.4).

2.2 General Buffers and Reagents

1. Phosphate buffered saline (PBS): 137 mM NaCl, 2.7 mM KCl, 10 mM Na_2HPO_4, 1.8 mM KH_2PO_4, pH 7.2 (*see* **Note 2**).
2. HEPES buffered salt solution (BSS): 174 mM NaCl, 3 mM KCl, 2.4 mM $CaCl_2$, 1.24 mM $MsS0_4$, 1.26 mM KH_2PO_4, 0.84 mM K_2HPO_4, 14.78 mM HEPES, 7.3 mM NaOH, pH 7.2, mouse isotonic (*see* **Notes 3** and **4**).
3. Staining medium (SM): mouse tonicity HEPES BSS at pH 7.2 supplemented with 3.5% newborn calf serum, 0.02% sodium azide, and 1 mM ethylenediaminetetraacetic acid (EDTA). Sterilize by filtering through a 0.22 μm pore size filter (*see* **Note 5**).
4. Fc block solution: monoclonal anti-mouse CD16/CD32 (clone 2.4G2) antibody diluted at 10 μg/mL in SM.
5. 70% ethanol cleaning solution and 99% ethanol.
6. *Auto*MACS rinsing buffer: 2 mM EDTA in PBS, pH 7.2. Sterilize by filtering through a 0.45 μm pore size filter. Store at 4 °C and use at room temperature (*see* **Note 6**).
7. *Auto*MACS running buffer: 2 mM EDTA in PBS with 0.5% bovine serum albumin (BSA), pH 7.2. Sterilize by filtering through a 0.45 μm pore size filter. Store at 4 °C, use at room temperature. Take a small aliquot to keep sterile for microbead labeling.
8. MACS anti-biotin microbeads (Miltenyi).
9. Sorting buffer: 50% fetal bovine serum (FBS) in SM.

2.3 Equipment

1. *Auto*MACS cell separator (Miltenyi Biotec) (*see* **Note 6**).
2. *Auto*MACS column (Miltenyi Biotec).
3. 1 l waste bottle.
4. Sterile autoclaved glass Pasteur pipettes (5 ¾ inch) and bulb or sterile 5 mL syringe with sterile blunt needle (19 gauge).
5. 15 or 50 mL conical tubes for sample collection.
6. Sterile autoclaved surgical scissors and forceps.
7. Carbon dioxide chamber.
8. Dissection board and pins.
9. Flow cytometer with sorting capabilities.
10. Cell strainers and FACS tubes.

Table 1
Antibodies for B-1 cell enrichment

Specificity*	Fluorochrome	mAb clone
CD90.2 (T cells)	Biotin	53–2.1
F4/80 (macrophages)	Biotin	F4/80
Gr-1 (granulocytes)	Biotin	RB6-9C5
CD49b (NK cells)	Biotin	DX-5
CD23 (B-2 cells)	Biotin	B3.B4

Table 2
Antibodies for B-1 cell purity check

Specificity*	Fluorochrome	mAb clone
Streptavidin	Qdot 605	
CD19 (B cells)	Cy5 PE	1D3
IgD	Cy7 PE	11–26
IgM	Alexa Fluor 700	331

Table 3
Antibodies for FACS-sorting and characterization of B-1 cells. Part 1: Cell surface markers

Specificity*	Fluorochrome	mAb clone
CD5	Biotin	53–5.8.3.1
CD90.2 (Thy1.2)	Pac blue or Cy5 PE	53–2.1
F4/80	Pac blue or Cy5 PE	F4/80
CD23	FITC	B3.B4
CD43	PE	S7
CD19	Cy5 PE or Alexa Fluor 700	1D3
IgD	Cy7 PE	11–26
IgM	Alexa Fluor 700 or APC	331

2.4 Antibodies

1. Antibodies used for cell isolation (*see* Table 1) and for checking B-1 cell purity (*see* Table 2). All anti-mouse monoclonal antibodies must be diluted in SM and used at pre-determined optimal concentrations determined by antibody titration (*see* **Note 7**).
2. Antibodies used for fluorescence activated cell sorting (FACS) and for the characterization of B-1 cells (*see* Table 3 and

Table 4
Antibodies for characterization of B-1 cells. Part 2: Biotin-revealing agent and live/dead marker staining

Specificity	Fluorochrome
Streptavidin	Qdot 605
Live/dead	Violet (read on Pac blue)

Table 4). All anti-mouse monoclonal antibodies must be diluted in SM and used at pre-determined optimal concentrations determined by antibody titration (*see* **Note 7**).

3 Methods

3.1 Collection of Peritoneal cavity Cells (PerC)

1. Euthanize mice by overexposure to carbon dioxide. Do not use cervical dislocation as red blood cells from ruptured blood vessels may contaminate peritoneal cavity lavage. Process one mouse at a time as long exposure to air can dry out the peritoneal membrane and reduce elasticity.
2. Pin mouse to dissection board, tucking tail behind one of the hind legs (*see* Fig. 1a). Spray abdomen lightly with ethanol.
3. Make a small incision along the ventral midline just caudal to the sternum after lifting off skin from underlying serosa. Use blunt-ended scissors to carefully separate the skin away from the fragile peritoneal pleura (peritoneal membrane) underneath using blunt dissection. It is important not to cut. Extend incision down to the tail and up to the neck. Be very careful not to puncture the peritoneal membrane. If puncture does occur, *see* **Note 8** and Fig. 2.
4. Once the abdominal cavity has been fully exposed, pin the skin flaps to the side and continue to separate the skin from the pleura along the sides of the mouse (*see* Fig. 1b).
5. Orient the mouse with its body perpendicular to the table.
6. With sharp scissors or glass Pasteur pipette, make a very small incision in the pleural on the ventral midline, just proximal to the tail.
7. Fill pipette or syringe with SM, insert gently into cavity and dispense two pipette volumes of SM (approximately 5 mL total). Put an air bubble at the top of the fluid volume to force the fluid through the cavity (*see* Fig. 1c). If using the syringe with blunt needle, suck a bit of abdominal fat through the incision to plug the hole while mixing the medium and to indicate point of entry.

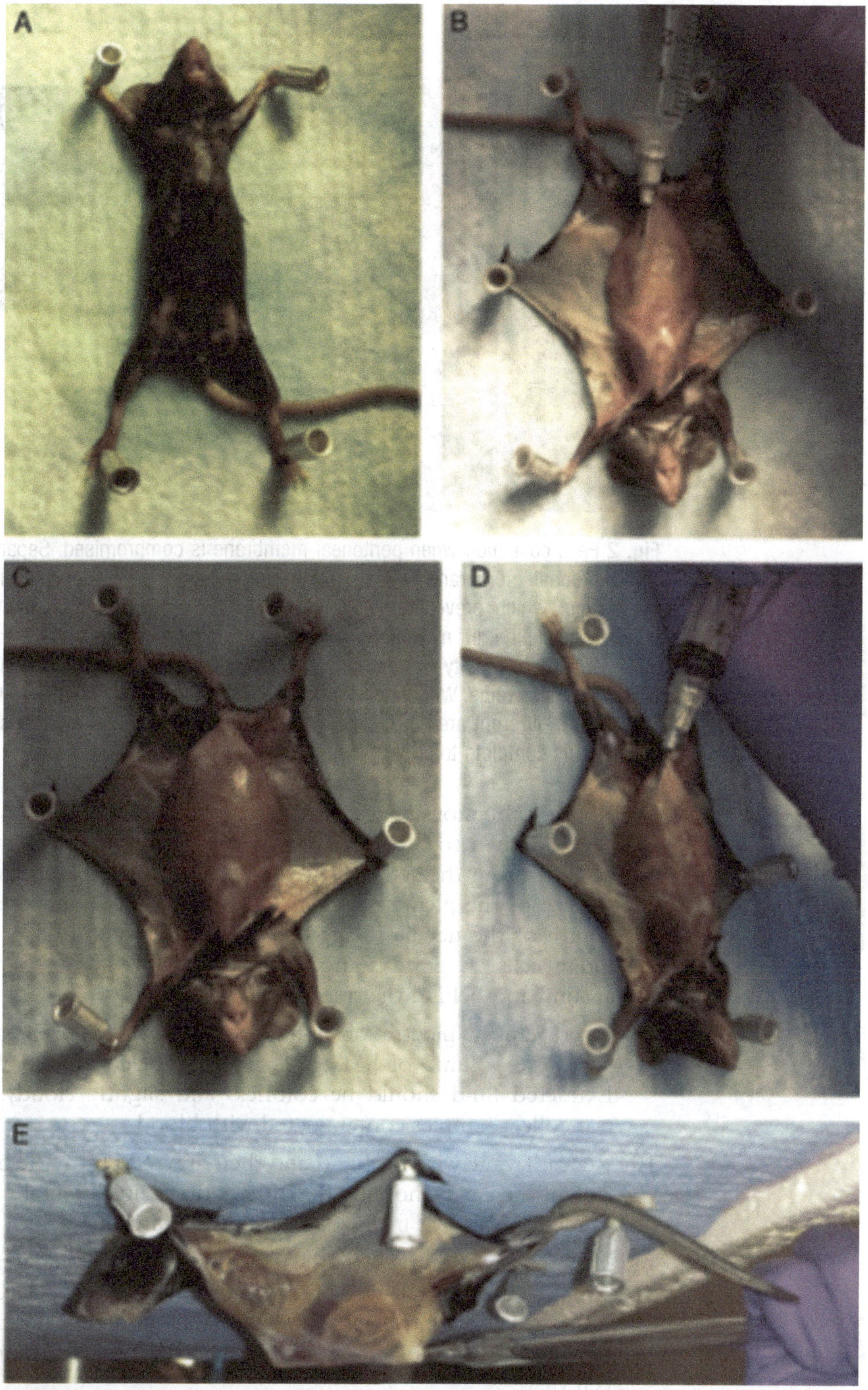

Fig. 1 PerC collection from C57Bl/6 mice. To collect cells from lavage washes of the peritoneal cavity, a series of steps must be followed. (**a**) Pin mouse to dissection board. (**b**) Separate skin from peritoneal pleura and pin down. Through a small incision, insert glass pipette or blunt-needled syringe. (**c**) Fill peritoneal cavity with SM so that it distends and massage SM to dislodge cells. (**d**) A good source of B-1 cells is from around and behind the spleen. (**e**) For final collection of cells, use a glass pipette. Invert mouse and collect remaining cells by drawing pipette along the pleural membrane

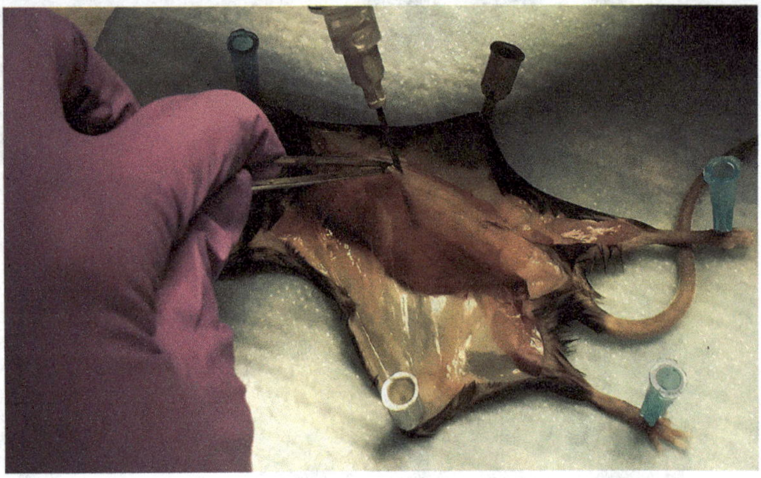

Fig. 2 PerC collection when peritoneal membrane is compromised. Separating the peritoneal membrane from the skin can result in a hole or tear in the membrane, which prevents the normal collection of PerC. With the mouse pinned and supine, lift membrane with forceps, holding both sides of the hole. Insert SM into the cavity and massage outer membrane with the tip of a pipette or with a blunt needle. Withdraw as much fluid as you can and repeat aiming the pipette at a different area of the cavity. Hold the membrane with forceps until collection is complete to prevent fluid and cells from leaking out

8. Keeping the mouse perpendicular to the table, gently massage the abdomen to mix the fluid inside the cavity and dislodge cells. If using the syringe with blunt needle, ensure the outer surface of the pleura is moist (with SM or PBS) and use the length of the needle to move SM and organs around to dislodge cells. A good source of peritoneal B-1 cells is from around and behind the spleen (*see* Fig. 1d).
9. Insert empty pipette or blunt-needled syringe and extract 1 pipette volume of SM. Collect into labeled conical tube. Extracted fluid should be colorless and slightly cloudy. Do not collect samples contaminated with blood.
10. Repeat lavage with fresh SM and then draw SM from the other side of the cavity, holding the pipette tip against pleural membrane to protect it from contact with the intestines.
11. The first two lavages of the peritoneum have the greatest concentration of cells and are therefore the most crucial. Continue to lavage and extract medium two or three more times until about 8 mL of cells has been collected. This will increase cell yield.
12. For the last lavage with glass pipette, invert mouse and draw the glass pipette along the pleural membrane, sucking up the

last of the cells from the cavity (*see* Fig. 1e). The same pipette/blunt-needled syringe may be used for multiple lavages as long as it remains sterile.

13. One female 8–15-week-old mouse can yield 5–six million cells.

3.2 Collection of Pleural Cavity Cells (PlerC)

1. Cells from pleural cavity can be collected after cells from the peritoneal cavity have been retrieved. Cut the peritoneum and reposition the major organs away from the pleural membrane.
2. Make a small incision on the right side of the pleura, so as to avoid the heart.
3. With a glass pipette or blunt-needled syringe, insert a small amount of air into the pleural space to separate the lungs from the walls of the cavity.
4. Insert a small volume of SM, hold mouse perpendicular to the table as before to swirl the medium around the pleural cavity space.
5. Withdraw the PlerC fluid and repeat, trying to direct the SM to a different part of the cavity to maximize the number of cells retrieved.
6. PlerC can be pooled for maximal cell numbers. Expected cell yield is approximately 2–three million cells per mouse.

3.3 Magnetic-Based Cell Isolation of B-1 Cells from Peritoneal and Pleural Cavities

Here below we describe a negative selection method to purify B-1 cells from the total peritoneal and pleural cavities cell pool by immunomagnetic cell separation using magnetic-activated cell sorting (MACS®, *see* **Note 6**). Compared to FACS purification of B-1 cells, magnetic-based isolation of B-1 cells has many practical advantages, including much greater speed of isolation, the ability to scale-up cell numbers, and favorable costs if hourly sorting rates are charged on flow cytometers. However, the suggested stains for B-1 cell enrichment by magnetic cell separation can also be used for FACS purification or with alternatives immunomagnetic sorting methods.

This procedure must be performed in a BSL-2 class hood if cells are to be used for cell culture or further in vivo work.

1. Centrifuge cells collected from the body cavities at 500 × *g* for 5 min at 4 °C and discard supernatant. Resuspend cells in 1 mL of SM and count cells using a hemocytometer.
2. Centrifuge again and resuspend the total number of cells required for isolation in Fc block solution as indicated in Table 5.
3. After an incubation of 15 min on ice, fill the tube with SM to wash cells. Centrifuge cells at 500 × *g* for 5 min at 4 °C and discard supernatant.

Table 5
Resuspension volume for staining cells

Number of cells for isolation	Volume of Fc Block in SM
1–5 × 10^7	100 µL per 1 × 10^7 cells
5 × 10^7–1 × 10^8	500 µL
≥1 × 10^8	1 mL

4. Resuspend the cell pellet in the complete mix of biotinylated antibodies listed in Table 1, in the same volume as used for Fc block solution. Mix well and incubate cells for 15 min on ice.
5. Fill the tube with sterile *auto*MACS running buffer to wash cells. Centrifuge cells at 500 × *g* for 5 min at 4 °C. Discard supernatant.
6. Resuspend the cell pellet with anti-biotin microbeads in sterile running buffer (*see* **Note 9**) and incubate cells for 30 min at 4 °C with continuous rotation.
7. Following incubation, fill the tube with sterile running buffer to wash cells and centrifuge at 500 × *g* for 5 min at 4 °C. Discard supernatant.
8. Filter cells through sterile nylon mesh at 1 × 10^7 cells/300 µL running buffer.
9. Remove 30 µL from the sample: 25 µL will be used to run a flow cytometry purity check (as PRE-*auto*MACS sample; *see* Subheading 3.4), while the remaining 5 µL will serve to count cells using a hemocytometer.
10. Prepare two 15 mL conical tubes for *auto*MACS collection: the positive fraction will contain unwanted biotinylated cells, while the negative fraction will contain enriched, non-labeled B-1 cells.
11. Pre-clean *auto*MACS as per manufacturer's instructions and choose "Separation" from menu on screen, select "DepleteS" and run per manufacturer's instructions (*see* **Note 10**).
12. Centrifuge positive and negative fractions at 500 × *g* for 5 min at 4 °C. Discard supernatant and resuspend expected fractions in SM at 7.5 × 10^5 cells/30 µL (expected yield of 1–two million B-1 cells per PerC).
13. Remove 30 µL from each fraction: 5 µL for cell count and 25 µL for purity check via flow cytometry analysis.

3.4 B-1 Cell Purity Check Via Flow cytometry Analysis

Below we list the steps required for checking the purity of B-1 cells via flow cytometry. In addition to the experimental samples, also a compensation sample for each fluorochrome utilized in the staining panel (i.e., a cell sample stained with only one of the antibody-conjugates used) should be prepared. This enables appropriate setting of compensation either directly on the machine or post data acquisition, using an appropriate analysis software such as FlowJo (BD).

1. Incubate the pre- and post-*auto*MACS cells with the previously titrated antibody mix listed in Table 2 for 15 min on ice in the dark. These cells have already been stained with Fc block solution (*see* Subheading 3.3).
2. In parallel, stain splenocytes (1.25×10^6 cells/50 μL) with Fc block solution (*see* Subheading 3.3) and then incubate with one fluorochrome-conjugated antibody per sample for 15 min on ice (*see* **Note 11**).
3. Wash cells with SM and centrifuge at 500 × *g* for 5 min at 4 °C. Discard supernatant and resuspend cells in 400 μL of SM.
4. Analyze both the experimental and compensation samples using a flow cytometer. Refer to Fig. 3 for gating strategy.
5. B-1 cell purity is calculated as the percentage of B-1$^+$ cells in the live cell population (this can be automatically performed by most flow cytometry analysis software).

3.5 FACS-Sorting of B-1a and B-1b Cells

Negative immunomagnetic cell separation methods have the great advantage that the cellular population of interest remains unbound by antibodies. However, compared to negative selection, positive isolation of B-1 cells has the added advantage of allowing the separation of B-1a and B-1b cells. The addition of an anti-CD5 antibody to the enrichment cocktail listed in Table 1 can yield relatively high purities of CD5$^-$ B-1b cells. However, because CD5 expression on B-1 cells can be very low, the purities achieved by this approach are usually lower than those achieved by negative selection of immunomagnetic cell separation. Below we describe the steps for fluorescence-activated cell sorting (FACS) of B-1a and B-1b cells.

1. Harvest cells from body cavities as described in Subheadings 3.1 and 3.2, and centrifuge the cell suspension at 500 × *g* for 5 min at 4 °C. Discard supernatant and count cells.
2. Incubate cells with Fc block solution for 15 min on ice as previously described. After the incubation, wash cells with SM and centrifuge at 500 × *g* for 5 min at 4 °C. Discard supernatant.
3. Resuspend cells with the previously titrated fluorochrome-conjugated antibodies listed in Table 3 and incubate for 15 min on ice. Following the incubation, wash cells with SM, centrifuge at 500 × *g* for 5 min at 4 °C and discard supernatant.

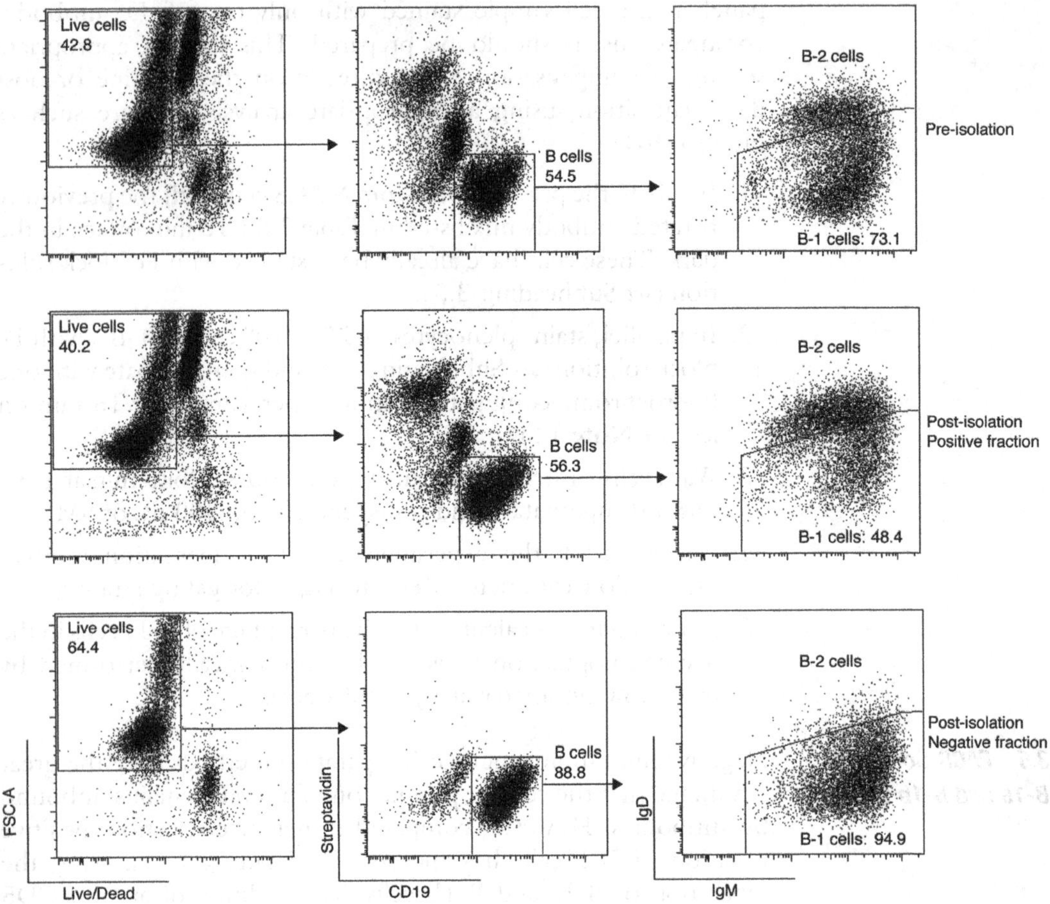

Fig. 3 Gating strategy for purity check of MACS-enriched B-1 cells in the pre-isolation and post-isolation positive and negative fractions. Flow cytometric analysis of body cavity cells. First gate on live cells. Forward scatter (FSC) indicates cell size and the Live/Dead fluorochrome marker distinguishes dead fluorochrome-positive cells (to the right in the first dot plots) from live cells. $CD19^+$ B cells within the live population are then gated as a separate population from the unwanted cells (labeled with biotinylated antibodies, Subheading 3.3). Unwanted cells, including T cells, macrophages, granulocytes, and NK cells, are detected with fluorochrome-conjugated streptavidin. B-1 cells within the $CD19^+$ population are distinguished from **B-2 cells** by their expression of IgM and IgD. B-1 cells are IgM^{hi} $IgD^{variable}$; **B-2 cells** are IgM^{lo} IgD^{hi}. B-1 cell purity is then calculated as a percentage of live cells, using a specific **flow cytometry** analysis software

4. Resuspend cells with streptavidin–Qdot 605 (titrated before use, *see* Table 4) and incubate for 15 min on ice. Following the incubation, wash cells with SM, centrifuge at 500 × *g* for 5 min at 4 °C and discard supernatant.
5. Resuspend cells at 1×10^7 cells/mL in SM and pass through filter-top FACS tubes to eliminate cell clumps that can block the cell sorter.

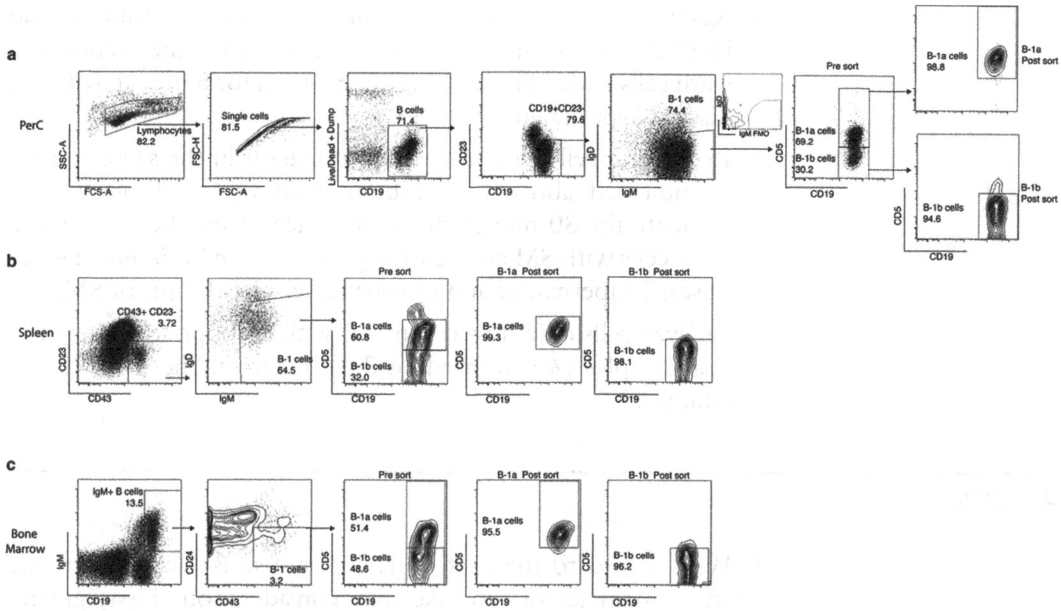

Fig. 4 Immune phenotyping and FACS-sorting of B-1 cells from PerC, spleen, and bone marrow. (**a**) Lymphocytes are gated according to their size (FSC-A) and granularity (SSC-A). Single cells are determined by using forward scatter area versus height (FSC-A and FSC-H), eliminating the presence of doublets and cell clumps, which fall off of the diagonal. Live single B cells are identified by the expression of CD19 and then the differential expression of the CD23, CD5, IgM, and IgD markers allows to distinguish between B-1a and B-1b cells. To set the correct gate for IgM$^+$ cells, an IgM FMO (sample stained with every fluorochrome-conjugated antibody within the antibody mix reported in Table 3, except for IgM), is run (smaller plot). Comparing the staining to the FMO allows for setting a precise gate at the point at which IgM$^+$ cells are detected above background, and thus identifies all IgM$^+$ cells. B-1a and B-b cells can be distinguished from one another according to their CD5 positivity. A similar analysis to identify B-1 cells among the spleen (**b**) and bone marrow (**c**) is reported although not showing live/singlet gates. Boxes indicate gating strategy; numbers represent frequencies of events within each gate. Shown are results from a representative FACS-sort

6. Perform a two-way sort of cells, collecting B-1a (CD5$^+$) and B-1b cells (CD5$^-$) in 15 mL collection tubes containing 1 mL of sorting buffer. Refer to Fig. 4a for gating strategy.
7. B-1 cells can be isolated from the spleen (*see* Fig. 4b) and bone marrow (*see* Fig. 4c) using the same method (*see* **Note 12**).

3.6 Immune Phenotyping of B-1a and B-1b Cells from Body Cavities

1. Incubate cells isolated as in Subheadings 3.1 and 3.2 with Fc block solution at a ratio of 6.25×10^5 cells/25 μL for 15 min in the dark on ice. Following the incubation, wash cells with SM, centrifuge at 500 × *g* for 5 min at 4 °C and discard supernatant.
2. Resuspend cells at 6.25×10^5 cells/25 μL in the antibody cocktail made of the antibodies listed in Table 3 and incubate for 20 min in the dark on ice. After the incubation, wash cells with SM and centrifuge at 500 × *g* for 5 min at 4 °C. Discard supernatant.

3. Resuspend cells with Streptavidin-Qdot 605 (*see* Table 4) and incubate for 20 min in the dark on ice. After the incubation, wash cells with SM, centrifuge at 500 × *g* for 5 min at 4 °C and discard supernatant.
4. Resuspend cells with a Live/Dead marker in the same volume as indicated above for antibody staining (*see* Table 4) and incubate for 30 min in the dark on ice. After the incubation, wash cells with SM and centrifuge at 500 × *g* for 5 min at 4 °C. Discard supernatant and resuspend cells in 400 μL of SM.
5. Analyze cells on a flow cytometer with appropriate compensation samples (*see* Subheading 3.4). Refer to Fig. 4 for gating strategy.

4 Notes

1. With regard to the best source of mouse B-1 cells, there are three main factors to take into consideration. First, greater numbers of B-1 cells can be retrieved from BALB/c compared to C57Bl/6 mice. Second, female mice have been found to contain more B-1 cells than their male counterparts ([50] and Waffarn, E and Baumgarth N, unpublished observations). Using the techniques outlined in this chapter, it is possible to collect at least 5–six million cells from the peritoneal cavity (PerC) of a female mouse and 2–three million cells from the pleural cavity (PlerC). Third, older mice yield more B-1 cells than younger ones; however, it is not recommended to use mice over 15 weeks of age as BALB/c mice in particular may spontaneously develop B-cell lymphomas [51, 52].
2. PBS solution can be generated as a 1× solution or a 10× stock solution. To prepare 1 l of a 1× solution, dissolve the following reagents in 800 mL of H_2O: 8 g NaCl, 0.2 g KCl, 1.44 g Na_2HPO_4, 0.24 g KH_2PO_4. Adjust pH to 7.2 using HCL. Add H_2O to make 1 l. Sterilize by autoclaving.
3. To prepare the mouse isotonic BSS, combine the following: 897 mL ddH20, 88 mL 1.68 M NaCl, 2.2 mL 1.68 M KCl, 2.2 mL 1.12 M $CaCl_2$ $2H_2O$, 740 μL 1.68 M $MgSO_4$ $7H_2O$, 1.5 mL potassium phosphate buffer mix, and 8.8 mL HEPES buffer to a total volume of 1 l. Sterilize by filtering through a 0.45 μm pore size filter. Do not autoclave as it would lead to precipitation. To generate the mouse tonicity BSS prepare (1) saline stock solutions in ddH_2O: 1.68 M NaCl, 1.68 M KCl, 1.12 M $CaCl_2$ $2H_2O$, 1.68 M $MgSO_4$ $7H_2O$; (2) potassium phosphate buffer mix in ddH_2O, pH 7.2: mix 1.68 M KH_2PO_4 and 1.12 M K_2HPO_4 together at a 1:1 ratio; (3) HEPES buffer in ddH_2O, pH 7.2: 1.68 M HEPES, 1.68 M NaOH.

4. The mouse tonicity buffer can be substituted with PBS. However, note that most PBS solutions are not mouse isotonic, and this will affect the survival rate of the harvested cells. We found mouse tonicity buffer to yield superior cell survival.
5. For magnetic cell separation-based isolation of B-1 cells and FACS-based sorting of B-1a and B-1b cells, use SM without sodium azide.
6. Our immunomagnetic cell separation protocols were optimized for use with an *auto*MACS "classic" and then also used for the *auto*MACS Pro (both Miltenyi). The system requires cells to be stained with antibodies conjugated to small magnetic beads, which are then passed over a magnetic column to trap stained cells. Following washes, the trapped cells are released by removal of the magnet. Depending on whether positive or negative enrichment is required, the cells that bound or are in the flow-through, respectively, contain the desired cell population. Due to the mechanical stress placed on the cells, negative enrichment reduces the risk of unnecessary cell activation. However, purity is usually somewhat lower than when bound cells are collected. Non-automatic systems from the same vendor, and numerous other commercial systems from other companies are available. Immunomagnetic cell separation with those other systems would be expected to yield very similar results using the protocols outlined here. Specifically, the buffers used for cell preparation and the antibody clones and staining procedures would not be affected by the choice of the magnetic cell separation system. Buffers for running cells over the column and their elution may require adjustment based on the manufacturer's recommendations.
7. Prior to start of the experiment, each fluorochrome-conjugated antibody is titrated for the optimal dilution by staining an appropriate tissue with increasing dilutions of the antibody. This is a critical step that should not be omitted. The distance between fluorochrome-positive and fluorochrome-negative fractions will change with the amount of antibodies (more antibodies do not necessarily equal better staining as they often increase background staining). Optimal dilution is determined to be the one that maximizes the distance between these positive and negative populations. The provided lists of fluorochrome-conjugated antibodies are guides, and alternative fluorochromes may be substituted as necessary and appropriate.
8. Here we report how to harvest peritoneal cavity cells in cases where the peritoneal membrane is accidentally punctured. (1) If the peritoneal membrane is ruptured during preparation, continue to prepare and pin back pleura as above. (2) Do not

orient the mouse perpendicular to the table; instead keep the mouse supine and use forceps to hold the pleural membrane near the point of puncture, pulling the membrane off the organs like a tent (*see* Fig. 2); this is crucial to keep the peritoneal fluid from draining out during lavage. (3) Proceed to lavage cavity through the puncture point as discussed above, but avoid swirling or excessive movement of organs with blunt-needled syringe; never let go of forceps or the lavage fluid will leak out. This will result in lower cell yield because you cannot adequately massage the SM around the peritoneal cavity, leaving cells unincorporated in your harvest.

9. Anti-biotin microbeads can be replaced with anti-streptavidin microbeads. However, we found the anti-biotin beads to remove labeled cells more efficiently, yielding higher purities. Microbeads should be titrated. We currently use anti-biotin beads at a dilution of 1:20 in running buffer.
10. Our protocol for B-1 cell enrichment is described for the use of an *auto*MACS "classic." For use of other magnetic cell separators, the exact conditions would need to be optimized by the user. However, both the antibody cocktails for purification and the FACS analysis procedure remain the same (*see* also **Note 6**).
11. In general, to prepare the compensation samples use the same cell antibody conjugate as the one used in the antibody staining mix. However, if the frequency of the cell population to be stained is low (<1–2%), it is preferable to use an antibody conjugated to the same fluorochrome but that has a specificity for a marker more commonly expressed in the spleen. This creates no problems if the fluorochrome is FITC, PE, or any other single molecule. However, when tandem dyes such as Cy5-PE and Cy-7-PE are used, differences in conjugation ratios may affect spillover and thus the compensation settings. Instead of using spleen cells, one can also use compensation beads conjugated with anti-mouse or anti-rat antibodies on which the conjugates are directly attached. The use of spleen cells represents a more cost-effective method.
12. For the isolation of B-1 cells from the bone marrow, the anti-CD23 antibody (used to identify B-2 cells) must be replaced with the anti-CD24 antibody.

Acknowledgments

Data for the B-1 cell FACS-sorts were kindly provided by Dr. Elizabeth E. Waffarn (Columbia University). This work was supported in part by NIH U19AI109962 and AI117890.

References

1. Baumgarth N (2011) The double life of a B-1 cell: self-reactivity selects for protective effector functions. Nat Rev Immunol 11(1):34–46. https://doi.org/10.1038/nri2901
2. Baumgarth N (2017) A hard(y) look at B-1 cell development and function. J Immunol 199 (10):3387–3394. https://doi.org/10.4049/jimmunol.1700943
3. Stall AM, Adams S, Herzenberg LA, Kantor AB (1992) Characteristics and development of the murine B-1b (Ly-1 B sister) cell population. Ann N Y Acad Sci 651:33–43
4. Savage HP, Klasener K, Smith FL, Luo Z, Reth M, Baumgarth N (2019) TLR induces reorganization of the IgM-BCR complex regulating murine B-1 cell responses to infections. elife 8. https://doi.org/10.7554/eLife.46997
5. Baumgarth N, Herman OC, Jager GC, Brown L, Herzenberg LA (1999) Innate and acquired humoral immunities to influenza virus are mediated by distinct arms of the immune system. Proc Natl Acad Sci U S A 96 (5):2250–2255
6. Hooijkaas H, Benner R, Pleasants JR, Wostmann BS (1984) Isotypes and specificities of immunoglobulins produced by germ-free mice fed chemically defined ultrafiltered "antigen-free" diet. Eur J Immunol 14 (12):1127–1130. https://doi.org/10.1002/eji.1830141212
7. Bos NA, Kimura H, Meeuwsen CG, De Visser H, Hazenberg MP, Wostmann BS, Pleasants JR, Benner R, Marcus DM (1989) Serum immunoglobulin levels and naturally occurring antibodies against carbohydrate antigens in germ-free BALB/c mice fed chemically defined ultrafiltered diet. Eur J Immunol 19 (12):2335–2339. https://doi.org/10.1002/eji.1830191223
8. Haury M, Sundblad A, Grandien A, Barreau C, Coutinho A, Nobrega A (1997) The repertoire of serum IgM in normal mice is largely independent of external antigenic contact. Eur J Immunol 27(6):1557–1563. https://doi.org/10.1002/eji.1830270635
9. Tornberg UC, Holmberg D (1995) B-1a, B-1b and B-2 B cells display unique VHDJH repertoires formed at different stages of ontogeny and under different selection pressures. EMBO J 14(8):1680–1689
10. Kantor AB, Merrill CE, Herzenberg LA, Hillson JL (1997) An unbiased analysis of V(H)-D-J(H) sequences from B-1a, B-1b, and conventional B cells. J Immunol 158(3):1175–1186
11. Notkins AL (2004) Polyreactivity of antibody molecules. Trends Immunol 25(4):174–179. https://doi.org/10.1016/j.it.2004.02.004
12. Stewart J (1992) Immunoglobulins did not arise in evolution to fight infection. Immunol Today 13(10):396–399. discussion 399-400
13. Bouvet JP, Dighiero G (1998) From natural polyreactive autoantibodies to a la carte monoreactive antibodies to infectious agents: is it a small world after all? Infect Immun 66(1):1–4
14. Baumgarth N, Tung JW, Herzenberg LA (2005) Inherent specificities in natural antibodies: a key to immune defense against pathogen invasion. Springer Semin Immunopathol 26 (4):347–362. https://doi.org/10.1007/s00281-004-0182-2
15. Chen Y, Park YB, Patel E, Silverman GJ (2009) IgM antibodies to apoptosis-associated determinants recruit C1q and enhance dendritic cell phagocytosis of apoptotic cells. J Immunol 182 (10):6031–6043. https://doi.org/10.4049/jimmunol.0804191
16. Chen GY, Tang J, Zheng P, Liu Y (2009) CD24 and Siglec-10 selectively repress tissue damage-induced immune responses. Science 323(5922):1722–1725. https://doi.org/10.1126/science.1168988
17. Zhang M, Alicot EM, Chiu I, Li J, Verna N, Vorup-Jensen T, Kessler B, Shimaoka M, Chan R, Friend D, Mahmood U, Weissleder R, Moore FD, Carroll MC (2006) Identification of the target self-antigens in reperfusion injury. J Exp Med 203 (1):141–152. doi:jem.20050390
18. Kulik L, Fleming SD, Moratz C, Reuter JW, Novikov A, Chen K, Andrews KA, Markaryan A, Quigg RJ, Silverman GJ, Tsokos GC, Holers VM (2009) Pathogenic natural antibodies recognizing annexin IV are required to develop intestinal ischemia-reperfusion injury. J Immunol 182(9):5363–5373. https://doi.org/10.4049/jimmunol.0803980
19. Smith FL, Baumgarth N (2019) B-1 cell responses to infections. Curr Opin Immunol 57:23–31. https://doi.org/10.1016/j.coi.2018.12.001
20. Baumgarth N, Herman OC, Jager GC, Brown LE, Herzenberg LA, Chen J (2000) B-1 and B-2 cell-derived immunoglobulin M antibodies are nonredundant components of the protective response to influenza virus infection. J Exp Med 192(2):271–280
21. Choi YS, Baumgarth N (2008) Dual role for B-1a cells in immunity to influenza virus infection. J Exp Med 205(13):3053–3064. https://doi.org/10.1084/jem.20080979
22. Jayasekera JP, Moseman EA, Carroll MC (2007) Natural antibody and complement mediate neutralization of influenza virus in

the absence of prior immunity. J Virol 81 (7):3487–3494. https://doi.org/10.1128/JVI.02128-06

23. Briles DE, Nahm M, Schroer K, Davie J, Baker P, Kearney J, Barletta R (1981) Antiphosphocholine antibodies found in normal mouse serum are protective against intravenous infection with type 3 streptococcus pneumoniae. J Exp Med 153(3):694–705

24. Boes M, Prodeus AP, Schmidt T, Carroll MC, Chen J (1998) A critical role of natural immunoglobulin M in immediate defense against systemic bacterial infection. J Exp Med 188 (12):2381–2386

25. Ochsenbein AF, Fehr T, Lutz C, Suter M, Brombacher F, Hengartner H, Zinkernagel RM (1999) Control of early viral and bacterial distribution and disease by natural antibodies. Science 286(5447):2156–2159

26. Zhou ZH, Zhang Y, Hu YF, Wahl LM, Cisar JO, Notkins AL (2007) The broad antibacterial activity of the natural antibody repertoire is due to polyreactive antibodies. Cell Host Microbe 1(1):51–61. https://doi.org/10.1016/j.chom.2007.01.002

27. O'Garra A, Chang R, Go N, Hastings R, Haughton G, Howard M (1992) Ly-1 B (B-1) cells are the main source of B cell-derived interleukin 10. Eur J Immunol 22 (3):711–717. https://doi.org/10.1002/eji.1830220314

28. Rauch PJ, Chudnovskiy A, Robbins CS, Weber GF, Etzrodt M, Hilgendorf I, Tiglao E, Figueiredo JL, Iwamoto Y, Theurl I, Gorbatov R, Waring MT, Chicoine AT, Mouded M, Pittet MJ, Nahrendorf M, Weissleder R, Swirski FK (2012) Innate response activator B cells protect against microbial sepsis. Science 335 (6068):597–601. https://doi.org/10.1126/science.1215173

29. Hayakawa K, Hardy RR, Herzenberg LA (1985) Progenitors for Ly-1 B cells are distinct from progenitors for other B cells. J Exp Med 161(6):1554–1568

30. Kawahara T, Ohdan H, Zhao G, Yang YG, Sykes M (2003) Peritoneal cavity B cells are precursors of splenic IgM natural antibody-producing cells. J Immunol 171 (10):5406–5414

31. Tumang JR, Frances R, Yeo SG, Rothstein TL (2005) Spontaneously Ig-secreting B-1 cells violate the accepted paradigm for expression of differentiation-associated transcription factors. J Immunol 174(6):3173–3177

32. Yang Y, Tung JW, Ghosn EE, Herzenberg LA (2007) Division and differentiation of natural antibody-producing cells in mouse spleen. Proc Natl Acad Sci U S A 104(11):4542–4546. https://doi.org/10.1073/pnas.0700001104

33. McIntyre TM, Holmes KL, Steinberg AD, Kastner DL (1991) CD5+ peritoneal B cells express high levels of membrane, but not secretory, C mu mRNA. J Immunol 146 (10):3639–3645

34. Choi YS, Dieter JA, Rothaeusler K, Luo Z, Baumgarth N (2012) B-1 cells in the bone marrow are a significant source of natural IgM. Eur J Immunol 42(1):120–129. https://doi.org/10.1002/eji.201141890

35. Martin F, Oliver AM, Kearney JF (2001) Marginal zone and B1 B cells unite in the early response against T-independent blood-borne particulate antigens. Immunity 14(5):617–629

36. Ohdan H, Swenson KG, Kruger Gray HS, Yang YG, Xu Y, Thall AD, Sykes M (2000) Mac-1-negative B-1b phenotype of natural antibody-producing cells, including those responding to gal alpha 1,3Gal epitopes in alpha 1,3-galactosyltransferase-deficient mice. J Immunol 165(10):5518–5529

37. Ha SA, Tsuji M, Suzuki K, Meek B, Yasuda N, Kaisho T, Fagarasan S (2006) Regulation of B1 cell migration by signals through toll-like receptors. J Exp Med 203(11):2541–2550

38. Cole LE, Yang Y, Elkins KL, Fernandez ET, Qureshi N, Shlomchik MJ, Herzenberg LA, Vogel SN (2009) Antigen-specific B-1a antibodies induced by Francisella tularensis LPS provide long-term protection against F. tularensis LVS challenge. Proc Natl Acad Sci U S A 106 (11):4343–4348. https://doi.org/10.1073/pnas.0813411106

39. Nisitani S, Tsubata T, Murakami M, Honjo T (1995) Administration of interleukin-5 or −10 activates peritoneal B-1 cells and induces autoimmune hemolytic anemia in anti-erythrocyte autoantibody-transgenic mice. Eur J Immunol 25(11):3047–3052. https://doi.org/10.1002/eji.1830251110

40. Murakami M, Tsubata T, Shinkura R, Nisitani S, Okamoto M, Yoshioka H, Usui T, Miyawaki S, Honjo T (1994) Oral administration of lipopolysaccharides activates B-1 cells in the peritoneal cavity and lamina propria of the gut and induces autoimmune symptoms in an autoantibody transgenic mouse. J Exp Med 180(1):111–121

41. Alugupalli KR, Leong JM, Woodland RT, Muramatsu M, Honjo T, Gerstein RM (2004) B1b lymphocytes confer T cell-independent long-lasting immunity. Immunity 21 (3):379–390. https://doi.org/10.1016/j.immuni.2004.06.019

42. Haas KM, Poe JC, Steeber DA, Tedder TF (2005) B-1a and B-1b cells exhibit distinct developmental requirements and have unique functional roles in innate and adaptive immunity to S. pneumoniae. Immunity 23(1):7–18. doi: 10.1016/j.immuni.2005.04.011
43. Gil-Cruz C, Bobat S, Marshall JL, Kingsley RA, Ross EA, Henderson IR, Leyton DL, Coughlan RE, Khan M, Jensen KT, Buckley CD, Dougan G, MacLennan IC, Lopez-Macias C, Cunningham AF (2009) The porin OmpD from nontyphoidal Salmonella is a key target for a protective B1b cell antibody response. Proc Natl Acad Sci U S A 106 (24):9803–9808. https://doi.org/10.1073/pnas.0812431106
44. Kroese FG, Butcher EC, Stall AM, Lalor PA, Adams S, Herzenberg LA (1989) Many of the IgA producing plasma cells in murine gut are derived from self-replenishing precursors in the peritoneal cavity. Int Immunol 1(1):75–84
45. Rosado MM, Aranburu A, Capolunghi F, Giorda E, Cascioli S, Cenci F, Petrini S, Miller E, Leanderson T, Bottazzo GF, Natali PG, Carsetti R (2009) From the fetal liver to spleen and gut: the highway to natural antibody. Mucosal Immunol 2(4):351–361. https://doi.org/10.1038/mi.2009.15
46. Savage HP, Yenson VM, Sawhney SS, Mousseau BJ, Lund FE, Baumgarth N (2017) Blimp-1-dependent and -independent natural antibody production by B-1 and B-1-derived plasma cells. J Exp Med. https://doi.org/10.1084/jem.20161122
47. Baumgarth N (2004) B-cell immunophenotyping. Methods Cell Biol 75:643–662
48. Wells SM, Kantor AB, Stall AM (1994) CD43 (S7) expression identifies peripheral B cell subsets. J Immunol 153(12):5503–5515
49. Herzenberg LA, Stall AM, Braun J, Weaver D, Baltimore D, Grosschedl R (1987) Depletion of the predominant B-cell population in immunoglobulin mu heavy-chain transgenic mice. Nature 329(6134):71–73. https://doi.org/10.1038/329071a0
50. Zeng Z, Surewaard BGJ, Wong CHY, Guettler C, Petri B, Burkhard R, Wyss M, Le Moual H, Devinney R, Thompson GC, Blackwood J, Joffe AR, McCoy KD, Jenne CN, Kubes P (2018) Sex-hormone-driven innate antibodies protect females and infants against EPEC infection. Nat Immunol 19 (10):1100–1111. https://doi.org/10.1038/s41590-018-0211-2
51. Kim KJ, Kanellopoulos-Langevin C, Merwin RM, Sachs DH, Asofsky R (1979) Establishment and characterization of BALB/c lymphoma lines with B cell properties. J Immunol 122(2):549–554
52. Pattengale PK, Frith CH (1983) Immunomorphologic classification of spontaneous lymphoid cell neoplasms occurring in female BALB/c mice. J Natl Cancer Inst 70 (1):169–179

Chapter 3

Purification and Immunophenotypic Characterization of Murine Plasma Cells

Van Duc Dang, Simon Fillatreau, and Andreia C. Lino

Abstract

B cells are primarily known for their capacity to differentiate into antibody-secreting cells (ASCs). ASCs are usually viewed as terminally differentiated cells sharing a unique phenotype. However, it lately became evident that ASCs exist in a variety of subsets differing by their lifespan, anatomic location, and immunological function. Thus, ASCs can exist as long-lived plasma cells (LLPC) that can persist for years in a nonproliferating state within particular niches in the bone marrow (BM), or as short-lived plasma cells (SLPC) that are primarily found in secondary lymphoid organs or inflamed tissues and wane upon the termination of the associated immune response. Another layer of ASC diversity was uncovered with the discovery of their capacity to produce various pro- or anti-inflammatory cytokines. Notably, a subset of natural regulatory plasma cells characterized by the distinctive expression of the inhibitory receptor lymphocyte activation gene (LAG)-3 and a unique capacity to produce interleukin (IL)-10 upon stimulation was recently identified. Here, we describe how to immunophenotypically characterize murine plasma cells as well as how to isolate them using cell sorting, with a special focus on these recently described natural regulatory plasma cells.

Key words Natural regulatory plasma cells, Plasma cells, IL-10, LAG-3, Purification of murine plasma cells, Immunophenotypic characterization of murine plasma cells

1 Introduction

B cells are unique in their capacity to differentiate into ASCs, which represents one of the most important features of immune responses. Indeed, primary immunodeficiencies resulting in a defect in antibody production are associated with a markedly increased susceptibility to infectious diseases [1]. Moreover, ASCs maintaining the production of specific antibodies after an immune challenge are the basis for the serological memory that underlies the beneficial effect of most successful vaccines [2, 3]. In addition to provide an essential layer of immune defense against pathogens, ASCs also play important roles in immune-mediated inflammatory diseases, in which they can act as pathogenic cells via the production of antibodies reacting against self-antigens or innocuous

Francesca Mion and Silvia Tonon (eds.), *Regulatory B Cells: Methods and Protocols*, Methods in Molecular Biology, vol. 2270, https://doi.org/10.1007/978-1-0716-1237-8_3,

environmental antigens leading to autoimmune or allergic disorders, respectively [4]. Understanding the biology of ASCs is therefore of primary importance in fundamental and clinical immunology.

The molecular mechanisms underlying the differentiation of activated B cells into ASCs, particularly the transcription network implicated, are progressively being elucidated [2]. However, these cells are heterogeneous, and the clinical implications of this diversity, as well as the molecular mechanisms underlying their differentiation, are only starting to emerge. ASCs differ according to their proliferative status and lifespan. Thus, activated B cells first give rise to plasmablasts, which start secreting antibodies while proliferating, and plasma cells, which are no longer proliferative and are considered as terminally differentiated. Plasma cells can be short-lived or long-lived, with a lifespan ranging from several days to decades [5]. In fact, the evaluation of the half-life of serum antibody titers to particular vaccine antigens indicated that some plasma cells might live for the entire life of the host, producing antibodies while remaining in a nonproliferative state [6].

ASCs can also perform antibody-independent functions through the production of cytokines [7]. These novel activities might be particularly relevant in inflammatory diseases since these cells often accumulate in large numbers in secondary lymphoid organs or inflamed tissues in these diseases. For instance, ASCs were found to suppress the progression of T cell-mediated autoimmune diseases through the production of IL-10 [8]. Recently, a subset of natural regulatory plasma cells showing an epigenome and transcriptome specialized for IL-10 expression, which distinctively expressed LAG-3 was identified [9]. This study provided proof of evidence that protective and pathogenic plasma cells might be distinguishable in autoimmune disorders. Here, we provide a detailed protocol describing how to immunophenotypically characterize murine plasma cells, and to purify them using cell sorting, with a special focus on recently described LAG-3$^+$ natural regulatory plasma cells.

2 Materials

2.1 Equipment

1. Pipette P1000, P200, P100, P10, P2.5, and multichannel pipette.
2. Centrifuge and microcentrifuge.
3. Laminar flow hood.
4. Cell incubator.
5. Instrument for automated separation of various cells types from a tissue (e.g., AutoMACS pro from Miltenyi Biotec).

6. Flow cytometer (e.g., FACSymphony, Fortessa, Canto, LSR II from BD Biosciences or MACSQuant® from Miltenyi Biotec) and cell sorter (e.g., Sorter Aria I and II from BD Biosciences).
7. EliSpot reader.

2.2 Consumables

1. Neubauer improved counting chamber.
2. 96-well microtiter plates (V-bottom).
3. 96-well tissue culture-treated microplates (U-bottom).
4. Petri dishes, polystyrene size 100 mm.
5. 15 mL and 50 mL conical polypropylene tubes.
6. 5, 2, 1.5, and 0.5 mL tubes.
7. Cell strainer (40–100 μm).
8. Pre-separation filters (30 μm).
9. Tips 1000, 200, 20, 10, 2.5 μL.
10. Needles (18G and 25G) and syringes (3 mL and 10 mL).
11. MultiScreen-IP Filter Plate, 0.45 μm, clear, sterile.

2.3 Animals

1. C57BL/6 mice were bred under specific pathogen-free conditions. Males or females older than 8 weeks of age were used (*see* **Note 1**).

2.4 Antibodies and Stimulation Agonists

Here below we provide the list of reagents we have been routinely using to perform the described protocols. However, based on the needs and availability of the laboratory, other reagents and companies may be used.

1. Monoclonal antibodies for flow cytometry analysis (*see* Table 1).
2. Anti-PE microbeads (Miltenyi Biotec).
3. Anti-mouse Ig(H + L) chain (capture antibody) and alkaline phosphatase (AP)-conjugated IgM, IgG, IgG1, IgG2b, IgG2c, IgG3, and IgA (detection antibody) for ELISPOT assay (Southern Biotechnology Associates).
4. Fc block solution: 30 μg/mL purified anti-mouse CD16/CD32 (clone 2.4G2) antibody in PBS/BSA solution.
5. LPS (*Escherichia coli* O55:B5).
6. Anti-IgM (Fab) antibody, cell culture grade.
7. Agonistic anti-CD40 antibody (clone FGK-45, produced in DRFZ, Berlin, Germany), cell culture grade.
8. IL-6 and IL-21 cytokines, cell culture grade.

2.5 Buffers and Media

1. Phosphate-buffered saline (PBS): 136.9 mM NaCl, 2.68 mM KCl, 1.47 mM KH_2PO_4, 7.9 mM Na_2HPO_4; pH 7.2–7.4.

Table 1
Antibodies used for flow cytometry

Target	Clone
B220 (CD45R)	RA3-6B2
CD1d	1B1
CD4	GK1.5/RM4–5
CD8	53–6.72/53–6.7
CD11b	M1/70.15.11/M1/70
CD11c	N418
CD19	6D5
CD40	FGK-45
CD43	S7
CD69	H1.2F3
CD71	RI7217
CD79α	F11–172
CD79β	HM79–12
CD81	Eat-2
CD138	281–2
CD200	OX-90
CXCR3	CXCR3–173
FAS (CD95)	O2
Foxp3	FJK-16 s
GL7	GL7
Ki-67	16A8
LAG-3 (CD223)	C9B7W
MHC-II	M5/114
PD-L1	MIH5
PD-L2	TY25
TCR-β	H57–597

2. PBS/BSA solution: 0.5% (w/v) bovine serum albumin (BSA) in PBS.
3. Red Blood Cell Lysis Buffer (RBC lysis): 0.155 M NH_4Cl, 0.01 M $KHCO_3$, 0.1 mM ethylenediamintetraacetate (EDTA); pH 7.5.

4. Complete RPMI medium: 50 μM ß-mercaptoethanol, 100 U/mL penicillin, 100 μg/mL streptomycin, and 10% fetal calf serum (FCS, v/v) in RPMI 1640 medium.
5. ELISPOT wash solution: 0.1% Tween-20 in PBS.

2.6 Other Reagents

1. Foxp3 staining kit.
2. Bio-Plex Pro Mouse Cytokine IL-10 Set, 1× 96 well.
3. 5-Bromo-4-chloro-3-indolyl phosphate (BCIP)/nitro blue tetrazolium (NBT) substrate for use with AP.
4. 4′,6-Diamidino-2-phenylindole (DAPI), Propidium Iodide (PI) and uncoupled Pacific Orange.
5. 0.5 M EDTA, pH 8.0.
6. 70% and 35% ethanol.
7. Deionized water.

3 Methods

In the following protocol, all centrifugations (spin down) are performed at 400 × *g* for 5–10 min at 4 °C, unless indicated otherwise.

3.1 Isolation of Splenocytes

1. Euthanize mice (*see* **Note 1**) by cervical dislocation and disinfect the animal with 70% ethanol. Carefully open underbelly skin with scissors (be careful to not injure intestines) and fix the mouse on a dissection board with needles (*see* **Note 2**).
2. Collect spleens and transfer into a 100-mm Petri dish with ice-cold PBS/BSA solution.
3. Mash spleens in the Petri dish to obtain a cell suspension. To this end, load the dissociated spleen through the cell strainer (70 μm) and obtain a single cell suspension using the plunger of a 3-mL syringe.
4. Collect the cell suspension in PBS/BSA solution using a 10-mL syringe with a large needle (18G) and transfer to a 50-mL tube using small needle (25G).
5. Rinse sieve with fresh PBS/BSA solution and collect all the cell suspension as in **Step 4** in the same 50 mL tube, then spin down and discard the supernatant.
6. Resuspend in RBC lysis buffer (1 mL/spleen) and incubate for 4 min at room temperature. Then fill up the tube with medium and spin down to block the lysis reaction.
7. Resuspend in PBS/BSA solution and count cells using a counting chamber or the MACSQuant® Flow Cytometer.

3.2 Identification and Immunophenotype Characterization of LAG-3+ Regulatory Plasma cells by Flow Cytometry

3.2.1 Surface Staining

1. To identify LAG-3^+ regulatory plasma cells, add 3–5 × 10^6 splenocytes/well into 96-well V-bottom plate and spin down. Then, remove the supernatant by flicking the plate and using paper towel.
2. Resuspend cells with 50 μL Fc block solution to block unspecific bindings. After a 15 min incubation at 4 °C, spin the cells down and remove the supernatant as described above.
3. Add 50 μL of the antibody staining mix made of anti-CD19, -CD138, –LAG-3, -CD4 and -CD8 antibodies diluted in PBS/BSA solution. Antibodies should be appropriately titrated to obtain optimal staining. Make sure to resuspend cells well by pipetting up and down and incubate 15 min at 4 °C (*see* **Note 3**). The antibodies of the antibody staining mix are required to identify regulatory plasma cells; however, antibodies relevant to characterize the phenotypes of regulatory plasma cells can also be added (*see* **Note 4**).
4. Following the incubation, wash twice by adding 250 μL of PBS/BSA solution and resuspending the cells well. Then, spin down and remove the supernatant as described above.
5. Repeat **steps 3–4** for staining with secondary staining reagent (if applicable) in 50 μL per well.
6. If samples are acquired within 5 h from the end of the extracellular staining protocol, then resuspend cells in 200–300 μL of PBS/BSA solution and store in the fridge protected from light (e.g., cover with aluminum foil) until acquisition. Otherwise, fix cells (*see* **Note 5**).
7. Before acquisition, add 0.1 μg/mL PI or 0.1 μg/mL DAPI or any other alternative to exclude dead cells.
8. At this point, samples can be acquired on the flow cytometer or further processed for intracellular staining. The flow cytometry data can be analyzed through an appropriate software. Figure 1 shows a gating strategy to identify the LAG-3^+ and LAG-3^- plasma cells.

3.2.2 Intracellular Staining of LAG-3^+ Regulatory Plasma Cells

After staining for surface markers as described above, splenocytes can be stained for intracellular markers. In this case, they are first stained with the uncoupled pacific orange dye or any alternative reagent that labels dead cells. Cells are then fixed and processed for staining with Ki-67 (marker expressed by proliferating cells) and/or other intracellular markers using a Foxp3 staining kit which has been formulated and optimized for cell staining with antibodies to transcription factors and nuclear proteins.

1. After removal of the supernatant, cells must be resuspended in 100 μL of fixation/permeabilization solution (prepared according to manufacturer's instructions) and incubated for

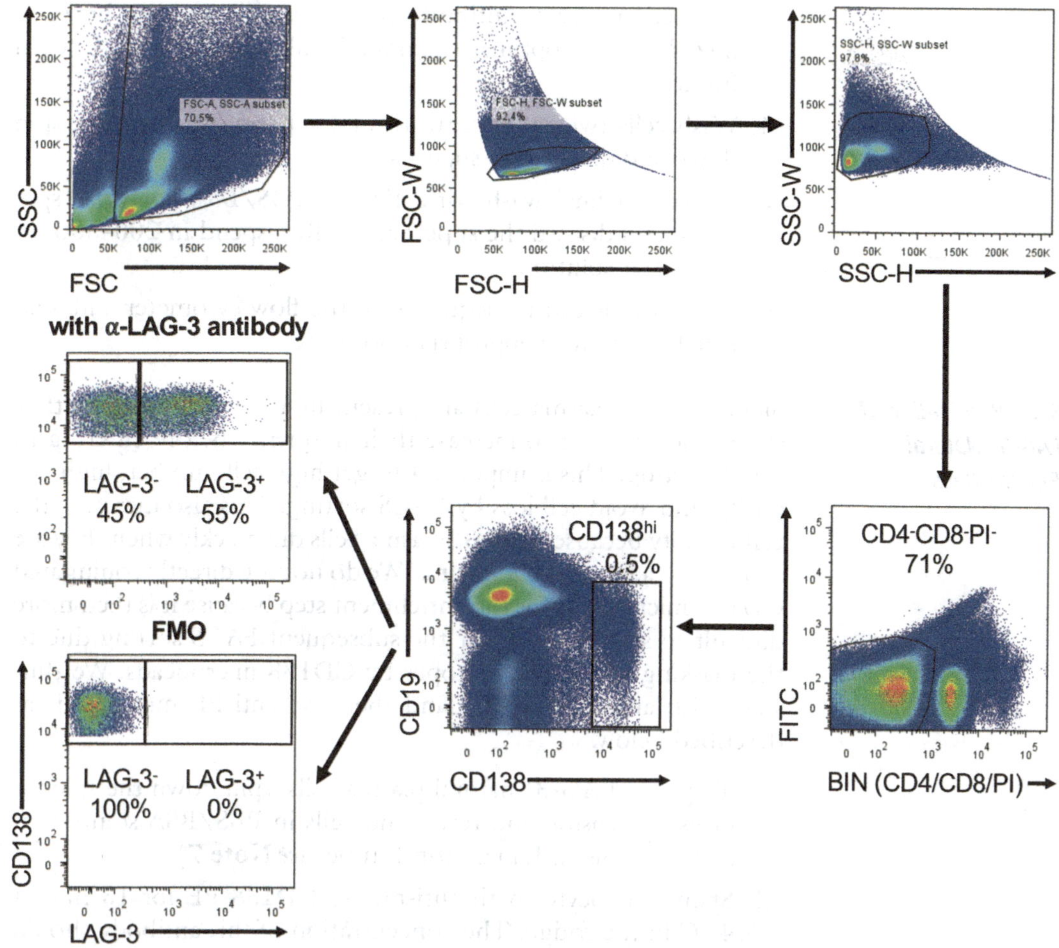

Fig. 1 Gating strategy to identify the LAG-3$^+$ regulatory plasma cell population. C57BL/6 splenocytes were surface stained with anti-CD19, -CD138, –LAG-3, -CD4, -CD8 antibodies and with propidium iodide (PI) and analyzed using flow cytometer. To identify LAG-3$^+$ regulatory plasma cells, cells were first gated based on the size and granularity using FSC and SSC to exclude debris (upper left). Then clumped cells were eliminated using FSC-W and FSC-H (upper middle) and SSC-W and SSC-H (upper right). Single cells were then gated as CD4$^-$CD8$^-$PI$^-$ live cells to exclude dead and T cells (bottom right). Subsequently plasma cells were gated as CD138^{hi} on the basis of the differential expression of the CD19 and CD138 surface molecules (bottom middle). Eventually, LAG-3 plasma cells were identified based on the expression of CD138 and LAG-3. Splenocytes from *Lag3*$^{-/-}$ mice or an FMO (fluorescence minus one) for LAG-3 were used to set the gate for LAG-3$^+$ cells

1 h at 4 °C. After incubation, spin down and discard the supernatant (*see* **Note 6**).

2. Wash samples twice by resuspending cells in 1× perm/wash buffer (prepared according to manufacturer's instructions). Spin down and remove the supernatant.
3. Add 50 μL/well of anti-Ki-67 and/or other intracellular markers antibody mix prepared in 1× perm/wash buffer and resuspend very well. Antibodies to other intracellular antigens can

be used similarly. Antibody concentrations have to be optimized to gain optimal staining. Incubate for 1 h at 4 °C in fridge.

4. Wash cells twice with 150 μL of 1× perm/wash buffer, spin down and discard the supernatant.
5. Perform a final wash with 250 μL PBS/BSA solution, spin down and discard the supernatant. Resuspend in 200–300 μL PBS/BSA solution.
6. Stained cells can be acquired on the flow cytometer and analyzed through an appropriate software.

3.3 Purification of LAG-3⁺ Natural Plasma Cells

Since LAG-3⁺ plasma cells are present in a low cell number, they should be enriched to increase their frequency before entering to FACS sorting. This is important to get high cell number, high cell purity, and avoid cell loss by FACS sorting. This also increases the cell viability because LAG-3⁺ plasma cells die quickly when they are exposed to a long FACS sorting. We do not use directly conjugated CD138 microbeads for the enrichment step because it is then more difficult to stain CD138 for the subsequent FACS sorting due to the masking of CD138 epitopes by CD138 microbeads. We thus stain with anti-CD138-PE, and then use anti-PE microbeads as described below.

1. To purify LAG-3⁺ natural plasma cells, spin down the splenocytes suspension and resuspend cells in PBS/BSA solution at 2×10^8 cells/mL in a 50-mL tube (*see* **Note 7**).
2. Stain splenocytes with anti-mouse CD138-PE for 15 min at 4 °C in the fridge. The concentration of this antibody should be optimized to obtain the best staining. After incubation fill up the tube with complete RPMI medium, spin down and discard the supernatant.
3. Following the wash, resuspend cells in PBS/BSA solution at 1×10^8 cells/mL and add magnetic anti-PE microbeads (according to manufacturer instructions).
4. After incubation at 4 °C in the fridge (according to manufacturer instructions), fill up with complete RPMI medium, spin down and discard the supernatant.
5. Resuspend cells in PBS/BSA solution at 2×10^8 cells/mL, remove cell clumps by pre-separation filter and process the sample with AutoMACS pro using the Posseld2 program (*see* **Note 8**).
6. After autoMACS enrichment, the obtained CD138⁺ cells are centrifuged to remove the supernatant and then resuspended at 1×10^8 cells/mL in the staining mix containing anti-CD19, -CD138, –LAG-3 antibodies and the "dump" CD11b/CD11c/TCR-β/DAPI.

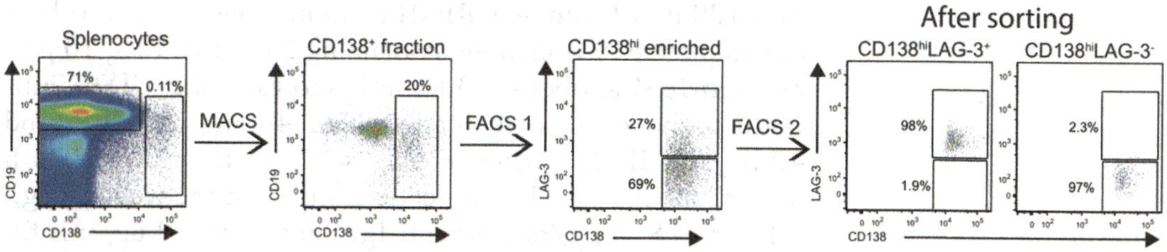

Fig. 2 Strategy to sort LAG-3$^+$ plasma cells. Splenocytes were stained with the anti-CD138-PE antibody, followed by labeling with magnetic anti-PE microbeads, and magnetic separation on autoMACS pro (Miltenyi Biotec). The obtained CD138-positive fraction was stained for CD19, CD138, LAG-3, and CD11b/CD11c/TCR-β/DAPI. After CD138^{hi} enrichment by a first round of sorting, CD138^{hi}LAG-3$^+$CD11b$^-$CD11c$^-$TCR-β$^-$DAPI$^-$ and CD138^{hi}LAG-3$^-$CD11b$^-$CD11c$^-$TCR-β$^-$DAPI$^-$ cells were then isolated by a secound round of sorting. Numbers in FACS plots indicate the percentages of gated cells before MACS, after MACS enrichment, after FACS 1 and FACS 2 (from left to right)

7. To highly purify LAG-3$^+$ natural plasma cells, two sequential FACS sorting are necessary (*see* **Notes 9** and **10**). First proceed with the isolation of CD138^{hi}CD11b$^-$CD11c$^-$TCR-β$^-$DAPI$^-$ cells using the enrichment procedure. Then separate CD138^{hi}LAG-3$^+$CD11b$^-$CD11c$^-$TCR-β$^-$DAPI$^-$ and CD138^{hi}LAG-3$^-$CD11b$^-$CD11c$^-$TCR-β$^-$DAPI$^-$ cells using the high purity procedure. Figure 2 illustrates a strategy to purify LAG-3$^+$ regulatory plasma cells (*see* **Note 11**).
8. If the researcher is interested in the analysis of other B cell subsets (e.g., to compare epigenome, transcriptome, and secretome with LAG-3$^+$ and LAG-3$^-$ plasma cell subsets) then do not discard the CD138-negative fraction resulting from autoMACS separation. Collect the CD138$^-$ population and stain with anti-CD19, -CD138, -CD1d antibodies and CD11b/CD11c/TCR-β/DAPI. At the end of incubation, sort CD19$^+$CD138$^-$CD11b$^-$CD11c$^-$TCRβ$^-$DAPI$^-$, CD19$^+$CD1d^{hi}CD11b$^-$CD11c$^-$TCR-β$^-$DAPI$^-$ and CD19$^+$CD1d^{low}CD11b$^-$CD11c$^-$TCR-β$^-$DAPI$^-$ (*see* **Note 12**).

3.4 Stimulation of LAG-3$^+$ Regulatory Plasma cells and Evaluation of Cytokine Production

After sorting, seed the different B cell subsets, e.g., CD19$^+$CD138$^-$, CD19$^+$CD1d^{hi}, CD19$^+$CD1d^{low}, CD138^{hi}LAG-3$^+$ and CD138^{hi}LAG-3$^-$, and/or any other B cell subset, to compare their ability to produce cytokines. LPS, anti-IgM and anti-CD40 antibodies are selected for plasma and B cell subset stimulation because they have been shown to trigger cytokine production. IL-6 and IL-21 are important for plasma cell survival.

1. Seed 1 × 10^5 CD138^{hi}LAG-3$^+$CD11b$^-$CD11c$^-$TCR-β$^-$DAPI$^-$ and CD138^{hi}LAG-3$^-$CD11b$^-$CD11c$^-$TCR-β$^-$DAPI$^-$ plasma cells and B cell subsets in 100 μL of complete RPMI medium per well in 96-well round bottom plates.

2. Add 100 μL of complete RPMI medium (negative control) or of complete RPMI medium containing 2 μg/mL LPS, 10 μg/mL anti-IgM antibody, 20 μg/mL agonistic anti-CD40 antibody, alone or in combination with 40 ng/mL IL-6 and 40 ng/mL IL-21. Incubate cells at 37 °C, 5% CO_2 for 24 h in a cell incubator. The final concentration in the well is 1 μg/mL for LPS, 5 μg/mL for anti-IgM antibody, 10 μg/mL for agonistic anti-CD40 antibody, 20 ng/mL for IL-6 and 20 ng/mL for IL-21.
3. Cytokine concentration secreted by plasma cell and B cell subsets is quantified in cell supernatant. To this end, following incubation, spin down the culture plate, collect 150 μL of cell supernatant and transfer into a new 96 well plate. Keep at −20 °C until further use. Cytokine concentration in the supernatant is determined by the Bio-Plex kit (Bio-Rad) according to manufacturer's instructions (*see* **Note 13**).

3.5 Detection of Antibody Production in LAG-3$^+$ Plasma cells by ELISPOT Assay

ELISPOT assay enables the detection and quantification of the frequency of protein-secreting cells at single cell level. In this method, proteins such as cytokines or antibodies secreted by cells in culture will be captured by specific antibody pre-coated on the plate surface. After incubation, cells are washed out and secreted molecules are detected using a detection antibody conjugated with an enzyme, followed by a substrate with a precipitating product. In the end, visible spots on the plate surface correspond to individual cytokine or ASCs. To determine the frequency of ASCs and identify the classes of immunoglobin, ELISPOT assay is applied for sorted LAG-3$^+$ and LAG-3$^-$ plasma cells.

1. Pre-wet each well of EIA/RIA high-binding plate with 15 μL of a 35% ethanol solution for 1 min and then rinse three times with 150 μL of PBS. Do not let wells dry out.
2. Coat plates with 50 μL of a 5 μg/mL solution of anti-IgH + L (heavy and light chain) antibody in PBS overnight at 4 °C.
3. Decant solution and wash twice with 150 μL of PBS.
4. To block unspecific binding, add 200 μL of complete RPMI medium and incubate 2 h at 37 °C.
5. Wash sorted CD138^{hi}LAG-3$^+$CD11b$^-$CD11c$^-$TCR-β$^-$DAPI$^-$ and CD138^{hi}LAG-3$^-$CD11b$^-$CD11c$^-$TCR-β$^-$DAPI$^-$ plasma cells by filling up with cold complete RPMI medium in 15 mL falcon tube to minimize background from soluble antibodies and resuspend to 10^6 cells/mL in complete RPMI medium.
6. Decant medium from plates and prefill all wells except for the top row of the plate with 200 μL of complete RPMI medium.

7. Fill top row with cell suspensions using 250 μL for the fivefold dilution series or 300 μL for the threefold dilution series. Transfer either 50 μL (for the fivefold dilution) or 100 μL (for the threefold dilution) from the top row to the one below and mix carefully by pipetting up and down. Continue the dilution series by transferring cells from the filled row to the one below.
8. Incubate for 3 h at 37 °C in a cell culture incubator (5% CO_2 and 95% H_2O), then decant cells and wash three to six times with the wash solution.
9. Prepare AP-conjugated antibodies, including IgM, IgA and IgG, IgG1, IgG2b, IgG2c, IgG3 by diluting 1:500 in wash solution. Add 100 μL to each well and incubate for 2 h at 37 °C.
10. After incubation, wash three times with deionized water.
11. Add 35 μL of BCIP/NBT (ready to use) per well starting with the highly diluted rows and wait for 5–10 min until spots become visible (from bottom).
12. Quickly stop development reaction under running deionized water and pull off plastic cover from the bottom of the plate. Carefully wash both sides of plates.
13. Let dry for several hours at 37 °C or overnight at room temperature. The plates are then ready for analysis using an EliSpot reader.

4 Notes

1. The older the animals are, the more plasma cells and LAG-3$^+$ plasma cells they have [9], therefore according to the purpose of this experiment this should be taken into consideration.
2. For the sterile isolation of plasma cells, every step should be performed under laminar hood.
3. We recommend using CD4 and CD8 in the same dump channel with PI (e.g., anti-CD4 and anti-CD8 antibodies in conjugation with PerCP) in order to save channels for other markers. Since CD4$^+$ and CD8$^+$ cells express LAG-3, they are excluded from the analysis to avoid any interference with the quantification and characterization of LAG-3$^+$ plasma cells.
4. Depending on the capacity of the flow cytometer in your laboratory, the anti-CD1d, -CD69, -CD81, -CD200, -IgM, -PD-L2, -PD-L1, -CD79α, -CD79β, -B220, -MHC-II, -CD43, -CD71, -FAS, and -CXCR3 antibodies can be combined with the required staining mix (CD19, CD138, LAG-3, CD4, and CD8) to characterize the immunophenotypes of

regulatory plasma cells. The CD1d, CD69, CD81, CD200, IgM, PD-L2, PD-L1, CD79α, CD79β molecules are upregulated on LAG3$^+$ ASCs, while the B220, MHC-II, CD43, CD71, FAS, and CXCR3 molecules are downregulated on LAG-3$^+$ ASCs.

5. If the operator is not able to acquire samples within 5 h from the ending of the extracellular staining protocol, then cells should be fixed with 2% paraformaldehyde. Resuspend cells in 200 μL PBS (or PBS/BSA) and add 200 μL of 4% paraformaldehyde. Incubate 15 min at room temperature on bench. Then spin down and carefully remove the supernatant (you might want to leave some residual wash buffer to not lose cells as pellets can be loose). Finally, resuspend in 200–400 μL of PBS/BSA solution. The PBS/BSA buffer should contain azide if samples are kept for several days.
6. The fixed cells could be nuclear stained in the next day. If so, resuspend cells in 100 μL PBS/BSA solution and store at 4 °C overnight.
7. Splenocytes from *Lag3*$^{-/-}$ mice (these mice can be purchased from the Jackson Laboratories) were used to identify the LAG-3$^+$ subsets. Alternatively, an FMO (fluorescence minus one) for LAG-3 can be used.
8. Instead of AutoMACS device, there are several available magnetic systems to enrich the cells of interest. There are LS and MS columns (Miltenyi) and correspondent magnetic supports. Also, there are column-free magnetic systems from stem cell technologies.
9. Since CD138$^+$ cells die quickly after AutoMACS separation, you should stain cells and perform next steps as fast as possible.
10. In order to yield high cell numbers and increase cell viability, coat FACS collection tubes with complete RPMI medium supplemented with 10% FCS and incubate at 37 °C for 30 min.
11. The cell purity is often ≥98% after FACS 2 sorting. In case the purity is not priority, LAG-3$^+$ and LAG-3$^-$ can be sorted without FACS enrichment procedure. In this case the purity is often ≥95%.
12. In case total B cells are used to compare with LAG-3$^+$ and LAG-3$^-$ plasma cells, the CD138-negative fraction resulting from separation is stained with anti-CD11b, -CD11c, and -CD43 microbeads (Miltenyi Biotec) according to manufacturer's instructions. Then total B cells can be obtained by magnetic isolation using depletion selection program on AutoMACS device or manual magnetic system.
13. Several IL-10 ELISA kits are commercially available and could be used to measure IL-10 concentration. Nevertheless, we

used the Bio-Plex kit (Bio-Rad) because it is able to measure several cytokines at the same time using a low volume (50 μL) of cell supernatant. Alternatively, ProcartaPlex kit (Thermo Fisher Scientific) can also be used.

Acknowledgments

V.D.D is supported by Vinmec grant ISC.19.11. S.F. lab is supported by ERC PREG-LAB 647696, AXA Chair Translational Immunology, Chair of Excellence (University Paris Descartes), Agence Nationale pour la Recherche (ANR), INSERM, and CNRS. DFG grant LI3540/1-1 to ACL.

References

1. Smith T, Cunningham-Rundles C (2019) Primary B-cell immunodeficiencies. Hum Immunol 80(6):351–362. https://doi.org/10.1016/j.humimm.2018.10.015
2. Nutt SL, Hodgkin PD, Tarlinton DM, Corcoran LM (2015) The generation of antibody-secreting plasma cells. Nat Rev Immunol 15(3):160–171. https://doi.org/10.1038/nri3795
3. Oracki SA, Walker JA, Hibbs ML, Corcoran LM, Tarlinton DM (2010) Plasma cell development and survival. Immunol Rev 237(1):140–159. https://doi.org/10.1111/j.1600-065X.2010.00940.x
4. Chang HD, Tokoyoda K, Hoyer B, Alexander T, Khodadadi L, Mei H, Dorner T, Hiepe F, Burmester GR, Radbruch A (2019) Pathogenic memory plasma cells in autoimmunity. Curr Opin Immunol 61:86–91. https://doi.org/10.1016/j.coi.2019.09.005
5. Radbruch A, Muehlinghaus G, Luger EO, Inamine A, Smith KG, Dorner T, Hiepe F (2006) Competence and competition: the challenge of becoming a long-lived plasma cell. Nat Rev Immunol 6(10):741–750. https://doi.org/10.1038/nri1886
6. Amanna IJ, Carlson NE, Slifka MK (2007) Duration of humoral immunity to common viral and vaccine antigens. N Engl J Med 357(19):1903–1915. https://doi.org/10.1056/NEJMoa066092
7. Shen P, Fillatreau S (2015) Antibody-independent functions of B cells: a focus on cytokines. Nat Rev Immunol 15(7):441–451. https://doi.org/10.1038/nri3857
8. Fillatreau S, Sweenie CH, McGeachy MJ, Gray D, Anderton SM (2002) B cells regulate autoimmunity by provision of IL-10. Nat Immunol 3(10):944–950. https://doi.org/10.1038/ni833
9. Lino AC, Dang VD, Lampropoulou V, Welle A, Joedicke J, Pohar J, Simon Q, Thalmensi J, Baures A, Fluhler V, Sakwa I, Stervbo U, Ries S, Jouneau L, Boudinot P, Tsubata T, Adachi T, Hutloff A, Dorner T, Zimber-Strobl-U, de Vos AF, Dahlke K, Loh G, Korniotis S, Goosmann C, Weill JC, Reynaud CA, Kaufmann SHE, Walter J, Fillatreau S (2018) LAG-3 inhibitory receptor expression identifies immunosuppressive natural regulatory plasma cells. Immunity 49(1):120–133 e129. https://doi.org/10.1016/j.immuni.2018.06.007

Chapter 4

Purification of Murine and Human IL-10-Producing B Cells from Different Anatomical Compartments

Francesca Mion, Eleonora Martinis, Carlo E. M. Pucillo, and Silvia Tonon

Abstract

IL-10 is the best known and most studied anti-inflammatory cytokine and, in the last 20 years, it has acquired even greater fame as it has been associated with the regulatory phenotype of B cells. Indeed, although great efforts have been made to find a unique marker, to date IL-10 remains the main way to follow both murine and human regulatory B cells, hence the need of precise and reproducible methods to identify and purify IL-10-producing B cells for both functional and molecular downstream assays. In this chapter, we present our protocols to isolate these cells from the murine spleen and peritoneum and from human peripheral blood. Since the production of IL-10 by B cells is not only a weapon to counteract the adverse effect of pro-inflammatory cytokines but also a response to cellular activation, we focused on those B cells that are prone to IL-10 production and detectable following a short-term stimulation with phorbol-12-myristate-13-acetate, ionomycin, and lipopolysaccharide (murine system) or CpG (human system).

Key words B cells, IL-10, Spleen, Peritoneum, Blood

1 Introduction

Under steady-state conditions, the balance between the regulatory and effector immune response maintains homeostasis. When this equilibrium is altered, we have the onset of pathological conditions that are the result of either an under- or over-reaction of the immune response [1]. In this perspective, the study of the biology and function of regulatory cells such as myeloid-derived suppressor cells and regulatory T and B cells becomes particularly relevant. The idea that B cells could perform a regulatory action besides antigen presentation and antibody production comes as a result of the study of pathological conditions such as autoimmune diseases, infection, and cancer where B cells were shown to negatively regulate the immune response [2]. Since then, there have been several attempts to identify a specific marker that could distinguish regulatory B cells, but the only result was that a variety of B cell subsets have been reported as being regulatory B cells. Some of these subsets

Francesca Mion and Silvia Tonon (eds.), *Regulatory B Cells: Methods and Protocols*, Methods in Molecular Biology, vol. 2270, https://doi.org/10.1007/978-1-0716-1237-8_4, © Springer Science+Business Media, LLC, part of Springer Nature 2021

share the expression of certain surface molecules such as, for example, CD1d and CD138, but the only real common factor is the production of the anti-inflammatory cytokine IL-10.

Initially described as a T helper 2-specific factor, it is now well established that IL-10 is instead produced by almost all leukocytes and also by nonimmune cells, such as epithelial cells and keratinocytes, and tumor cells. In addition to being an abundantly expressed cytokine, IL-10 is characterized by an expression profile which strictly depends on the specific context and cell type, and this is one of the reasons why to date no therapy having IL-10 as prime drug target has been approved although its relevancy for the treatment of autoimmune diseases, tissue damage, and cancer [3, 4]. These general considerations are particularly relevant in the case of B cells in which it was shown that IL-10 expression is under the control of various signal transduction pathways and transcriptional networks [5].

Although the production of IL-10 is one of the most effective weapons of regulatory B cells, linking the expression of this cytokine to the B-cell regulatory phenotype has generated further confusion in an already quite confused research area. Indeed, as discussed very clearly by Lighaam and coworkers, IL-10 may be secreted by B cells at specific stages of their developmental and differentiation fate, not only as a consequence of acting as immune regulators of the immune response but also as a result of B-cell activation and function toward humoral immunity [6]. In this regard, it becomes particularly important to specify, within the experimental study, the timing and the pathways of B-cell stimulation to study IL-10 production. Further stressing this concept, we recently demonstrated that, in the mouse, early IL-10-producing B cells (5-h stimulation with phorbol-12-myristate-13-acetate, ionomycin, and lipopolysaccharide, LPI) are characterized by the demethylation of the mCNS-4.5 region and partial demethylation of mCNS-9. However, this demethylation of mCNS-4.5 proved to be specific for early IL-10^{+} B cells: if IL-10^{-} B cells are re-stimulated with LPS for 24–48 h, they become able to produce IL-10 (delayed IL-10-producing B cells), but they do not demethylate mCNS-4.5 and undergo partial demethylation on mCNS-9 [7].

In this chapter, we present the detailed protocols for the isolation of B cells that are prone for IL-10 production and detectable following a 5-h stimulation with PMA, ionomycin, and LPS, in mice, or with PMA, ionomycin, and CpG, in humans. Since the identification of IL-10-producing B cells by flow cytometry requires cell membrane permeabilization, we also provide an alternative method based on the usage of the cytokine-reporter mice designated tiger (interleukin-ten ires gfp-enhanced reporter). The described protocols allow the inclusion of all the IL-10-producing B cells detectable after treatment with LPI, overcoming the problem of selecting a single population based on the analysis of surface marker expression.

2 Materials

2.1 General Equipment

1. Autoclave-sterilized forceps and scissors and disposable scalpels.
2. Conical 15- and 50-mL tubes.
3. 5 mL polypropylene tubes.
4. 70 μm cell strainer.
5. Petri dishes and 24-well flat-bottom culture plates.
6. 10 mL syringes and 0.5 mL insulin syringes.
7. 27G needles.
8. Cell incubator, maintained at 37 °C and 5% CO_2.
9. Flow cytometer and analysis software.
10. Cell sorter and analysis software.

2.2 Buffers, Solutions, and Media

1. Phosphate-buffered saline (PBS): 137 mM NaCl; 2.68 mM KCl; 8.1 mM Na_2HPO_4; 1.47 mM KH_2PO_4.
2. 70% ethanol in water.
3. 0.192 M sodium citrate in PBS. Filter-sterilize. This stock solution should be diluted 10× in the final medium.
4. Red blood cell (RBC) lysing buffer.
5. Wash medium: 10% fetal bovine serum (FBS, *see* **Note 1**), 20 mM HEPES, 2 mM L-glutamine, 100 U/mL penicillin, 100 μg/mL streptomycin in RPMI 1640.
6. Culture medium: 10% FBS (*see* **Note 1**), 20 mM HEPES, 2 mM L-glutamine, 1 mM sodium pyruvate, 1× nonessential amino acids (from 100× mix), 100 U/mL penicillin, 100 μg/mL streptomycin, and 50 μM β-mercaptoethanol in RPMI 1640.
7. MACS buffer: 0.5% bovine serum albumin (BSA), 2 mM ethylenediaminetetraacetic acid (EDTA) in PBS. Filter-sterilize and store at 4 °C.
8. Peritoneal lavage buffer: 3% FBS in PBS.
9. 1.5% PFA in PBS.

2.3 Mice and Biological Material

1. 6- to 12-week-old female C57BL/6 mice as source of spleen for B-cell isolation.
2. 6- to 12-week-old female Il10^{tm1Flv} mice (IL-10 reporter GFP knock-in *tiger*).
3. Peripheral blood of healthy donors with informed consent.

1. Kit for immunomagnetic isolation of murine B cells (*see* **Note 2**).

2.4 Reagents for B Cell Isolation and Culture

2. Kit for immunomagnetic/immunodensity isolation of human B cells (*see* **Note 3**).
3. Kit for immunomagnetic isolation of regulatory B cells (Miltenyi, *see* **Note 4**).
4. Immunomagnetic separation system (e.g., magnets, columns).
5. Density gradient medium such as Ficoll or Lymphoprep (*see* **Note 5**).
6. LPI stimulation cocktail: 10 μg/mL lipopolysaccharide (LPS from *Escherichia coli* O55:B5), 50 ng/mL phorbol 12-myristate 13-acetate (PMA), and 500 ng/mL ionomycin resuspended in culture medium (*see* **Note 6**).
7. LPIM stimulation cocktail: LPI stimulation cocktail with the addition of 2 μM monensin (*see* **Note 6**).
8. CPIB stimulation cocktail: 10 μg/mL CpG (ODN 2006), 50 ng/mL PMA, 1 μg/mL ionomycin, 10 μg/mL brefeldin A resuspended in culture medium (*see* **Note 6**).

2.5 Reagents for Cell Staining

1. Anti-mouse CD19 (clone 6D5) and IL-10 (clone JES5-16E3) antibodies for flow cytometry (*see* **Note 7**).
2. Anti-human CD19 (clone HIB19) and IL-10 (clone JES3-19F1) antibodies for flow cytometry (*see* **Note 7**).
3. Dead-cell dye for flow cytometry, compatible with cell fixation (e.g., Invitrogen LIVE/DEAD Fixable Dead Cell Stain Kits). Use according to specific manufacturer's instructions.
4. Unconjugated anti-mouse CD16/CD32 mAb (FcBlock, clone 2.4G2). Use according to specific manufacturer's instructions.
5. Human Fc Block. Use according to specific manufacturer's instructions.
6. Fixation/permeabilization buffers for intracellular staining. Choose a kit containing a fixation/permeabilization solution and a washing buffer which allow to maintain cells permeabilized. Follow manufacturer's instruction for volumes and timing.

3 Methods

As already outlined in the introduction, although IL-10 production has been extensively used to define regulatory B cells, IL-10^{+} B cells might include B cells with different functions and at different stages of differentiation. In this chapter, we present the detailed protocols for the isolation of B cells that are prone for IL-10 production and detectable following a 5-h stimulation with PMA, ionomycin, and LPS, in mice, or with PMA, ionomycin, and CpG, in humans.

However, depending on the aim of the study, the timing and stimulation protocol can be changed and induced, rather than prone, IL-10-producing B cells can be analyzed.

3.1 Splenic Murine IL-10+ B Cell Isolation

3.1.1 Isolation of Splenic IL-10-Secreting B Cells from Wild-Type Mice

The procedure presented here below outlines the steps required to purify splenic IL-10-secreting B cells by coupling the Regulatory B-cell isolation kit from Miltenyi and fluorescence-activated cell sorting (FACS). The combination of these two methodologies allows to purify approximately 100.000 IL-10-secreting B cells from 100×10^6 splenocytes, with a purity >95%. Importantly, the CD19$^+$IL-10$^+$ cells obtained at the end of the procedure are viable and can be used for functional assays.

1. Sacrifice mice in accordance with the ethical standards of the Animal Care Committee of the home Institution. Lay the animal on its right side and wet the left side with a 70% ethanol solution. Using scissors and forceps, perform an incision that allows to expose the spleen.
2. Collect the spleen in a conical 15-mL tube previously filled with PBS supplemented with 0.0192 M sodium citrate, and move to a laminar flow hood.
3. Place the spleen in a Petri dish and dissociate the organ in sterile PBS supplemented with 0.0192 M sodium citrate, by gently scraping with a blade. Collect the splenocytes suspension in a 50-mL tube. Alternatively, directly mesh the spleen on a cell strainer allocated on a 50-mL tube with the plumber of a 5-mL syringe. Centrifuge at $300 \times g$ for 5 min and decant the supernatant.
4. Resuspend the cell pellet in 2 mL of RBC lysing buffer and incubate for 1–2 min at room temperature. Mix gently. At the end of incubation, add 50 mL of wash medium to block the reaction. Determine cell number and centrifuge at $300 \times g$ for 5 min. Decant the supernatant.
5. The first step of the Regulatory B cell isolation protocol is the pre-enrichment of the B cell population. Follow manufacturer's instruction to isolate B cells and then determine the cell number.
6. In order to isolate the B cells that are prone for IL-10 production, IL-10 secretion must be induced. To this purpose, seed the enriched B cell fraction at 1.6×10^6 cells/mL in culture medium and add the LPI stimulation cocktail. Culture for 5 h at 37 °C and 5% of CO_2 (*see* **Note 8–10**).
7. Following the incubation, carefully collect cells by pipetting up and down and rinsing wells with cold MACS buffer. Use either a 15- or 50-mL collection tube depending on the specific cell number (collect approximately 10^7 cells in a 15-mL tube or 30×10^7 cells in a 50-mL tube).

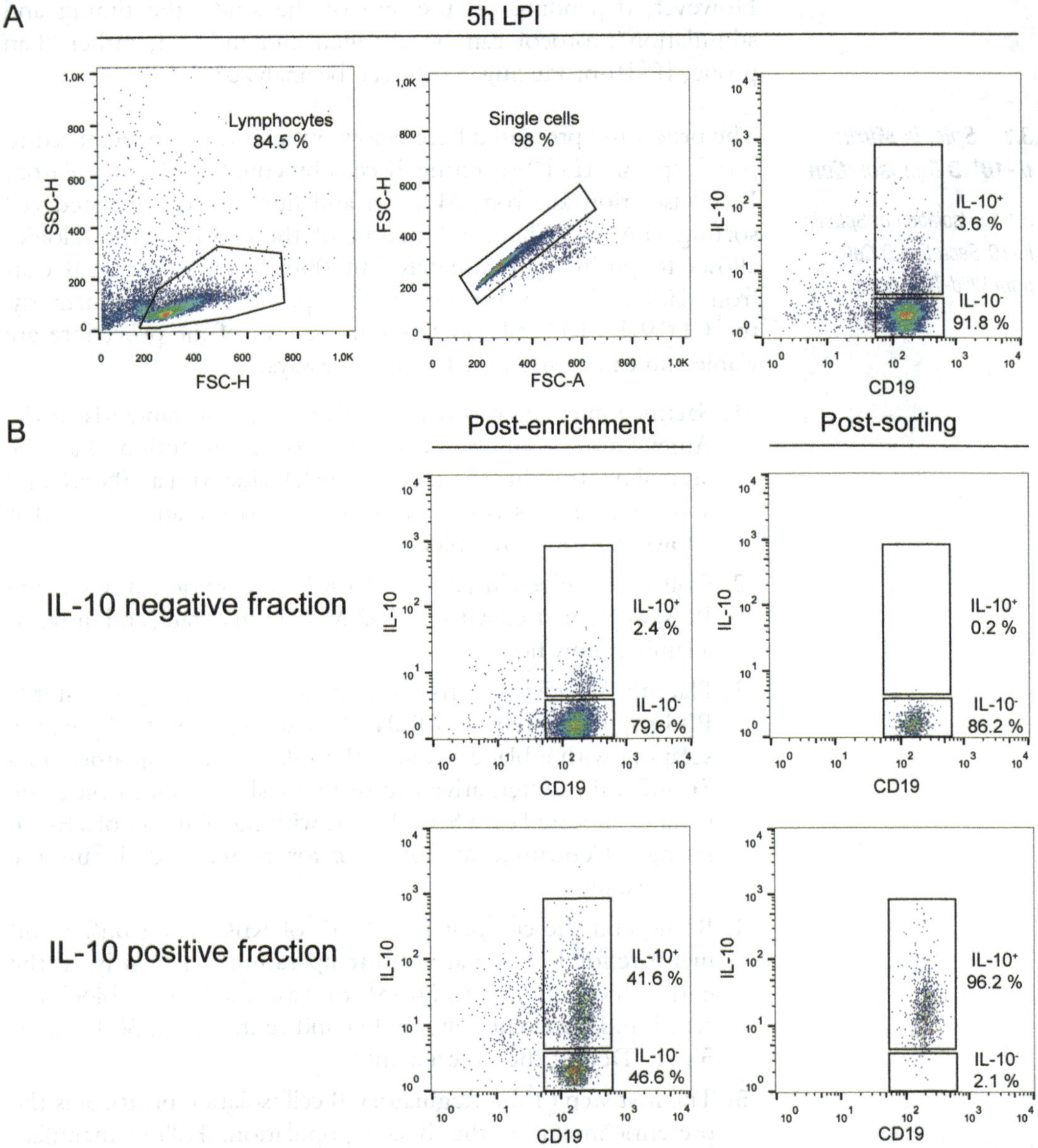

Fig. 1 Isolation of IL-10-secreting B cells from the spleen of wt mice. The gating strategy followed for the cell sorting of IL-10-secreting B cells is made of multiple steps. (**a**) First, viable cells are selected on the base of their morphology ("lymphocytes" gate), and doublets are excluded ("single cells" gate). Finally, the percentage of IL-10-secreting B cells before the enrichment protocol is determined by the CD19 versus IL-10 dot plot. (**b**) The purity of IL-10 secreting (IL-10^{+}) and non-secreting (IL-10^{-}) B cells is shown for both magnetic enrichment only (post-enrichment) and for magnetic enrichment combined with cell sorting (post-sorting)

8. Wash cells twice with cold MACS buffer by centrifuging at $300 \times g$ for 5 min at 4 °C.
9. Resuspend the cell pellet in 10 mL of warm culture medium if you are working in a 15-mL tube, or in 45 mL if cells were

collected in a 50-mL tube. Label the collected B cells with the Regulatory B cells catch reagent following manufacturer's instruction and incubate for 45 min at 37 °C and 5% CO_2. This is a crucial step of the protocol since IL-10 secretion occurs and IL-10-producing B cells are captured. Moreover, it is absolutely crucial to turn tubes at least every 5 min to prevent the settling of cells (*see* **Note 11**).

10. After the secretion step, follow manufacturer's instruction to perform the labeling with the Regulatory B Cell Detection Antibody. We recommend to add any antibody for cell surface staining (e.g., anti-CD19 Ab) during this step (the exact moment in which the antibody should be added is indicated in the manufacturer's instruction).
11. Proceed with the enrichment of IL-10-secreting B cells, following manufacturer's instruction. Perform a single round of magnetic separation through the column and then proceed with the cell sorting of IL-10^+ and IL-10^- cells through FACS (*see* **Note 12**). Before sorting, coat collection tubes with FBS and resuspended cells at a concentration compatible with the characteristics of the specific cell sorter available.
12. Sort according to the gating strategy shown in Fig. 1a. The combination of the Regulatory B cell isolation kit and FACS allows to significantly increase the purity of the populations of interest (*see* Fig. 1b and **Note 13**).

3.1.2 Isolation of Splenic GFP+ B Cells from IL-10 Reporter GFP Knock-in Tiger Mice

Although the method described in Subheading 3.1.1 allows to obtain a highly pure IL-10^+ B cell population, it is a quite long procedure. An alternative to the combination of the Regulatory B-cell isolation kit and FACS is represented by the usage of IL-10 reporter mouse strains which were born from the necessity to track and subsequently investigate the role of IL-10-producing cells [8]. Among the available IL-10 reporter mouse strains, we used IL10-IRES-EGFP (*tiger*) mice, which are characterized by the peculiarity that IL-10 and GFP are produced simultaneously as two separate proteins, since the coding sequence for the reporter protein is cloned after the 3′-UTR of the *il-10* gene [9]. This allows to follow IL-10 production without the need of performing an intracellular cytokine staining, a procedure which implies cell death: the production of IL-10 goes together with GFP synthesis, but while IL-10 is secreted, the reporter protein is retained inside the cell, enabling the detection of IL-10-producing B cells by flow cytometry without the need to fix and permeabilize the cells.

1. Collect and process the spleen from the IL-10 reporter GFP knock-in *tiger* mouse and from the sex- and age-matched wild-type (wt) counterpart, as described in steps 1–4 of Subheading 3.1.1 (*see* **Note 14**). Determine the cell number.

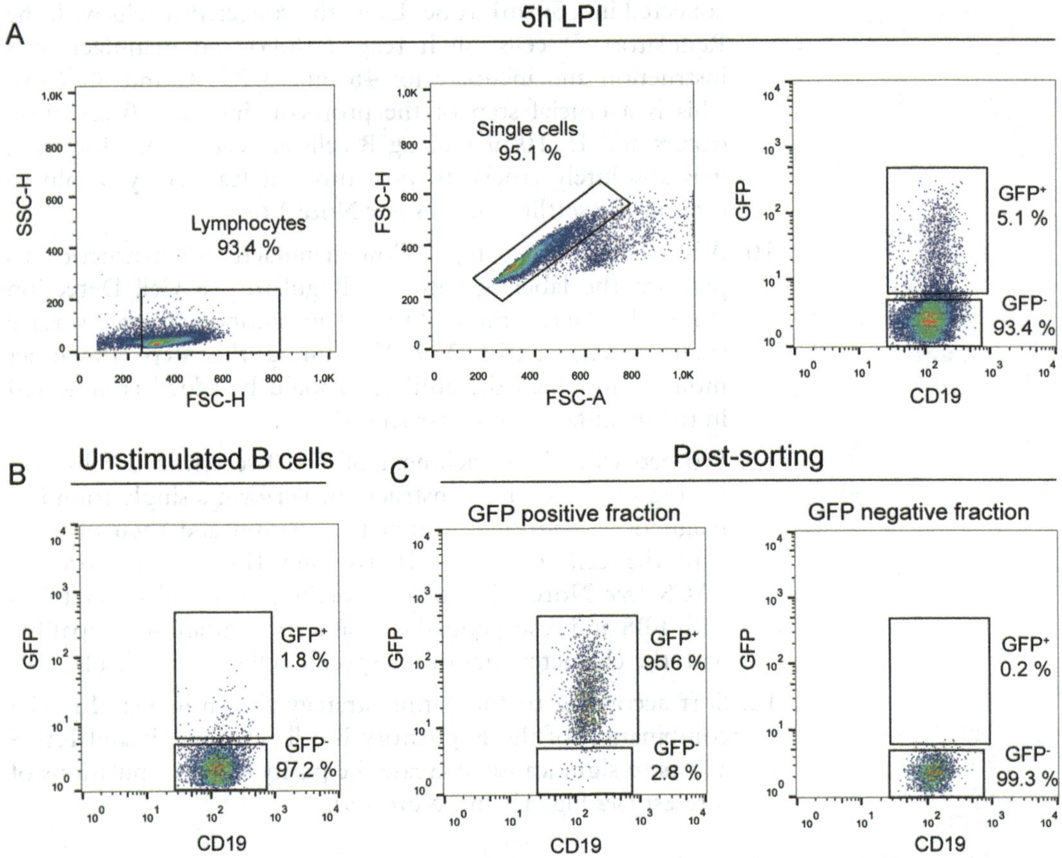

Fig. 2 Isolation of GFP$^+$ B cells from the spleen of IL-10 reporter GFP knock-in *tiger* mice. (**a**) Viable B cells are selected based on their morphology ("lymphocytes" gate), and doublets are excluded from the sorting ("single cells" gate). The comparison of LPI-treated B cells (**a**) with the unstimulated B-cell sample (**b**) allows to set the gates for the GFP$^+$ and GFP$^-$ populations on the CD19 versus GFP dot plot. (**c**) The purity of the two fractions after sorting is shown

2. Proceed to B-cell isolation following the instructions of the specific employed kit (*see* **Note 2**). We recommend to process the totality of isolated splenocytes. At the end of the isolation protocol, determine the cell number and resuspend the B cells at 1.6×10^6 cells/mL in culture medium.
3. In order to isolate the B cells that are prone for IL-10 production, wt and *tiger* B cells must be cultured for 5 h at 37 °C and 5% of CO_2 in the presence of the LPI stimulation cocktail (*see* **Notes 8–10**).
4. At the end of the incubation, carefully collect all the cells by pipetting up and down and rinsing each well with PBS or culture medium. Centrifuge at 300 × *g* for 5 min and discard the supernatant.

5. After washing once with PBS, proceed with the surface staining of CD19 by incubating the cells with a specific anti-CD19 antibody for 15 min in wet ice in the dark (*see* **Note 15**). Wash once with PBS, centrifuge at 300 × *g* for 5 min, and resuspend the cell pellet in PBS (*see* **Note 13**).
6. Proceed with the cell sorting of $CD19^{+}GFP^{+}$ and $CD19^{+}GFP^{-}$ cells. Before sorting, cells should be resuspended at a concentration compatible with the cell sorter performance, and collection tubes should be coated with FBS. Sort according to the gating strategy shown in Fig. 2 (*see* **Note 12**).

3.2 Isolation of Peritoneal IL-10+ B Cells

It is widely known that, in the murine system, IL-10 is mainly produced by peritoneal B-1a lymphocytes [10]. Moreover, Tedder and coworkers demonstrated that the fraction of peritoneal cavity B cells that respond to LPI stimulation by producing IL-10 is much larger compared to the spleen [11, 12]. Although the regulatory B-cell isolation kit from Miltenyi Biotec is designed to isolate IL-10-secreting B cells from mouse spleen or peritoneal cavity cells, we have never tested this product on peritoneal cavity B cells. Here below, we describe how to isolate the peritoneal cavity of B-cell population prone for IL-10 production by FACS. Since IL-10 staining requires to fix and permeabilize the cells, the reader should keep in mind that this method does not allow to obtain viable peritoneal $IL\text{-}10^{+}$ B cells, and therefore cannot be used for downstream functional assays (*see* **Note 16**).

1. Sacrifice mice in accordance with the ethical standards of the Animal Care Committee of the home Institution. Lay the animal supine and wet the skin and fur with 70% ethanol. Cut the skin at the level of the abdomen and inject 5–10 mL of peritoneal lavage buffer with a syringe (27G needle). Gently massage to dislodge cells.
2. Carefully recover the cell suspension, avoiding to puncture the intestine or break blood vessels (*see* **Note 17**). Wash cells with PBS and centrifuge at 300 × *g* for 5 min.
3. Do not proceed with B-cell isolation but rather directly stimulate the total peritoneal population with the stimulation cocktail that allows to select the B cells that are prone for IL-10 production. To this aim, culture total peritoneal cells for 5 h at 37 °C and 5% of CO_2 in the presence of the LPIM stimulation cocktail. Resuspend the cell suspension at 1.6×10^6 cells/mL in culture medium, seed 10^6 cells per well and add the LPIM stimulation cocktail (*see* **Note 8–10**).
4. At the end of the 5-h incubation, carefully collect all the cells in 5 mL polypropylene tubes by pipetting up and down and by rinsing the wells with PBS or culture medium (*see* **Note 18**).

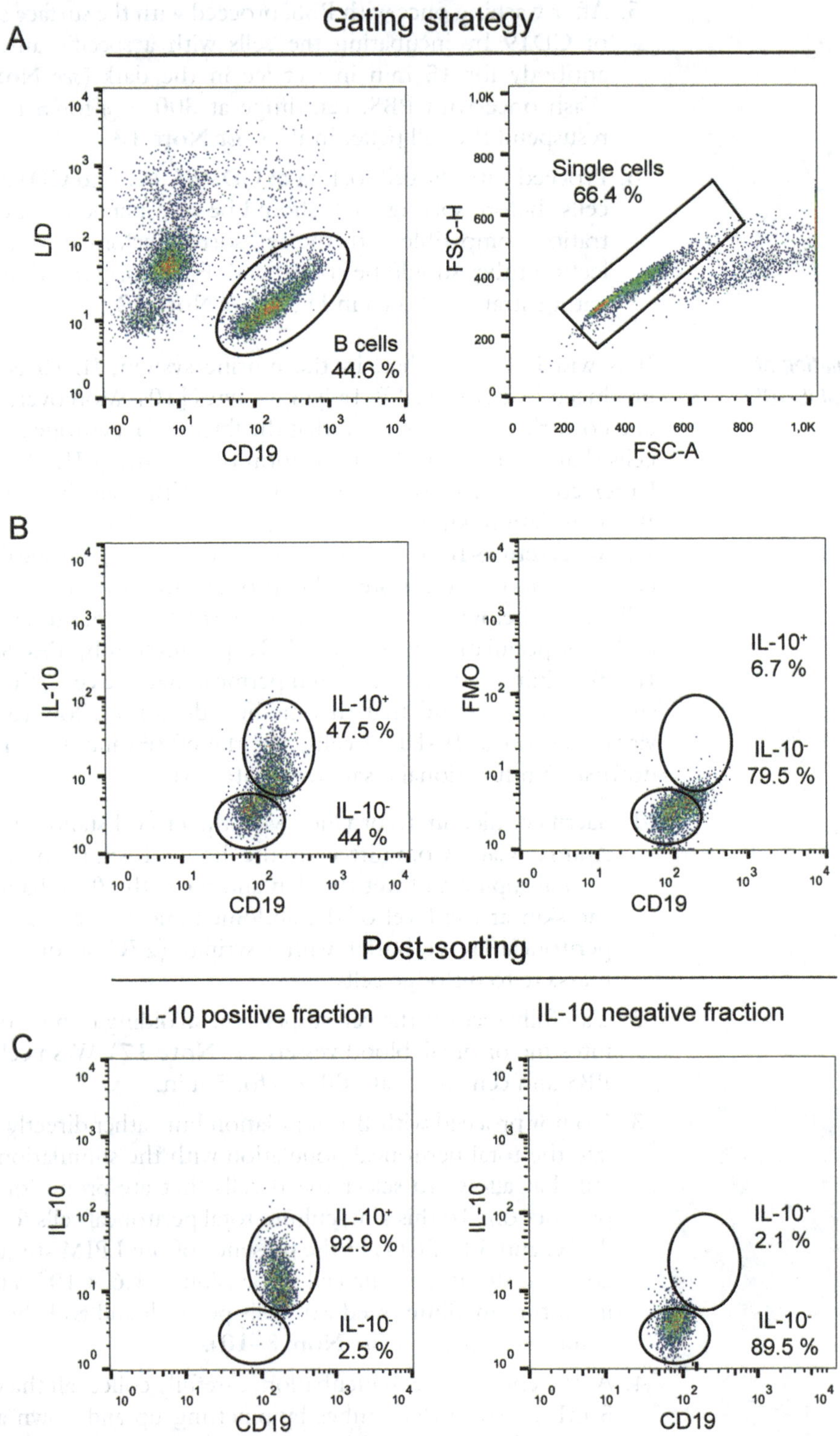

Fig. 3 Isolation of IL-10$^+$ B cells from the peritoneum of wt mice. (**a**) Viable B cells are selected based on their positivity for the CD19 molecule and negativity for the LIVE/DEAD fluorescent dye (L/D). Doublets are excluded from the sorting. (**b**) Gates for positivity/negativity to IL-10 are set on the basis of the fluorescence minus one (FMO) control for IL-10 staining. (**c**) The purity of the IL-10$^+$ and IL-10$^-$ fractions after sorting is shown

5. Wash once with PBS, centrifuge at 300 × *g* for 5 min and proceed with LIVE/DEAD staining. Briefly vortex each sample tube and immediately add murine Fc block diluted in PBS according to supplier's instructions. Incubate for 15 min in wet ice in the dark.
6. Wash with 2 mL of cold PBS and centrifuge at 300 × *g* for 5 min. Remove the supernatant and proceed with surface staining for CD19 incubating for 15 min in wet ice in the dark (*see* **Note 15**).
7. After washing, proceed with cell fixation and permeabilization using appropriate fixation/permeabilization buffers for intracellular staining. If using a commercial kit, follow manufacturer's instruction for volumes and timing and incubate in wet ice in the dark. Wash cells twice with 2 mL of cold permeabilization wash buffer and centrifuge at 300 × *g* for 5 min.
8. Stain cells for intracellular IL-10 by resuspending the appropriate antibody in the permeabilization wash buffer and incubating for 30 min in wet ice in the dark (*see* **Note** 7). Remember to include an unstained control to set gate for sorting of IL-10^+ and IL-10^- B cells.
9. After incubation, pull together the content of all tubes, add 2 mL of cold permeabilization wash buffer and centrifuge for 5 min at 300 × *g*. Discard the supernatant and resuspend the cell pellet in PBS (*see* **Note 19**).
10. Proceed with cell sorting following the gating strategy shown in Fig. 3 (*see* **Note 13**). In order to obtain approximately 500.000 IL-10^+ B cells, we recommend to pull together the peritoneal lavage from six mice.

3.3 Isolation of Human IL-10^+ B Cells from the Peripheral Blood

The need of reliable protocols to detect and analyze human regulatory B cells comes from multiple studies demonstrating an association between abnormalities in regulatory B-cell numbers or function and immune-related pathologies, such as autoimmune diseases, cancers, and chronic infections [2, 13]. To our knowledge, a kit for the immunomagnetic/immunodensity isolation of human regulatory B cells has not been developed yet. For this reason, here below we present the procedure to isolate the human B cell population prone for IL-10 production by FACS. Since IL-10 staining requires cell fixation and permeabilization, the reader should keep in mind that this method does not allow to obtain viable human IL-10^+ B cells, and therefore cannot be used for downstream functional assays (*see* **Note 16**). However, if one is interested in obtaining viable cells, a possible solution could be the combination of a total human B-cell isolation kit with the human IL-10 secretion assay detection kit which was developed by Miltenyi Biotec for the sensitive detection of human IL-10-secreting cells.

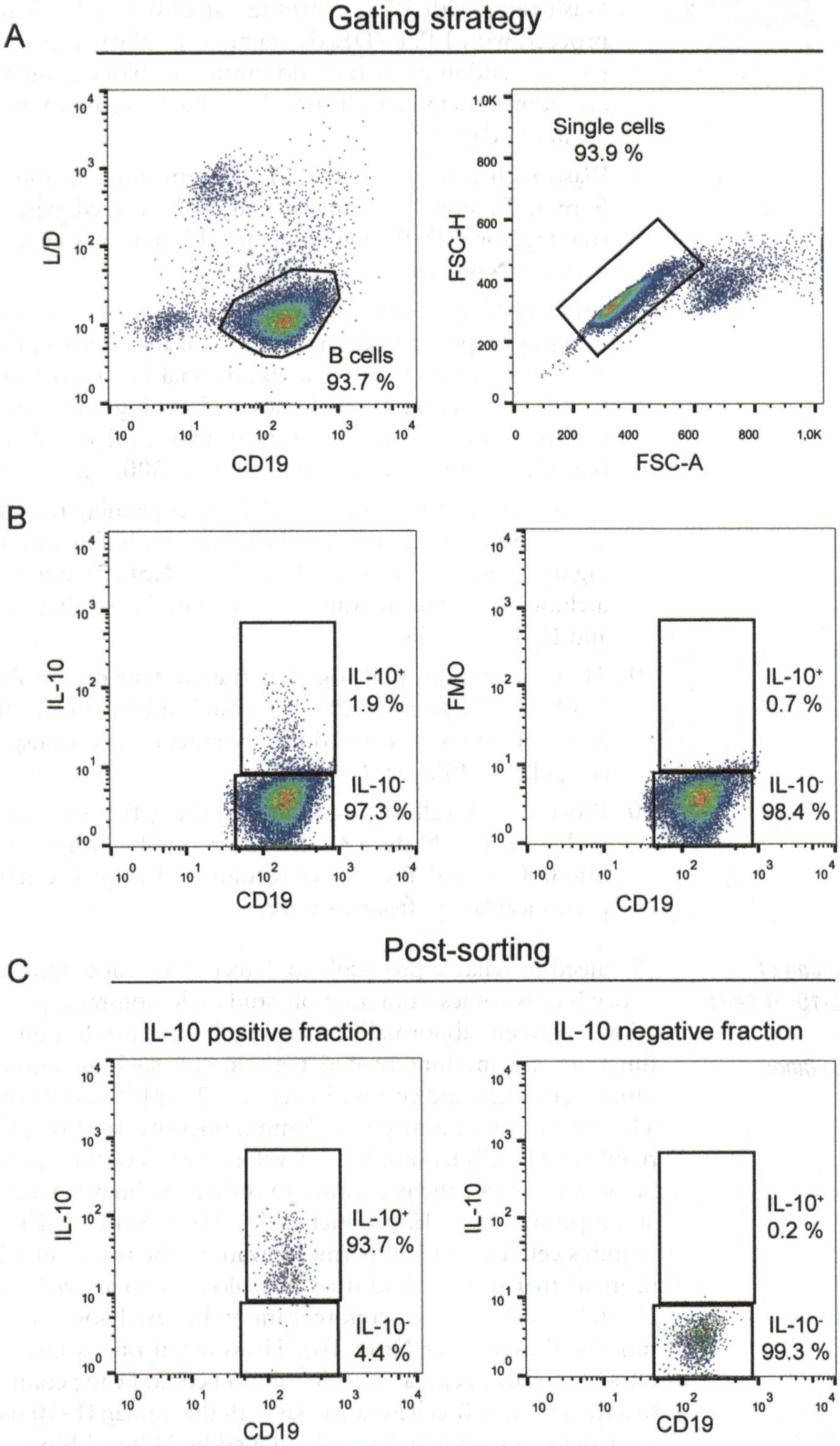

Fig. 4 Isolation of human peripheral blood IL-10$^+$ B cells. (**a**) Viable B cells are selected based on their positivity for the CD19 molecule and negativity for the LIVE/DEAD fluorescent dye (L/D). Doublets are excluded from the sorting. (**b**) Gates for positivity/negativity to IL-10 are set on the basis of the fluorescence minus one (FMO) control for IL-10 staining. (**c**) The purity of the IL-10$^+$ and IL-10$^-$ fractions after sorting is shown

1. In order to obtain a sufficient number of human IL-10$^+$ B cells, collect 40 mL of peripheral blood from each healthy volunteer who had given informed consent (*see* **Note 20**).
2. Isolate B cells according to the manufacturer's instruction of the chosen kit. Usually, the starting material of kits for the immunomagnetic isolation of human B cells is peripheral blood mononuclear cells (PBMCs), and therefore a processing of blood on a density gradient medium will be necessary.
3. Determine the cell number and select the B cells that are prone for IL-10 production. To this aim, culture total human B cells for 5 h at 37 °C and 5% of CO_2 in the presence of the CPIB stimulation cocktail. Resuspend the cell suspension at 1.6×10^6 cells/mL in culture medium, seed 10^6 cells per well, and add the CPIB stimulation cocktail (*see* **Note 8–10**).
4. At the end of the 5-h incubation, carefully collect all the cells in 5 mL polypropylene tubes by pipetting up and down and rinsing each well with PBS or culture medium (*see* **Note 18**). Centrifuge at 300 × *g* for 5 min.
5. Wash once with PBS and proceed with LIVE/DEAD staining following manufacturer's instructions. Briefly vortex the tube and immediately add Fc block previously diluted in PBS according to supplier's instructions. Incubate for 15 min in wet ice in the dark.
6. Wash with 2 mL of cold PBS and centrifuge at 300 × *g* for 5 min. Remove the supernatant and proceed with surface staining for CD19 incubating for 15 min in wet ice in the dark (*see* **Note 15**).
7. After washing, proceed with cell fixation and permeabilization using appropriate fixation/permeabilization buffers for intracellular staining. If using a commercial kit, follow manufacturer's instruction for volumes and timing and incubate in wet ice in the dark. Wash cells twice by using 2 mL of cold permeabilization wash buffer and centrifuge at 300 × *g* for 5 min.
8. Stain cells for intracellular IL-10 by resuspending the appropriate antibody in the permeabilization wash buffer and incubating for 30 min in wet ice in the dark. Remember to include an unstained control to set the gate for sorting IL-10$^+$ and IL-10$^-$ B cells.
9. After incubation, pull together all tubes, wash with 2 mL of cold permeabilization wash buffer, and centrifuge for 5 min at 300 × *g*.

10. Resuspend the cell pellet in PBS and proceed with cell sorting following the gating strategy shown in Fig. 4 (*see* **Note 13**). Remember to resuspend cells at a concentration compatible with the cell sorter performance and to coat the collection tubes with FBS.

4 Notes

1. FBS was heated at 56 °C for 30 min to inactivate complement.
2. There are several kits on the market that allow to isolate murine B cells from total splenocytes with high degrees of purity. However, we recommend the choice of a kit based on a negative selection method that leaves the B cells untouched, avoiding a possible activation of the population of interest. Specifically, we routinely use the "B cell isolation kit" from Miltenyi Biotec which removes non-B cells coupling a labeling with a cocktail of biotin-conjugated antibodies against CD43, CD4, and Ter-119, and with anti-biotin microbeads.
3. There are several kits on the market that allow to isolate human B cells from peripheral blood with high degrees of purity. As for murine B cells, also in this case we suggest using a kit based on a negative selection method. For our experiments, we used the "RosetteSep Human B cell Enrichment cocktail" from StemCell, which is based on an immunodensity-negative selection method and which works on whole blood.
4. To our knowledge, this is the only available ready-made commercial kit.
5. If performing an immunodensity isolation of human B cells using the "RosetteSep Human B cell Enrichment cocktail," then the density medium is required to generate the density gradient and pellet the non-B cells along with the red blood cells. Otherwise, immunomagnetic kits are designed to isolate B cells from peripheral blood mononuclear cells (PBMCs) and, in this case, the density gradient medium is required to isolate PBMCs from whole blood.
6. Dissolve LPS at 1 mg/mL in sterile PBS and CpG at 10 μg/mL in H_2O. Store at −20 °C in 10 μL aliquots. Dissolve PMA at 1 mg/mL in dimethyl sulfoxide (DMSO) and store at −20 °C in 100 μg/mL aliquots. Dissolve ionomycin at 1 mg/mL in DMSO and store at −20 °C in 10 μL aliquots. Monensin and Brefeldin A are necessary to block cytokine secretion.
7. The final concentration of each antibody should be optimized before use through titration, starting from the indications provided by the manufacturer.

8. If the research interest is the analysis of induced, rather than prone, IL-10-producing B cells, the timing and stimulation protocol must be changed accordingly (e.g., 48 h stimulation with LPS, 48 h stimulation with anti-CD40 mAb plus 5 h stimulation with LPI).
9. Although one could stimulate all B cells together, using appropriate supports for the number of total cells (25- or 75-cm^2 cell culture flasks, 15- or 50-mL tubes), in our experience, seeding cells in 24-well plates leads to an increased efficiency in the induction of IL-10$^+$ B cells. We usually seed 10^6 cells in 600 μL and add 70 μL of the LPI/LPIM/CPIB cocktail in cell culture medium. Remember to calculate the final concentration of the LPI/LPIM/CPIB components on the final volume of 670 μL.
10. Remember to always include in the experimental plan the negative control in which cells are cultured in the absence of the IL-10-inducing stimulation cocktail.
11. If available, a tube rotator can be placed inside the incubator to keep cells in the suspended state.
12. The protocol of the Regulatory B cell isolation kit highly suggests to perform two consecutive column runs to increase the purity of IL-10-secreting B cells. Nevertheless, the purity obtained by enriching the eluted fraction over a second column is not equal to that obtained by replacing the second round in column with cell sorting through FACS. Depending on the type of downstream assay and on the necessary grade of cell purity, the operator must choose the best option.
13. We recommend checking the purity of sorted samples at the end of every single FACS experiment.
14. In this experiment, wt B cells represent the technical control for the analysis of GFP expression by flow cytometry.
15. Depending on the aim of the experiment, other surface markers, in addition to CD19, can be assessed.
16. The downstream assay must keep in mind the treatment to which the cells were subjected. As an example, we performed the methylation analysis of the *il-10* gene *locus* of peritoneal cavity IL-10-secreting B cells as described in [7]. Since the IL-10 staining protocol includes a fixation step with PFA, samples should be decross-linked (65 °C for 1 h) before being processed.
17. The rupture of blood vessels leads to a contamination of the peritoneal sample with peripheral blood circulating cells. The peritoneal cavity cell pellet should not contain red blood cells.
18. When collecting the stimulated cells, transfer the content of 3 wells of the 24-well plate in a single 5 mL polypropylene tube. In this way, a total of 3×10^6 cells will be present in each tube and stained together.

19. The protocol can be stopped at this point and cells can undergo FACS the day after. In that case though, the cell pellet should be resuspended in PBS supplemented with 1.5% PFA and not in PBS only.
20. We usually collect the sample from blood donors and then process it the day after. The only trick we take is to keep the blood at 37 °C under slight shaking.

References

1. Peng B, Ming Y, Yang C (2018) Regulatory B cells: the cutting edge of immune tolerance in kidney transplantation. Cell Death Dis 9 (2):109. https://doi.org/10.1038/s41419-017-0152-y
2. Mauri C, Menon M (2017) Human regulatory B cells in health and disease: therapeutic potential. J Clin Invest 127(3):772–779. https://doi.org/10.1172/JCI85113
3. Iyer SS, Cheng G (2012) Role of interleukin 10 transcriptional regulation in inflammation and autoimmune disease. Crit Rev Immunol 32(1):23–63. https://doi.org/10.1615/critrevimmunol.v32.i1.30
4. Wang X, Wong K, Ouyang W, Rutz S (2019) Targeting IL-10 family cytokines for the treatment of human diseases. Cold Spring Harb Perspect Biol 11(2). https://doi.org/10.1101/cshperspect.a028548
5. Baba Y, Matsumoto M, Kurosaki T (2015) Signals controlling the development and activity of regulatory B-lineage cells. Int Immunol 27(10):487–493. https://doi.org/10.1093/intimm/dxv027
6. Lighaam LC, Unger PA, Vredevoogd DW, Verhoeven D, Vermeulen E, Turksma AW, Ten Brinke A, Rispens T, van Ham SM (2018) In vitro-induced human IL-10(+) B cells do not show a subset-defining marker signature and plastically co-express IL-10 with pro-inflammatory cytokines. Front Immunol 9:1913. https://doi.org/10.3389/fimmu.2018.01913
7. Tonon S, Mion F, Dong J, Chang HD, Dalla E, Scapini P, Perruolo G, Zanello A, Dugo M, Cassatella MA, Colombo MP, Radbruch A, Tripodo C, Pucillo CE (2019) IL-10-producing B cells are characterized by a specific methylation signature. Eur J Immunol 49(8):1213–1225. https://doi.org/10.1002/eji.201848025
8. Bouabe H (2012) Cytokine reporter mice: the special case of IL-10. Scand J Immunol 75 (6):553–567. https://doi.org/10.1111/j.1365-3083.2012.02695.x
9. Kamanaka M, Kim ST, Wan YY, Sutterwala FS, Lara-Tejero M, Galan JE, Harhaj E, Flavell RA (2006) Expression of interleukin-10 in intestinal lymphocytes detected by an interleukin-10 reporter knockin tiger mouse. Immunity 25 (6):941–952. https://doi.org/10.1016/j.immuni.2006.09.013
10. O'Garra A, Chang R, Go N, Hastings R, Haughton G, Howard M (1992) Ly-1 B (B-1) cells are the main source of B cell-derived interleukin 10. Eur J Immunol 22 (3):711–717. https://doi.org/10.1002/eji.1830220314
11. Yanaba K, Bouaziz JD, Haas KM, Poe JC, Fujimoto M, Tedder TF (2008) A regulatory B cell subset with a unique CD1dhiCD5+ phenotype controls T cell-dependent inflammatory responses. Immunity 28(5):639–650. https://doi.org/10.1016/j.immuni.2008.03.017
12. Yanaba K, Bouaziz JD, Matsushita T, Tsubata T, Tedder TF (2009) The development and function of regulatory B cells expressing IL-10 (B10 cells) requires antigen receptor diversity and TLR signals. J Immunol 182(12):7459–7472. https://doi.org/10.4049/jimmunol.0900270
13. Miyagaki T, Fujimoto M, Sato S (2015) Regulatory B cells in human inflammatory and autoimmune diseases: from mouse models to clinical research. Int Immunol 27 (10):495–504. https://doi.org/10.1093/intimm/dxv026

Chapter 5

Purification and Immunophenotypic Characterization of Human $CD19^+CD24^{hi}CD38^{hi}$ and $CD19^+CD24^{hi}CD27^+$ B Cells

Hannah F. Bradford and Claudia Mauri

Abstract

Regulatory B cells (Bregs) have immunosuppressive capacity, primarily via the production of IL-10. IL-10 expression and immunosuppression have been described in a number of human B cell subsets, two of which include the $CD19^+CD24^{hi}CD38^{hi}$ and $CD19^+CD24^{hi}CD27^+$ populations. In this chapter, we describe how to identify and isolate these subsets from peripheral blood B cells via flow cytometry. We also explain how to expand Bregs in culture and how to identify them based on intracellular expression of IL-10.

Key words Regulatory B cells, IL-10, Autoimmunity, Immune regulation, Phenotyping, Flow cytometry

1 Introduction

Regulatory B cells (Bregs) have been described in a range of B cell subsets in mice and humans, with the primary effect of inhibiting differentiation of pro-inflammatory T-cell subsets, and inducing Treg differentiation [1, 2]. While human Bregs are less well understood compared to their murine counterparts, two of the better characterized human B cell subsets in which Bregs are enriched are the $CD19^+CD24^{hi}CD38^{hi}$ (immature) and $CD19^+CD24^{hi}CD27^+$ subsets [1, 3]. Moreover, impaired function of Bregs within both of these subsets has been demonstrated in autoimmunity, allergy, and cancer [4, 5].

The $CD19^+CD24^{hi}CD38^{hi}$ subset represents the immature B-cell population newly emerged from the bone marrow and entering circulation [6]. Previous work by our laboratory demonstrated that this subset produces large quantities of IL-10 following TLR9 and CD40 stimulation [1]. $CD19^+CD24^{hi}CD38^{hi}$ Bregs have the capacity to inhibit the differentiation of naïve $CD4^+$ T cells into pro-inflammatory Th1 and Th17 T cells, inhibit effector $CD4^+$ T-cell production of IFNγ and TNFα, and promote the differentiation of $CD4^+CD25^+$ regulatory T cells (Tregs) [2]. In addition to

Francesca Mion and Silvia Tonon (eds.), *Regulatory B Cells: Methods and Protocols*, Methods in Molecular Biology, vol. 2270, https://doi.org/10.1007/978-1-0716-1237-8_5,

CpGC stimulation, IFNα expands Bregs from this subset; in this context plasmacytoid dendritic cells (pDCs) represent the source of IFNα following TLR9 stimulation. The CD19^{+}CD24^{hi}CD38^{hi}-derived Breg subset participates in a regulatory feedback loop restraining further production of IFNα by pDCs, representing an important homeostatic mechanism to prevent excessive inflammation [7]. Reduced frequencies of CD19^{+}CD24^{hi}CD38^{hi} Bregs and impaired regulatory capacity have been observed in a number of conditions including systemic lupus erythematosus (SLE) [1, 7], rheumatoid arthritis [2], atopic dermatitis [8], and psoriasis [9]. In SLE, CD19^{+}CD24^{hi}CD38^{hi} Bregs produce less IL-10 on a per-cell basis and have impaired ability to suppress CD4^{+} T-cell pro-inflammatory cytokine production, defects which are more pronounced with high disease activity [1, 7].

The CD19^{+}CD24^{hi}CD27^{+} memory B-cell population is also appreciated for its regulatory potential. A rare subset of CD19^{+}CD24^{hi}CD27^{+} IL-10^{+} B cells, termed B10 cells, has been described in humans [3]. B10 cells are observed in newborn cord blood at very low frequencies and in adult blood, spleen, and tonsils. B10 precursors (B10pro) are enriched within the CD19^{+}CD24^{hi}CD27^{+} subset; B10pro B cells acquire the capacity to express IL-10 (intracellularly and at the transcriptional level) following 48 h stimulation in vivo with dual CD40 and TLR stimulation, with the phorbol ester PMA, ionomycin, and Brefeldin A stimulation for the final 5 h of culture. Unique to the CD19^{+}CD24^{hi}CD27^{hi} B10 subset is the capacity to suppress monocyte TNFα production, which is IL-10-dependent [3]. In RA patients, reduced frequencies of CD19^{+}CD27^{+} have been observed which is associated with impaired capacity to inhibit CD4^{+} T-cell IFNγ production [10]. Conversely, Breg inhibition of CD4^{+} IFNγ production is detrimental in patients with gastric cancer. Frequencies of gastric tissue CD19^{+}CD24^{hi}CD27^{+} Bregs are elevated in these patients, inhibiting CD4^{+} proliferation and IFNγ production, and higher frequencies of these cells are associated with a poor prognosis [11].

The significance of aberrant Breg function in the pathogenesis of autoimmune disease, allergy, and cancer highlights a requirement for in-depth characterization and functional understanding of Bregs. However, the marked heterogeneity of the Breg populations in terms of surface phenotype, regulatory function, and expansion stimuli is a major complicating factor in understanding their origin and immunological role. Unlike in Tregs, where FoxP3 is the hallmark transcription factor for these cells, no such transcription factor or surface marker has been identified for Bregs, and at present, IL-10 expression remains the defining factor in humans, emphasizing a need to identify surrogate Breg markers.

Flow cytometry can be used to comprehensively characterize the phenotype of B-cell subsets, and to measure the intracellular expression of IL-10, thus allowing identification of Bregs. Here we illustrate how to isolate B cells from whole blood and distinguish the $CD19^{+}CD24^{hi}CD38^{hi}$ and $CD19^{+}CD24^{hi}CD27^{+}$ subsets ex vivo. We also describe how to prepare B cells for isolation via fluorescence-activated cell sorting (FACS) of the $CD19^{+}CD24^{hi}CD38^{hi}$ and $CD19^{+}CD24^{hi}CD27^{+}$ subsets, which can be subsequently cultured to expand Bregs and investigate their developmental fate and IL-10 expression under different culture environments. Finally, we designate how to expand Bregs in culture using a range of stimuli to allow exploration of their phenotype, potentially beyond the $CD19^{+}CD24^{hi}CD38^{hi}$ and $CD19^{+}CD24^{hi}CD27^{+}$ subsets described here, and also to facilitate functional assays to assess their suppressive capacity in a range of immunological contexts.

2 Materials

2.1 General Equipment

1. 5 mL round-bottom polystyrene tubes (with filter cap).
2. 5 mL round-bottom polypropylene capped tubes.
3. Cell sorter (e.g., BD FACS Aria).
4. Flow cytometer (e.g., BD LSRII).
5. Sodium heparin-containing vacutainer tubes.
6. Round-bottom 96-well culture plates.
7. 50 mL tubes.
8. 10 mL serological pipets.

2.2 Buffer and Reagents

1. RPMI 1640 culture medium.
2. Complete medium: RPMI 1640 culture medium supplemented with 10% fetal calf serum (FCS) and 100 IU/mL penicillin and streptomycin.
3. Phosphate-buffered saline (PBS), with $MgCl_2$ and $CaCl_2$, sterile-filtered, pH 6.9–7.1.
4. Collection media: 50% FCS in RPMI 1640.
5. Staining buffer: 2% FCS and 0.01% sodium azide in PBS.
6. Density gradient medium for the isolation of mononuclear cells from peripheral blood (e.g., Ficoll-Paque, density 1.077 g/mL).
7. Red Blood Cell Lysing Buffer.
8. Human B Cell Enrichment Kit and magnet (*see* **Note 1**).

2.3 Reagents for B Cell Culture and Flow cytometry Analysis

1. CpGC ODN 2395.
2. Recombinant human IFN-α.

Table 1
Fluorescent mAbs against B-cell surface markers and IL-10

Target	Fluorochrome	Clone	Concentration	Isotype
CD19	BV785	HIB19	2 μg/mL	Mouse IgG1, κ
CD24	APCeFluor780	SN3A52H10	2 μg/mL	Mouse IgG1, κ
CD38	PerCPeFluor710	HB7	2 μg/mL	Mouse IgG1, κ
CD27	PE/dazzle	M-T271	2 μg/mL	Mouse IgG1, κ
IgM	BV510	MHM-88	2 μg/mL	Mouse IgG1, κ
IgD	BV605	IA6–2	2 μg/mL	Mouse IgG2a, κ
IL-10	APC	JES3-19F1	4 μg/mL	Rat IgG2a, κ

3. Human megaCD40L.
4. PIB cocktail: 50 ng/mL phorbol 12-myristate 13-acetate (PMA), 250 ng/mL ionomycin, and 5 μg/mL Brefeldin A in complete medium. Used to maximize intracellular IL-10 production.
5. 4′,6-Diamidino-2-phenylindole (DAPI). Working dilutions of DAPI should be prepared in sterile water (*see* **Note 2**).
6. Dye for the discrimination of viable from nonviable cells in multicolor flow cytometric applications (e.g., LIVE/DEAD Fixable Blue Dead Cell Dye). Reconstitute the dye according to manufacturer's instructions (*see* **Note 2**).
7. FcR blocking reagent: unconjugated anti-CD16/CD32 (clone 2.4G2) monoclonal antibody diluted in staining buffer according to manufacturer's instructions.
8. Fluorescently conjugated monoclonal antibodies (mAbs) for detection of surface molecules and intracellular cytokines (*see* Table 1).
9. Intracellular (IC) Fixation buffer.
10. Permeabilization buffer.
11. Anti-Mouse Ig, κ/Negative Control Compensation Particles.

3 Methods

3.1 Isolation of Peripheral Blood Mononuclear Cells from Whole Human Blood

The following method is to isolate PBMC from human peripheral blood samples. For healthy donors, 50 mL of whole blood yields on average approximately 6–7 × 10^7 PBMC. Directions in this section are based on whole blood volume of 50 mL. Scale up or down according to your sample volume.

1. Collect human blood in sodium heparin-containing vacutainer tubes.
2. Pool 50 mL whole blood into two 50 mL tubes (25 mL each) and dilute 1:1 with pure RPMI 1640 medium (*see* **Note 3**).
3. Pipette 15 mL Ficoll-Paque into three 50 mL tubes.
4. Using a 10-mL serological pipet, slowly layer diluted whole blood over the Ficoll-layer (33 mL per tube). Hold the pipette at approximately 70° to the inside of the tube to ensure full control of layering and minimal mixing of the blood and Ficoll layers.
5. Centrifuge layered tubes at 800 × *g* for 25 min at room temperature with minimal acceleration and brake.
6. Collect the resulting PBMC layers at the Ficoll interface into one 50 mL tube using a Pasteur pipette. Do not collect any red blood cell (*see* **Note 4**).
7. Make tube volume to 50 mL with complete medium.
8. Wash PBMC by centrifuging 500 × *g* for 10 min at 4 °C, and then resuspend cell pellet in 25 mL complete medium.
9. Count PBMC and estimate sample viability (*see* **Note 5**).
10. Make tube volume up to 50 mL with complete medium and centrifuge at 500 × *g* for 10 min at 4 °C. Resuspend cell pellet in the appropriate volume for ex vivo staining or for B-cell isolation (Subheading 3.2.) and culture (Subheading 3.3). Alternatively, cells can be frozen for future use (*see* **Note 6**).

3.2 B-Cell Isolation from Total Peripheral Blood Mononuclear Cells

The following method is to isolate CD19$^+$ B cells from PBMC samples using the human B-cell enrichment kit that best meets the operator's needs (*see* **Note 1**). Refer to the provided protocol for this kit for details of all applications. This method starts from freshly isolated PBMC but can be performed also on previously frozen PBMC (*see* **Note 7**).

1. Wash PBMC in separation buffer by topping up the tube volume to 50 mL with separation buffer and centrifuging at 500 × *g* for 10 min at 4 °C.
2. Resuspend the cell pellet at 5 × 10^7 cells/mL in separation buffer (*see* **Note 8**) into a 5-mL round-bottom polystyrene tube.
3. Proceed with B-cell enrichment, following manufacturer's instructions (*see* **Note 9**). Once the B-cell population has been isolated, proceed with the cell count (*see* **Note 5**).
4. Wash B cells by making tube volume up to 15 mL with complete medium and centrifuging at 500 × *g* for 10 min at 4 °C.

5. Resuspend B cells at 1×10^8 cells/mL in separation buffer for cell sorting, at 2.5×10^6 cells/mL in staining buffer for immediate ex vivo staining for flow cytometry, or at $1.25–2.5 \times 10^6$ cells/mL in complete medium for B-cell cultures (*see* **Note 10**).
6. For immediate ex vivo staining for flow cytometry, continue to Subheading 3.5, **steps 1–10**). For the setup of B-cell cultures, continue to Subheading 3.4.

3.3 Preparation of B Cells for Isolation of CD24^hi^CD38^hi^ and CD24^hi^CD27^+^ B Cells Using FACS

The following method is to prepare B cells for isolation of the $CD24^{hi}CD38^{hi}$ and $CD24^{hi}CD27^{+}$ B-cell subsets using FACS. Alternatively, cell sorting can be performed on total PBMC (*see* **Note 11**).

1. Wash isolated B cells twice with separation buffer by fuging at $500 \times g$ for 10 min at 4 °C.
2. Resuspend B cells at 1×10^8 cells/mL in separation buffer in 5 mL round-bottom polystyrene tubes. Set aside approximately 1×10^5 cells for a DAPI single-stained compensation sample.
3. Add anti-human CD19 BV785, CD24 APCeFluor780, CD38 PerCPeFluor710, and CD27 PE/Dazzle 594 mAbs (*see* Table 1) at the optimal concentration per tube as determined by titration (*see* **Note 12**). Incubate for 20 min on ice in the dark.
4. Wash cells twice by filling each tube with separation buffer and centrifuging at $500 \times g$ for 5 min at 4 °C. Resuspend cells at $30–50 \times 10^6$ cells/mL for sorting.
5. Remove cell clumps by pipetting each sample through the filter cap of a filter-top 5-mL round-bottom polystyrene tube.
6. Add DAPI at 0.05 μg/mL to each sample, in order to stain dead cells. At this step, also stain with DAPI the single-stained compensation sample.
7. Sort B cells according to the expression of subset-specific markers (*see* Fig. 1a).
8. Collect sorted B-cell subsets in 5-mL round-bottom capped polypropylene tubes containing 2 mL collection medium.

3.4 Culturing B Cells for Breg Expansion

This method describes the process for setting up a culture of isolated B cells or sorted B-cell subsets in order to expand the $IL\text{-}10^{+}$ population. CpGC, IFN-α, and megaCD40L have all been demonstrated to expand IL-10-producing B cells in culture [1, 7]. We recommend using CpGC as a minimum stimulus for IL-10 production and survival in culture, but Breg expansion can be increased further with addition of IFN-α or megaCD40L (*see* **Note 13**). For reference, the example stain in Fig. 2 shows IL-10 production by isolated B cells stimulated with CpGC alone.

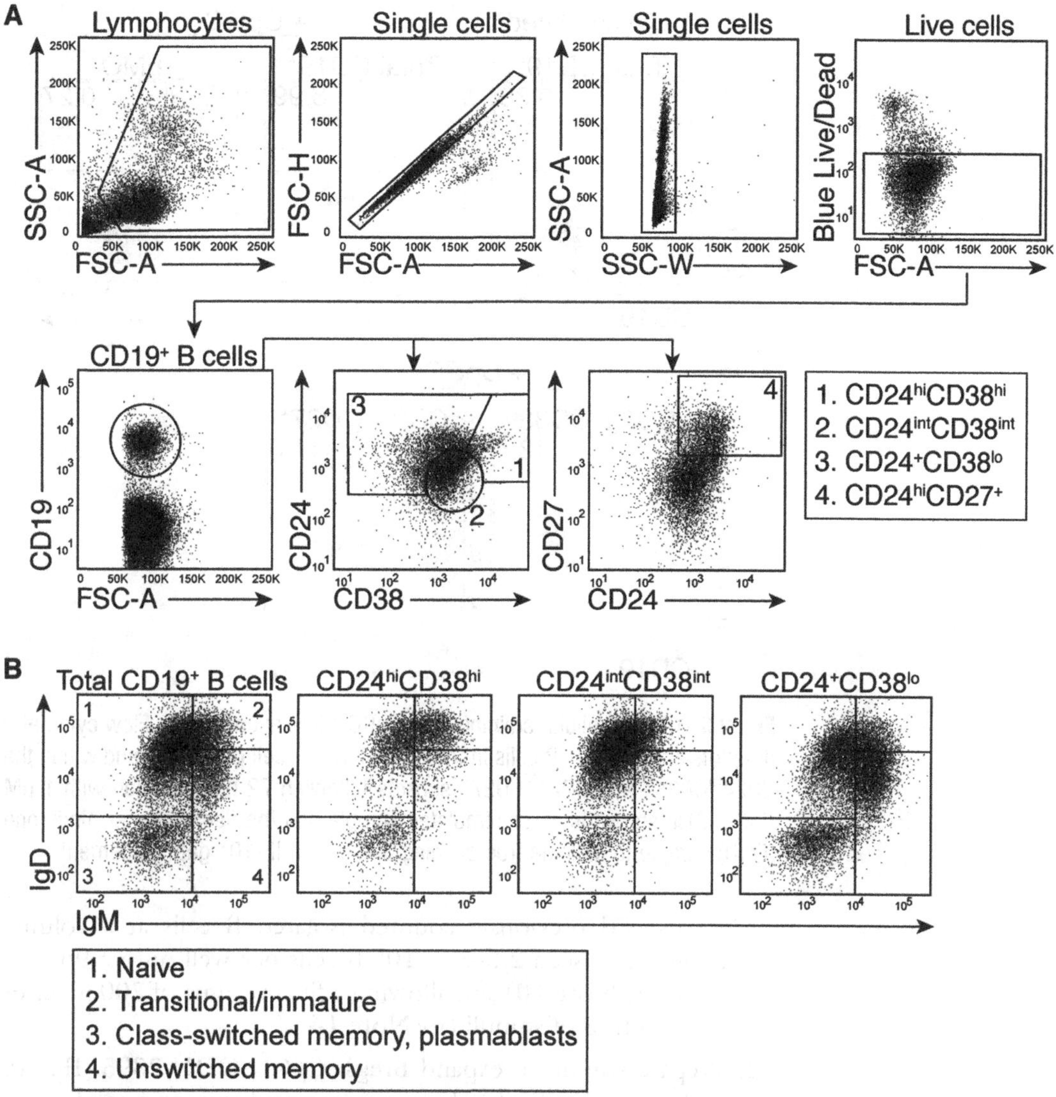

Fig. 1 Gating strategy for ex vivo identification of CD24^{hi}CD38^{hi} and CD24^{hi}CD27^{+} B cell subsets. Isolated healthy human PBMCs were stained for flow cytometry according to the protocol described in Subheading 3.5. Dot plots show gating strategies for ex vivo identification of CD24^{hi}CD38^{hi} and CD24^{hi}CD27^{+} B-cell subsets. In addition, expression of IgM and IgD can be used to validate gates set for CD24^{hi}CD38^{hi} and CD24^{hi}CD27^{+} subsets. (**a**) Flow cytometry dot plots show the gating strategy for ex vivo identification of live, CD19^{+}CD24^{hi}CD38^{hi} and CD24^{hi}CD27^{+} B-cell subsets from a total PBMC population. PBMC sample is gated on lymphocytes, then to include single cells and exclude doublets, then to include live cells only. B cells are then identified by the expression of CD19. The markers CD24 and CD38 are used to identify CD24^{hi}CD38^{hi} B cells, while CD24 and CD27 allow identification of CD24^{hi}CD27^{+} B cells. (**b**) Flow cytometry dot plots show IgM and IgD expression within the total B-cell population, and within the CD24^{hi}CD38^{hi}, CD24^{int}CD38^{int}, and CD24^{+}CD38^{lo} subsets. Labels 1–4 indicate the B-cell phenotype within each quadrant

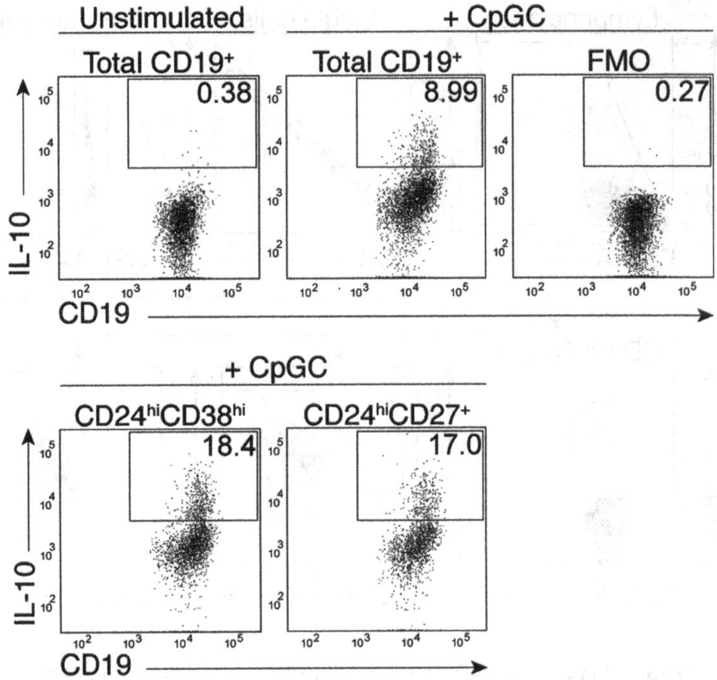

Fig. 2 IL-10 intracellular staining post-CpGC stimulation in vitro. Flow cytometry dot plots show IL-10^+ B cells in the total $CD19^+$ B-cell population and within the $CD24^{hi}CD38^{hi}$ and $CD24^{hi}CD27^+$ subsets following 72 h stimulation with 1 μM CpGC. Also shown is an unstimulated sample and the fluorescence-minus-one (FMO) sample to indicate true staining and inform IL-10^+ gate placement

1. Resuspend previously counted isolated B cells at a volume allowing to seed 2.5–5 × 10^5 B cells per well onto a 96-well plate (*see* **Note 10**) and allowing a final volume of 200 μL after the addition of stimuli (*see* **Note 14**).
2. Prepare stimuli to expand Bregs. CpGC ODN 2395, IFN-α, and megaCD40L should be resuspended in complete medium to produce a final concentration of 1 μM, 1000 U/mL, and 1 μg/mL, respectively (*see* **Note 15**).
3. Add required stimuli for Breg induction to relevant wells. If used in conjunction, CpGC, IFN-α, and megaCD40L can be added at the same time.
4. Fill the empty wells surrounding samples with complete medium (*see* **Note 16**).
5. Incubate at 37 °C, 5% CO_2 for 72 h.
6. During the final 5 h of culture, decant supernatants (*see* **Note 17**) and resuspend cells in 100 μL of PIB cocktail (*see* **Note 18**). Incubate for 5 h at 37 °C, 5% CO_2.
7. At the end of incubation, proceed to Subheading 3.5 for staining of cells for analysis by flow cytometry.

3.5 Fluorescent Staining for the Analysis of Surface Markers and Intracellular Cytokines by Flow Cytometry

The following method describes how to use fluorescently conjugated mAbs to stain surface markers and intracellular cytokines for analysis by flow cytometry. For surface marker staining alone (either ex vivo or post-culture), follow **steps 1–10**.

1. B cells will have been prepared in 96-well plates for ex vivo staining as per Subheading 3.2, **step 11** or post-culture as per Subheading 3.4.
2. Wash plate twice in PBS by centrifuging at 600 × *g* for 5 min at 4 °C.
3. Resuspend cells in 50 μL of staining buffer containing LIVE/DEAD Fixable Blue Dead Cell Stain, diluted according to manufacturer's instructions. Incubate for 20 min at room temperature in the dark.
4. Wash cells twice with staining buffer by centrifuging at 800 × *g* for 3 min at 4 °C.
5. Resuspend cells in 20 μL FcR blocking reagent per 10^7 cells in the well. Incubate for 10 min in the dark at 4 °C.
6. Wash cells twice in staining buffer by centrifuging at 800 × *g* for 3 min at 4 °C.
7. Resuspend cells in 50 μL of staining buffer containing anti-human CD19 BV785, CD24 APCeFluor780, CD38 PerCPeFluor710, CD27 PE/Dazzle 595, IgM BV510, IgD BV605 mAbs diluted at optimal concentrations determined by titration (*see* **Note 12**). Incubate for 30 min in the dark at 4 °C.
8. Wash plate twice in staining buffer, centrifuging at 800 × *g* for 3 min at 4 °C.
9. Resuspend cells in 100 μL intracellular (IC) fixation buffer. Incubate for 10 min in the dark at 4 °C. Wash cells twice with staining buffer, centrifuging at 800 × *g* for 3 min at 4 °C.
10. If staining for cell surface markers only (ex vivo or after culture), resuspend cells in 200 μL staining buffer in 5 mL polystyrene round-bottom tubes. Store in the dark at 4 °C until analyzing by flow cytometry. If additionally staining for intracellular cytokines, continue with this section.
11. Wash cells twice with permeabilization buffer, centrifuging at 800 × *g* for 3 min at 4 °C. Resuspend cells in 50 μL permeabilization buffer, incubate for 5 min in the dark at 4 °C.
12. On top of the 50 μL permeabilization buffer, add 50 μL of permeabilization buffer containing anti-IL-10 APC mAb at the optimal concentration as determined by titration (*see* **Note 12**). For the IL-10 FMO control, add 50 μL permeabilization buffer instead of IL-10 mAb. Incubate for 40 min in the dark at 4 °C.

13. Wash cells twice with staining buffer, centrifuging at 800 × *g* for 3 min at 4 °C. Resuspend cells in 200 μL staining buffer in 5 mL round-bottom polystyrene tubes. If samples are not immediately analyzed by flow cytometry, store samples in the dark at 4 °C prior to analysis (*see* **Note 19**).
14. Prepare Anti-Mouse Ig, κ/Negative Control Compensation Particles as per manufacturer's instructions for each fluorochrome used.
15. Proceed to flow cytometry acquisition. Gate on lymphocytes, exclude doublets and dead cells and gate on the $CD19^+$ population. Within the $CD19^+$ population, use CD24 and CD38 expression to gate on the $CD24^{hi}CD38^{hi}$ subset, and use CD24 and CD27 expression to gate on the $CD24^{hi}CD27^+$ subset. Gate on the $IL\text{-}10^+$ B-cell population (within individual subsets or as part of the total $CD19^+$ population), using the unstimulated sample and fluorescence-minus-one (FMO) control as guidelines (*see* Subheading 3.6 and Fig. 2).

3.6 Guidelines for the Analysis of Stained Cells by Flow Cytometry

Peripheral B-cell subsets can be broadly identified by their expression of the surface markers CD24, CD38, and CD27. Immature B cells are identified as $CD24^{hi}CD38^{hi}$, mature B cells as $CD24^{int}CD38^{int}$, and memory B cells as $CD24^+CD38^{hi}$. CD27 is typically a marker of post-germinal center B cells and thus together with CD24 expression may be used as a memory B-cell marker (plasmablasts and plasma cells have low/negative CD24 expression). Note that not all memory B cells are $CD27^+$, for example, a $CD27^-IgD^-$ double-negative memory B-cell population has been described [12]. Ex vivo surface expression of CD24, CD38, and CD27 is sufficient to identify the $CD24^{hi}CD38^{hi}$ and $CD24^{hi}CD27^+$ subsets (*see* Fig. 1a).

Following stimulation and in vitro culture, delineation between individual B-cell subsets is not always clear due to the spread of surface marker expression by B cells during differentiation. For example, discriminating between the $CD24^{hi}CD38^{hi}$ immature and $CD24^{int}CD38^{int}$ mature subsets is not always evident as both of these markers are expressed as a spectrum. Analyzing the expression of surface IgM and IgD (*see* Fig. 1b) can validate B-cell subset gate placement compared to CD24, CD38, and CD27 expression alone. For example, $CD24^{hi}CD38^{hi}$ immature B cells are $IgM^{hi}IgD^{hi}$, whereas $CD24^{int}CD38^{int}$ B cells are IgM^+IgD^+. Therefore, within the gated $CD24^{hi}CD38^{hi}$ subset the high expression of IgM and IgD increases confidence of correct $CD24^{hi}CD38^{hi}$ gate placement. Additionally, IgM and IgD expression provides greater resolution into the memory B-cell compartment by delineating between IgM^+ non-class-switched memory and IgM^-IgD^- class-switched memory.

Figure 2 shows an example of gate positioning for the identification of IL-10$^+$ cells within the total B-cell, CD24^{hi}CD38^{hi} and CD24^{hi}CD27$^+$, populations. Also shown is the FMO control and the unstimulated B-cell condition. Following Breg expansion, there may not be a clear delineation between IL-10$^+$ and IL-10$^-$ populations. Therefore, we recommend using the unstimulated sample as an additional guideline for IL-10 gate placement. Indeed, isolated B cells cultured for 72 h without stimulation will produce very little IL-10 (0–3%) (*see* Fig. 2).

4 Notes

1. We recommend the STEMCELL EasySep B-cell enrichment kit as the isolated B-cell fraction has 95–99% purity.
2. For cell sorting we recommend using DAPI for staining dead cells as it can be added immediately prior to cell sorting thus minimizing incubation times. Differently, we recommend using the LIVE/DEAD™ Fixable Blue Dead Cell Stain Kit (ThermoFisher) for staining dead cells for flow cytometry as this is compatible with cell fixation. Prepare a 1:500 dilution of reconstituted stock in PBS and add to cells. Although other similar dyes to LIVE/DEAD Blue are available, we recommend this dye since it is excited by a UV laser and is compatible with the fluorescent mAb panel described in this protocol.
3. To retrieve the maximum amount of blood from the vacutainer tube, use a Pasteur pipette to rinse out any remaining sample with RPMI 1640 medium.
4. Following centrifugation of harvested PBMC, there may be residual red blood cell contamination (the pellet will be red in color). In this event, resuspend the pellet in 5 mL Red Blood Cell Lysis Buffer and incubate for 5 min at room temperature before washing in complete medium and continuing with the protocol.
5. We suggest using a trypan blue exclusion assay to count cells and assess viability.
6. B-cell isolation is optimally performed immediately following PBMC isolation as this avoids cell death occurring during the freezing/thawing process. However, it may be required that PBMC are stored in advance. In this case, prepare freezing medium (10% DMSO in FCS) for a volume allowing 1×10^7 PBMCs/mL. Store freezing medium on ice until use. Following cell count and centrifugation, resuspend the cell pellet in 1 mL of cold freezing medium, then pour in the remaining medium. Rapidly aliquot resuspended cells at 1 mL per cryovial. DMSO is toxic to cells, so minimize the length of time

cells are in contact with DMSO. Store cryovials in a Mr. Frosty™ container (ThermoFisher) with propan-2-ol in a -80 °C freezer to allow freezing at -1 °C per minute. Transfer cryovials to liquid nitrogen storage after no longer than 3 days at -80 °C storage. If cells are left any longer cell viability declines.

7. Thaw and wash cells rapidly to minimize cell exposure to DMSO (which is toxic to cells) and to optimize viability. Minimize the length of time cryovials are on ice following removal from liquid nitrogen storage.
8. Following centrifugation, aspirate as much supernatant as possible without disturbing the cell pellet before resuspending in the appropriate separation buffer volume. This is because the efficacy of the B-cell Enrichment Kit is volume-sensitive.
9. At the final step of the B-cell enrichment protocol when extracting the B-cell fraction, after 2–3 s of tube inversion, there will be droplets attached to the tube edge. Do not dislodge these into the B-cell fraction as these may contain non-B cells which will decrease the purity of the isolated B-cell sample.
10. The number of B cells plated per well may vary depending on the numbers of B cells isolated and the number of wells intended to include per sample. We recommend plating between 2–5 × 10^5 B cells per well since B cells proliferate more and tend to have higher viability at lower cell densities. Ensure number of B cells plated per well is consistent across conditions/repeats.
11. The time required to sort a sample will be greatly reduced by starting from isolated B cells rather than total PBMC.
12. While in this protocol we describe to use 2 μg/mL mAb for extracellular marker staining and 4 μg/mL mAb for IL-10 intracellular staining (*see* Table 1), we suggest titrating mAbs to find the optimal concentrations for individual laboratories.
13. We recommend using CpGC as a minimum stimulus for IL-10 production and survival in culture, but Breg expansion can be increased further with addition of IFN-α or megaCD40L. Consider the context in which wishing to investigate Bregs when selecting the stimuli to include. Indeed, CpGC stimulates B-cell-specific TLR9, whereas IFN-α is predominantly derived from activated pDCs, and megaCD40L simulates co-stimulatory signals provided to B cells by $CD4^+$ Th cells.
14. Include an unstimulated B-cell sample, and a sample to be used as an FMO for IL-10 staining. These can both be used as guidelines for correct IL-10 gate placement (*see* Subheading 3.6 and Fig. 2).

15. Titrate stimuli to find optimum concentration for the needed application. Although our given concentrations were found to maximally induce Bregs, we recommend titrating each stimulus in order to find optimal concentrations for individual laboratories.
16. During incubation, some medium may evaporate from wells and this can reduce cell viability. Filling the empty wells surrounding samples with medium is a way to limit evaporation from the samples and therefore reduce cell death.
17. Cell culture supernatants can be decanted into a 96-well plate and stored at -80 °C for further analysis, such as ELISA. ELISA measures secreted cytokine in cell supernatants, and this could be of interest since flow cytometry measures the intracellular expression of cytokines, which may not be representative of secreted IL-10.
18. PMA and ionomycin activate B cells and induce cytokine production. Brefeldin A inhibits cytokine secretion so in combination with PMA and ionomycin increases intracellular cytokine levels, maximizing intracellular IL-10 detection by flow cytometry.
19. To maintain optimal sample and staining quality, we recommend analyzing samples by flow cytometry no longer than 48 h after surface marker staining, and no longer than 24 h after for intracellular cytokine staining. Optimally, samples should be run soon after staining. Some tandem fluorochromes (for example, PE-Cy5) can degrade and separate into differentially fluorescing components.

Acknowledgments

This work is funded by an Arthritis Research UK program grant (ref. 21786) awarded to Claudia Mauri. Hannah Bradford is funded by a UCB BIOPHARMA SPRL/BBSRC PhD Studentship (ref. BB/P504725/1). We would like to thank Dr. Diego Catalan for his constructive criticisms on the manuscript.

References

1. Blair PA, Noreña LY, Flores-Borja F et al (2010) CD19+CD24hiCD38hi B cells exhibit regulatory capacity in healthy individuals but are functionally impaired in systemic lupus erythematosus. Immunity 32:129–140
2. Flores-Borja F, Bosma A, Ng D et al (2013) CD19+CD24hiCD38hi B cells maintain regulatory T cells while limiting TH1 and TH17 differentiation. Sci Transl Med 5:173ra23. https://doi.org/10.1126/scitranslmed.300540
3. Iwata Y, Matsushita T, Horikawa M et al (2011) Characterisation of a rare IL-10-competent B-cell subset in humans that parallels mouse regulatory B10 cells. Blood 117:530–541

4. Mauri C, Menon M (2017) Human regulatory B cells in health and disease: therapeutic potential. J Clin Invest 127:772–779
5. Candado KM, Lykken JM, Tedder TF (2014) B10 cell regulation of health and disease. Immunol Rev 259:259–272
6. Weill J, Weller S (2009) Human marginal zone B cells. Annu Rev Immunol 27:267–287
7. Menon M, Blair PA, Isenberg DA et al (2016) A regulatory feedback between Plasmacytoid dendritic cells and regulatory B cells is aberrant in systemic lupus erythematosus. Immunity 44:683–697
8. Yoshihara Y, Ishiuji Y, Yoshizaki A et al (2019) IL-10-producing regulatory B cells are decreased in patients with atopic dermatitis. J Invest Dermatol 139:475–478
9. Hayashi M, Yanaba K, Umezawa Y et al (2016) IL-10-producing regulatory B cells are decreased in patients with psoriasis. J Dermatol Sci 81:93–100
10. Bankó Z, Pozsgay J, Szili D et al (2017) Induction and differentiation of regulatory B cells from healthy blood donors and rheumatoid arthritis patients. J Immunol 198:1512–1520
11. Murakami Y, Saito H, Sakabe T et al (2019) Increased regulatory B cells are involved in immune evasion in patients with gastric cancer. Sci Rep 9:1–9
12. Wei C, Anolik J, Cappione A et al (2007) A new population of cells lacking expression of CD27 represents a notable component of the B cell memory compartment in systemic lupus erythematosus. J Immunol 178:6624–6633

Part II

Mechanisms of Immune Suppression by B Cells

Chapter 6

Detection of IL-10 in Murine B Cells: In Vitro and In Vivo Techniques

Xiang Lin, Xiaohui Wang, and Liwei Lu

Abstract

With the ever-increasing understanding of the roles of B cells in immune response and autoimmune pathogenesis, various techniques have been optimized for the detection of IL-10 production in B cells. In this chapter, we describe several commonly used methods for the effective detection of IL-10 in B cells at both mRNA and protein levels, including quantitative PCR analysis, intracellular staining of IL-10 in live B cells by flow cytometry, ELISA for secreted IL-10 detection, and ELISPOT assay for enumerating IL-10-producing B cells. We have further co-stained IL-10 with other cytokines and examined the staining efficiency. Moreover, we provide a detailed protocol for the detection of IL-10-producing B cells in situ by immunofluorescence microscopy. Since emerging evidence has suggested the promising strategy of cell therapy, we also provide a protocol to determine $CD19^{+}CD1d^{hi}CD5^{+}$ B-cell distribution upon adoptive transfer using tile-scan imaging. Together, the application of the described methods for the detection of IL-10 will facilitate the characterization of B-cell subsets with regulatory functions and enhance our current understanding of the critical roles of B cells in immune response and autoimmune development.

Key words IL-10, Regulatory B cells, Adoptive transfer, In situ detection, Tile scan

1 Introduction

B cells play a critical role in the regulation of immune responses by producing antigen-specific antibodies, presenting antigens to $CD4^{+}$ T cells and secreting cytokines [1–3]. Apart from being well characterized as an effector arm in adaptive immunity, B cells have been increasingly recognized to play either a protective or pathogenic role in the development of autoimmune diseases by producing immunosuppressive or proinflammatory cytokines, respectively. B cells were found to produce IL-6 during experimental autoimmune encephalomyelitis (EAE) development, while elimination of IL-6-producing B cells can ameliorate disease course [4]. Interestingly, it has been shown that IL-17-secreting B cells play critical roles in infection with *Trypanosoma cruzi* [5]. Moreover, the protective role of B cells in regulating autoimmunity and

Francesca Mion and Silvia Tonon (eds.), *Regulatory B Cells: Methods and Protocols*, Methods in Molecular Biology, vol. 2270, https://doi.org/10.1007/978-1-0716-1237-8_6,

inflammation via the production of IL-10 has been reported in several mouse models [6–9]. Various B-cell subsets with different phenotypes have been shown to possess regulatory functions in both the murine and human systems. In mice, splenic marginal zone (MZ) B cells ($CD1d^{hi}CD21^{hi}CD23^{-}CD24^{hi}IgM^{hi}IgD^{lo}$) and T2-MZP B cells ($CD1d^{hi}CD21^{hi}CD23^{hi}CD24^{hi}IgM^{hi}IgD^{hi}$) have been demonstrated to delay autoimmune disease development [9, 10]. In humans, $CD19^{+}CD24^{hi}CD38^{hi}CD5^{+}CD1d^{hi}$ B cells have been detected in the peripheral blood and were shown to inhibit Th1 cell responses in systemic lupus erythematosus (SLE) patients [11]. $CD25^{hi}CD27^{hi}CD86^{hi}CD1d^{hi}IL\text{-}10^{hi}TGF\text{-}\beta^{hi}$ B cells were shown to suppress effector $CD4^{+}$ T-cell responses but to enhance Foxp3 and CTLA-4 expressions in Treg cells [12]. Among the diverse regulatory B-cell subsets, IL-10-producing B cells have been extensively studied [3, 13, 14]. IL-10-producing B cells in vitro generated via activation of CD40, BAFF receptor, toll-like receptor, B cell receptor, and CD80/CD86 signaling pathways, respectively, have exhibited potent protective roles under pathological conditions such as EAE, lupus, rheumatoid arthritis, hepatitis, carcinogenesis, graft-versus-host disease, intestinal injury, allergic airway disease, and experimental Sjögren's syndrome [15–22]. Notably, Tedder and colleagues have developed a highly efficient method for expanding IL-10-producing B cells in culture, which elicit marked inhibitory effects on suppressing autoimmune inflammation in animal models [23]. Thus, effective expansion of IL-10-producing B cells in culture could be potentially applied for the development of new cell therapies in the treatment of autoimmune diseases.

The following section focuses on various techniques currently used for the detection of IL-10 in murine B cells both in culture and in situ detection, by quantitative polymerase chain reaction (qPCR), flow cytometry, enzyme-linked immunosorbent assay (ELISA), enzyme-linked immunosorbent spot (ELISPOT) assay, and immunofluorescence microscopy.

2 Materials

All procedures are to be carried out using sterile tissue/cell culture techniques with sterile solutions/buffers and equipment and are conducted in biosafety containment hoods.

2.1 Equipment

1. Equipment and device-specific reagents for quantitative PCR with double-stranded DNA-binding dyes as reporters (*see* **Note 1**).
2. Fluorescence-activated cell sorter (FACS) and flow cytometer.
3. Confocal laser-scanning microscope.

4. Humidified incubator maintained at 37 °C and 5% CO_2.
5. Magnetic separation apparatus.
6. Refrigerated centrifuge.
7. 15 and 50 mL conical tubes.
8. 1.5 mL and microcentrifuge tubes.
9. 100 μm mesh filter.
10. ELISA plate reader with appropriate filter for peroxidase substrate employed.

2.2 Media and Buffers

1. Phosphate-buffered saline (PBS): 137 mM NaCl, 2.7 mM KCl, 10 mM Na_2HPO_4 and 1.8 mM KH_2PO_4. Add distilled water to a total volume of 1 l and adjust the pH to 7.4.
2. R10 medium: 2 mM L-Glutamine, 10% fetal bovine serum (FBS), 10 mM HEPES pH 7.5, 100 U/mL penicillin and 100 μg/mL streptomycin, 100 μM 2-mercaptoethanol in complete RPMI 1640 culture medium.
3. RNA extraction reagent for cells and tissues (*see* **Note 2**).
4. RNase-free water (DEPC-H_2O): 0.05% diethyl pyrocarbonate dissolved in water.
5. 75% ethanol solution: 75% ethanol dissolved in DEPC-H_2O.
6. Reverse transcription buffer (10×): 100 μg/mL bovine serum albumin (BSA), 10 mM dithiothreitol (DTT), 25 mM KCl, 3.5 mM $MgCl_2$, 50 mM Tris–HCl (pH 7.5).
7. PCR buffer (10×): 500 mM KCl, 100 mM Tris–HCl (pH 8.3).
8. Staining medium: 2% FBS (v/v), 10 mM NaN_3, 10 mM HEPES (pH 7.2) in Hank's Buffered Salt Solution (HBSS).
9. B cell isolation buffer: 0.5% BSA, 2 mM ethylenediaminetetraacetic acid (EDTA) in PBS.
10. Ammonium-chloride-potassium (ACK) lysis buffer: 0.15 M NH_4Cl, 10 mM $KHCO_3$, 0.1 mM Na_2EDTA in double distilled water.
11. Intracellular cytokine staining stimulation mixture stock solutions (1000×): 50 μg/mL phorbol myristate acetate (PMA); 1 μg/μL ionomycin dissolved in DMSO; 2 μM monensin solution.
12. FACS buffer: 0.5–1% BSA or 5–10% FBS, 0.1% sodium azide (NaN_3) in PBS.
13. Fixation buffer: 4% paraformaldehyde in PBS.
14. Permeabilization buffer: 0.1% saponin, 1 mM $CaCl_2$, 1 mM $MgSO_4$, 0.05% NaN_3, 0.1% BSA, 10 mM HEPES (pH 7.2) in PBS. Store up to 6 months at 4 °C.
15. PBST: 0.05% Tween in PBS.

16. ELISA blocking solution: 0.5% gelatin, 0.5% BSA in PBST.
17. Streptavidin-alkaline phosphatase solution: 1 mg/mL streptavidin-alkaline phosphatase dissolved in 100 mM Tris–HCl (pH 9.5).
18. 5-Bromo-4-chloro-3-indolylphosphate/nitro blue tetrazolium (BCIP/NBT) solution containing 0.15 mg/mL BCIP, 0.3 mg/mL NBT, 100 mM Tris buffer, and 5 mM $MgCl_2$; pH 9.5.
19. ELISA stop solution: 2 M H_2SO_4.
20. Optimal cutting temperature compound (OCT).
21. 0.25% Triton X-100 in PBS.

2.3 Cytokines, Antibodies, and Other Reagents

1. Lipopolysaccharide (LPS, Escherichia coli F583) dissolved in DMSO. Filter and store at −80 °C.
2. Purified anti-mouse CD16/32 (clone 2.4G2) antibody.
3. Monoclonal antibodies (mAbs): anti-mouse CD19 (clone 6D5); CD5 (clone 57–5.3); CD1d (clone 1B1); CD11c (clone N418); IL-10 (clone JES5-16E3); IL-6 (clone MP5-20F3) antibodies, and fluorochrome-conjugated Rat IgG2b isotype control.
4. IL-10 capture (reconstitute at 0.5 mg/mL in sterile PBS) and detection (reconstitute at 0.2 mg/mL in sterile PBS) antibodies for ELISA (*see* **Note 3**).
5. IL-10 reference standard: reconstitute at 100 μg/mL in sterile PBS (*see* **Note 3**).
6. Peroxidase-conjugated streptavidin (HRP).
7. 3,3′,5,5′-Tetramethylbenzidine (TMB).
8. Nuclei staining dye, 4′,6-diamidino-2-phenylindole (DAPI) in mounting medium.
9. Live/dead cell staining dye.
10. Fluorescence cell-tracking dye (e.g., carboxyfluorescein succinimidyl ester or seminaphtharhodafluor).

2.4 Reagents for IL-10 mRNA Measurement

1. Chloroform.
2. Isopropanol.
3. Reagents for cDNA synthesis (*see* Table 1). All reagents used for reverse transcription are widely available commercially.
4. IL-10 primers (*see* Tables 2 and 3).
5. Reagents for Taq DNA polymerase PCR (*see* Table 4). All reagents used for PCR are widely available commercially.
6. Reagents for quantitative PCR (*see* Table 5). SYBR green is reported as an example of dsDNA intercalating dye.

Table 1
Reagents for mRNA reverse transcription

Components	Volume
Reverse transcriptase	1 μL (200 U)
Reverse transcriptase buffer	4 μL
dNTP (a mixture of 2 mM dATP, dCTP, dGTP, dTTP)	5 μL
Random primer (oligo-dT18–20)	2 μL
RNA sample	Up to 2.5 μg
DEPC-H_2O	Up to 20 μL

Table 2
PCR primer design of IL-10 detection set 1

	Sequence (5′- > 3′)	Length	Tm	GC%
Forward	GTAGAAGTGATGCCCCAGGC	20	60.5	60.00
Reverse	GAGAAATCGATGACAGCGCC	20	59.4	55.00
Product length	117 bp			

Table 3
PCR primer design of IL-10 detection set 2

	Sequence (5′- > 3′)	Length	Tm	GC%
Forward	GCCGGGAAGACAATAACTGC	20	59.3	55.00
Reverse	GCCTGGGGCATCACTTCTAC	20	60.5	60.00
Product length	223 bp			

Table 4
Mixture for Taq DNA polymerase PCR

Components	Volume
10× PCR buffer	5 μL
10 mM dNTPs	1 μL
50 mM $MgCl_2$	1.5 μL
Primer mix (10 μM each)	1 μL
Template DNA	≥1 μL (200 ng)
Taq DNA polymerase	0.2 μL
Autoclaved, distilled water	Up to 50 μL

Table 5
Recipe for qPCR

Components	Volume
SYBR green dissolved in PCR buffer	25 μL
Forward primer, 10 μM	1 μL
Reverse primer, 10 μM	1 μL
cDNA generated from 10 pg to 1 μg of total RNA	≤ 10 μL
DEPC-H_2O	Up to 50 μL

2.5 Reagents for B-Cell Isolation

1. Biotin-labeled anti-B220 monoclonal antibody (clone RA3-6B2).
2. Anti-biotin magnetic beads.

2.6 Mice

1. C57BL/6 female mice, between 6 and 8 weeks of age, are used in all experiments.

3 Methods

This section begins with a brief description of the method used for B-cell purification. It then moves to the specific topic of the chapter which summarizes the protocols for the detection of IL-10-producing B cells and for the measurement of IL-10 secreted by murine B cells in culture. The mRNA levels of IL-10 are measured by quantitative PCR, while protein levels are measured by ELISA, ELISPOT, immunofluorescence microscopy, and flow cytometry. Finally, fluorescence-labeled $CD19^{+}CD1d^{hi}CD5^{+}$ B-cell distribution is visualized by tile-scan confocal microscopy.

3.1 B Cell Purification and $CD19^{+}CD1d^{hi}CD5^{+}$ Cell Isolation

1. Harvest lymphocytes from mouse spleen and remove erythrocytes by incubating 3 min on ice with ACK lysis buffer. Prepare the single-cell suspension by filtering through 100 μm mesh. For every 10^6 B cells, add 0.5 μg of biotin-labeled anti-B220 monoclonal antibody (0.5 mg/mL) in B-cell isolation buffer and incubate for 10 min at 4 °C.
2. Wash cells with B-cell isolation buffer to remove the unbound antibody and centrifuge at 300 × *g* for 5 min at 4 °C.
3. Discard the supernatant and resuspend the cells with anti-biotin magnetic beads (8 × 10^5 beads per 10^5 B cells) for 10 min at 4 °C.
4. Wash cells with B-cell isolation buffer and separate the magnetic beads antibody-conjugated cells using the magnetic separation apparatus. Allow 5 min for the beads (and attached cells) to accumulate adjacent to the magnet.

5. Count isolated B cells and resuspend in R10 medium at the final concentration of 5×10^6/mL.
6. The obtained B cells can be further stained in order to purify the $CD19^+CD1d^{hi}CD5^+$ and $CD19^+CD1d^{low}CD5^-$ B-cell populations by fluorescence-activated cell sorting (FACS). First incubate the B cells with the appropriate quantities of isotype controls, anti-CD1d, anti-CD5, and anti-CD19 antibodies on ice for 30 min. Wash cells and resuspend in R10 medium at the final concentration of 10^6/mL. Upon alignment of a cell sorter equipped with a sterile cartridge system, load the cells stained with isotype controls to define the gating strategy. Further, load single-stained cells to define the color compensation strategy. Based on the above settings, $CD19^+CD1d^{hi}CD5^+$ and $CD19^+CD1d^{low}CD5^-$ populations can be determined among the total purified B cell sample.

3.2 IL-10 mRNA Measurement

The conventional reverse transcription polymerase chain reaction (RT-PCR) has often been applied to detect relatively rare mRNA transcripts. However, the amplified PCR products cannot be truly quantitative and only give a crude ratio between samples. The quantitative real-time PCR (qPCR), one of the best developed molecular technologies of the last decade, has shown a higher accuracy by probing fluorescent tag for detection. The following protocol describes the measurement of IL-10 gene expression by comparison with the housekeeping gene 18S ribosomal RNA (18S rRNA).

3.2.1 mRNA Extraction

1. mRNA samples from tissues or purified cells are prepared with RNA extraction reagent: tissues (50–100 mg) or cells ($0.5–3 \times 10^6$) are suspended with 0.5–1.0 mL of phenol and guanidine isothiocyanate solution on ice.
2. Add 0.2 mL of chloroform to the phenol and guanidine isothiocyanate solution, mix thoroughly with vortexer, and incubate at room temperature for 10 min.
3. Centrifuge the sample at $12,000 \times g$ for 10 min at 4 °C.
4. Carefully transfer the colorless supernatant to a new 1.5 mL tube (*see* **Note 4**).
5. Precipitate the RNA by adding equal volume of 100% isopropanol. Samples are thoroughly mixed with vortexer and incubated on ice for 10 min.
6. Centrifuge at $12,000 \times g$ for 10 min at 4 °C.
7. Discard the supernatant cautiously, without disrupting the RNA pellet.
8. Wash the RNA pellet with 1 mL of 75% ethanol solution.

9. Centrifuge at 7500 × *g* for 5 min at 4 °C and discard the supernatant.
10. Vacuum or air-dry the RNA pellet for 5–10 min at room temperature.
11. Resuspend the RNA pellet in DEPC-H_2O; incubate at 56 °C for 5 min to dissolve the RNA.
12. Measure RNA concentration. RNA samples with A260/280 ratios between 1.8 and 2.0 are used for cDNA synthesis.
13. Store RNA samples at −80 °C till analysis.

3.2.2 Complementary DNA (cDNA) Preparation

1. cDNA is synthesized from mRNA by using reverse transcription: to synthesize first-strand cDNA, mix the reagents reported in Table 1 in a sterile microcentrifuge tube on ice.
2. Gently mix reaction contents and centrifuge all the remaining solution to the bottom of the tube.
3. RT-PCR is performed by using the following recycling protocol: 25 °C for 10 min, 42 °C for 60 min. Terminate the reaction at 85 °C for 5 min.
4. Store cDNA samples at −80 °C till use.

3.2.3 Design and Control of Primers for IL-10 cDNA Amplification

1. Forward and reverse primers for mouse *il10* gene can be designed using different protocols. Primers should have a GC content of no more than 50%, an annealing temperature between 57 and 63 °C and a length of 20 ± 2 bp. Typically, primers designed among the CDS region (68–604 bp) are suitable for qPCR assay. Two sets of primers designed using the NCBI Primer-BLAST program are reported in Tables 2 and 3.
2. Before being used for qPCR, the designed primers are tested by Taq DNA polymerase PCR with the reaction mixture reported in Table 4.
3. To verify the specificity of designed primers, perform 25–35 cycles of PCR amplification with the following settings: 2 min at 94 °C, 30 s at 94 °C, 45 s at 60 °C, and 50 s at 72 °C. The reaction is terminated with an elongation step of 10 min at 72 °C. PCR products can be stored at 4 °C before analysis. Cycle numbers should be optimized for each primer pair.
4. Analyze the PCR products by 1.5% agarose gel electrophoresis (*see* Fig. 1).

3.2.4 Quantitative Real-Time PCR (qPCR)

1. The mRNA expression is measured by quantitative PCR with double-stranded DNA-binding dyes as reporters. Mix thoroughly the reagents listed in Table 5, and load the samples in 96-well or 384-well PCR plate.

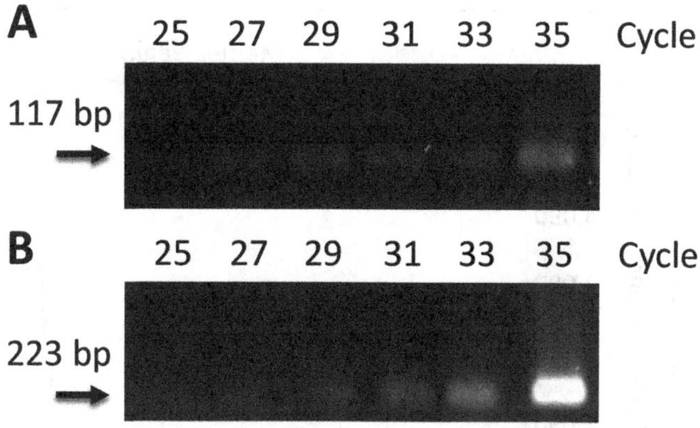

Fig. 1 Detection of IL-10 gene expression using RT-PCR. This method was used to evaluate the specificity of two IL-10 primer sets. PCR amplification of primer set 1 (**a**) and set 2 (**b**) was performed for 25–35 cycles

Table 6
Reaction setup protocol for qPCR

Steps		Time
50 °C (UDG incubation)		2 min
95 °C		2 min
40 cycles of:	95 °C	15 s
	60 °C	1 min
60 °C		15 s
90 °C		15 s

2. qPCR is performed by using the protocol reported in Table 6, and melting curves are analyzed as initial step of gene expression analysis (*see* Fig. 2 and **Note 5**).
3. Cycling threshold (CT) values of *il10* and of the housekeeping gene *18S rRNA* are obtained. The relative expression of *il10* to *18S rRNA* is calculated by $2^{-\Delta\Delta Ct}$ method [24].

3.3 Intracellular IL-10 Measurement by Flow Cytometry

The levels of gene transcripts are usually correlated with protein expression that can be readily examined by flow cytometry. As cytokine production has been shown to be heterogeneous even within cell subpopulations, multiple cell surface markers are therefore used to identify the cytokine-producing cell subsets among various cell populations by flow cytometric analysis. This protocol is applicable for measuring the intracellular production of IL-10 and of other cytokines in B cells by flow cytometric analysis.

1. Stimulate B cells (1×10^6 cells/mL) for 4 h with 1× intracellular cytokine staining stimulation mixture. At the end of the

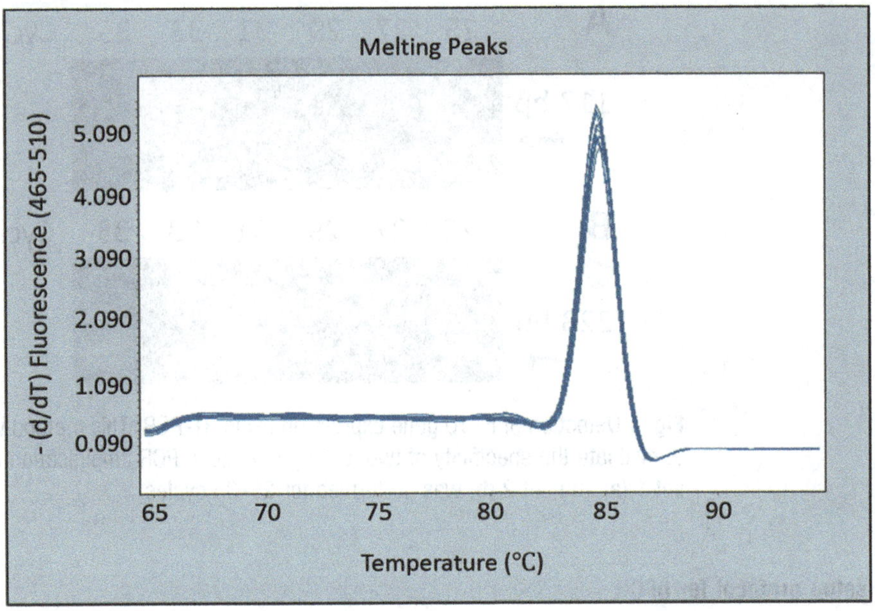

Fig. 2 Melting curve analysis. Representative curve of a reference gene. The single peak is typically representing a pure, single amplicon

4 h incubation, collect cells and distribute to 1.5 mL tubes or microwell plates for immunofluorescent staining.

2. Centrifuge cell suspension at 300 × *g*, 4 °C for 5 min. Cautiously remove supernatant without disrupting the cell pellet and resuspend cells with ice-cold PBS.
3. For each condition, prepare live/dead cell staining dye (propidium iodide, Zombie Aqua™, etc.) using ice-cold staining medium in accordance with manufacture instructions. Incubate the cell suspension for 15 min at 4 °C.
4. Wash cells with ice-cold PBS and centrifuge at 300 × *g* for 5 min at 4 °C.
5. For each condition, prepare 2 μL of anti-mouse CD16/32 antibody into 98 μL of ice-cold staining medium and incubate the cell suspension for 15 min at 4 °C (*see* **Note 6**).
6. Wash cells with ice-cold PBS and centrifuge at 300 × *g* for 5 min at 4 °C. Carefully discard supernatant without disrupting the cell pellet.
7. Resuspend the cell pellet with 100 μL of staining medium containing fluorochrome-conjugated monoclonal antibodies directed against the CD1d, CD5, and CD19 surface molecules. The quantity of each mAbs must be calculated following manufacturer's instructions. Moreover, distinguishable fluorochrome must be chosen for the three mAbs. Incubate at 4 °C in the dark for 30 min.

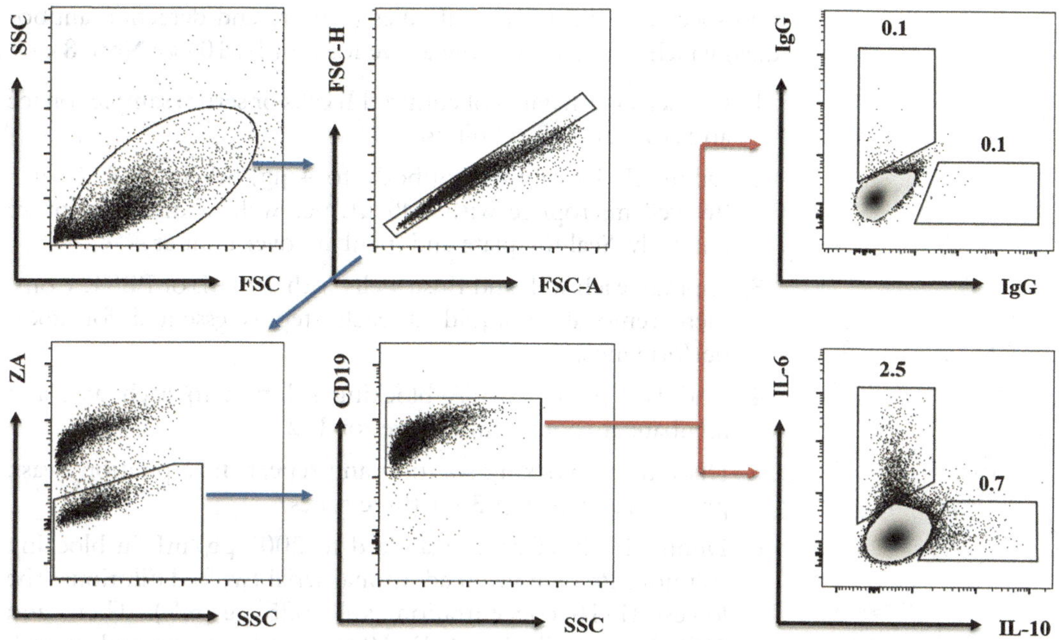

Fig. 3 Intracellular staining of IL-10-producing B cells analyzed by flow cytometry. B cells were stimulated with PMA, ionomycin, and monensin for 4 h and stained for the detection of IL-10- and IL-6-producing B cells by flow cytometric analysis. The gating strategy requires a first step in which cells are gated based on the size and granularity using FSC and SSC (upper left) to exclude debris, and then on FSC-A versus FSC-H (upper middle) for getting singlets. The Zombie Aqua (ZA) dye (bottom left) was used to discriminate between viable and dead cells, while CD19 staining (bottom middle) allows the gating on B cells only. Staining with specific isotype controls (upper right) was necessary to set the gates for CD19$^+$IL-6$^+$ and CD19$^+$IL-10$^+$ cells (bottom right)

8. Wash cell suspension twice with ice-cold PBS, centrifuge by 300 × *g* for 5 min at 4 °C.
9. Discard the supernatant, resuspend cells with 100 μL of fixation buffer by repeat pipetting, and incubate at 4 °C for 20 min.
10. Wash cell suspensions with 400 μL of permeabilization buffer and centrifuge for 5 min at 300 × *g* and at 4 °C.
11. Thoroughly resuspend cells in 50 μL of permeabilization buffer containing fluorochrome-conjugated anti-mouse IL-10 mAb or isotype control Ab (*see* **Note** 7). Antibody quantity must be calculated following manufacturer's instructions Incubate at 4 °C for 30 min in the dark.
12. Wash cells two times with permeabilization buffer (500 μL/wash) and resuspend in FACS buffer prior to flow cytometric analysis (*see* Fig. 3).

3.4 Detection of Secreted IL-10 by ELISA

The following described method allows the measurement of IL-10 levels in B-cell culture supernatants or in serum samples. IL-10 levels are detected with an ELISA bioassay, which is based on the usage of two specific monoclonal antibodies (capture and detection antibodies) which can recognize the active form of IL-10 (*see* **Note 8**).

1. Collect supernatants of cultured B cells or serum samples on ice and store at −80 °C till use.
2. Dilute IL-10 capture antibody to 4 μg/mL in PBS. Coat a 96-well microplate with 100 μL per well of diluted capture antibody. Seal the plate and incubate overnight at 4 °C.
3. Aspirate each well and rinse wells with 200 μL of PBST. Complete removal of liquid at each step is essential for good performance.
4. Add 100 μL of ELISA blocking solution to each well and incubate at room temperature for 1–2 h.
5. Discard the blocking solution and repeat the aspiration/wash procedure as in **step 3** for three times.
6. Dilute IL-10 reference standard to 2000 pg/mL in blocking solution. Prepare seven additional serial twofold dilutions (the lowest IL-10 concentration is 15.625 pg/mL). Then, add 100 μL per well of each IL-10 standard dilution and of each sample in analysis. All samples and IL-10 standard dilutions should be prepared and tested in triplicate.
7. Seal with a new adhesive strip and incubate at room temperature for 2 h.
8. Repeat the aspiration/wash procedure as in **step 3** for three times.
9. Dilute IL-10 detection antibody to 300 ng/mL in blocking solution. Add 100 μL of diluted detection antibody to each well. Seal with a new adhesive strip and incubate 2 h at room temperature.
10. Repeat the aspiration/wash procedure as in **step 3** for three times.
11. Dilute peroxidase-conjugated streptavidin to the concentration of 500 ng/mL. Add 100 μL of diluted peroxidase-conjugated streptavidin to each well, seal the plate with new adhesive strip, and incubate at room temperature for 20 min. Avoid placing the plate in direct light.
12. Repeat the aspiration/wash procedure as in **step 3** for four times.
13. Add 100 μL of TMB, the chromogenic substrate for peroxidase detection, to each well. Incubate at room temperature for 20 min. Avoid placing the plate in direct light.
14. Add 50 μL of ELISA stop solution to each well, and gently tap the plate to ensure thorough mixing.
15. Measure the optical density of each well immediately by using a microplate reader at 450 nm wavelength.

3.5 Measuring of IL-10 Secreting B Cells by ELISPOT Assay

The basic ELISPOT protocol is designed to quantify the number of cells within a specific population secreting a given cytokine or chemokine. To accomplish this goal, viable cells of interest are cultured in a microtiter plate which is coated with a high concentration of high-affinity anti-cytokine antibody. The cytokines secreted by the cells are immediately bound by the coated antibody lying below each cell. The following protocol describes the determination of IL-10 secreted by B cells. Similar to ELISA, the specific pair of anti-IL-10 antibodies is applied to form the enzyme-link immune complex (*see* **Note 8**).

1. Coat the microtiter plate with 100 μL of 10 μg/mL anti-IL-10 capture antibody in sterile PBS. Seal the plate with adhesive strip and incubate overnight at 4 °C.
2. Aspirate each well and wash with 200 μL of sterile PBST.
3. Add 100 μL of R10 medium as blocking solution and incubate at 37 °C for 2 h.
4. Discard the supernatant and repeat the aspiration/wash procedure as in **step 2** for three times.
5. FACS sorted $CD19^{+}CD1d^{hi}CD5^{+}$ and $CD19^{+}CD1d^{low}CD5^{-}$ cells are seeded into separated wells of the microtiter plate. Typically, the cells are serially diluted additional two- to four-fold starting from 10^4 to 10^6 cells per well to ensure that at least one dilution yields a quantifiable number of ELISPOTs. Each dilution should be studied in triplicate or quadruplicate to ensure consistency and generate a statistically valid result.
6. Incubate the microtiter plate in a humidified 37 °C, 5% CO_2 incubator. Initial optimization experiments should evaluate incubation periods of 6, 12, and 24 h.
7. Repeat the aspirate/wash procedure for three times as in **step 2**.
8. Add 100 μL of biotinylated anti-IL-10 detection antibody (2 μg/mL) into each well and incubate overnight at 4 °C or 2 h at room temperature.
9. Repeat the aspirate/wash procedure for three times as in **step 2**.
10. Dilute alkaline phosphatase-conjugated streptavidin with blocking solution to the concentration of 2 μg/mL. Add 100 μL of diluted streptavidin-alkaline phosphatase to each well, seal the plate with new adhesive strip, and incubate at room temperature for 60 min. Avoid placing the plate in direct light.
11. Add 100 μL of BCIP/NBT solution, the chromogenic substrate for alkaline phosphatase detection to each well and incubate in the dark at room temperature for 20 min until bluish/purple spots develop.

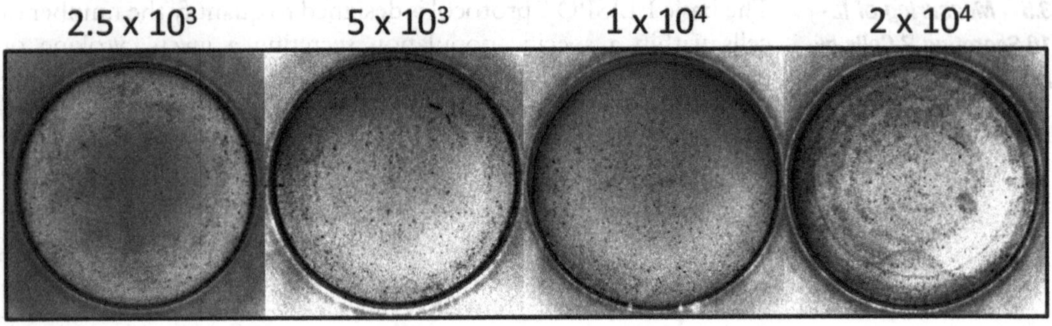

Fig. 4 Representative results of ELISPOT assay. IL-10-producing $CD19^{+}CD1d^{hi}CD5^{+}$ B cells were detected by ELISPOT assay. Serial diluted seedings of 2.5×10^3, 5×10^3, 1×10^4, and 2×10^4 cells per well are shown

12. Repeat the aspirate/wash for three times as in **step 2**.
13. Spots can be quantified using a 10× to 30× dissecting microscope or using a specific ELISPOT reader (*see* Fig. 4).

3.6 IL-10 Detection by Immunofluorescence Microscopy

This protocol is applicable to identify IL-10-producing B cells in situ. For example, IL-10-secreting B cells in frozen sections of spleen, draining lymph nodes and tissues can be observed by microscopy after immunofluorescence counterstains.

1. Frozen sections of lymphoid organs and tissues can be prepared after decalcification, embedded in OCT, and serial sections (5–10 μm) are prepared under cryostat. Slides can be stored at −80 °C till analysis.
2. Place frozen sections in a humidified chamber and maintain at room temperature for 10 min to warm up slides.
3. Fix slides in 4% paraformaldehyde in PBS for 15 min at room temperature.
4. Wash slides by gently rinsing with PBS for three times.
5. Permeabilize slides with 0.25% Triton X-100 in PBS for 10 min at room temperature (*see* **Note 9**).
6. Wash slides as in **step 4**.
7. Block slides with the incubation of 1% BSA in PBST for 30 min (*see* **Note 10**).
8. Wash slides as in **step 4**.
9. Prepare antibodies mixture of fluorochrome-conjugated anti-CD19 and anti-IL-10 antibodies in 98 μL of 1% BSA in PBST in a humidified chamber. The quantity of each antibody must be calculated following manufacturer's instructions. Incubate for 2 h at room temperature or overnight at 4 °C. Alternatively, primary antibodies (e.g., rabbit anti-mouse IL-10 or biotinylated anti-mouse IL-10) can be used.
10. Wash slides as in **step 4**.

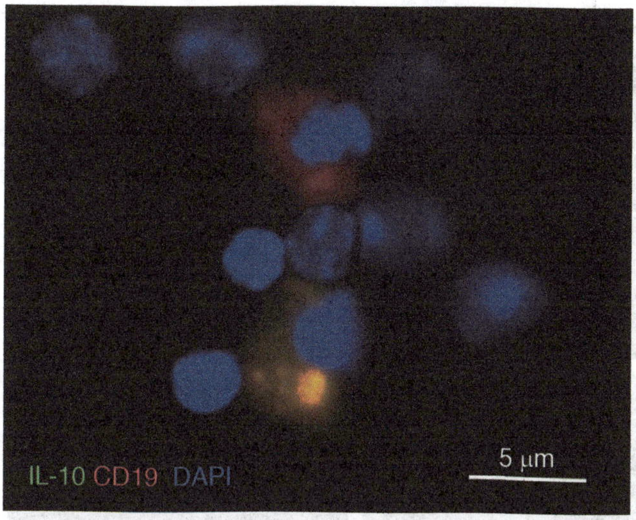

Fig. 5 Visualization of IL-10^+ B cells. For confocal microscopic analysis of IL-10^+ B cells, frozen sections of murine spleen were fixed and stained with DAPI (blue), anti-IL-10 (green), and anti-CD19 (red) antibodies (bar = 5 µm)

11. (Optional) If the antibodies used in **step 9** are not fluorochrome-conjugated, prepare the mixture of secondary antibodies which are raised in different species (multiple fluorescent dyes) against primary antibodies to avoid cross-reaction.
12. Wash slides as in **step 4**. Avoid placing the slides in direct light.
13. Coverslip with aqueous mounting medium containing DAPI.
14. Acquire images in a standard immunofluorescence microscope or a confocal microscope, using the filters/laser corresponding to each color (*see* Fig. 5).

3.7 Immunofluorescence Microscopy for the Detection of the Anatomical Distribution of CD19 + CD1dhiCD5+ B Cells In Situ

It has been reported that adoptive transfer cell therapy serves as a novel and promising strategy in treating various pathologies including cancer and autoimmune diseases [25, 26]. To determine the functional in vivo interactions between regulatory and effector immune cell subsets, we present a protocol which is applicable for visualizing the anatomical distribution of adoptively transferred $CD19^+CD1d^{hi}CD5^+$ B cells in the spleen.

1. Wash FACS sorted $CD19^+CD1d^{hi}CD5^+$ B cells twice with PBS at room temperature and centrifuge at 300 × *g* for 5 min.
2. Resuspend the cell pellet with 1 mL of PBS and label $CD19^+CD1d^{hi}CD5^+$ B cells with a fluorescence cell-tracking dye (e.g., the red fluorescence cell-tracking dye seminaphtharhodafluor, SNARF-1) in the dark for 10 min at 37 °C.

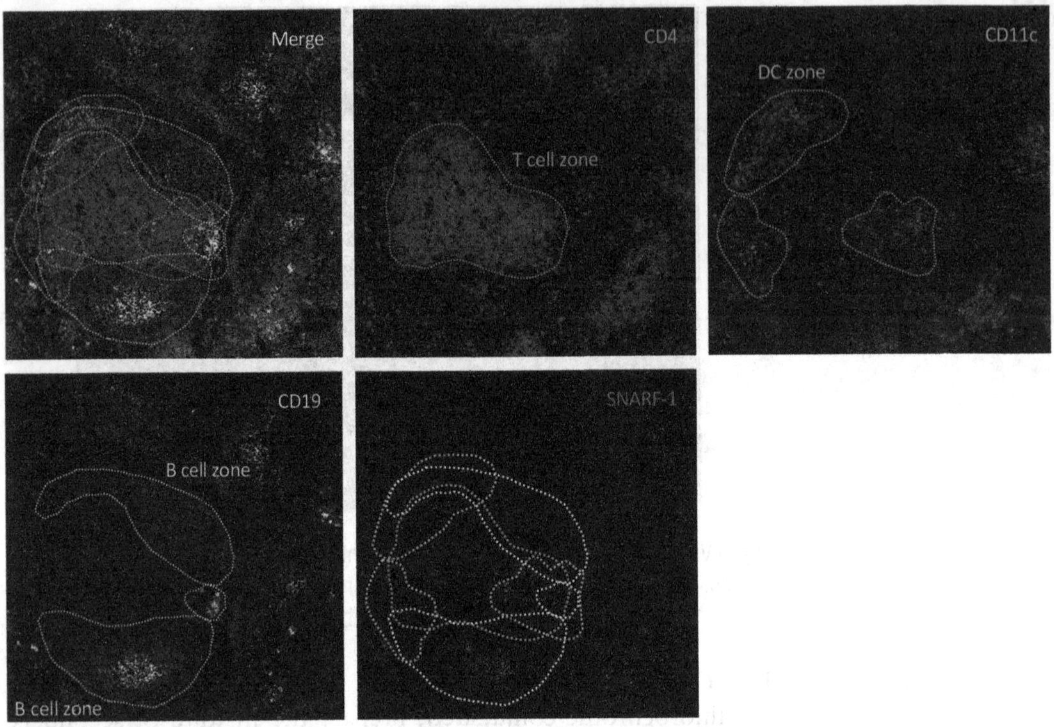

Fig. 6 Visualization of CD19$^+$CD1d^{hi}CD5$^+$ B-cell distribution in the spleen. FACS sorted CD19$^+$CD1d^{hi}CD5$^+$ B cells were labeled with the red fluorescence cell-tracking dye seminaphtharhodafluor (SNARF-1) and intravenously transferred into naïve recipient mice. The spleen was collected 24 h post-transfer, and sections from this tissue were stained with anti-CD19 (yellow), anti-CD4 (blue), and anti-CD11c (green) antibodies (bar = 100 μm). The merged panel shows that transferred CD19$^+$CD1d^{hi}CD5$^+$ B cells (red) can be detected in the T-cell zone, suggesting their potential interactions with CD4$^+$ T cells

3. Wash cells twice with 10 mL of R10 medium and centrifuge at 300 × *g* for 5 min at room temperature.
4. Resuspend the cell pellet with ice-old PBS and intravenously inject 5 × 10^5 cells in 200 μL PBS per mouse into the tail vein.
5. Sacrifice mice using a euthanasia agent 24 h post-adoptive transfer. Surgically remove spleens for frozen section preparation as described in Subheading 3.6.
6. In order to determine the anatomical distribution of transferred cells, stain splenic sections with fluorochrome-conjugated anti-CD11c, anti-CD19, and anti-CD4 antibodies as described in Subheading 3.6 (*see* **Note 11**).
7. Wash slides as described in Subheading 3.6 and cover with aqueous mounting medium containing DAPI.
8. Acquire tile-scan images in a standard immunofluorescence microscope or a confocal microscope, using the filters/laser corresponding to each color (*see* Fig. 6). As the borders of

$CD19^+$ B-cell zone, $CD4^+$ T-cell zone and $CD11c^+$ dendritic cell zone in the single follicle are indicated by the fluorescence staining, SNARF-1-labeled $CD19^+CD1d^{hi}CD5^+$ B cells can be detected mainly in the $CD4^+$ T-cell zone and B-cell zone.

4 Notes

1. Quantitative PCR instruments are commercially available and used for amplifying and detecting DNA. Based on the thermal cycler and fluorimeter, DNA can be probed with fluorescence dyes (e.g., SYBR Green) and amplified for detection.
2. A phenol and guanidine isothiocyanate-based solution such as TRIzol® (Invitrogen), or an equivalent from other suppliers, can be used for RNA extraction. Moreover, reliable RNA extraction kits are commercially available and produce good-quality RNA for downstream applications such as sequencing and qPCR.
3. Many different suppliers provide pairs of antibodies of sufficient quality to be used in these techniques.
4. All procedures for RNA extraction must be performed in RNase-free conditions. Use sterile tips, tubes, and solutions.
5. The analysis of the melting point curve indicates the presence and identity of single-nucleotide polymorphisms. A single peak represents a single PCR product and testifies the specificity of primers.
6. CD16 and CD32 are also known as FcγIII and FCγII, respectively, and bind to epitopes located in the constant region domain of IgG. In the mouse system, the purified anti-CD16/CD32 antibody directly blocks FcγII/III receptors from non-specific binding with fluorochrome-conjugated antibodies.
7. Contextually to IL-10 staining, the production of other cytokines can be followed by intracellular cytokine staining. Figure 3 shows the co-staining of $CD19^+IL\text{-}10^+$ and $CD19^+IL\text{-}6^+$ cells.
8. In the ELISA and ELISPOT assays, the capture and detection antibodies bind to IL-10, forming a sandwich-like complex.
9. Triton X-100 is a strong detergent that improves the penetration of the antibody. Alternative permeabilization reagents can be used, such as 100 μM digitonin or 0.5% saponin.
10. Alternative blocking solutions can be used, such as 1% gelatin or 10% serum from the species from which the secondary antibody was generated.

11. Particular attention must be given to the choice of the fluorochromes conjugated to the anti-CD19, -CD4, and -CD11c antibodies, which indicate the borders of B-cell zones, $CD4^+$ T-cell zones, and dendritic cell zones, respectively. Indeed, the excitation of fluorochromes should be distinct from the fluorescence of the cell-tracking dye used to stain $CD19^+CD1d^{hi}CD5^+$ cells.

Acknowledgments

This work was supported by grants from the National Natural Science Foundation of China (No. 82071817 and 91842304), Chongqing International Institute for Immunology (2020YJC10), Hong Kong Research Grants Council (27111820 and 17149716) and Hong Kong Croucher Foundation (260960116).

References

1. Shlomchik MJ, Craft JE, Mamula MJ (2001) From T to B and back again: positive feedback in systemic autoimmune disease. Nat Rev Immunol 1:147–153
2. Harris DP, Haynes L, Sayles PC, Duso DK, Eaton SM, Lepak NM, Johnson LL, Swain SL, Lund FE (2000) Reciprocal regulation of polarized cytokine production by effector B and T cells. Nat Immunol 1:475–482
3. Mauri C, Bosma A (2012) Immune regulatory function of B cells. Annu Rev Immunol 30:221–241
4. Barr TA, Shen P, Brown S, Lampropoulou V, Roch T, Lawrie S, Fan B, O'Connor RA, Anderton SM, Bar-Or A, Fillatreau S, Gray D (2012) B cell depletion therapy ameliorates autoimmune disease through ablation of IL-6-producing B cells. J Exp Med 209:1001–1010
5. Bermejo DA, Jackson SW, Gorosito-Serran M, Acosta-Rodriguez EV, Amezcua-Vesely MC, Sather BD, Singh AK, Khim S, Mucci J, Liggitt D, Campetella O, Oukka M, Gruppi A, Rawlings DJ (2013) Trypanosoma cruzi trans-sialidase initiates a program independent of the transcription factors RORgammat and Ahr that leads to IL-17 production by activated B cells. Nat Immunol 14:514–522
6. Fillatreau S, Sweenie CH, McGeachy MJ, Gray D, Anderton SM (2002) B cells regulate autoimmunity by provision of IL-10. Nat Immunol 3:944–950
7. Matsushita T, Yanaba K, Bouaziz JD, Fujimoto M, Tedder TF (2008) Regulatory B cells inhibit EAE initiation in mice while other B cells promote disease progression. J Clin Invest 118:3420–3430
8. Mizoguchi A, Mizoguchi E, Takedatsu H, Blumberg RS, Bhan AK (2002) Chronic intestinal inflammatory condition generates IL-10-producing regulatory B cell subset characterized by CD1d upregulation. Immunity 16:219–230
9. Yanaba K, Bouaziz JD, Haas KM, Poe JC, Fujimoto M, Tedder TF (2008) A regulatory B cell subset with a unique CD1dhiCD5+ phenotype controls T cell-dependent inflammatory responses. Immunity 28:639–650
10. Evans JG, Chavez-Rueda KA, Eddaoudi A, Meyer-Bahlburg A, Rawlings DJ, Ehrenstein MR, Mauri C (2007) Novel suppressive function of transitional 2 B cells in experimental arthritis. J Immunol 178:7868–7878
11. Blair PA, Norena LY, Flores-Borja F, Rawlings DJ, Isenberg DA, Ehrenstein MR, Mauri C (2010) CD19(+)CD24(hi)CD38(hi) B cells exhibit regulatory capacity in healthy individuals but are functionally impaired in systemic lupus erythematosus patients. Immunity 32:129–140
12. Kessel A, Haj T, Peri R, Snir A, Melamed D, Sabo E, Toubi E (2012) Human CD19(+) CD25(high) B regulatory cells suppress proliferation of CD4(+) T cells and enhance Foxp3

and CTLA-4 expression in T-regulatory cells. Autoimmun Rev 11:670–677

13. Kalampokis I, Yoshizaki A, Tedder TF (2013) IL-10-producing regulatory B cells (B10 cells) in autoimmune disease. Arthritis Res Ther 15 (Suppl 1):S1
14. Yang M, Rui K, Wang S, Lu L (2013) Regulatory B cells in autoimmune diseases. Cell Mol Immunol 10:122–132
15. Mauri C, Jury EC (2010) Could the expression of CD86 and FcgammaRIIB on B cells be functionally related and involved in driving rheumatoid arthritis? Arthritis Res Ther 12:133
16. Schioppa T, Moore R, Thompson RG, Rosser EC, Kulbe H, Nedospasov S, Mauri C, Coussens LM, Balkwill FR (2011) B regulatory cells and the tumor-promoting actions of TNF-alpha during squamous carcinogenesis. Proc Natl Acad Sci U S A 108:10662–10667
17. Le Huu D, Matsushita T, Jin G, Hamaguchi Y, Hasegawa M, Takehara K, Tedder TF, Fujimoto M (2013) Donor-derived regulatory B cells are important for suppression of murine sclerodermatous chronic graft-versus-host disease. Blood 121:3274–3283
18. Yanaba K, Yoshizaki A, Asano Y, Kadono T, Tedder TF, Sato S (2011) IL-10-producing regulatory B10 cells inhibit intestinal injury in a mouse model. Am J Pathol 178:735–743
19. Tedder TF, Matsushita T (2010) Regulatory B cells that produce IL-10: a breath of fresh air in allergic airway disease. J Allergy Clin Immunol 125:1125–1127
20. Yang M, Sun L, Wang S, Ko KH, Xu H, Zheng BJ, Cao X, Lu L (2010) Novel function of B cell-activating factor in the induction of IL-10-producing regulatory B cells. J Immunol 184:3321–3325
21. Yang M, Deng J, Liu Y, Ko KH, Wang X, Jiao Z, Wang S, Hua Z, Sun L, Srivastava G, Lau CS, Cao X, Lu L (2012) IL-10-producing regulatory B10 cells ameliorate collagen-induced arthritis via suppressing Th17 cell generation. Am J Pathol 180:2375–2385
22. Lin X, Wang X, Xiao F, Ma K, Liu L, Wang X, Xu D, Wang F, Shi X, Liu D, Zhao Y, Lu L (2019) IL-10-producing regulatory B cells restrain the T follicular helper cell response in primary Sjogren's syndrome. Cell Mol Immunol 16:921–931
23. Yoshizaki A, Miyagaki T, DiLillo DJ, Matsushita T, Horikawa M, Kountikov EI, Spolski R, Poe JC, Leonard WJ, Tedder TF (2012) Regulatory B cells control T-cell autoimmunity through IL-21-dependent cognate interactions. Nature 491:264–268
24. Livak KJ, Schmittgen TD (2001) Analysis of relative gene expression data using real-time quantitative PCR and the 2(−Delta Delta C (T)) method. Methods 25:402–408
25. Christoffersson G, von Herrath M (2019) Regulatory immune mechanisms beyond regulatory T cells. Trends Immunol 40:482–491
26. Romano M, Fanelli G, Albany CJ, Giganti G, Lombardi G (2019) Past, present, and future of regulatory T cell therapy in transplantation and autoimmunity. Front Immunol 10:43

Chapter 7

Detection and Quantification of Transforming Growth Factor-β1 Produced by Murine B Cells: Pros and Cons of Different Techniques

Yoshiyuki Mishima, Akihiko Oka, and Shunji Ishihara

Abstract

Transforming growth factor (TGF)-β1 is one of the regulatory cytokines produced by B cells and has a pivotal role in intestinal homeostasis. TGF-β1 can determine the fate of naive T cells, such as differentiation, proliferation, and apoptosis, which are relevant to the pathogenesis of autoimmunity, infection, inflammation, allergy, and cancer. Here, we describe detailed methods for detection and quantification of TGF-β1 secreted by B cells using ELISA, flow cytometry, and real-time PCR.

Key words TGF-β, Regulatory B cells, LAP, Intracellular staining

1 Introduction

Regulatory B cells (Bregs) have protective roles in inflammatory, autoimmune, allergic, and infectious diseases [1–4]. Bregs suppress an excessive immune reaction, and also prevent disease onset or decrease disease activity by producing the anti-inflammatory cytokines interleukin (IL)-10, transforming growth factor (TGF)-β1, and IL-35 [4, 5]. We and others have reported the importance of bacterial-stimulated Bregs in inflammatory bowel diseases (IBD) [6–8], while the absence of B cells or IL-10-secretion by B cells has been shown to result in deterioration of mucosal inflammation in murine experimental T-cell-mediated colitis [7, 8]. In humans, B-cell depletion by anti-CD20 antibodies is considered to be potentially associated with development and worsening of IBD [9, 10]. Moreover, Bregs have also been shown to contribute to carcinogenesis [1, 11]. Bregs reduce anti-tumor effects by stimulating regulatory T cells (Tregs) [1], and suppressing activated B cells and natural killer cells, which have cytotoxic responses toward tumors [12, 13]. Together, these findings indicate that Bregs are key immune cells in physiological conditions as well as in a variety of

Francesca Mion and Silvia Tonon (eds.), *Regulatory B Cells: Methods and Protocols*, Methods in Molecular Biology, vol. 2270, https://doi.org/10.1007/978-1-0716-1237-8_7,

refractory diseases. Investigation of IL-10 secreted by B cells has mainly been conducted in Bregs studies [14, 15], though B-cell-produced TGF-β1 is also known to play important roles in T-cell immunity, mucosal homeostasis, and tumorigenesis [1, 16–18].

TGF-β1, the main isoform of the TGF-β family, is predominantly secreted by hematopoietic cells, including a certain subpopulation of Tregs, Bregs, macrophages, dendritic cells, megakaryocytes, endothelial cells, chondrocytes, and platelets, and was shown to have pleiotropic effects on a variety of biological processes, such as inflammation, immune reactions, fibrosis, tissue regeneration/remodeling, and carcinogenesis [19, 20]. In the context of immune disorders, TGF-β1 appears to be protective, as it develops and maintains Foxp3$^+$ Tregs, and inhibits proliferation and differentiation of effector T cells [21, 22]. However, when in the presence of another inflammatory cytokine, TGF-β1 can promote Th17 response, which is potentially pathogenic in some types of inflammatory disorders [23]. Thus, it is considered that the function of TGF-β1 may depend on disease phenotype, timing, and other modifications.

TGF-β is initially synthesized as pro-TGF-β, then processed in the Golgi apparatus by a furin-like peptidase, which separates the mature C-terminal pro-region from the N-terminal latency-associated peptide (LAP). LAP combines with the bioactive C-terminal region to form a small latent TGF-β complex, which is further linked to the latent-TGF-β-binding protein (LTBP) to become a large latent TGF-β complex. This large complex is then deposited into the extracellular matrix and becomes extracellularly dissociated when activated by further multi-factorial regulatory factors, such as proteases, integrins, pH, temperature, and reactive oxygen species [19, 20, 24]. Finally, released free active TGF-β binds with its receptor and then functions.

Using a mouse model of autoimmune encephalomyelitis, B-cell-specific TGF-β1-deficient mice were shown to develop severe neural inflammation [17]. Also, neutralization of TGF-β1 in LPS-stimulated B cells has been found to decrease the level of IgA class switching [25, 26]. Those results indicate that TGF-β1 is an important immune mediator for facilitating the regulatory function of B cells in physiological and immune disorders. However, there are few studies of TGF-β1 in B cells as compared with IL-10, possibly due to technical issues and difficulties, or complicated measurement methods. While it is obvious that quantification of the active form alone secreted by B cells is required in order to elucidate its function, B cells produce relatively low levels of pro- and active-TGF-β under physiological conditions [27], with "total" (latent + active form) TGF-β alternatively measured in B-cell studies. Regarding this point, PCR, ELISA, ELISPOT, intracellular staining, and immunohistochemistry have been used to detect and/or quantify the various forms of TGF-β [24], each of which features pleiotropic pros and cons. For example, TGF-β mRNA levels do not always correlate with the amount of secreted protein due to multi-factorial modifications after gene upregulation. Resting human B cells express a relatively high level of TGF-β1 mRNA but secrete low amounts of TGF-β1 protein. Upon stimulation with LPS or an anti-IgM antibody, B cells produce relatively high amounts of TGF-β1 protein with little alteration of TGF-β1 mRNA [28]. Those findings suggest that post-transcriptional/translational regulation of TGF-β1 has effects on protein levels. Other indirect methods for investigating TGF-β1 activity include measurement of LAP, examination of cell lines that express luciferase under the control of a TGF-β responsive promoter, immunohistochemical assays of phosphorylated-Smad, and experiments with TGF-β^{GFP} mice [29–31], though the effectiveness of those techniques remains to be verified.

There is increasing demand for effective methods to investigate B-cell-specific TGF-β1 in a variety of diseases. We previously reported basic techniques for measuring TGF-β produced by B cells [24]. In the present chapter, those contents are updated, and detailed instructions for detection and quantification of B-cell-derived TGF-β using PCR, ELISA, and flow cytometry are provided.

2 Materials

2.1 B-Cell Isolation

1. Specific pathogen-free raised C57BL/6 or BALB/c mice.
2. Red blood cell lysing buffer: 150 mM ammonium chloride, 10 mM potassium bicarbonate, and 0.1 mM ethylenediamine-tetraacetic acid (EDTA).
3. 70 μm cell strainer.
4. Immunomagnetic separation system for B-cell isolation (*see* **Note 1**).
5. MACS buffer: 0.5% bovine serum albumin (BSA) and 2 mM EDTA in phosphate-buffered saline (PBS). Degas before use and keep cold (2–8 °C).

2.2 B Cell Culture

1. Complete culture medium: RPMI 1640 containing 10% heat-inactivated fetal bovine serum (FBS) (*see* **Note 2**), 100 U/mL penicillin/streptomycin, 1 mM sodium pyruvate, and 50 μM 2-mercaptoethanol (β-ME).
2. Activation components: lipopolysaccharide from *E. coli K12* (LPS, stock 1 mg/mL) and CpG oligonucleotide 1826 (CpG-ODN, stock 500 μM).
3. Cytokine stimulation cocktail: phorbol 12-myristate 13-acetate (PMA, stock solution: 2.5 mg/mL in DMSO at −80 °C),

Table 1
Conjugated antibodies for TGF-β1 detection by flow cytometry

Target	Conjugate	Clone
CD19	BV605	6D5
B220	Pacific blue	RA3-6B2
CD45	Pacific Orange	30-F11
TGF-β1	AF488	IC240G
LAP (option)	PE	Tw7-16B4
CD1d (option)	PerCP-cy™5.5	1B1
CD5 (option)	PerCP	53–7.3

ionomycin (stock solution: 2.5 mg/mL in DMSO at −80 °C), and a protein transport inhibitor (e.g., GolgiStop, monensin).

4. Aqueous, nontoxic tissue storage reagent that rapidly permeates tissues to stabilize and protect cellular RNA such as RNA-later solution.

2.3 Flow Cytometry

1. Antibodies for extracellular and intracellular staining (*see* Table 1).
2. Dye for the discrimination of viable from nonviable cells in multicolor flow cytometric applications (e.g., LIVE/DEAD® Fixable Near-IR Dead Cell Stain Kit).
3. Fc block reagent: anti-CD16/CD32 antibody.
4. Staining buffer: 2% FBS in PBS (*see* **Note 3**).
5. Fixation/permeabilization solution and permeabilization buffer for intracellular staining.
6. Flow cytometer instrument and software.

2.4 Elisa

1. Mouse TGF-β1 ELISA kit.
2. 1 N HCl.
3. 1.2 N NaOH, 0.5 M HEPES in water.
4. Wash buffer: 0.05% tween-20 in PBS.
5. Stop solution: 2 M H_2SO_4.
6. Microplate reader.

2.5 Real-Time PCR

1. RNA isolation kit.
2. 70% ethanol and RNase-free water (*see* **Note 4**).
3. cDNA Synthesis Kit with a range from 3 pg to 3 μg.
4. SYBR® Green PCR Master Mix.

5. Primers: *Tgfb1*; 5'-TGCTTCAGCTCCACAGAGAA-3′, 5'-TACTGTGTGTCCAGGCTCCA-3′, and *Gapdh*; 5'-ACCCAGAAGACTCTGGATGG-3′, 5'-GGTCCTCAGTGTAGCCCAAG-3′.
6. Thermal cycler.
7. Real-time PCR detection system.

3 Methods

3.1 B-Cell Isolation

1. Euthanize mice and collect the spleen and mesenteric lymph nodes (MLNs).
2. Prepare single cell suspensions from these organs. Crush MLNs with the plunger of a syringe through a 70-μm cell strainer into MACS buffer. Spleens are mechanically dissociated, and red blood cells are lysed in 5 mL red blood cell lysing buffer for 10 min.
3. Wash the cells twice with MACS buffer and determine the cell number of cell suspensions. Centrifuge for 5 min at 300 × *g* (*see* **Note 5**).
4. Resuspend cell pellets in 35 μL MACS buffer per 10^7 cells and proceed to B cells isolation following the instructions provided by the manufacturer of the employed B cell isolation kit (*see* **Notes 6** and **7**).
5. Once the isolated B-cell population is obtained, check purity and viability by flow cytometry. The expected percentage of the $CD19^+$ fraction is greater than 97%, while cell viability is greater than 90% according to eosin Y-exclusion test (*see* **Note 8**).

3.2 B-Cell Culture

1. Plate 1×10^6 isolated B cells in 200 μL of complete culture medium in a 96-well plate for 48 h (37 °C, 5% CO_2). Culture B cells in the presence of 100–200 ng/mL LPS, 0.1–1 nM CpG-DNA, or without stimuli.
2. For intracellular cytokine staining, add 100 ng/mL PMA, 1 μg/mL ionomycin, and a protein transport inhibitor (follow manufacturer's instructions for the concentration) into medium during the last 4 h of the culture period.
3. Following cell culture, collect supernatants for measurements of TGF-β by ELISA (*see* **Note 9**). Cells will be used for flow cytometry or PCR assays. For RNA assays, harvested cells should be immediately stored in RNAlater stabilization solution.

3.3 Detection of TGF-β1 by Flow Cytometry

Flow cytometry is useful for detecting cell-specific TGF-β1 production. Results obtained using this method are reliant on cell number, antibody concentration, and incubation temperature/time. Therefore, it is important to apply the same culture conditions and staining procedures/settings to all samples for reliable and reproducible results.

1. Wash cultured B cells three times in cold staining buffer.
2. Incubate samples 15 min at 4 °C with Fc block reagent diluted in 50 μL staining buffer according to manufacturer's instructions.
3. Incubate samples 20 min at 4 °C with a dye for the discrimination of viable from nonviable cells in multicolor flow cytometric applications and with antibodies directed against CD19, B220, and CD45 in a final volume of 100 μL (*see* **Note 10**). According to the scope of the experiment, other antibodies can optionally be added [14] (*see* Table 1 and **Note 11**).
4. Wash cells twice with staining buffer by centrifuging for 5 min at 300 × *g*.
5. Fix and permeabilize cells with the appropriate fixation and permeabilization solutions following the manufacturer's instructions of the specific kit (*see* **Note 12**).
6. Stain intracellular TGF-β1 for 45 min at 4 °C (*see* Table 1).
7. Wash cells twice with staining buffer and analyze samples on a flow cytometer. To assess the percentage of TGF-β1$^+$ B cells, use the following gating strategy. First, the dead cell population is excluded using the staining of the dye for the discrimination of viable from nonviable cells. Then, white blood cells are determined based on the positive expression of the CD45 marker, and B lymphocytes are identified as B220$^+$CD19$^+$ cells among the live CD45$^+$ population. Finally, TGF-β-producing B cells are quantified by comparing the stimulated samples with the control condition, and further characterized by the use of optional markers (*see* Table 1). The gating strategy and representative experimental results are shown in Fig. 1.

3.4 Measurement of TGF-β1 Level in Cell Supernatant

ELISA is a sensitive and reproducible technique. Under certain conditions, the amount of active TGF-β1 produced by B cells is quite low (non-detectable). Therefore, the latent TGF-β1 in such samples should be activated by acid, as described below, to increase detectability. Moreover, it is important to pay attention that the complete culture medium contains bovine TGF-β1, which can be detected by the use of a mouse-TGF-β ELISA kit (*see* **Notes 2** and **13**).

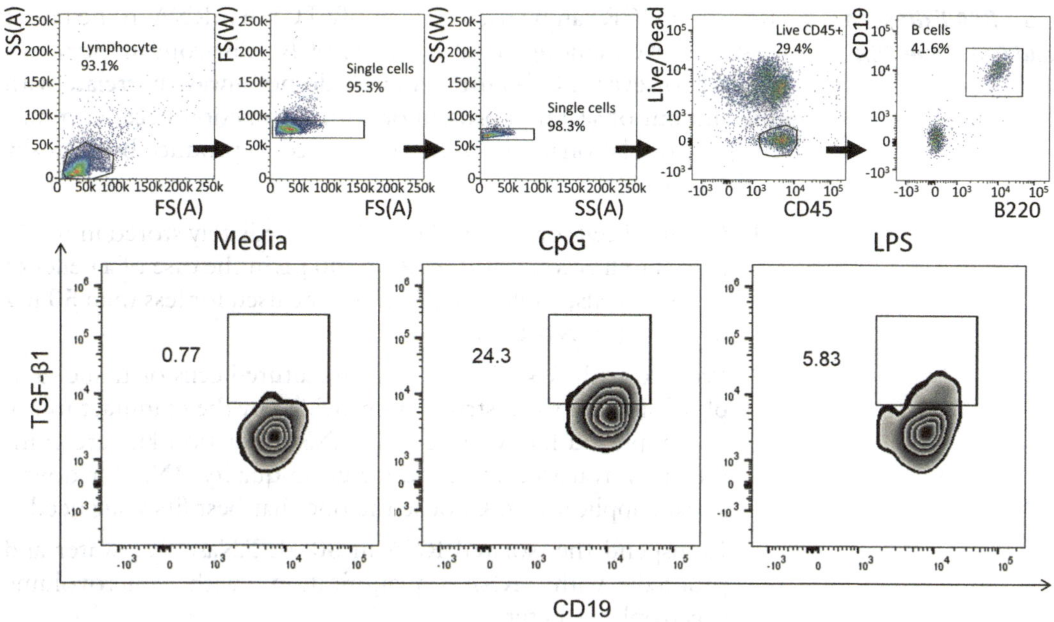

Fig. 1 Intracellular staining for the detection of TGF-β1 in TLR-activated B cells. Splenic B cells (5×10^5) were cultured in a final volume of 200 μL in a 96-well plate for 48 h with 200 ng/mL LPS, 1 nM CpG-DNA, or control medium. GolgiStop, 100 ng/mL PMA, and 1 μg/mL ionomycin were added during the final 4 h of the culture period. Cells were stained with a live/dead dye and with anti-CD19, -B220, -CD45, and -TGF-β1 antibodies, and then were subjected to flow cytometric analysis. A representative analysis of TGF-β1$^+$ cells among live CD45$^+$B220$^+$CD19$^+$-gated cells is shown

1. To activate latent TGF-β to an immunoreactive form, 100 μL supernatant from each sample is acidified and neutralized by incubation with 20 μL of 1 N HCl, followed by 20 μL of 1.2 N NaOH/0.5 M HEPES (*see* **Note 14**).
2. Transfer samples into wells of anti-TGF-β1-coated micro-titer strips and incubate for 2 h at room temperature (*see* **Note 15**).
3. Wash 3–5 times with wash buffer (*see* **Note 16**).
4. Add TGF-β1 conjugate to each well and incubate at room temperature for 2 h.
5. Wash five times, as in **step 3**.
6. Add substrate solution and incubate for 30 min at room temperature.
7. Add stop solution (*see* **Note 17**).
8. Determine the optical density of each well using a microplate reader set to 450 nm (with 570 nm used as the reference wavelength) and analyze with an appropriate software. A standard curve is generated to calculate the concentration of TGF-β in each set of samples.

3.5 RNA Extraction and Real-Time PCR

Real-time PCR can be used to quantify TGF-β mRNA in the target tissue or even among small numbers of B cells from in vitro cultures. However, TGF-β mRNA levels do not always correlate with the amount of secreted protein or with its function because multiple posttranslational processes are required to produce biologically active TGF-β.

1. Cultured cells or tissues should be immediately stored in RNAlater stabilization solution. Add 200 μL in the case of a pellet of cultured cells, while 500 μL should be used for less than 50 mg of tissue (*see* **Note 18**).
2. Proceed with RNA isolation from cultured cells or tissue samples following the instructions provided by the manufacturer of the employed kit. Very reliable RNA extraction kits are commercially available and produce good-quality RNA for downstream applications. Choose the one that best fits your needs.
3. Resuspend the isolated RNA in 30 μL RNase-free water and proceed with RNA quantification with microvolume spectrophotometer.
4. Once RNA has been quantified, proceed to cDNA synthesis from mRNA by using reverse transcription: prepare first-strand cDNA synthesis reaction in a microcentrifuge tube following the instructions provided by the manufacturer of the employed cDNA synthesis kit. Consider transcribing 100 ng of RNA.
5. Set the thermocycler accordingly to the instructions of the cDNA synthesis kit. Usually, the recycling protocol is made of an initial incubation step of 5 min at 25 °C for primer annealing, followed by the cDNA synthesis step at 42 °C for 15 min and a final step of 5 min at 95 °C to terminate the cDNA synthesis reaction. Once the reaction is ended, place samples on ice for immediate use for PCR. For long-term storage, store reaction samples at −30 °C.
6. Prepare real-time PCR reagents. Mix 12.5 μL SYBR® Green PCR Master Mix, 1 μL of 10 nM forward and reverse primers of TGF-β1 or GAPDH, 2 μL of the template (no dilution), and 8.5 μL water in PCR reaction tubes.
7. Perform quantitative real-time PCR using the Real-Time PCR System with the following settings: 95 °C for 10 min, then 40 cycles of 95 °C for 15 sec plus 60 °C for 1 min. At the end, a melting curve should be set (*see* **Note 19**).
8. Normalize mRNA expression level of TGF-β1 to that of GAPDH using sequence detector software. Results of a representative experiment are shown in Fig. 2.

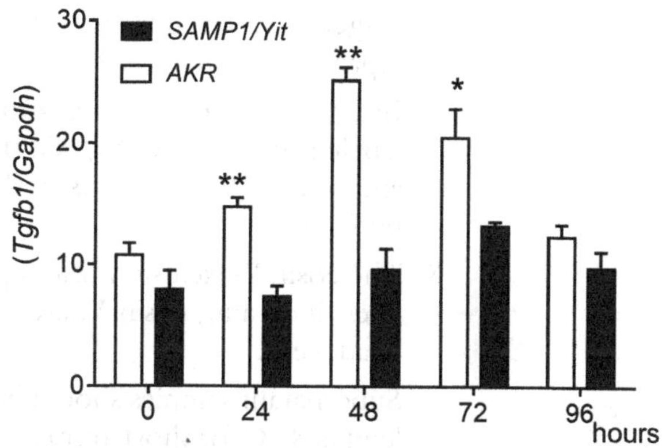

Fig. 2 *Tgfb1* gene expression in activated B cells from a murine model of Crohn's disease. 5×10^5 MLN B cells from 15-week-old SAMP1/Yit mice (murine model of Crohn's disease) and AKR/J mice (control) were cultured in a final volume of 200 μL in a 96-well plate for 24, 48, 72, or 96 h with 100 nM CpG-DNA or control medium. The level of *Tgfb1* in CpG-DNA-activated B cells was determined by real-time PCR and normalized according to Gapdh. Triplicate experiments were performed. Mean ± SD $*p < 0.05$, $**p < 0.01$

4 Notes

1. In our hands the MACS Miltenyi Biotec system (MACS buffer, LS columns, MACS separator and Pan B Cell Isolation Kit II, mouse) worked very well. We highly recommend using this upgraded system since it allows to obtain B cells with high purity and yield in a short time. Moreover, due to the negative selection isolation strategy employed by the Pan B Cell Isolation Kit II, isolated B cells do not contain any residual microbeads, which could influence downstream applications.
2. FBS contains abundant bovine TGF-β that can be detected by a mouse-TGF-β ELISA kit. Therefore, culture medium containing FBS should be acidified and neutralized before being tested through ELISA to quantify the basal level of bovine TGF-β. This value can be subtracted from any sample diluted in this medium after analysis to quantify murine TGF-β.
3. The use of FBS helps to prevent cell damage and increases the viability of B cells.
4. Depending on the RNA extraction kit used, these regents may or may not be included among the supplied reagents.
5. Use precooled solutions, work fast, and keep cells cold to improve viability and avoid nonspecific cell labeling during the isolation steps.
6. If using the Pan B Cell Isolation Kit II from Miltenyi Biotec, the protocol has an incubation step with an FcR blocking

reagent which improves the yield and purity for MACS separation.

7. In alternative to the biotin antibody cocktail, non-B cells can be labeled with anti-CD4, -CD11c, -CD49b, -CD90.2, –Gr-1, and -Ter-119 antibodies and immunomagnetically separated by B cells.
8. The eosin Y-exclusion test depends on the evidence that many dyes, including eosin Y, are excluded by viable, but not from dead, cells.
9. Supernatant samples should be immediately used for ELISA or kept at 4 °C for short-term or at −30 °C for long-term storage. A repeated freeze–thaw process may cause activation of latent TGF-β.
10. Titration of the optimal staining amount of the fluorescent antibody and optimization of staining time may be required, depending on the application.
11. The mix of anti-CD1d and anti-CD5 antibodies can be optionally used to identify a specific subset of regulatory B cells [14, 15]. The anti-LAP antibody can be also added for indirect measurement of TGF-β, as described in the introduction.
12. Cells can be stored overnight in fixation buffer at 4 °C.
13. FBS-free culture medium (TGF-β completely absent) can be used to measure the concentration of the active form of TGF-β by ELISA without the need of acid treatment. However, this culture condition significantly decreases B-cell viability, resulting in low or non-detectable TGF-β in supernatant.
14. Using representative samples, ensure that the test samples reach pH 3.0 or lower after the acidification step, and are between pH 7.2 and 7.6 after neutralization.
15. Incubating the ELISA samples at 4 °C overnight will increase assay sensitivity.
16. To increase the effectiveness of the washes, allow time for soaking (30–60 sec) during each wash step.
17. The volumes of samples and reagents and the incubation time may change depending on the specific TGF-β ELISA kit employed.
18. Ensure that the sample volume is within the capacity described in the datasheet of the employed RNA isolation kit. An excessive sample volume decreases purity and yield.
19. Melting curve analysis can provide information regarding the characteristics of the amplification products. Ensure that the PCR products show a single peak in this analysis. Multiple peaks indicate nonspecific products or contamination.

References

1. Cai X, Zhang L, Wei W (2019) Regulatory B cells in inflammatory diseases and tumor. Int Immunopharmacol 67:281–286
2. Mauri C, Menon M (2015) The expanding family of regulatory B cells. Int Immunol 27:479–486
3. Braza F, Chesne J, Castagnet S et al (2014) Regulatory functions of B cells in allergic diseases. Allergy 69:1454–1463
4. Rosser EC, Mauri C (2015) Regulatory B cells: origin, phenotype, and function. Immunity 42:607–612
5. Huang A, Cheng L, He M et al (2017) Interleukin-35 on B cell and T cell induction and regulation. J Inflamm (Lond) 14(16)
6. DeGruttola AK, Low D, Mizoguchi A, Mizoguchi E (2016) Current understanding of Dysbiosis in disease in human and animal models. Inflamm Bowel Dis 22:1137–1150
7. Mishima Y, Oka A, Liu B et al (2019) Microbiota maintain colonic homeostasis by activating TLR2/MyD88/PI3K signaling in IL-10-producing regulatory B cells. J Clin Invest 130:3702–3716
8. Mishima Y, Liu B, Hansen JJ, Sartor RB (2015) Resident bacteria-stimulated IL-10-secreting B cells ameliorate T cell-mediated colitis by inducing Tr-1 cells that require IL-27-signaling. Cell Mol Gastroenterol Hepatol 1:295–310
9. El Fassi D, Nielsen CH, Kjeldsen J et al (2008) Ulcerative colitis following B lymphocyte depletion with rituximab in a patient with graves' disease. Gut 57:714–715
10. Goetz M, Atreya R, Ghalibafian M et al (2007) Exacerbation of ulcerative colitis after rituximab salvage therapy. Inflamm Bowel Dis 13:1365–1368
11. Sarvaria A, Madrigal JA, Saudemont A (2017) B cell regulation in cancer and anti-tumor immunity. Cell Mol Immunol 14:662–674
12. Li Q, Teitz-Tennenbaum S, Donald EJ et al (2009) In vivo sensitized and in vitro activated B cells mediate tumor regression in cancer adoptive immunotherapy. J Immunol 183:3195–3203
13. Jones HP, Wang Y-C, Aldridge B, Weiss JM (2008) Lung and splenic B cells facilitate diverse effects on in vitro measures of antitumor immune responses. Cancer Immun 8(4)
14. Mizoguchi A, Mizoguchi E, Takedatsu H et al (2002) Chronic intestinal inflammatory condition generates IL-10-producing regulatory B cell subset characterized by CD1d upregulation. Immunity 16:219–230
15. Candando KM, Lykken JM, Tedder TF (2014) B10 cell regulation of health and disease. Immunol Rev 259:259–272
16. Dedobbeleer O, Stockis J, van der Woning B et al (2017) Cutting edge: active TGF-β1 released from GARP/TGF-β1 complexes on the surface of stimulated human B lymphocytes increases class-switch recombination and production of IgA. J Immunol 199:391–396
17. Bjarnadóttir K, Benkhoucha M, Merkler D et al (2016) B cell-derived transforming growth factor-β1 expression limits the induction phase of autoimmune neuroinflammation. Sci Rep 6:34594
18. Mishima Y, Ishihara S, Aziz MM et al (2010) Decreased production of interleukin-10 and transforming growth factor-β in toll-like receptor-activated intestinal B cells in SAMP1/Yit mice. Immunology 131:473–487
19. Batlle E, Massagué J (2019) Transforming growth factor-β signaling in immunity and Cancer. Immunity 50:924–940
20. Nolte M, Margadant C (2020) Controlling immunity and inflammation through integrin-dependent regulation of TGF-β. Trends Cell Biol 30:49–59
21. Iboshi Y, Nakamura K, Fukaura K et al (2017) Increased IL-17A/IL-17F expression ratio represents the key mucosal T helper/regulatory cell-related gene signature paralleling disease activity in ulcerative colitis. J Gastroenterol 52:315–326
22. Josefowicz SZ, Lu L-F, Rudensky AY (2012) Regulatory T cells: mechanisms of differentiation and function. Annu Rev Immunol 30:531–564
23. Omenetti S, Pizarro TT (2015) The Treg/Th17 Axis: a dynamic balance regulated by the gut microbiome. Front Immunol 6:639
24. Mishima Y, Ishihara S, Hansen JJ, Kinoshita Y (2014) TGF-β detection and measurement in murine B cells: pros and cons of the different techniques. Methods Mol Biol 1190:71–80
25. Zan H, Cerutti A, Dramitinos P et al (1998) CD40 engagement triggers switching to IgA1 and IgA2 in human B cells through induction of endogenous TGF-beta: evidence for TGF-beta but not IL-10-dependent direct S mu-->S alpha and sequential S mu-->S gamma, S gamma-->S alpha DNA recombination. J Immunol 161:5217–5225
26. Gros MJ, Naquet P, Guinamard RR (2008) Cell intrinsic TGF-beta 1 regulation of B cells. J Immunol 180:8153–8158

27. Wang M, Gu Z, Yang J et al (2019) Changes among TGF-β1+ Breg cells and helper T cell subsets in a murine model of allergic rhinitis with prolonged OVA challenge. Int Immunopharmacol 69:347–357
28. Kehrl JH, Roberts AB, Wakefield LM et al (1986) Transforming growth factor beta is an important immunomodulatory protein for human B lymphocytes. J Immunol 137:3855–3860
29. Areström I, Zuber B, Bengtsson T, Ahlborg N (2012) Measurement of human latent transforming growth factor-β1 using a latency associated protein-reactive ELISA. J Immunol Methods 379:23–29
30. Rogier E, Durrbach A, Abecassis L et al (2005) A novel biological assay to detect the active form of TGF-beta in urine to monitor renal allograft rejection. Kidney Int 68:1875–1883
31. Jurukovski V, Dabovic B, Todorovic V et al (2005) Methods for measuring TGF-b using antibodies, cells, and mice. Methods Mol Med 117:161–175

Chapter 8

IL-35 Detection in B Cells at the mRNA and Protein Level

Bhalchandra Mirlekar, Daniel Michaud, and Yuliya Pylayeva-Gupta

Abstract

Emerging research suggests that IL-35-producing regulatory B cells accumulate in patients and mouse models of pancreatic cancer, one of the most lethal cancers, characterized by late diagnosis, high mortality, and morbidity. Identification of IL-35-producing B cells can be challenging due to the heterodimeric nature of IL-35 and diversity of cell surface markers that define regulatory B-cell subsets across spectrum of diseases. In this chapter, we describe the methods for the isolation of splenic and tumor-infiltrating murine regulatory B cells and subsequent detection of IL-35 by RT-qPCR and intracellular staining, as well as detection of circulating IL-35 by ELISA. We also describe methods for the detection of IL-35-producing human B cells by flow cytometry, RT-qPCR, and immunofluorescence in the context of pancreatic cancer. This chapter should facilitate the study of regulatory IL-35$^+$ B cells in cancer, autoimmunity, and inflammation.

Key words Pancreatic cancer, Regulatory B cells, IL-35, Intracellular cytokine staining, Immunosuppression

1 Introduction

B cells are well-known to positively regulate adaptive immune response through antibody production and to enhance T-cell activation and function through MHC class II antigen presentation. However, more recently, the existence of different subsets of B cells with immune regulatory functions was demonstrated by many studies in both humans and mice. Some subsets of regulatory B (Breg) cells have the capacity to maintain immune tolerance and suppress auto-inflammatory immune responses through the production of regulatory cytokines such as IL-10 and/or IL-35 [1–6]. Bregs may play a role in autoimmune and infectious diseases and cancer by suppression of effector T-cell responses through the release of the anti-inflammatory cytokine IL-35. IL-35 is a member of the IL-12 cytokine family, first described over 20 years ago

Authors Bhalchandra Mirlekar and Daniel Michaud contributed equally to this work.

Francesca Mion and Silvia Tonon (eds.), *Regulatory B Cells: Methods and Protocols*, Methods in Molecular Biology, vol. 2270, https://doi.org/10.1007/978-1-0716-1237-8_8,

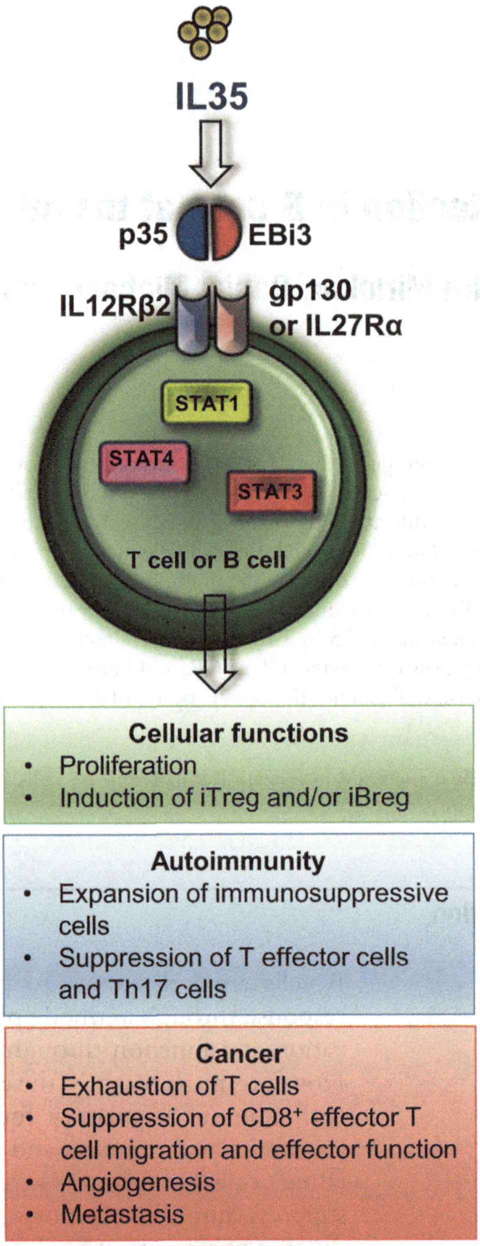

Fig. 1 Proposed functional role for IL35 in immune cells

[7]. As shown in Fig. 1, this heterodimeric cytokine is comprised of one p35 subunit, which is also a subunit of IL-12, and one EBi3 subunit, which is also a subunit of IL-27 [7, 8]. A decrease in IL-35-mediated regulatory function, although not essential for normal survival, leads to exacerbated autoimmunity and reduced cancer growth [4, 5, 9–13]. IL-35 has now been reported to be expressed in several distinct cell types such as Treg, B cells, dendritic

cells, myeloid cells and, more recently, tumor cells [6, 14], and the expression of IL-35, at least in immune cells, appears to be induced by inflammatory cues, such as Toll-like receptor ligands [15].

Pertinent to this chapter, IL-35-secreting Breg cells were shown to exhibit immune suppressive properties, as seen in infection and autoimmune models such as experimental autoimmune encephalomyelitis (EAE), where the presence of IL-35^+ Breg cells was associated with suppressed inflammatory immune populations and reduced disease severity [5]. Though past research has mostly focused on the role of Breg cells in the field of autoimmunity, a new wave of research provided novel insights into the potential involvement of Breg cells in anti-tumor immunity and cancer progression and, in this regard, IL-35^+ Breg cells have been reported to promote tumor growth in pancreatic cancer [10, 16–18]. In this light, there is an acute need to better characterize tumor-associated mouse and human Breg cells in order to improve our current understanding of the role of these cells in the cancer context. The difficulty in identifying IL-35^+ Breg cells may lie in the strategies that were employed up to date, such as the use of only mRNA and/or staining for single subunits of IL-35. IL-35 expression is one of the functional indicators of Breg cells, thus intracellular identification of IL-35 and the functional ex vivo and in vivo potential of IL-35^+ Breg cells both in the human and mouse setting should serve as a vital standard in studies of tumor-associated IL-35^+ Breg cells.

We recently identified a subset of Breg cells that facilitate the growth of pancreatic ductal adenocarcinoma (PDAC) in C57Bl/6 J mice, and we observed that tumor-associated Breg cells produce the immune suppressive cytokines IL-10 and IL-35 [10, 12, 13]. Additionally, we determined that PDAC growth is uniquely influenced by B-cell-secreted IL-35, and tumor-associated IL-35^+ Breg cells promote tumor growth by inhibiting cytotoxic $CD8^+IFN\text{-}\gamma^+$ T cells [13]. In human PDAC, $CD19^+CD24^{hi}CD38^{hi}$ lymphocytes emerged as the B-cell subset that produces the highest amount of IL-35 among peripheral blood mononuclear cells (PBMCs) [13, 19, 20]. In this chapter, we describe protocols that allow the identification of tumor-promoting IL-35-producing Breg cells in both mouse and human. Specifically, we provide methods needed for the isolation and characterization of pancreatic tumor-infiltrating $CD19^+CD21^{hi}CD5^+CD1d^{hi}$ Breg cells from mice and $CD19^+CD24^{hi}CD38^{hi}$ immature B cells from human peripheral blood. Furthermore, we provide the detailed protocols for the isolation, culture, and in vitro stimulation of pancreatic tumor-associated Breg cells. Finally, we describe how to identify IL-35-producing Breg cells by RT-qPCR, intracellular staining, immunofluorescence, as well as the detection of circulating IL-35 by ELISA.

2 Materials

2.1 Equipment

1. Scientific balances.
2. 15 mL and 50 mL conical tubes.
3. 5 mL syringes.
4. 40 μm and 70 μm cell strainers.
5. 5 mL polystyrene test tubes for fluorescence-activated cell sorting (FACS tubes).
6. Sterile 5 mL, 10 mL, and 25 mL serological pipettes.
7. Sterile 96-well tissue culture plates.
8. Cryovials.
9. Hemocytometer or automated cell counter.
10. Refrigerated centrifuge.
11. Biosafety cabinet/hood for tissue culture.
12. Vortexer.
13. 37 °C cell culture incubator with 5% CO_2.
14. Wet ice to maintain cells and reagents at ~4 °C.
15. Dissecting forceps and scissors.
16. Hemostat.
17. Razor blades.
18. Petri dishes.
19. Spectrophotometer for RNA quantification (e.g., Nanodrop).

2.2 General Buffers and Reagents

1. 70% (v/v) ethanol in sterile water.
2. 1× phosphate-buffered saline (PBS): 137 mM NaCl, 2.7 mM KCl, 10 mM Na_2HPO_4, 1.8 mM KH_2PO_4. pH 7.4.
3. 0.4% Trypan blue solution for cell counting.
4. Magnetic activated cell sorting (MACS) buffer: 0.5% bovine serum albumin (BSA) and 2 mM EDTA in 1× PBS. Filter-sterilize using a 0.2-μm vacuum filter and store at 4 °C.
5. Freezing medium: 90% heat-inactivated fetal calf serum (FCS) and 10% dimethyl sulfoxide (DMSO).
6. DMEM medium.
7. RPMI 1640 medium.
8. 0.05% Trypsin-EDTA.

2.3 Induction of the PDAC Mouse Model and Isolation of Splenic and Pancreatic Tumor-Infiltrating B Cells

1. C57Bl/6 J mice (7- to 8-week-old, either gender).
2. Murine pancreatic ductal adenocarcinoma cell line. Originally derived from primary pancreatic tumor of *Kras*$^{G12D/+}$; *TP53*$^{R172H/+}$;*p48*$^{Cre/+}$ (KPC) mice, and orthotopically injected into pancreas of syngeneic C57Bl/6 J mice [12, 21].
3. Matrigel (Corning).
4. Ketamine and xylazine for mouse surgical anesthesia.
5. Buprenorphine.
6. 5–0 Vicryl RAPIDE sutures (Ethicon).
7. 5–0 PROLENE sutures (Ethicon).
8. Red Blood Cell (RBC) lysis buffer: 155 mM NH_4Cl, 12 mM $NaHCO_3$, 0.1 mM EDTA.
9. Density gradient medium such as OptiPrep Density Gradient Medium (*see* **Note 1**).
10. Complete DMEM medium: 10% heat-inactivated FCS and 1× penicillin-streptomycin in DMEM.
11. Pancreatic tumor digestion buffer: 1.25 mg/mL collagenase IV, 1 mg/mL hyaluronidase, 0.1% trypsin inhibitor from soybean (STI), 1:10 DNase 1 (1 mg/mL stock) in DMEM.
12. Complete RPMI medium: 10% heat-inactivated FCS and 1× penicillin-streptomycin in RPMI 1640.
13. Anti-mouse CD45 microbeads and specific equipment (e.g., columns and magnets) for immunomagnetic separation.

2.4 Isolation of Human B Cells

1. Peripheral blood.
2. Yellow top glass blood collection tubes with Acid Citrate Dextrose (*see* **Note 2**).
3. Lymphoprep (*see* **Note 3**).
4. 0.9% NaCl solution.

2.5 In Vitro Culture of Murine and Human B Cells

1. B-cell culture medium: 10% heat-inactivated FCS, 0.01% penicillin-streptomycin, and 50 μM 2-mercaptoethanol in supplemented RPMI 1640 (with L-Glutamine and $NaHCO_3$). Filter-sterilize through 0.22 μm filter.
2. Agonistic anti-CD40 antibody (clone HM40–3).
3. Lipopolysaccharide (LPS, O111:B4).
4. Phorbol 12-myristate 13-acetate (PMA).
5. Ionomycin.

2.6 ELISA-Based Detection of IL-35

1. Purple top EDTA blood collection tubes.
2. Mouse IL-35 Heterodimer ELISA Kit (*see* **Note 4**).
3. ELISA plate reader.

Table 1
Primers for the detection of IL-35 by RT-qPCR

Mouse	Forward Primer (5′-3′)	Reverse Primer (5′-3′)
Il12a	catcgatgagctgatgcag	cagatagcccatcaccctgt
Ebi3	tgctcttcctgtcacttgcc	cgggataccgagaagcatg
Actb	ggctgtattcccctccatcg	ccagttggtaacaatgccatgt
Human		
IL12A	gatgagctgatgcaggcc	agtcctccacctcgttgtccgtga
EBI3	gcagacgccaacgtccac	ccagtcactcagttccccgt
HPRT	cctgctggattacatcaaagcactg	tccaacacttcgtggggtcct

4. Multichannel pipettor.
5. Wash bottle or automated microplate washer.
6. Adhesive plate sealers.

2.7 RT-qPCR Based Detection of IL-35

1. Micropipettors and tips.
2. Multichannel pipettor.
3. RNA extraction kit for low number of cells (*see* **Note 5**).
4. cDNA synthesis kit (*see* **Note 6**).
5. SYBR green master mix (*see* **Note 6**).
6. Primers for murine and human IL-35 (both the p35 and EBi3 subunits) and for the housekeeping genes β-Actin (*Actb*) and hypoxanthine guanine phosphoribosyl transferase (*HPRT*) (*see* Table 1).
7. RT-qPCR thermocycler and suitable plates.

2.8 Immunofluorescence

All the materials reported in this section are from Leica Biosystems. Although other platforms are commercially available, we recommend the Leica Bond-Rx system as it preserves tissue morphology quite well and allows for multiplex immunofluorescence, even in the case of primary antibodies derived from same species.

1. Leica Bond-Rx fully automated staining platform (Leica Biosystems).
2. Bond™ Dewax solution (Leica Biosystems).
3. Bond Wash solution (Leica Biosystems).
4. Bond-epitope retrieval solution 1, pH 6.0 (Leica Biosystems).
5. Bond-epitope retrieval solution 2, pH 9.0 (Leica Biosystems).
6. Bond peroxide blocking solution (Leica Biosystems).
7. Hoechst 33258.

Table 2
Antibodies for the detection of human IL-35 by immunofluorescence

Primary antibody	Clone
CD20	MJ1
CD8	4B11
CD4	4B12
EBi3	HPA046635
Cytokeratin (CK)	Zo622
IL-12a (p35)	HPA001886
Secondary antibody	
EnVision+ system- HRP Anti-mouse #K4001	N/A
ImmPRESS HRP Anti-rabbit polymer #MP-7401-15	N/A

8. ProLong Gold Antifade Mountant (Life Technologies).
9. Primary and secondary antibodies for immunofluorescence (*see* Table 2).

2.9 Flow Cytometry

1. FACS buffer: 2% heat-inactivated FCS and 0.05% sodium azide in 1× PBS.
2. Sorting buffer: 1% heat-inactivated FCS in 1× PBS. Filter-sterilize using a 0.2 μm filter.
3. Sort collection medium: 10% FBS and 1× penicillin/streptomycin in 1× RPMI.
4. Fluorescently conjugated antibodies for the detection of surface and intracellular molecules (*see* Table 3). Antibodies should be diluted in the appropriate buffer according to manufacturer's indications and/or to titration experiments.
5. Fixable cell viability reagent (*see* **Note** 7).
6. Brefeldin A.
7. Fixation/permeabilization solution and permeabilization buffer for intracellular cytokine staining. Use according to manufacturer's instructions.
8. Fc Block reagent: unconjugated anti-CD16/CD32 (clone 2.4G2) monoclonal antibody diluted in FACS buffer according to manufacturer's instructions.
9. Compensation beads.
10. Cell sorter with multiparameter cytometry capability.

Table 3
Antibodies for the detection of IL-35-producing B cells by flow cytometry

Target	Clone	Conjugate
Mouse		
CD45	30-F11	AF700
CD19	6D5	FITC
CD21	7E9	PerCP
CD5	53–7.3	PECy7
CD1d	1B1	BV421
IL-35 (p35)	27,537	PerCP
IL-35 (EBI3)	355,022	APC
Human		
CD19	HIB19	AF700
CD24	ML5	PerCP
CD38	HB-7	PE/Cy7
IL-35 (p35)	SNKY35	eFluor660
IL-35 (EBI3)	B032F6	PE

11. Flow cytometer with multiparameter cytometry capabilities for the acquisition of stained samples.
12. Flow cytometry software for data analysis.

3 Methods

3.1 Induction of Murine Pancreatic Tumors

Syngeneic mouse modeling of cancer allows for the study of the immune infiltrate into various tumor types. Orthotopic injection of tumor cells can recapitulate the tumor microenvironment in the hosts. Using a substrate matrix such as Matrigel better allows for the retention and growth of the cancer cells within the injection site by providing a strong and supportive scaffold. The aim of this section is to describe how to establish orthotopic pancreatic murine tumors from syngeneic pancreatic ductal adenocarcinoma (PDAC) cells.

1. Culture murine PDAC cells in complete DMEM medium. Wash adherent cells twice in 1× PBS and detach cells with 2 mL trypsin for 5 min at 37 °C. Centrifuge the suspended cells at 300 × *g* for 5 min, resuspend in ice-cold 1× PBS, and proceed to cell count.

2. Prepare tumor cell injection aliquots by mixing 25 μL of ice-cold PBS containing 75,000 PDAC cells with 25 μL of ice-cold Matrigel in a sterile 1.7 mL microcentrifuge tube. This is sufficient for the injection of one mouse. Always keep aliquots on ice prior to injection (*see* **Note 8**).
3. Anesthetize mice with an intraperitoneal injection of a 100 mg/kg ketamine/10 mg/kg xylazine cocktail.
4. Make a small incision with dissecting scissors into the left flank and gently externalize the pancreas with sterile dissecting forceps.
5. Inject a tumor cell suspension aliquot using a 28-gauge needle into the tail of the pancreas.
6. Close the wound by running 5–0 Vicryl RAPIDE sutures for the peritoneum and 5–0 PROLENE sutures for the skin with a hemostat.
7. Provide appropriate pain relief, such as by injecting 0.1 mg/kg buprenorphine subcutaneously.
8. Euthanize the mouse approximately 3 weeks post-injection and isolate the needed samples.

3.2 Isolation of Tumor-Infiltrating Lymphocytes

The isolation of tumor-infiltrating lymphocytes (TILs) is a useful approach to study anti-tumor immune responses. TILs can be isolated by density gradient centrifugation followed by enrichment of $CD45^+$ leukocytes by immunomagnetic separation. Below we describe the methods to dissociate fresh pancreatic tumors and generate a single-cell suspension.

3.2.1 Murine Pancreatic Tumors Harvest and Digestion

1. Collect the pancreatic tumor from tumor-bearing mice using sterile dissection equipment.
2. Place the isolated tumor in a 15-mL conical tube containing RPMI 1640 medium on ice to achieve maximum yield and viability of tumor-infiltrating immune cells (*see* **Note 9**).
3. Mince the isolated tumor samples into a homogenous mash using a sterile single edge razor blade in a sterile Petri dish containing 5 mL of pancreatic tumor digestion buffer (*see* **Note 10**).
4. Using a sterile 10 mL serological pipet, transfer the minced tumor homogenate and pancreatic tumor digestion buffer into a 15-mL sterile conical tube. Rinse the plate with an additional 2–3 mL of digestion buffer to collect remaining minced tissue (~7–8 mL total volume of digestion medium per tube).
5. Incubate the tissue-containing conical tubes at 37 °C in a water bath for 30 min while briefly vortexing the tubes after every 10 min.

6. After incubation, filter the digested tumor suspension by pouring through a 70-μm cell strainer into a new sterile 50 mL conical tube.
7. Rinse the strainer with 5 mL of FACS buffer and centrifuge the tube at 300 × *g* for 5 min at 4 °C.
8. After centrifugation, decant the supernatant and resuspend pellet vigorously using 5 mL of FACS buffer with a serological pipet. Centrifuge the tube at 300 × *g* for 5 min at 4 °C and decant the supernatant.
9. Lyse the red blood cells by resuspending the pellet in 5 mL of RBC lysis buffer and incubate at room temperature for 5 min. Add 25 mL of 1× PBS to the tube to quench lysis buffer and spin the tubes at 300 × *g* for 5 min at 4 °C.
10. Decant the supernatant and resuspend the cell pellet in 7 mL of RPMI 1640. Mix well with a sterile 10 mL serological pipet. Samples can be left on ice if needed at this step for a maximum of 30–40 min.

3.2.2 Isolation of Tumor-Infiltrating Immune Cells

1. In a new 15 mL conical tube, add 5 mL of density gradient medium and carefully layer the pancreatic tumor cell suspension by inverting the tube sideways and slowly dispensing the suspension. Avoid mixing layers and make sure no bubbles are present between the cell suspension and the density gradient medium.
2. Centrifuge the tubes for 30 min at 950 × *g* at room temperature. Reduce acceleration speed and shut off centrifuge brakes for this step to maintain layer separation.
3. After centrifugation, the mononuclear immune cells will form a distinct white band at the medium interface between the RPMI 1640 medium and the density gradient medium.
4. Remove cells from the interface using a sterile 1000 μL pipet tip without removing the upper RPMI 1640 layer. Transfer the cells into sterile 15 mL conical tubes containing 5 mL complete RPMI 1640 medium and mix gently.
5. Centrifuge at 300 × *g* for 5 min at 4 °C. Decant supernatant and wash again with 3 mL complete RPMI 1640 medium. Transfer the suspension to a sterile 5 mL polystyrene FACS tube. Spin at 300 × *g* for 5 min at 4 °C.
6. Decant the supernatant and resuspend the cell pellet in MACS buffer. Proceed with the isolation of tumor-infiltrating $CD45^+$ leukocytes using mouse CD45 microbeads and following manufacturer's instructions (*see* **Note 11**).
7. Wash the collected $CD45^+$ leukocytes with ice-cold PBS by centrifugation at 300 × *g* for 5 min at 4 °C and resuspend cells in 1 mL of FACS buffer. Proceed to cell staining for sorting of Breg cells (*see* Subheading 3.4.1).

3.3 Isolation of Splenocytes from Tumor-Bearing Mice

1. Dissect the spleen out of the tumor-bearing mouse using sterile forceps and scissors and place it into a 15-mL conical tube containing 5 mL of RPMI 1640 medium. Pour the spleen-containing tube over a 70-μm strainer placed on a sterile 50 mL conical tube.
2. Break up the spleen into a single-cell suspension by pressing with the rubber end of a sterile 5 mL syringe. Using 10 mL of RPMI 1640 medium with 10% FBS, rinse the strainer to force remaining cells through the strainer.
3. Centrifuge cell suspension at 300 × *g* for 5 min at 4 °C and decant the supernatant.
4. Resuspend the pellet in 5 mL of 1× RBC lysis buffer and incubate for 5 min at room temperature.
5. Stop the lysis reaction by adding 25 mL of 1× PBS into the same tube and centrifuge immediately at 300 × *g* for 5 min at 4 °C. Decant the supernatant.
6. Resuspend the cell pellet in 1 mL of MACS buffer and perform a cell count and viability analysis with trypan blue and a hemocytometer. Suspension may need to be diluted further with MACS buffer if sample concentration is very high.
7. Centrifuge cell suspension at 300 × *g* for 5 min at 4 °C and decant the supernatant.
8. Resuspend the cell pellet in an appropriate volume of MACS buffer so that the final cell concentration is 1 × 10^7 cells/mL. Freshly isolated mononuclear cells can be immediately used for downstream assays or frozen using freezing medium for future experiments (*see* **Note 12**).

3.4 Detection of Murine IL-35-Producing Breg Cells

B cells are generally known to positively regulate the immune response by producing antigen-specific antibodies and inducing $CD4^+$ T-cell activation. However, specific B-cell subsets, i.e., Breg cells, can also have an immunosuppressive function, indicating their critical role in controlling effector immune responses. In the context of cancer, the expansion of Breg cells likely depends on the specific tumor model or cancer cell line that is used in the experimental study. In this regard, particular attention should be paid to select the most appropriate model that will allow the study of this functional B-cell subtype. The aim of this section is the description of the methods and protocols required to isolate regulatory (Breg, $CD19^+CD21^{hi}CD5^+CD1d^{hi}$) and conventional (Bcon, $CD19^+CD21^{lo}CD5^-CD1d^-$) B cells from the tumors and spleens of pancreatic tumor-bearing mice.

3.4.1 Cell Staining for Sorting of Breg Cells

1. Adjust the concentration of splenocytes (*see* Subheading 3.3) or of tumor-infiltrating leukocytes (*see* Subheading 3.2.2) to 1 × 10^7 cells/mL in PBS in a sterile 5 mL FACS tube (*see* **Note 13**).

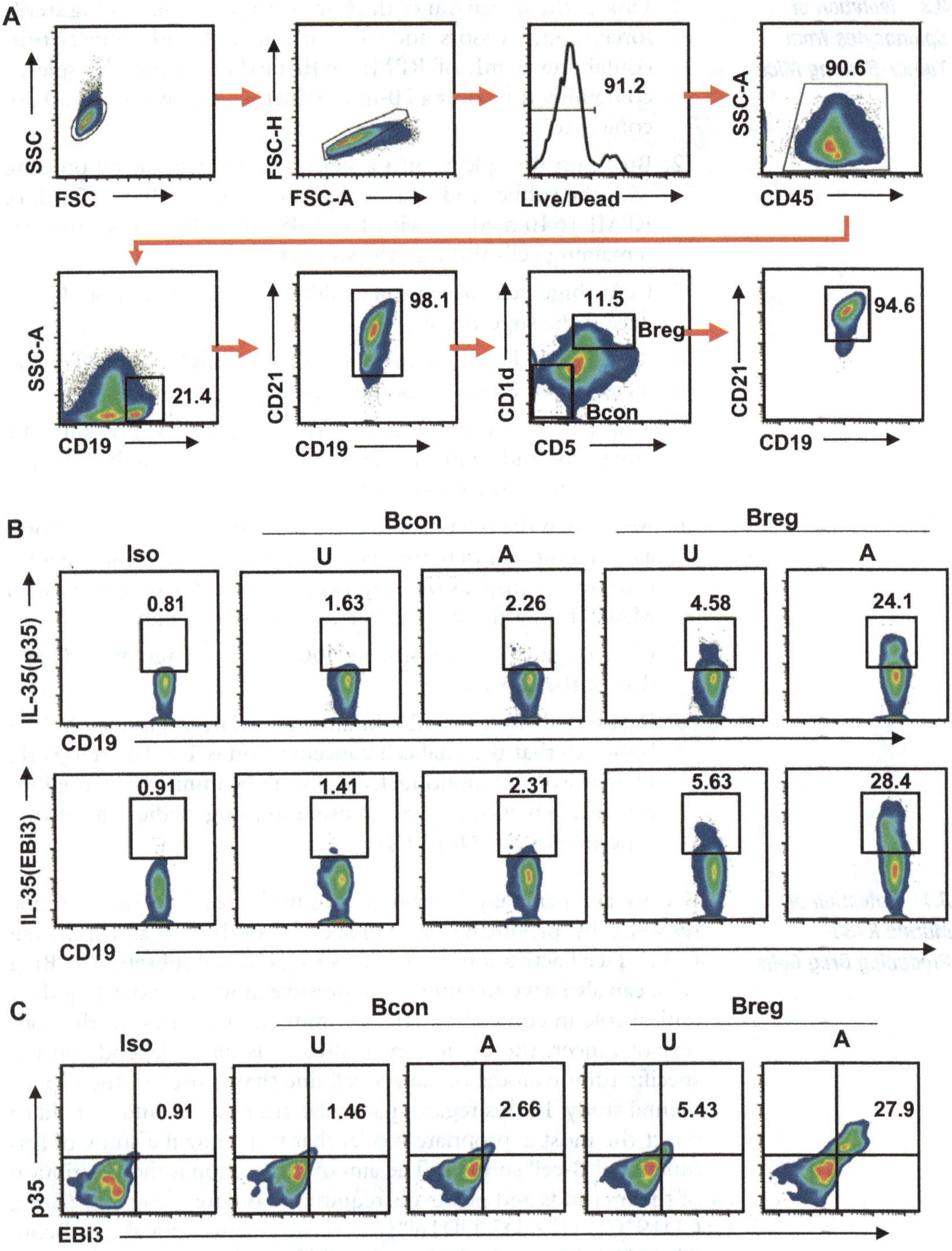

Fig. 2 Analysis of tumor-infiltrating regulatory and conventional murine B cells. Within the total tumor-infiltrating B-cell population, IL-35-producing suppressive Breg cells express the highest levels of CD21 and CD1d markers. (**a**) Intratumoral B cells were isolated by mechanical disruption followed by enzymatic digestion, density gradient, and magnetic separation. B cells were stained for cell surface CD45, CD19, CD21, CD5, and CD1d along with LIVE/DEAD Aqua viability dye. $CD19^{+}CD21^{hi}CD5^{+}CD1d^{hi}$ Breg and

2. To exclude dead cells during sorting, stain samples by adding the chosen fixable cell viability reagent, according to manufacturer's instructions. Incubate for 10 min at room temperature in the dark. Wash with 2 mL of PBS and centrifuge the cell suspension at 300 × *g* for 5 min at 4 °C. Decant supernatant.
3. Resuspend the cells in 1 mL of FACS buffer containing Fc Block reagent and incubate for 15 min on ice. Wash with 2 mL of PBS and centrifuge at 300 × *g* for 5 min at 4 °C. Discard the supernatant.
4. Resuspend the cell pellet in 1 mL of FACS buffer containing the anti-CD45, -CD19, -CD21, -CD5, and -CD1d antibodies (*see* Table 3) diluted in the mix as recommended by the manufacturer. Incubate for 20 min in the dark at 4 °C. Prepare single color compensation controls by using compensation beads according to manufacturer's protocol.
5. Wash the cells once with 2 mL of cell sorting buffer (*see* **Note 14**). Decant supernatant.
6. Resuspend cells in FACS buffer at a concentration of 1 × 10^7 cells/mL, which will ensure a sorting speed of approximately 18,000–20,000 events per second at the optimal pressure.
7. Proceed with the cell sorting of Breg and Bcon cells using the gating strategy described in Fig. 2a. Approximate yields of Breg cells are 3.0–4.7 × 10^6 and 5–6 x10^5 from mouse spleen and tumor, respectively.
8. Collect the sorted cells in 5 mL FACS tubes or 15 mL conical tubes containing 1 mL and 3 mL of complete RPMI medium, respectively (*see* **Note 15**).

3.4.2 In Vitro Culture and Stimulation of Sorted B Cells

1. Resuspend sorted Breg ($CD19^+CD21^{hi}CD1d^{hi}CD5^+$) and Bcon ($CD19^+CD21^{lo}CD1d^-CD5^-$) cells at the final concentration of 5 × 10^5 cells/mL in sterile pre-warmed B-cell culture medium containing 1 μg/mL anti-CD40 antibody and 2 μg/mL LPS or in B-cell culture medium alone as a control.
2. Culture B cells in a 96-well plate, at 100,000 cells/well, in a cell culture incubator at 37 °C with 5% CO_2 for 48 h. During the

Fig. 2 (continued) $CD19^+CD21^{lo}CD5^-CD1d^-$ Bcon cells were purified by FACS sorting. (**b**, **c**) $CD19^+CD21^{hi}CD5^+CD1d^{hi}$ Breg and $CD19^+CD21^{lo}CD5^-CD1d^-$ Bcon cells were left unstimulated (U) or activated (A) in the presence of anti-CD40 and LPS for 48 h. The PMA plus ionomycin cell stimulator cocktail and Brefeldin A were added during the last 5 h of culture. After 48 h, the cultured cells were fixed, permeabilized, and stained for detection of intracellular p35 and EBi3 by flow cytometry. The representative flow cytometry plots show the expression of p35 and EBi3 (**b**) as well as $CD19^+$ B cells double positive for p35 and EBi3 (**c**). The numbers in the quadrants represent the frequency of each population. The frequency of Breg and Bcon cells that express IL-35 increases significantly after B-cell stimulation through CD40 and TLR4 compared to unstimulated cells

final 5 h of culture, add 50 ng/mL PMA, 250 ng/mL Ionomycin, and 5 μg/mL Brefeldin A to the appropriate cell cultures to accumulate the induced cytokines and block their secretion.

3. At the end of the 48-h stimulation with LPS and anti-CD40 antibody, harvest the B cells and proceed with the downstream assays for the evaluation of IL-35 production.

3.5 Analysis and Quantification of IL-35 Production by B Cells

IL-35 is a heterodimeric cytokine made up of p35 and EBi3 subunits, mainly produced by Breg and CD4$^+$ regulatory T-cell types. B-cell-specific IL-35 is essential for pancreatic tumorigenesis by inhibiting CD8$^+$ T-cell effector functions and infiltration into the tumor microenvironment. Decreased frequency of IL-35-producing B cells correlates with smaller tumor size in murine models; therefore, it is important to detect and quantify IL-35 production. Here we describe how to analyze and quantify IL-35 production by B cells by flow cytometry, QPCR, and ELISA.

3.5.1 Intracellular Cytokine staining for the Detection of IL-35-Producing B Cells

1. Harvest the medium containing the stimulated B cells from the cell culture plate by pipet mixing (*see* Subheading 3.4.2) and dispense cells into a 5-mL FACS tube or 1.7 mL microcentrifuge tube. Centrifuge the cells at 300 × *g* for 5 min at 4 °C and carefully aspirate all the medium from the tube without touching the cell pellet. Resuspend the cells in PBS.
2. Repeat the wash procedure and then resuspend the cells in 100 μL PBS containing the chosen fixable cell viability reagent, diluted according to manufacturer's instructions.
3. Wash cells in 500 μL FACS buffer, centrifuge at 300 × *g* for 5 min at 4 °C and discard supernatant.
4. Resuspend the cells in FACS buffer containing Fc Block reagent for 10 min on ice. Centrifuge at 300 × *g* for 5 min at 4 °C and discard supernatant.
5. Resuspend the cells with 1 mL of cold FACS buffer and wash cells at 300 × *g* at 4 °C for 5 min and discard supernatant.
6. Add 100 μL of diluted anti-CD19 antibody in FACS buffer (*see* Table 3) and incubate for 20 min in the dark on ice. Wash cells twice with cold FACS buffer and centrifuge at 300 × *g* for 5 min at 4 °C.
7. Resuspend the cell pellet with 100 μL of fixation buffer and incubate for 20 minutes in the dark on ice. Centrifuge the cells at 500 × *g* for 5 min at 4 °C.
8. Resuspend the pellet with 1 mL of ice-cold 1× permeabilization buffer and wash the cells by centrifugation at 500 × *g* for 5 min at 4 °C. Remove the supernatant and repeat step twice.

9. Resuspend the cell pellet in 100 μL of ice-cold 1× permeabilization buffer containing either fluorochrome labeled at α-p35 and α-EBi3 antibodies (*see* Table 3) or their respective isotype control antibodies (*see* **Note 16**). Incubate cells for 60 min in the dark on ice.
10. Wash the cells twice with 1 mL of permeabilization buffer and twice with 1 mL of FACS buffer by centrifugation at 500 × *g* for 5 min at 4 °C and discard supernatant.
11. Resuspend cells in 350 μL of FACS buffer in a 5 mL FACS tube. Samples are ready to be acquired on a flow cytometer. Figure 2b, c show representative FACS plots for both unstimulated (U) and activated (A) Breg and Bcon cells.

3.5.2 Real-Time Quantitative PCR for the Detection of IL-35 Transcripts

1. Isolate RNA from sorted (*see* Subheading 3.4.1) or in vitro activated (*see* Subheading 3.4.2) murine Breg and Bcon cells by using a RNA extraction kit reliable for RNA purification also from very small numbers of cells. Follow manufacturer's instructions.
2. Quantify total isolated RNA using a spectrophotometer and proceed with reverse transcription (RT) of 1 μg RNA to cDNA by using an appropriate kit (*see* **Note 5**). Follow manufacturer's instructions for reaction setup.
3. Keep the reaction tubes on ice until you are ready to load them in the thermocycler. Load the reaction tubes into the thermal cycler and start the program. Table 4 summarizes the steps of the program adopted in our lab thermocycler.
4. Once the reverse transcription reaction is over, proceed with the qPCR reaction. Starting from the SYBR green master mix (*see* **Note 5**), prepare a reaction master mix for each primer set by adding all required components listed in Table 5, except for the cDNA template. Mix the reaction master mix thoroughly and dispense 8 μL into each PCR well of the PCR plate. Add 2 μL of the cDNA template to each well containing the reaction mix. Seal the plate with optically transparent film and briefly centrifuge the plate to remove air bubbles and to collect reaction mixture at the bottom of the well.

Table 4
cDNA Synthesis PCR Program

Parameter	Step 1: incubation	Step 2: extension	Step 3: termination	Step 4: hold
Temperature (°C)	25	37	85	4
Time (min)	10	120	5	∞

Table 5
SYBR reaction setup

Component	Concentration
SYBR green supermix (2×)	1× (5 μL)
Forward and reverse primer (10 uM each)	500 nM (1 μL each)
cDNA template	100 ng
Nuclease-free H_2O	Adjust to total reaction volume 10 μL

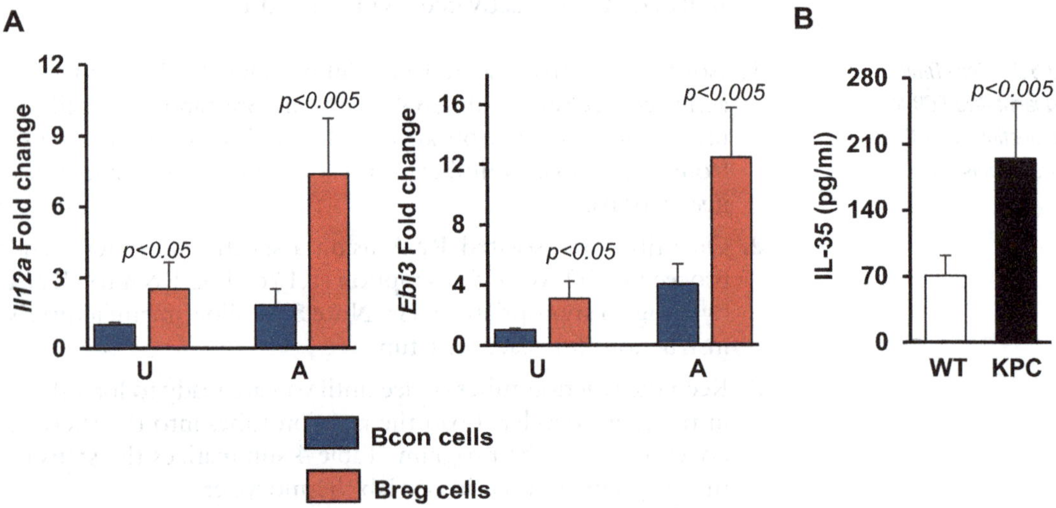

Fig. 3 Detection of IL-35 gene expression by qPCR and quantification of circulating IL-35 by ELISA. (**a**) Mouse pancreatic tumor-infiltrating Breg and Bcon cells were isolated by FACS. After stimulation, Breg and Bcon cells were processed for RNA isolation followed by cDNA synthesis and qPCR. Quantification of *Il12a* and *Ebi3* gene expression from activated (A) and unstimulated (U) Breg and Bcon cells is shown, with β-Actin used as endogenous control. (**b**) Circulating IL-35 levels were detected in serum samples of wild-type and pancreatic cancer-bearing mice by ELISA

5. Load the PCR plate into the RT-qPCR instrument and start the run. Figure 3a shows the fold change expression of the *Il12a* and *Ebi3* genes in unstimulated and activated mouse Breg and Bcon cells (*see* **Note 17**).

3.5.3 Detection of Circulating Murine IL-35 by ELISA

1. Collect mouse peripheral blood in EDTA blood collection tubes using animal protocol-approved methods.
2. Isolate the plasma from the blood by centrifuging tubes at 1000 × *g* for 10 min at 4 °C. Plasma can be immediately tested or can be stored at −80 °C until subsequent use. Keep plasma on ice if using immediately.

3. Determine circulating IL-35 quantity using a mouse IL-35 heterodimer ELISA kit, according to manufacturer's instructions. During the incubation steps of the assay, cover and seal the microtiter plate wells with adhesive plate sealers in order to reduce sample evaporation and avoid contamination.
4. Analyze the assay by reading the absorbance of each sample at 450 nm through an ELISA plate reader. Figure 3b shows the result of an experiment in which circulating IL-35 was detected in plasma samples of healthy and pancreatic tumor-bearing mice.

3.6 Identification and Detection of IL-35-Producing Human B Cells

3.6.1 Isolation of PBMCs from Human Peripheral Blood

1. Collect human whole blood samples into acid citrate dextrose-coated tubes. Dilute the blood by adding an equal volume of 0.9% NaCl.
2. Carefully layer 20 mL of diluted blood over 10 mL of Lymphoprep in a 50-mL centrifuge tube. Avoid the mixing of blood and Lymphoprep to maximize isolation yield of blood mononuclear cells (*see* **Note 18**).
3. Centrifuge the tube at 800 × *g* for 25 min at room temperature. For this step, the centrifuge acceleration and brake need to be turned off to maintain layer separation.
4. After centrifugation, the PBMCs form a distinct band at the sample/medium interface. The cells are best removed by using a 1000-μL pipet tip from the interface without removing the upper layer. Collect cell suspension into a sterile 15 mL conical tube.
5. Dilute the harvested fraction 1:1 with RPMI-1640 medium to reduce the density of the solution and pellet the cells by centrifugation at 300 × *g* for 5 min at room temperature.

3.6.2 Isolation and Activation of Human Breg Cells

1. Wash the isolated PBMCs two times with 1 mL of RPMI 1640 medium by centrifugation at 300 × *g* for 5 min at 4 °C. Transfer the PBMCs to sterile 5 mL FACS tubes.
2. Resuspend cells at a concentration of 1 × 10^7 cells/mL in FACS buffer. Incubate the cells for 20 min on ice and in the dark with fluorochrome-conjugated antibodies against CD19, CD24, and CD38 (*see* Table 3). In parallel, prepare single color compensation controls using compensation beads according to manufacturer's instructions.
3. Wash cells twice with 1 mL of FACS buffer and centrifuge at 300 × *g* for 5 min at 4 °C. Decant supernatant.
4. Resuspend the cells at a concentration of 1 × 10^7 cells/mL in FACS buffer and filter the samples through a 40-μm cell strainer before proceeding with sorting.

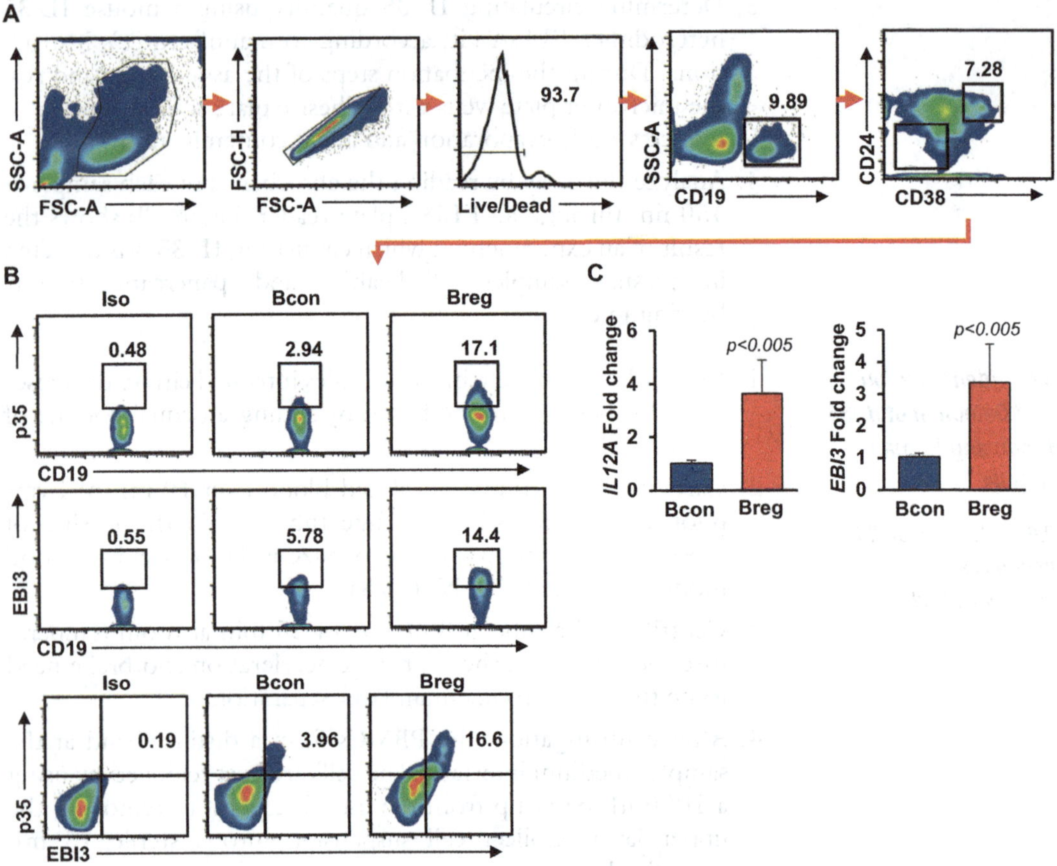

Fig. 4 Strategy for isolation of human Breg cells and quantification of IL-35 expression by intracellular flow cytometry and qPCR. (**a**) Gating strategy for the isolation of Breg cells from human PBMCs. PBMCs were isolated from blood samples of PDAC patients by Lymphoprep and stained with LIVE/DEAD Aqua viability dye and anti-CD19, anti-CD24 and anti-CD38 antibodies for FACS sorting. Representative flow cytometry plots show the gating strategy for the purification of Breg (immature B) and Bcon cells. (**b**) Representative flow cytometry plots for intracellular staining of single positive p35 and EBi3 cells as well as double positive p35 and EBi3 cells among the activated Breg and Bcon subsets isolated from PDAC patient PBMCs. Breg and Bcon cells were activated with 50 ng/mL PMA, 250 ng/mL Ionomycin, and 5 ug/mL Brefeldin A for 5 h. The numbers in the quadrants indicate the frequency of each population. (**c**) qPCR analysis for quantification of *Il12A* and *EBi3* gene expression from peripheral Breg and Bcon cells of pancreatic cancer patients

5. Sort the PBMCs. Use the differential expression of the CD19, CD24, and CD38 surface molecules to distinguish between immature B cells (Breg, $CD19^{+}CD24^{hi}CD38^{hi}$) and mature B cells (Bcon, $CD19^{+}CD24^{-}CD38^{-}$). Follow the gating strategy described in Fig. 4a to discriminate between immature and mature B cells.
6. Collect the sorted B-cell subsets in sterile 15 mL conical tubes containing 3 mL of RPMI medium. The approximate yield of immature B cells from 20 mL of human peripheral blood is 2×10^5–6×10^5.

7. Wash the sorted B-cell subsets twice with 5 mL of RPMI 1640 medium and centrifuge at 300 × *g* for 5 min at 4 °C.
8. Seed 100,000 B cells/well in a 96-well cell culture plate and stimulate the B-cell subsets by adding 50 ng/mL PMA, 250 ng/mL Ionomycin and 5 ug/mL Brefeldin A in 200 μL of B-cell culture medium. Culture for 5 h in an incubator at 37 °C, 5% CO_2.
9. After incubation, transfer media-containing cell suspension to sterile 5 mL FACS tubes and centrifuge the suspension at 300 × *g* for 5 min at 4 °C. Decant the supernatant and wash the cells once with 1 mL of 1× PBS.

3.6.3 Detection of IL-35-Expressing Human B Cells through Flow Cytometry

1. Stain the cells with 100 μL of PBS containing the chosen fixable cell viability reagent, diluted according to manufacturer's instructions. Incubate for 10 min at 4 °C in the dark. Centrifuge the B cells at 300 × *g* for 5 min at 4 °C and discard the supernatant.
2. Resuspend the cells with 1 mL of cold FACS buffer and centrifuge cells at 300 × *g* at 4 °C for 5 min.
3. Dilute the anti-CD19 antibody in FACS buffer (*see* Table 3), according to manufacturer's indications and/or to titration experiments. Add 100 μL of diluted antibody and incubate for 20 min in the dark on ice. Wash twice with ice-cold FACS buffer and centrifuge the cells at 300 × *g* for 5 min at 4 °C.
4. Resuspend the cell pellet with 100 μL of fixation buffer and incubate for 20 min in the dark on ice. Centrifuge the cells at 500 × *g* for 5 min at 4 °C.
5. Resuspend the pellet with 1 mL of ice-cold 1× permeabilization buffer and pellet the cells by centrifugation at 500 × *g* for 5 min at 4 °C. Remove the supernatant and repeat this step.
6. Resuspend the cell pellet in 100 μL of ice-cold permeabilization buffer containing either α-p35 and α-EBI3 fluorochrome labeled antibodies (*see* Table 3) or their respective isotype control antibodies. Incubate cells for 60 min in the dark on ice.
7. Centrifuge the cells at 500 × *g* for 5 min at 4 °C and discard supernatant. Wash the cells twice with 1 mL of permeabilization buffer and twice with 1 mL of FACS buffer.
8. Transfer the cells to FACS tubes, acquire the samples with a flow cytometer and analyze data using a flow cytometry analysis software. Representative FACS plots for IL-35-producing Breg and Bcon cells are shown in Fig. 4b.

3.6.4 Detection of IL-35 Expression by Immunofluorescence in Human Pancreatic cancer Lesions

1. Cut 6-μm-thick sections from Formalin-Fixed Paraffin-Embedded (FFPE) blocks containing human PDAC lesions.
2. Use the Leica Bond-Rx fully automated staining platform for triple immunofluorescence staining.
3. Dewax the slides using Bond™ Dewax solution and hydrate in Bond Wash solution. Retrieve the epitope for all targets using Bond-epitope retrieval solution 1 pH 6.0 or solution 2 pH 9.0 for 20 min followed by 10 min of endogenous peroxidase blocking using Bond peroxide blocking.
4. Apply primary and secondary antibodies (*see* Table 2) diluted in incubation buffer according to manufacturer's instructions (*see* **Note 19**).
5. Stained slides are counterstained with Hoechst 33258 for nucleic acid visualization and mounted with ProLong® Gold Antifade Mountant.

4 Notes

1. For the isolation of tumor-infiltrating lymphocytes from pancreatic tumors we find that Ficoll is a suitable alternative for OptiPrep. In the case in which the use of Ficoll is preferable, we recommend a protocol published by Tan and Lei [22].
2. We find that Acid Citrate Dextrose-coated tubes are suitable for the collection of peripheral blood because of the ability for long storage time (6–7 hours) at room temperature without significant decreases in cell viability. Alternatively, EDTA- or heparin-coated tubes can also be used.
3. We recommend Lymphoprep because it allows for maximal isolation of mononuclear cells from human blood samples. Indeed, we have also tested Ficoll and OptiPrep with human peripheral blood, but Lymphoprep gives a better yield.
4. We used the Mouse IL-35 Heterodimer ELISA Kit from BioLegend.
5. We recommend using the RNeasy Micro kit (Qiagen) or a similar kit for the isolation of RNA since it gives consistent RNA yields from very small number of cells, which may be the case for tumoral B cells. Kits with a low elution volume (<15 μL) will work better for this step.
6. We used Maxima First Strand cDNA Synthesis Kit (Thermo Fisher) for cDNA synthesis. This kit gives very high quality, single-stranded cDNA from 0.02 to 2 μg total RNA. Equivalent commercially available kits can be used for this purpose. Additionally, for RT-qPCR we routinely use SsoAdvanced™ Universal SYBR from BioRad.

7. We utilize LIVE/DEAD™ Aqua fluorescent reactive dye (Thermo Fisher) for defining viable cells but have also used 7-AAD and other viability dyes with this protocol. LIVE/DEAD Aqua works very well with the antibodies listed in Table 3 for both sorting and analysis of IL-35.
8. It is essential to keep the Matrigel-cell suspensions for orthotopic injections on ice. Matrigel polymerizes as it warms and will not be injectable through a syringe once polymerized.
9. All media, solutions, and tubes should be kept sterile, and all tumor-processing steps should be performed in a biological safety cabinet.
10. After mincing of tumor, keep the cell suspension on ice to prevent potential loss of cell viability while processing other samples.
11. The enrichment of $CD45^+$ leukocytes by immunomagnetic selection is to reduce the chances of contamination of non-leukocytes and to shorten the time for sorting of B-cell subsets by flow cytometry. While immunomagnetic isolation is not entirely required, we highly recommend it to prevent downstream assay issues.
12. The mononuclear cells ($1–3 \times 10^6$ cells) can be stored in sterile cryovials with 1 mL of freezing medium per sample at −80 °C or in liquid nitrogen [23].
13. For cell staining prior to sorting, the cells should be kept on ice to maintain cell viability.
14. Cells must be kept in a buffer with a low protein concentration (1% FCS or 1% BSA) to help prevent the sorters from clogging.
15. Collection medium can be supplemented with additional 10% FBS to offset the sheath fluid that will dilute the collection medium as cells are collected.
16. We recommend diluting the fluorochrome-conjugated anti-p35 and anti-EBi3 antibodies in ice-cold 1× permeabilization buffer to maintain cellular membrane permeabilization and achieve the maximum antibody binding for intracellular staining.
17. The protocol for IL-35 detection by quantitative PCR can also be used on human Breg cells. Indeed, Fig. 4c shows the fold change expression of *Il12a* and *EBi3* genes in Breg and Bcon cells isolated from human PBMCs.
18. The ratio of blood to Lymphoprep should be 2:1. In the case in which a volume of blood inferior than 20 mL is available, adjust Lymphoprep volume in order to maintain the 2:1 ratio.
19. Positive and negative (without primary antibodies) controls as well as single stain controls are necessary in immunofluorescence to make sure that cross reactivity between the antibodies

did not occur. We typically stain sections for cytokeratin (CK), CD4, CD8, and/or CD20 in addition to EBI3/p35 to show colocalization of cytokine and each specific cell type. CK will stain all PDAC cells and allow for the visualization of the different IL-35-producing immune cells within the pancreatic tumor microenvironment.

Acknowledgments

This work was supported in part by R37 CA230786 (Y. P.-G.), University Cancer Research Fund at the University of North Carolina at Chapel Hill, V Scholar Plus Award (Y. P.-G.), Concern Foundation Conquer Cancer Now Award (Y.P.-G), and F31 CA239494-01A1 Ruth L. Kirschstein Predoctoral Individual National Research Service Award (D.M.). The UNC Flow Cytometry Core Facility, the UNC Translational Pathology Laboratory, and the UNC Lineberger Animal Studies Core are supported in part by P30 CA016086 Cancer Center Core Support Grant to the UNC LCCC.

References

1. Rosser EC, Mauri C (2015) Regulatory B cells: origin, phenotype, and function. Immunity 42 (4):607–612. Epub 2015/04/23. https://doi.org/10.1016/j.immuni.2015.04.005
2. Kalampokis I, Yoshizaki A, Tedder TF (2013) IL-10-producing regulatory B cells (B10 cells) in autoimmune disease. Arthritis Res Ther 15 (Suppl 1):S1. https://doi.org/10.1186/ar3907
3. Banko Z, Pozsgay J, Szili D, Toth M, Gati T, Nagy G, Rojkovich B, Sarmay G (2017) Induction and differentiation of IL-10-producing regulatory B cells from healthy blood donors and rheumatoid arthritis patients. J Immunol 198(4):1512–1520. Epub 2017/01/15. https://doi.org/10.4049/jimmunol.1600218
4. Shen P, Roch T, Lampropoulou V, O'Connor RA, Stervbo U, Hilgenberg E, Ries S, Dang VD, Jaimes Y, Daridon C, Li R, Jouneau L, Boudinot P, Wilantri S, Sakwa I, Miyazaki Y, Leech MD, McPherson RC, Wirtz S, Neurath M, Hoehlig K, Meinl E, Grutzkau A, Grun JR, Horn K, Kuhl AA, Dorner T, Bar-Or A, Kaufmann SHE, Anderton SM, Fillatreau S (2014) IL-35-producing B cells are critical regulators of immunity during autoimmune and infectious diseases. Nature. 507 (7492):366–370. https://doi.org/10.1038/nature12979
5. Wang RX, Yu CR, Dambuza IM, Mahdi RM, Dolinska MB, Sergeev YV, Wingfield PT, Kim SH, Egwuagu CE (2014) Interleukin-35 induces regulatory B cells that suppress autoimmune disease. Nat Med. 20(6):633–641. https://doi.org/10.1038/nm.3554
6. Pylayeva-Gupta Y (2016) Molecular pathways: Interleukin-35 in autoimmunity and Cancer. Clin Cancer Res 22(20):4973–4978. Epub 2016/09/02. https://doi.org/10.1158/1078-0432.CCR-16-0743
7. Devergne O, Birkenbach M, Kieff E (1997) Epstein-Barr virus-induced gene 3 and the p35 subunit of interleukin 12 form a novel heterodimeric hematopoietin. Proc Natl Acad Sci U S A. 94(22):12041–12046. https://doi.org/10.1073/pnas.94.22.12041
8. Collison LW, Workman CJ, Kuo TT, Boyd K, Wang Y, Vignali KM, Cross R, Sehy D, Blumberg RS, Vignali DA (2007) The inhibitory cytokine IL-35 contributes to regulatory T-cell function. Nature 450(7169):566–569. Epub 2007/11/23. https://doi.org/10.1038/nature06306
9. Egwuagu CE, Yu CR (2015) Interleukin 35-Producing B Cells (i35-Breg): A New Mediator of Regulatory B-Cell Functions in CNS Autoimmune Diseases. Crit Rev Immunol. 35(1):49–57. https://doi.org/10.1615/critrevimmunol.2015012558

10. Pylayeva-Gupta Y, Das S, Handler JS, Hajdu CH, Coffre M, Koralov SB, Bar-Sagi D (2016) IL35-Producing B Cells Promote the Development of Pancreatic Neoplasia. Cancer Discov. 6 (3):247–255. https://doi.org/10.1158/2159-8290.CD-15-0843
11. Turnis ME, Sawant DV, Szymczak-Workman AL, Andrews LP, Delgoffe GM, Yano H, Beres AJ, Vogel P, Workman CJ, Vignali DA (2016) Interleukin-35 Limits Anti-Tumor Immunity. Immunity. 44(2):316–329. https://doi.org/10.1016/j.immuni.2016.01.013
12. Mirlekar B, Michaud D, Searcy R, Greene K, Pylayeva-Gupta Y (2018) IL35 Hinders Endogenous Antitumor T-cell Immunity and Responsiveness to Immunotherapy in Pancreatic Cancer. Cancer Immunol Res. 6 (9):1014–1024. https://doi.org/10.1158/2326-6066.CIR-17-0710
13. Mirlekar B, Michaud D, Lee SJ, Kren NP, Harris C, Greene K, Goldman EC, Gupta GP, Fields RC, Hawkins WG, DeNardo DG, Rashid NU, Yeh JJ, McRee AJ, Vincent BG, Vignali DAA, Pylayeva-Gupta Y (2020) B cell-Derived IL35 Drives STAT3-Dependent CD8 (+) T-cell Exclusion in Pancreatic Cancer. Cancer Immunol Res. 8(3):292–308. https://doi.org/10.1158/2326-6066.CIR-19-0349
14. Huang C, Li N, Li Z, Chang A, Chen Y, Zhao T, Li Y, Wang X, Zhang W, Wang Z, Luo L, Shi J, Yang S, Ren H, Hao J (2017) Tumour-derived Interleukin 35 promotes pancreatic ductal adenocarcinoma cell extravasation and metastasis by inducing ICAM1 expression. Nat Commun. 8:14035. https://doi.org/10.1038/ncomms14035
15. Collison LW, Chaturvedi V, Henderson AL, Giacomin PR, Guy C, Bankoti J, Finkelstein D, Forbes K, Workman CJ, Brown SA, Rehg JE, Jones ML, Ni HT, Artis D, Turk MJ, Vignali DA (2010) IL-35-mediated induction of a potent regulatory T cell population. Nat Immunol. 11(12):1093–1101. https://doi.org/10.1038/ni.1952
16. Schwartz M, Zhang Y, Rosenblatt JD (2016) B cell regulation of the anti-tumor response and role in carcinogenesis. J Immunother Cancer 4:40. https://doi.org/10.1186/s40425-016-0145-x
17. Sarvaria A, Madrigal JA, Saudemont A (2017) B cell regulation in cancer and anti-tumor immunity. Cell Mol Immunol. 14 (8):662–674. https://doi.org/10.1038/cmi.2017.35
18. Tsou P, Katayama H, Ostrin EJ, Hanash SM (2016) The emerging role of B cells in tumor immunity. Cancer Res 76(19):5597–5601. Epub 2016/09/17. https://doi.org/10.1158/0008-5472.CAN-16-0431
19. Blair PA, Norena LY, Flores-Borja F, Rawlings DJ, Isenberg DA, Ehrenstein MR, Mauri C (2010) CD19(+)CD24(hi)CD38(hi) B cells exhibit regulatory capacity in healthy individuals but are functionally impaired in systemic lupus erythematosus patients. Immunity 32 (1):129–140. Epub 2010/01/19. https://doi.org/10.1016/j.immuni.2009.11.009
20. Flores-Borja F, Bosma A, Ng D, Reddy V, Ehrenstein MR, Isenberg DA, Mauri C (2013) CD19+CD24hiCD38hi B cells maintain regulatory T cells while limiting TH1 and TH17 differentiation. Sci Transl Med. 5 (173):173ra23. https://doi.org/10.1126/scitranslmed.3005407
21. Bayne LJ, Beatty GL, Jhala N, Clark CE, Rhim AD, Stanger BZ, Vonderheide RH (2012) Tumor-derived granulocyte-macrophage colony-stimulating factor regulates myeloid inflammation and T cell immunity in pancreatic cancer. Cancer Cell. 21(6):822–835. https://doi.org/10.1016/j.ccr.2012.04.025
22. Tan YS, Lei YL (1960) Isolation of Tumor-Infiltrating Lymphocytes by Ficoll-Paque Density Gradient Centrifugation. Methods Mol Biol. 2019:93–99. https://doi.org/10.1007/978-1-4939-9167-9_8
23. Riedhammer C, Halbritter D, Weissert R (2016) Peripheral blood mononuclear cells: isolation, freezing, thawing, and culture. Methods Mol Biol 1304:53–61. Epub 2014/08/06. https://doi.org/10.1007/7651_2014_99

Chapter 9

Characterization and Activation of Fas Ligand-Producing Mouse B Cells and Their Killer Exosomes

Steven K. Lundy, Sophina H. Taitano, and Luciën E. P. M. van der Vlugt

Abstract

B lymphocytes make several contributions to immune regulation including production of antibodies with regulatory properties, release of immune suppressive cytokines, and expression of death-inducing ligands. A role for Fas ligand (FasL)-expressing "killer" B cells in regulating T helper (T_H) cell survival and chronic inflammation has been demonstrated in animal models of schistosome worm and other infections, asthma, autoimmune arthritis, and type 1 diabetes. $FasL^+$ B cells were also capable of inducing immune tolerance in a male-to-female transplantation model. Interestingly, populations of B cells found in the spleen and lungs of naïve mice constitutively expresses FasL and have potent killer function against T_H cells that is antigen-specific and FasL-dependent. Epstein-Barr virus-transformed human B cells constitutively express FasL and package it into exosomes that co-express MHC Class II molecules and have killer function against antigen-specific T_H cells. $FasL^+$ exosomes with markers of B-cell lineage are abundant in the spleen of naïve mice. Killer B cells therefore represent a novel target for immune modulation in many disease settings. Our laboratory has published methods of characterizing $FasL^+$ B cells and inducing their proliferation in vitro. This updated chapter will describe methods of identifying and expanding killer B cells from mice, detecting FasL expression in B cells, extracting $FasL^+$ exosomes from spleen and culture supernatants, and performing functional killing assays against antigen-specific T_H cells.

Key words B lymphocytes, Exosomes, Fas ligand, Immune regulation, Apoptosis, Interleukin-10

1 Introduction

Fas ligand (FasL, CD178) was first discovered to function as a death-inducing ligand during the characterization of mice on the C3H strain background that had developed a spontaneous, autosomal recessive, generalized lymphoproliferative disorder [1, 2]. A point mutation in the FasL gene in these C3H gld/gld mice was later shown to result in a structural change to the protein, which inhibits its ability to bind the death receptor Fas (CD95) [3–5]. Reciprocally, an insertion into an intron of the gene encoding Fas in MRL lpr/lpr mice drastically reduces expression of the Fas receptor and results in the mice having a lymphoproliferative disorder similar to that seen in C3H gld/gld mice [6, 7]. Both strains of

Francesca Mion and Silvia Tonon (eds.), *Regulatory B Cells: Methods and Protocols*, Methods in Molecular Biology, vol. 2270, https://doi.org/10.1007/978-1-0716-1237-8_9, © Springer Science+Business Media, LLC, part of Springer Nature 2021

mice are prone to splenomegaly and lymphadenopathy that begins around 12 weeks of age, and which is associated with elevated levels of neutrophils, and the presence of T cells in the periphery with aberrant surface marker expression. Increased levels of serum antibodies against double-stranded DNA in these mice have led to their characterization as having a lupus-like syndrome [8]. Subsequently it was found that patients diagnosed with autoimmune lymphoproliferative syndrome (ALPS) have mutations that also affect the FasL-Fas signaling axis with the most frequent mutations being in the Fas receptor [9–11]. Because of the homotrimeric structure of the Fas membrane complex, these mutations can be inherited as autosomal dominant alleles since a conformational change to only one of the three proteins in the trimer can lead to functional loss of the entire complex [12]. Patients with ALPS have enlarged secondary lymphoid organs and the accumulation of circulating CD4 and CD8 double-negative T lymphocytes that has been used as a diagnostic feature of ALPS [13, 14]. Mutations in human Fas (ALPS type 1a) can result in a range of symptoms and severity even within the same family, the most common being hemolytic anemia and autoimmune thrombocytopenia [12, 15]. In contrast, a mutation in the human FasL gene (ALPS type 1b) has only been infrequently reported in patients with systemic lupus erythematosus [16, 17].

The above findings highlight the importance of induction of T- and B-cell apoptosis via the FasL-Fas signaling pathway as a mechanism of regulating lymphocyte homeostasis and maintaining tolerance toward self-antigens. Cytotoxic T lymphocytes (CTL) and natural killer (NK) cells are well-recognized for their specialized functions as killer/effector immune cells that utilize FasL to induce cell death of virus-infected cells and tumor cells [18, 19]. Although FasL expression by B lymphocytes was first reported by Hahne et al. in 1996, and enough evidence has been documented to support these initial findings, relatively little attention has been given to characterizing $FasL^+$ B cells and their roles in the immune system [20, 21]. Work from our laboratory has demonstrated that B cells, particularly the $CD5^+$ B-cell subset in the mouse spleen and lung, express FasL and mediate T_H cell apoptosis in mouse models of schistosome infection, chronic cockroach allergen-induced asthma, and collagen-induced arthritis [22–25]. Other laboratories have studied FasL expression by B cells in mouse models of type 1 diabetes, systemic lupus erythematosus, *T. cruzi* infection, and transplant tolerance [26–30]. There have also been multiple reports of FasL expression by human B cells, particularly in multiple myeloma and B-CLL patients, and also on non-transformed B cells (reviewed in reference 21).

Outside of the immune system, expression of FasL is restricted to specialized cell types at specific anatomical locations, where it plays an important function in maintaining tissue immune privilege [31]. In the eye, FasL is expressed by corneal epithelial and endothelial cells as well as retinal pigment epithelial cells [32–34]. Ovarian epithelial cells and testicular Leydig cells express FasL, which is thought to maintain immune tolerance of these reproductive organs [35, 36]. Another important role of FasL in reproduction is its expression by placental trophoblast cells which protect the fetus from the mother's immune system [37, 38]. FasL expression is also relatively common among cancer cells of many types and provides a mechanism of escape from immune surveillance [39, 40]. Although the cell-type-specific mechanisms of controlling FasL expression could be of high importance for understanding immune privilege and tumor control, the majority of studies focused on FasL gene and protein expression have been conducted by activating CTL through the T-cell receptor signaling axis [41–44].

Originally it was thought that FasL was primarily expressed on the cell surface and that, similarly to many other surface proteins, its expression was regulated at the mRNA transcription level after cell activation. It has subsequently been found that the transcription of the FasL gene is low in most cell types, even upon activation [45]. Accumulating evidence suggests that the majority of FasL protein possessed by cells that express it is preformed and transported into the lysosomal/endosomal compartment through mechanisms involving mono-ubiquitylation [46]. FasL protein is then integrated into small secretory vesicles (exosomes) that are transported to the cell surface and/or released upon stimulation [47–51]. In fact, cells that have forced surface expression of FasL through genetic engineering have been shown to activate innate inflammatory responses that can lead to destruction of the FasL-expressing cells and loss of immune privilege [52–54]. Thus, transient expression of FasL on the cell surface, which is maintained by a combination of low gene transcription, intracellular protein sequestration in the endosomal-lysosomal compartment, and rapid cleavage of membrane FasL by matrix metalloproteinases, seems to be the preferred mechanism for inducing immune suppression without causing overt inflammation [55–57]. For this reason, we believe that the constitutive cell surface expression of FasL that we have observed in a small number of B cells in the spleens and lungs of naïve mice is an immunologically significant circumstance that deserves further attention. At the same time, the more prevalent packaging of FasL into B-cell exosomes that also express MHC class II, which are capable of inducing T_H cell death, is an exciting area for further studies [58].

Many factors contribute to making the study of FasL expression by B cells technically challenging. Foremost is the scarcity of surface $FasL^+$ B cells in easily accessible anatomical locations. In our experience, the best source is the spleen, where the $CD5^+$ B-cell subset is the dominant lymphocyte population with constitutive surface FasL expression above background. As shown in Fig. 1a,

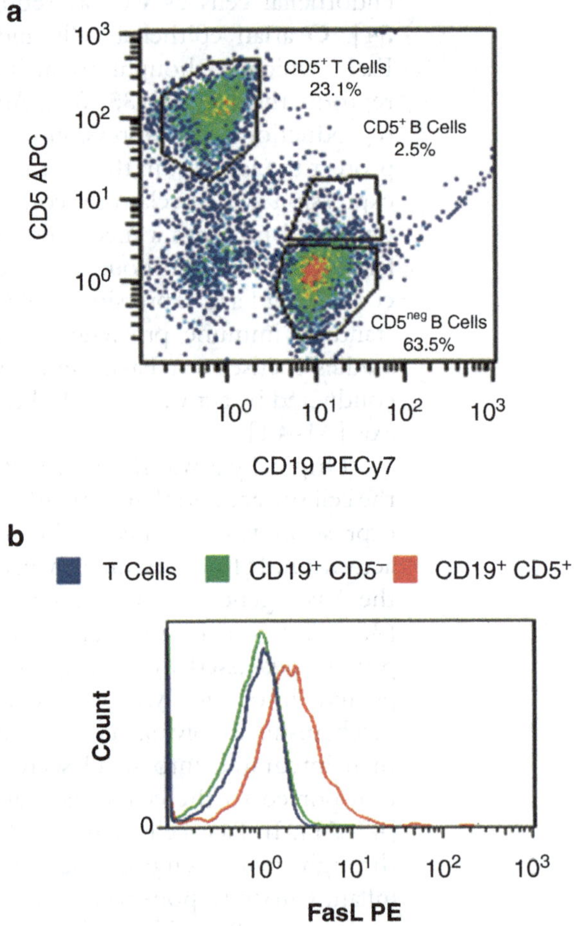

Fig. 1 FasL expression is enriched within the splenic CD5$^+$ B lymphocyte subset. Splenocytes isolated from the spleen of a naïve DBA/1 mouse were stained with antibodies that bind mouse CD5, CD19, and FasL (CD178). Flow cytometry was performed, and the cells were pre-gated for forward scatter area (FSC-A) versus side scatter area (SSC-A) to identify lymphocytes. A second gating step was used to select single cells (FSC-A versus FSC-height). (**a**) Dot plot of CD5 versus CD19 showing gates used for panel (B). (**b**) FasL expression on the gated lymphocyte populations

three different populations can be distinguished among splenocytes from naïve DBA/1 mice by staining with anti-CD19 and anti-CD5 antibodies. Cells that are gated as CD5^{high}/CD19^{neg} (T cells) and CD5^{neg}/CD19$^+$ (B cells) have no surface expression of FasL, while CD5$^+$/CD19$^+$ B cells have a shift of the entire population toward higher FasL expression on the cell surface (*see* Fig. 1b). Similar results have been consistently found using spleens from other mouse strains including CBA/1, C57BL/6, and BALB/c [[23, 24] and unpublished results]. Further characterization of the surface marker phenotype of splenic FasL$^+$ B cells has recently been published [59].

Other than the relatively rare population found in the spleen, $CD5^+$ B cells are primarily located in mucosal tissues where they are known to have important functions in producing natural antibodies [60, 61]. It is extremely rare to find $CD5^+$ B cells in the lymph nodes or blood of naïve mice. The majority of peripheral $CD5^+$ B cells are not thought to be derived from bone marrow precursor cells, but rather come from cells produced in the fetal liver that then divide to form daughter cells [62, 63]. This suggests that bone marrow may not be a good source for stem cells that could be differentiated into $CD5^+$ B cells. However, Montandon et al. recently reported the presence of pro-B cells in the bone marrow of NOD mice that were elicited by activation through Toll-like receptor 9 and interferon gamma that expressed FasL and regulated type 1 diabetes [27].

As shown in Fig. 2 and Table 1, a low but consistent number of $FasL^+$ B cells can be found in the lungs of naïve BALB/c mice. These lung $FasL^+$ B cells have relatively high expression of CD5 and surface IgM compared with the total B-cell population, which is similar to the surface marker expression found on splenic $FasL^+$ B cells.

Another impediment to studying $FasL^+$ B cells has been the lack of cell culture methods that favor their survival and growth. Our laboratory has recently discovered a cell culture system that expands $FasL^+$ B cells in vitro that can mediate antigen-specific, and FasL-dependent T_H cell apoptosis [59]. Interestingly, the same culture conditions also induce IL-10-producing B-cell survival and cytokine release [59]. In the current chapter, we provide detailed protocols for the isolation, culture, and phenotypic and functional characterization of $FasL^+$ B cells used by our laboratory. Also included is a protocol for efficient isolation of exosomes from whole mouse spleen and characterization of their FasL protein expression. We hope to foster collaboration, help troubleshoot, and broaden interest in the study of killer B lymphocytes and their relationship to B cells with other immune suppressive functions [64].

2 Materials

2.1 General Equipment

1. Surgical scissors and forceps.
2. 15 mL centrifuge tubes.
3. 70 μm cell strainers.
4. Disposable syringes and needles (18 and 25 G).
5. Pipet tips ranging from 0.2 mL to 10 mL with appropriate pipettors and pipet aids.
6. 6-well culture plates.

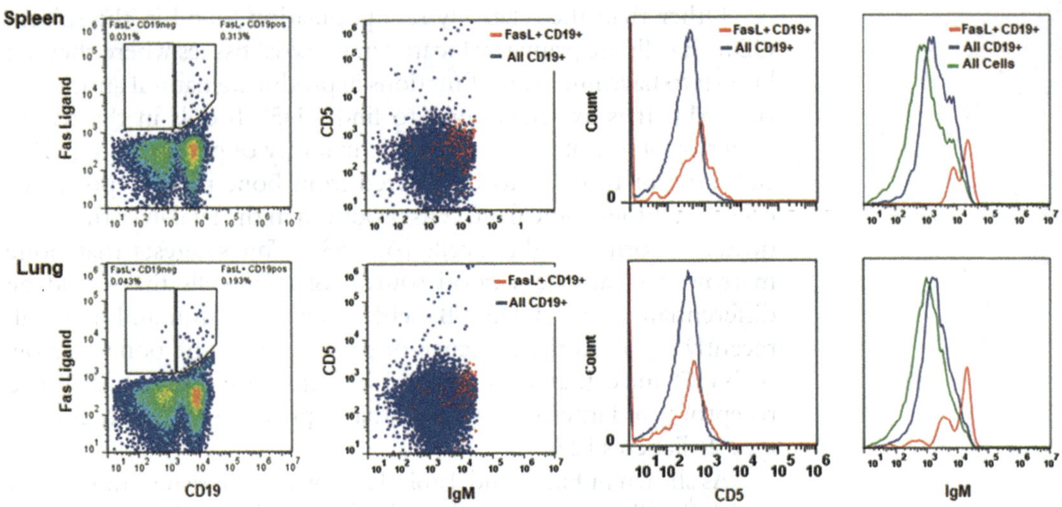

Fig. 2 The majority of FasL$^+$ lymphocytes from naïve BALB/c mouse spleen and lung are CD19$^+$IgM^{high}CD5^{int} B cells. Lymphocytes isolated from the spleens or lungs of individual naïve BALB/c mice (n = 5 mice) were gated as live (propidum iodide negative), single (FSC-H versus FSC-A), lymphoid (FSC-A versus SSC-A) cells and then plotted for CD19 versus FasL staining as shown (left panels). The FasL$^+$ cells were mostly CD19$^+$ and the remaining figures show CD5 and IgM levels of the FasL$^+$CD19$^+$ cells (red) overlain on the total CD19$^+$ cell population (blue). There was a marked enrichment of IgM^{high}CD5^{int} cells in the FasL$^+$CD19$^+$ subset. The data shown are representative dot and histogram plots from one mouse out of five. Statistical analyses can be found in Tables 1 and 3

7. 1, 3, and 10 mL syringes.
8. 0.22 μm filters for fitting to syringes.
9. Centrifuge tubes or bottle tops.
10. Columns and magnet for immunomagnetic separation.
11. Ultracentrifuge.
12. Sterile flasks, flat-bottom culture plates, and other sterile liquid handling supplies.
13. Flat-bottomed 96-well EIA plates.
14. Multichannel pipettors and tips.
15. Plastic film plate covers.
16. Plate reader equipped for absorbance measurements at 450 nm.

2.2 Mice

All procedures outlined in this chapter involving mice were approved by the University Committee for the Use and Care of Animals of the University of Michigan. Prior to performing any of these procedures, researchers should obtain approval from their institutional review board.

1. Wild-type BALB/cJ and DBA-1/J mice.

Table 1
Quantification of FasL+ subsets in dispersed spleen and lung tissue

BALBc Tissue ($n = 5$ mice)	Avg. cell # total (million) ± st. dev	%CD19 + ± st. dev	%FasL + CD19 + ± st. dev	%FasL + CD19neg ± st. dev	*t*-test Value $t =$	*P* Value	Per Mouse Ratio of %FasL + CD19+ vs CD19^{neg}	Est. Cell # FasL + CD19+ ± st. deviation
Spleen	72.8 ± 5.1	57.0 ± 3.0	0.244 ± 0.048	0.025 ± 0.200	10.2	<0.001	9.9 ± 2.0	180,010 ± 54,529
Lung	14.8 ± 1.1	51.6 ± 5.1	0.212 ± 0.031	0.047 ± 0.011	11.2	<0.001	4.7 ± 1.4	31,622 ± 6232

2. D1Lac.Cg-Tg (TCRa,TCRb)24Efro/J mice. Transgenic (Tg) mice on DBA-1 background that express a T-cell receptor (TCR) specific to an antigenic peptide of type II collagen ($cII_{259-273}$). Therefore, immunization with $cII_{259-273}$ can potentially stimulate all of the Th cells within the mouse.
3. C.Cg-Tg(DO11.10)10Dlo/J mice. Transgenic DO11.10 mice on BALB/c background that express a TCR specific to an antigenic peptide of ovalbumin ($OVA_{323-339}$).

2.3 Media and Liquid Reagents

1. Sterile 1× phosphate buffered saline (PBS): 137 mM sodium chloride, 2.7 mM potassium chloride, 10 mM sodium monophosphate, 1.8 mM potassium diphosphate, pH 7.2.
2. Standard Dulbecco's Modified Eagle Medium (DMEM) culture medium: 10% heat-inactivated fetal calf serum (FCS), 100 U/mL penicillin, 100 μg/mL streptomycin, and 2 mM L-glutamine in DMEM.
3. Standard RPMI medium: 10% heat-inactivated FCS, 100 U/mL penicillin, 100 μg/mL streptomycin.
4. Ammonium-Chloride-Potassium (ACK) red blood cell lysis buffer: 155 mM ammonium chloride, 10 mM potassium carbonate, 0.1 mM ethylenediaminetetraacetic acid (EDTA).
5. Tissue dispersal medium: 0.2% Type IV collagenase in serum-free DMEM.
6. Magnetic bead separation buffer: 2 mM EDTA, 0.5% bovine serum albumin (BSA), 0.01% sodium azide in 1× PBS. pH 7.4; degassed.
7. Collection medium: 20% fetal bovine serum (FBS) in RPMI.
8. Fibroblast culture medium: 10% non-heat inactivated adult bovine serum, 100 U/mL penicillin, 100 μg/mL streptomycin, and 2 mM L-glutamine in DMEM.
9. Trypsin buffer: 0.25% Trypsin in 1 × PBS supplemented with 0.53 mM EDTA.
10. Mouse B-cell culture medium: 10% heat-inactivated FCS, 50 μg/mL transferrin, 5 μg/mL insulin, 100 U/mL penicillin, 100 μg/mL streptomycin, and 2 mM L-glutamine in DMEM.
11. An approved mouse anesthetic such as isoflurane, ketamine/xylazine, or other.

2.4 Materials for B-Cell Culture and exosomes Purification

1. Magnetic bead-purified mouse $CD19^+$ B cells.
2. Non-transduced NIH3T3 fibroblasts (ATCC).
3. NIH3T3 fibroblasts stably transduced with the gene encoding mouse CD40 ligand (a kind gift of Kevin McDonagh and David Fox [65]).
4. IL-4 and IL-5 recombinant mouse cytokines.

5. Phorbol 12-myristate 13 acetate (PMA).
6. Ionomycin.
7. Lipopolysaccharide (LPS).
8. A protein transport inhibitor such as GolgiStop.
9. Cesium irradiator or other methods of stopping proliferation of NIH3T3 fibroblasts (*see* **Note 1**).

2.5 Western Blot Reagents

1. SDS lysis buffer: 62.5 mM Tris-HCl, 2% w/v SDS, 10% glycerol, 50 mM DTT, 0.01% w/v bromophenol blue.
2. Precasted SDS-PAGE gels: 4–20% Tris-Glycine 12-well gels.
3. Prestained protein molecular weight standard.
4. Running buffer: 50 mM MOPS, 50 mM Tris Base, 0.1% w/v SDS, 1 mM EDTA, pH 7.7.
5. Polyvinylidene difluoride (PVDF) membrane.
6. Transfer buffer: 20% methanol, 25 mM Tris, 192 mM glycine, pH 8.0.
7. Wash buffer: 0.05% Tween-20 in 1× PBS.
8. Blocking buffer: 5% w/v non-fat dry milk in wash buffer.
9. Blocking buffer: 5% w/v BSA in wash buffer.
10. Antibodies used for western blot: polyclonal rabbit anti-FasL, polyclonal rabbit anti-beta actin, and anti-rabbit IgG-HRP as secondary antibody.
11. Enhanced chemiluminescence (ECL) substrate: luminol-based substrate for the horseradish peroxidase (HRP) label conjugated to secondary antibodies.

2.6 Flow Cytometry Reagents

1. Flow cytometry buffer: 0.2% BSA, 0.1% sodium azide in 1× PBS.
2. FACS buffer: 0.2% BSA in 1× PBS.
3. Streptavidin-coated polystyrene beads (10–12 μm diameter) for exosome analysis.
4. Biotinylated anti-mouse antibodies for exosome capture.
5. 1 mg/mL propidium iodide in deionized water.
6. Antibodies for flow cytometry (*see* Table 2) and their relative fluorochrome-conjugated isotype control antibodies (PE-Hamster IgG1,κ; APC-Rat IgG2a,κ; PECy7-Rat IgG2a,κ and FITC-Rat IgG2b,κ).
7. FcBlock: unconjugated anti-CD16/CD32 antibody.
8. Saponin buffer: 0.2% w/v BSA, 0.5% w/v saponin in 1× PBS.

Table 2
Antibodies used to identify markers found on killer B cells

Antibody	Isotype	Conjugate	Clone
FasL	Hamster IgG1,k	PE	MFL3
CD19	Rat IgG2a,k	FITC	1D3
CD19	Rat IgG2a,k	APC	1D3
CD19	Rat IgG2a,k	PECy7	1D3
CD1d	Rat IgG2b,k	FITC	1B1
CD5	Rat IgG2a,k	APC	53-7.3
CD24	Rat IgG2b,k	FITC	M1/69
IgM	Rat IgG2a,k	PECy7	RMM-1
IL-10	Rat IgG2b,k	FITC	JES5-16E3

2.7 Reagents for B-Cell Cytokines and FasL ELISA

1. Carbonate coating buffer: 0.1 M Sodium bicarbonate, 0.1 M Sodium carbonate, pH 9.5.
2. ELISA wash buffer: 0.05% Tween20 in 1× PBS.
3. ELISA blocking buffer: 10% heat-inactivated FCS in 1× PBS.
4. Mouse IL-6 and IL-10 ELISA kits with cytokine standards.
5. Mouse FasL ELISA kits with standard (R and D Systems).
6. TMB substrate reagents A and B.
7. ELISA stop solution: 2 N sulfuric acid.

2.8 Measurement of Peptide-Specific Killing of Mouse T_H Cells by Killer B Cells

1. Splenocytes from the D1Lac.Cg-Tg (TCRa,TCRb)24Efro/J transgenic mouse strain.
2. Concanavalin A.
3. Kit for mouse $CD4^+$ T-cell-negative isolation through immunomagnetic separation.
4. Purified anti-mouse FasL (clone MFL3) antibody and its relative isotype control.
5. Annexin buffer: 10 mM HEPES, 140 mM NaCl, 2.5 mM anhydrous $CaCl_2$, pH 7.4.
6. PE-conjugated anti-mouse CD4 (clone H129.19) antibody.
7. FITC-Annexin V.
8. Propidium iodide solution: 1 mg/mL propidium iodide in deionized water.

3 Methods

3.1 Isolation of Purified B Lymphocytes and Exosomes from Mice

3.1.1 Preparation of Single-Cell Suspensions from Mouse Spleen (See Note 2)

1. Surgically remove the spleen from an euthanized mouse being careful to eliminate the pancreatic tissue and omentum (attached soft white tissues).
2. Make two or three small snips in the spleen capsule to facilitate the extraction of cells and place in 5 mL of 1× PBS in a labeled 15 mL centrifuge tube.
3. Pour the contents of the tube into a sterile 70-μm cell strainer that has been placed in a 6-well plate or small Petri dish (*see* Fig. 3).
4. Using the plunger of a 3- or 5-mL disposable syringe, gently crush the spleen pushing the cells through the pores of the cell strainer until all of the tissue remaining above the filter is white. Transfer the cell suspension back to the original tube.
5. Wash the cell strainer with an additional 5 mL of fresh 1× PBS and transfer the cell suspension to the original tube.
6. Pellet the spleen cells by centrifugation at 450 × *g* for 5 min.

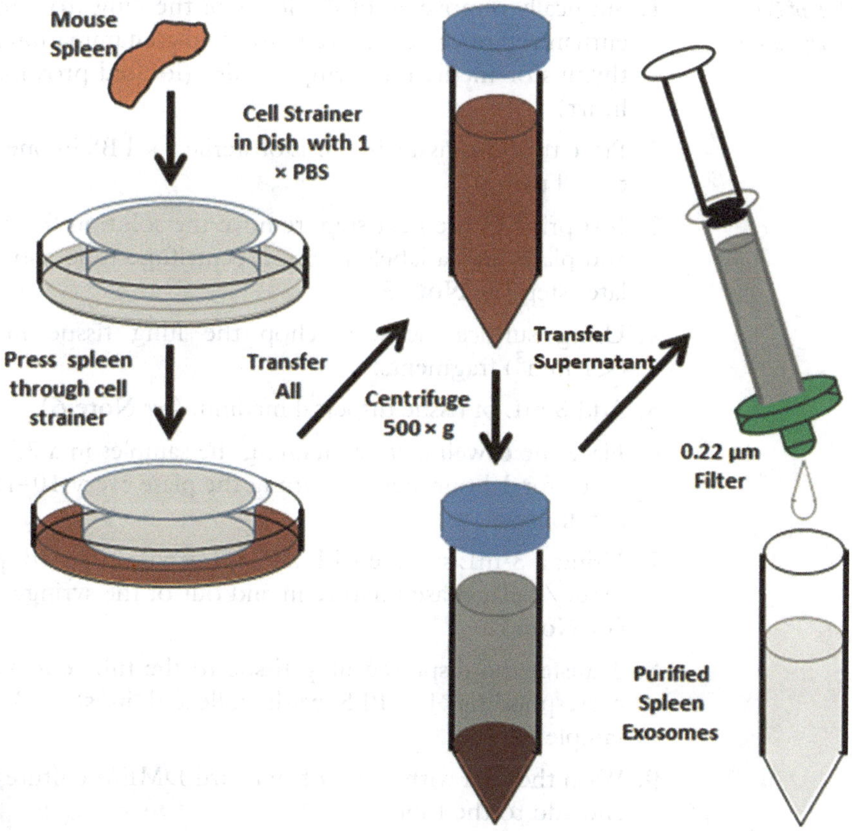

Fig. 3 Schematic diagram for the rapid isolation of cells and exosomes from mouse spleen

7. Remove the supernatant and resuspend the red pellet of spleen cells in the remaining PBS. This supernatant may be saved at 4 °C for up to 1 week for isolation of exosomes (*see* Subheading 3.1.6).
8. Add 3 mL of ACK red blood cell lysis buffer and incubate for 1–2 min (*see* **Note 3**).
9. Add 10 mL of standard DMEM culture medium to stop the lysis (*see* **Note 4**).
10. Perform a quick spin to remove the dead cell debris by allowing the cells to spin up to 200 × *g* and then immediately stopping the centrifuge.
11. Transfer the non-pelleted cells to a clean tube and centrifuge at 450 × *g* for 5 min to pellet the splenic leukocytes.
12. Discard the supernatant and resuspend the off-white cell pellet in the remaining medium.
13. Add 10 mL of DMEM culture medium or 1× PBS and count cells using preferred method.
14. Proceed to the desired assay(s).

3.1.2 Isolation of Cells from Mouse Lung Tissue

1. Surgically remove all of the lobes of the lung from individual euthanized mice being careful to avoid contamination from the thymus or mediastinal lymph nodes (located proximal to the heart).
2. Place the lung tissue in 3 mL of sterile 1× PBS in one well of a 6-well plate.
3. Just prior to the next step, remove the solution from the well and place into a labeled 15 mL centrifuge tube and store for later step (*see* **Note 5**).
4. Using surgical scissors, chop the lung tissue into small (<1 mm^3) fragments.
5. Add 3 mL of tissue dispersal medium (*see* **Note 6**).
6. Place the 6-well plate containing the samples in a 37 °C incubator for 1 hour, gently swirling the plate every 10–15 min to aid dispersal.
7. Using a 3-mL syringe with an 18G needle attached, pipet the tissue/collagenase mixture in and out of the syringe 20 times (*see* **Note 7**).
8. Transfer the dispersed lung tissue to the tube containing the corresponding 1× PBS wash collected in **step 3** for that sample.
9. Wash the well with 6 mL of standard DMEM culture medium and add to the tube.
10. Pellet the lung cells by centrifugation at 450× g for 5 min.

11. Remove the supernatant and wash cells once with 1× PBS.
12. Proceed with red blood cell lysis following **steps 7–10** of Subheading 3.1.1 to obtain single-cell suspensions of lung leukocytes.

3.1.3 Collection of Peritoneal Cells by Abdominal Lavage

1. Anesthetize mice with isoflurane, ketamine/xylazine, or other preferred method that will ensure the mouse will be alive but under anesthetic throughout the lavage procedure.
2. Using a 10 mL syringe filled with sterile 1× PBS and fitted with a 23 or 25G needle, insert the needle bevel up into the abdominal cavity being careful to avoid critical organs (*see* **Note 8**).
3. Slowly inject 8–10 mL of PBS, stopping if and when the liquid pressure begins to force solution to exit through the needle hole. Remove the syringe.
4. While still holding the mouse abdomen up, insert a sterile 18G needle into the side of the abdomen being careful that the open end of the needle is over an open 15 mL centrifuge tube to collect the lavage fluid (*see* **Note 9**).
5. Allow the injected fluid to continue dripping into the collection tube while turning the mouse abdomen down and allowing gravity to assist with the collection (*see* **Note 10**).
6. Pellet the peritoneal cells by centrifugation at 450 × *g* for 5 min (*see* **Note 11**).
7. Resuspend the pelleted peritoneal leukocytes in 2 mL of desired medium or buffer for counting.
8. Proceed with desired assays.

3.1.4 Immunomagnetic Purification of Mouse B Lymphocytes

Depending on the study, B cells can be purified from the cell populations obtained by processing one of the organs described above.

1. Wash cells by centrifugation with 10 mL of 4 °C magnetic bead separation buffer.
2. Proceed to MACS positive isolation of $CD19^+$ B cells using anti-CD19 microbeads. Follow the manufacturer's instructions.
3. Resuspend the obtained cell pellet in 10 mL of cell culture medium and count cells using preferred method.
4. Proceed to cell culture or flow cytometric analysis or sorting of purified $CD19^+$ B cells (*see* Table 3).

3.1.5 FACS Sorting $FasL^+$ B Cells

1. Euthanize 20–30 mice and collect spleens in pools of 5 in 50 mL centrifuge tubes containing 10 mL sterile PBS.

Table 3
Analysis of FasL+ subsets after magnetic bead positive selection with CD19 MACS beads (Miltenyi Biotech)

BALBc Tissue ($n = 5$ mice)	Avg. cell # (millions) ± st. dev	Mean %CD19 + ± st. dev	%FasL+ CD19 + ± st. dev	MFI CD5 All CD19+	MFI CD5 FasL+ CD19+	*P* value	MFI IgM All CD19+ ± st. dev	MFI IgM FasL+ CD19+ ± st. dev	*P* Value
Spleen	29.3 ± 5.1	93.9 ± 3.8	0.619 ± 0.079	451 ± 14	706 ± 114	<0.01	3914 ± 147	14,627 ± 2177	<0.001
Lung	3.3 ± 0.8	97.1 ± 1.1	0.741 ± 0.055	460 ± 30	644 ± 92	<0.01	3352 ± 105	14,017 ± 1887	<0.001

2. Prepare single-cell suspensions of splenocytes in PBS using scaled up amounts of buffers as those described in Subheading 3.1.1.
3. At the end of splenocytes isolation, combine cells into one sample and count.
4. Wash cells in FACS buffer and proceed to cell staining (*see* **Note 12**). Stain cells for 10 min at 4 °C with 1 μg of FcBlock for every one million cells.
5. Add 1 μg each of PE-anti-FasL and APC-anti-CD19 for every one million cells and incubate for 30 min at 4 °C.
6. Wash and resuspended cells in FACS buffer at the highest cell concentration recommended for the cell sorter to be used.
7. Immediately sort cells into 12 mL collection tubes containing 6 mL of collection medium. Coat the inside surface of each collection tube with collection medium prior to sorting.
8. Sort cells as fast as possible to ensure a sufficient yield. The expected yield of FasL$^+$ B cells from 20 to 30 mouse spleens is 1–two million cells.
9. Wash sorted cells with PBS and resuspend in B-cell culture medium for functional assays.

3.1.6 Isolation of Exosomes from Cell-Free spleen Extracts

1. The supernatant resulting from centrifugation of dispersed spleen cells described in **step 7** of Subheading 3.1.1 contains exosomes, including FasL$^+$ exosomes (*see* Fig. 3).
2. To remove the larger quantity of cellular debris from this cell-free spleen extract, spin the supernatant at 10,000 × *g* at 4 °C for 1 hour.
3. Transfer the supernatant to an open (plunger-removed) 1, 3, or 10 mL syringe pre-fitted with a 0.22-μm syringe filter.
4. Force the liquid through the filter with the plunger and collect the flow through, which contains a semi-purified exosome population that is suitable for high-sensitivity ELISA, flow cytometry, imaging, and some functional assays.
5. For greater purification and concentration of exosomes, transfer the supernatant to clean ultracentrifuge tubes and adjust the volumes so that the tubes opposite each other will be highly balanced.
6. Place the tubes containing spleen extract into a fixed-angle ultracentrifuge rotor and spin the samples at 110,000 × *g* at 4 °C for 2 h.
7. Discard the supernatant and partially resuspend the pellet in the remaining 1× PBS by repeated vortexing (*see* **Note 13**).
8. Refill the ultracentrifuge tube with fresh 1× PBS and repeat the centrifugation as described in **step 6**.

9. Discard the supernatant. Depending on the downstream assay, add 300 μl of 1× PBS, SDS lysis buffer, or another desired diluent (*see* **Note 14**).
10. Resuspend the pellet by repeated vortexing and transfer the resuspended exosomes to a clean 1.5 mL centrifuge tube.

3.1.7 Isolation of Exosomes from Culture Supernatants

1. Collect culture supernatant in the appropriate number and size of centrifuge tubes and spin the tubes at 500 × *g* for 10 min to pellet cells.
2. Transfer the supernatant to fresh centrifuge tubes and spin at 10,000 × *g* for 30 min to remove large debris.
3. Transfer the supernatant to an appropriate-sized filtration vessel (bottle top, centrifuge flip top, syringe) fitted with a 0.22-μ m filter.
4. Filter the supernatant collecting the flow through portion containing exosomes.
5. Proceed with ultracentrifugation as described above, in Subheading 3.1.6, **steps 5–6**.

3.2 Expansion of Mouse FasL$^+$ B Cells by In Vitro Cell Culture

The cell culture system proposed to expand mouse FasL$^+$ B cells (*see* Fig. 4a) was adapted from the one originally described by Schultze et al. for the in vitro culture of human B cells [66]. This model is made of two steps: the first requires the maintenance of NIH3T3 fibroblasts stably transduced with the gene encoding mouse CD40 ligand (*see* **Note 15**), while in the second one a coculture of murine B cells and irradiated mCD40L-NIH3T3 fibroblasts is set up.

3.2.1 Culture of Mouse CD40 Ligand-Transduced NIH3T3 Fibroblasts

Maintenance of a cell culture stock of mCD40L-Fb and NIH3T3 is performed in T75cm^2 flasks by passage of 0.5 million cells at confluency to a new flask containing the medium recommended by ATCC for the growth of NIH3T3 fibroblasts (*see* **Note 16**).

1. When cells reach confluency, remove culture medium and wash adherent cells with 20 mL of 1× PBS.
2. Add 3 mL of Trypsin buffer to the flask and rotate to wet the entire surface. Let stand 2–3 min at room temperature. Vigorously smack the side of the flask to release the adherent cells.
3. Add 10 mL of fibroblast culture medium to stop the enzymatic reaction from destroying the cells and then transfer fibroblasts to a 15-mL centrifuge tube.
4. Pellet cells by centrifugation at 450 × *g* for 5 min.
5. Resuspend pellet in 10 mL of medium and repeat centrifugation to wash the cells.
6. Resuspend fibroblasts in 5 mL, count, and place 0.5 million cells in a T75cm^2 flask to continue culture (*see* **Note 17**).

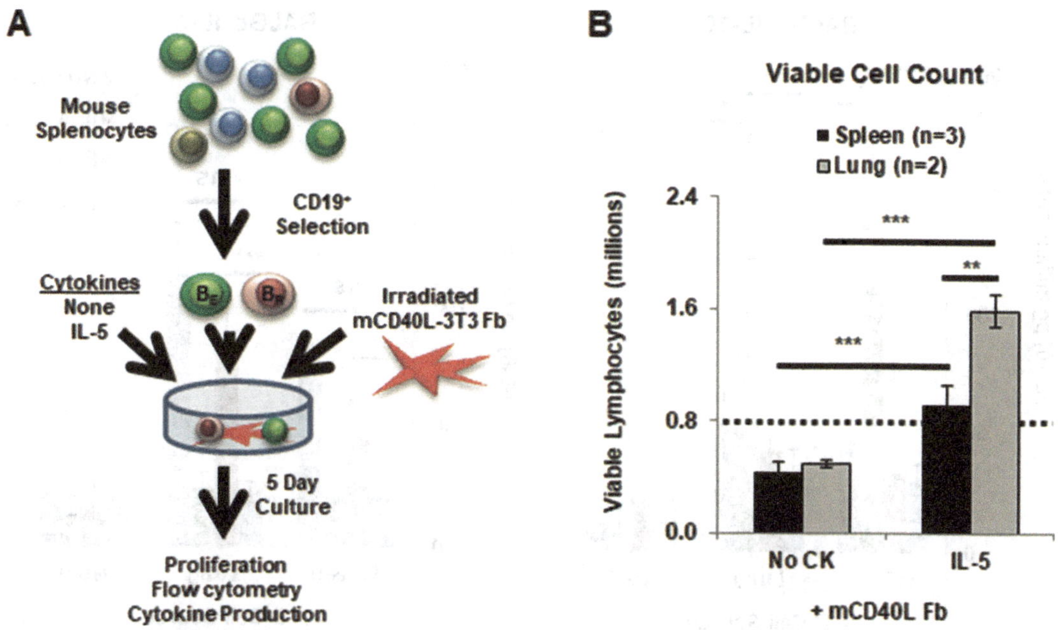

Fig. 4 CD40L-transduced fibroblasts and IL-5 induce proliferation of cultured B cells. (**a**) Schematic diagram of the B cell culture system. (**b**) Representative experiment in which B cells were positively selected by magnetic separation using CD19 beads from individual naïve BALB/c mouse spleens (n = 3 mice) or lungs (n = 2 mice). Purified B cells from each mouse were cultured in triplicate on a confluent monolayer of irradiated mCD40L-Fb in the presence or absence (no CK) of 100 ng/mL IL-5 for 5 days. Cells were harvested and viable B cells counted by trypan blue method. The dotted line indicates the number of B cells/well at the start of culture. Data are mean ± standard deviation of all wells: n = 9 for the spleen, n = 6 for the lung. $^{**}P < 0.02$, $^{***}P < 0.01$

3.2.2 Cell Culture Recommendations for the Expansion of FasL$^+$ B Cells

1. Obtain CD19$^+$ B cells by magnetic bead separation as described in Subheading 3.1.4. Wash cells by centrifugation at 450 × *g* two times in B-cell culture medium and count viable B cells by trypan blue exclusion method. Adjust concentration of B cells to eight million/mL.
2. Irradiate fibroblasts at 300 Gray (3000 Rad) and then wash fibroblasts two times in B-cell culture medium. Adjust fibroblast concentration to 10^6 cell/mL prior to coculture with B cells (*see* **Note 1**).
3. Dilute sterile recombinant IL-5 in B-cell culture medium to a 4× working concentration of 100–400 ng/mL. Cytokine addition to culture medium increases B-cell viability and proliferation (*see* Fig. 4b).
4. Add equal volumes of B cells, irradiated fibroblasts, medium, and/or cytokine(s) to replicate wells of flat-bottomed culture plates such that each component is diluted 1–4 in the final volume (*see* **Note 18**).

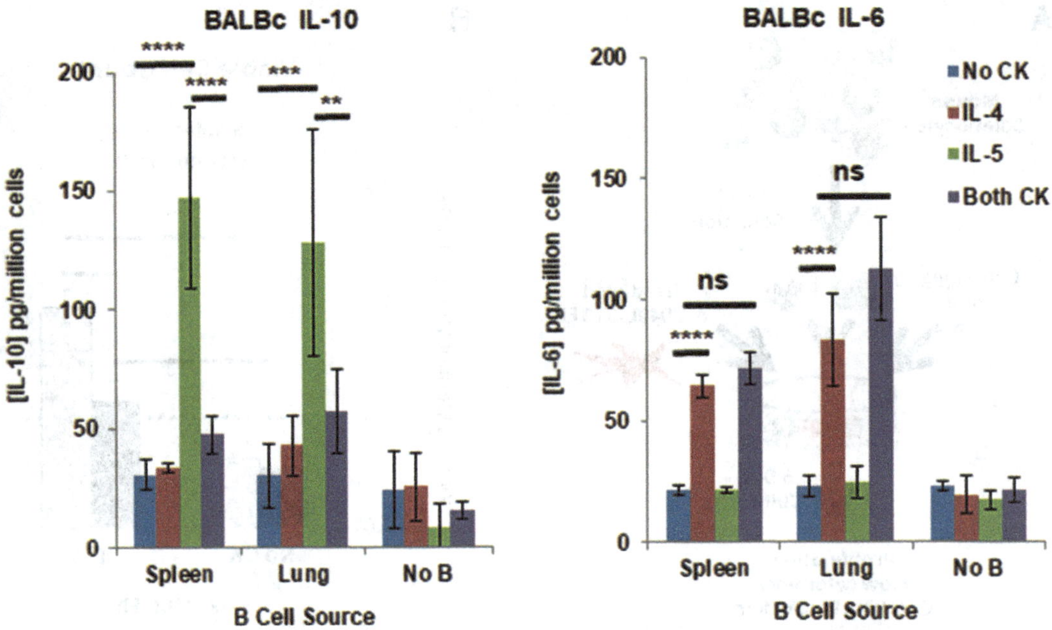

Fig. 5 IL-5 induces B-cell IL-10 production but is antagonized by IL-4. Purified $CD19^+$ B cells from the indicated sources were cultured on mCD40L Fb with or without (no CK) 50 ng/mL of the indicated cytokines. Culture supernatants were collected on day 5, and the IL-6 and IL-10 cytokines were quantified by ELISA using a standard curve. Cultures were performed in duplicate for n = 5 individual mice (10 wells/condition). "No B" refers to mCD40L Fb cells cultured with cytokines. Data are mean ± standard deviation. $^{**}P < 0.02$, $^{***}P < 0.01$, $^{****}P < 0.001$, ns = not significant

5. Place the plate in a humidified 37 °C incubator that has a supply of 5% CO_2 for the desired length of culture, which is optimally 5 days in our experience.
6. At the end of culture, cells are removed for counting, flow cytometry, and functional assays. Supernatants are instead collected for the analysis of IL-6 and IL-10 release by ELISA (*see* **Note 19**). An example of cytokine production by purified B cells from the spleens and lungs of naïve BALB/c mice is shown in Fig. 5, and more information can be found in reference [67].

3.3 Phenotypic Analysis of Killer B Cells

3.3.1 Flow Cytometric Characterization of $FasL^+$ B Cells

1. Prepare single-cell suspensions of cells in PBS as described in Subheading 3.1. or use cells that have come from cultures described in Subheading 3.2.2.
2. Distribute one million cells into flow cytometry tubes. Centrifuge tubes for 5 min at 450 × *g* and remove supernatant, then resuspend the cell pellet with a vortex.
3. Wash cells two times with flow cytometry buffer by centrifuging for 5 min at 450 × *g*. Pour off supernatant and resuspend cell pellets in small volume of buffer left behind.

4. Add 1 μg of FcBlock antibody to each sample and incubate for 10 min at 4 °C.
5. Prepare the desired antibody staining solutions from the list in Table 2 (1 μg of each antibody/million cells) for multi-color staining in flow cytometry buffer containing manufacturer suggested amount of propidium iodide (*see* **Note 20**). Adjust volume of staining mix to 50 μl per sample, then add antibody solution to each tube and incubate at 4 °C for 30 min.
6. Wash cells two times in flow cytometry buffer by centrifuging for 5 min at 450 × *g* and resuspend the final pellet in 300 μl of flow buffer.
7. Read samples as soon as possible on an appropriate flow cytometer that has been precalibrated for voltage and compensation settings using cells that are labeled with a single color and can collect fluorescence data for FITC, PE, PECy7, and APC. Analyze the flow data using an appropriate software package (*see* **Note 21**).
8. A representative analysis of the phenotypic characterization of $FasL^+$ B cells is shown in Fig. 2. The positioning of gates identifying specific populations is based on staining with an isotype control antibody. Additional data on the phenotype of cultured B cells can be found in reference [59].

3.3.2 Western Blot Analysis for Cellular FasL Expression

1. Expand mouse $FasL^+$ B cells in vitro as described in Subheading 3.2.2.
2. Remove stimulated B cells from culture plates and transfer to 15 mL centrifuge tubes for 5 min at 450 × *g*.
3. Wash stimulated B cells three times with 10 mL of PBS. Resuspend cells to five million cells/mL in PBS and move 1 mL of cell suspension to a 1.5-mL centrifuge tube.
4. Centrifuge cells at 350 × *g* for 10 min and remove PBS by aspiration. Disrupt cell pellet by agitating the centrifuge tubes with a vortex. Add 300 μl of SDS lysis buffer to cells and immediately mix thoroughly.
5. Heat lysed cells to 100 °C for 15 min. Make sure caps are secured to prevent sample loss. Samples can then be stored for several months at −80 °C or cooled on ice for immediate use.
6. Centrifuge lysed samples for 5 min at 2000 × *g* and move supernatant to a new tube.
7. Assemble gel box for electrophoresis using 4–20% Tris-Glycine 12-well gels. Fill with 1 × SDS running buffer. Make sure the gel box is properly assembled and that buffer is not leaking from the upper chamber.

8. With a syringe and needle, gently remove any bubbles from each well by squirting SDS running buffer into the wells.
9. Add 20 μl of cell lysate or protein standards to each well using gel-loading pipette tips.
10. Connect to power source and run at 175 volts for 60–90 min. Stop electrophoresis when the leading edges of the samples are just reaching the bottom of the gel.
11. Fill transfer box spacer with water and freeze to −80 °C prior to protein transfer.
12. For each gel, cut four pieces of extra-thick, highly absorbent paper and one piece of PVDF membrane. Each should be slightly larger than the gel.
13. In trays, soak sponges and paper in 1× transfer buffer and pre-wet the membrane with methanol prior to assembling transfer cassettes.
14. Assemble transfer cassettes, ensuring that no bubbles exist between any of the internal layers. Place assembled cassettes into transfer box, along with the frozen spacer. Fill with transfer buffer until the cassettes are submerged. Proteins will move toward the anode (red side) of the transfer box, so arrange the cassette so that the proteins will transfer toward the membrane.
15. Place transfer box in an ice bucket and cover with ice. Connect to power source and run for 1 h at 100 volts.
16. Briefly allow the transfer box to cool and then remove cassettes from the transfer box. Disassemble each cassette carefully, using a small forceps to remove the membrane from the gel.
17. Place membranes in trays "protein-side" up. Add 15 mL of milk blocking buffer to membranes and incubate at room temperature with gentle agitation for 1 h.
18. Remove milk blocking buffer and wash the membrane three times with 15 mL of wash buffer. For each wash, incubate membranes at room temperature for 5 min with gentle agitation. Do not allow the membrane to dry out.
19. Prepare the polyclonal rabbit anti-FasL primary antibody at the recommended concentration in BSA blocking buffer. Incubate membrane with the primary antibody overnight at 4 °C with gentle agitation.
20. Remove primary antibody solution and wash the membrane three times with 15 mL of wash buffer. For each wash, incubate membranes at room temperature for 15 min with gentle agitation. Do not allow the membrane to dry out.
21. Prepare secondary antibody at recommended concentration in milk blocking buffer. Incubate membrane with the secondary antibody for 1 h at room temperature with gentle agitation.

22. Remove secondary antibody solution and wash the membrane as in **step 20**.
23. Prepare ECL reagent according to manufacturer's specification. Dry membranes briefly and add 500 μl of ECL to each membrane. Wait 1 min and remove any excess ECL from the membrane before developing.
24. In a dark room, place a radiographic film on the membrane for between 1 and 30 min. Remove film and develop (*see* **Note 22**). After development, membranes can be stripped and re-probed for another protein (*see* **Note 23**).
25. Representative western blot data of FasL from cultured mouse B cells have been published [59].

3.4 Phenotypic Analysis of FasL$^+$ Exosomes

In the course of our studies looking at FasL expression by Epstein-Barr virus-transformed human B lymphoblastoid cells, it was found that the cells had intracellular stores of FasL in the form of exosomes [68]. The following methods were developed to measure FasL expression in exosomes extracted from mouse spleen and to determine if non-transformed mouse B cells were a likely source of FasL$^+$ exosomes. To determine the effects of antigen-specific activation on levels of FasL$^+$ exosomes in mouse spleen, we used a standard method of subcutaneous in vivo peptide immunization in two strains of T-cell receptor transgenic mice [25]. Exosomes of immunized and unimmunized mice can then be isolated using the method outlined in Fig. 3 and presented in Subheadings 3.1.6 or 3.1.7, and the levels of FasL on these exosomes can be analyzed by the following protocols.

3.4.1 Western Blot for FasL Protein in Exosomes

1. Starting with the filtered spleen extract (*see* Subheading 3.1.6, **step 4**) or culture supernatant (*see* Subheading 3.1.7, **step 4**), transfer cell-free fluid to ultracentrifuge tubes making sure to balance them carefully.
2. Centrifuge for 2 h at 110,000 × *g* to pellet the exosomes. Remove the supernatant and resuspend the pellet in 100–300 μL of SDS lysis buffer.
3. Proceed with the standard Western blot protocol described in Subheading 3.3.2.
4. Western blot results from an experiment in which total exosomes were purified from spleen extracts of unimmunized and collagen-immunized mice (day 28) are shown in Fig. 6a.

3.4.2 FasL ELISA of Exosome Protein Extracts

1. ELISA for FasL can be performed directly on the cell-free extracts of mouse spleen or culture supernatants of mouse B cells without ultracentrifugation.

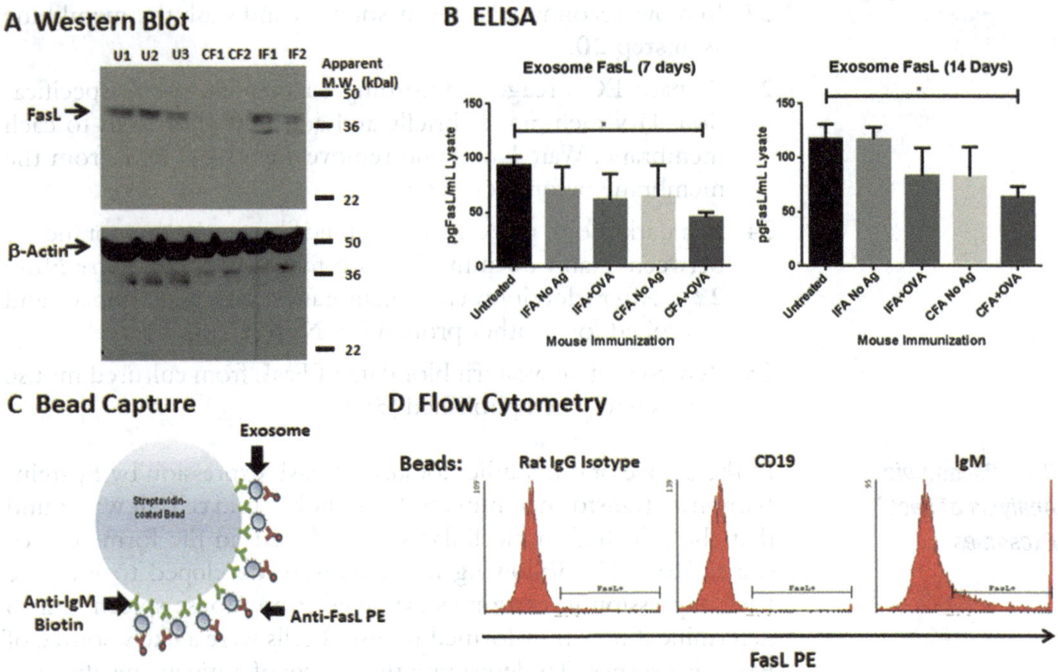

Fig. 6 Assays used to detect FasL$^+$ exosomes present in the mouse spleen. (**a**) Whole spleens were removed 28 days after immunization of DBA/1 mice with type II collagen emulsified in complete (CF1 & CF2) or incomplete (IF1 & IF2) Freund's adjuvant, or unimmunized mice (U1 to U3). Cell-free supernatant was collected as described, while exosomes were isolated by ultracentrifugation and then Western blot was performed. (**b**) Exosomes were isolated by ultracentrifugation method from spleens of DO11.10 mice after immunization with adjuvants with or without OVA peptide. ELISA was performed with commercial kits. (**c**) Scheme of exosome bead capture using biotin anti-IgM capture antibody and PE-conjugated anti-mouse FasL antibody. (**d**) Representative flow cytometry data of FasL$^+$ exosomes captured by anti-IgM but not with anti-CD19 or isotype control antibodies

2. If further purification or concentration is desired, proceed to ultracentrifugation at 110,000 × *g* for 2 h, and then resuspend the pellet in 1 × RIPA buffer containing protease inhibitors.
3. ELISA can be performed using a commercially available kit and following manufacturer's protocol. Figure 6b shows the results of an experiment in which OVA TCR-transgenic DO11.10 mice were immunized with incomplete Freund's adjuvant (IFA) or complete Freund's adjuvant (CFA) emulsified with either $OVA_{323-339}$ peptide or vehicle (1× PBS) control. Cell-free spleen extracts were prepared as shown in Fig. 3 on day 7 and day 14 after immunization using 3 mL of 1× PBS buffer.

3.4.3 Bead Capture of Exosomes for Flow Cytometric Analysis

Exosome analysis by flow cytometry is difficult due to their very small size. Therefore, it is necessary to first capture the exosomes on a larger substrate. An example is depicted in Fig. 6c and d in which 10–12 μm streptavidin-coated polystyrene beads were used.

1. Label beads with biotinylated anti-mouse CD19, anti-mouse IgM, or isotype control antibodies at 1 μg/mL for 1 h at room temperature.
2. Unbound capture antibody is washed away using 1× PBS by pelleting the beads at 500 × *g* for 5 min and by removing the supernatant. Repeat this step twice.
3. Incubate one million capture antibody-coated beads with cell-free extract from each spleen overnight at 4 °C with gentle rotation.
4. Wash away unbound exosomes from the beads by centrifuging at 500 × *g* for 5 min with two repeated washes in 1× PBS.
5. Perform a final wash using flow cytometry buffer. Add PE-conjugated anti-mouse FasL antibody diluted in flow cytometry staining buffer according to manufacturer's instruction and/or titration assays. Incubate at 4 °C for 30 min.
6. Wash twice in flow cytometry buffer and resuspend the final pellet in 300 μl of flow cytometry buffer. Flow cytometry can then be performed on the bead-captured exosomes using methods similar to those used for cells.

3.5 Functional Assays

3.5.1 Measurement of IL-10 Production by FasL$^+$ B Cells Using Intracellular Staining

1. Isolate FasL$^+$ B cells from splenocytes by FACS as described in Subheading 3.1.5 (*see* **Note 24**). Wash sorted B cells twice with PBS by centrifuging for 5 min at 450 × *g* and resuspend in B-cell culture medium.
2. In a 24-well plate, culture two million B cells with 50 ng/mL PMA, 1 μg/mL ionomycin, 5 μg/mL LPS, and GolgiStop at manufacturer's recommended concentration, in a final volume of 500 μl. For control conditions, prepare a triplicate set of wells in which B cells are treated with just monensin, or in which PMA, ionomycin, and LPS are added in the absence of monensin in culture medium.
3. After 5 h in culture, collect B cells and wash three times with PBS by centrifuging for 5 min at 450 × *g*. Then, fix in 4% paraformaldehyde for 20 min at room temperature.
4. Wash fixed cells three times with cold PBS, and twice with FACS buffer by centrifuging for 5 min at 450 × *g*. Permeabilize cells with saponin buffer for 15 min at room temperature. Spin down permeabilized cells and remove supernatant.
5. Prepare antibody solutions diluting the FITC-conjugated anti-IL-10 antibody and an appropriate isotype control antibody in saponin buffer according to manufacturer's instructions and/or titration assay. Add antibody solutions to permeabilized cells and incubate for 30 min in the dark at room temperature.

6. Wash cells once in permeabilization buffer, and then twice with flow cytometry buffer. Resuspend cells in 300 μL flow cytometry buffer and analyze using an appropriate flow cytometer.

3.5.2 Measurement of Peptide-Specific, FasL-Dependent Killing of Mouse T_H Cells by Killer B Cells

The following protocol describes in detail the method that was used in a published study which demonstrated that the severity of collagen-induced arthritis was inversely correlated with the presence of $CD5^+$ B lymphocytes expressing FasL [25]. The method can be adapted to any strain of mice in which the interaction between B and T lymphocytes is peptide-specific.

1. Harvest splenocytes from TCR-transgenic mice following protocol in Subheading 3.1.1.
2. Stimulate splenocytes at the final concentration of 5×10^6 cell/mL in 24-well plates in standard RPMI medium supplemented with 2 μg/mL Concanavalin A for 3 days.
3. Remove stimulated splenocytes from culture plates and wash once with PBS centrifuging for 5 min at 450 × *g*. Determine cell number.
4. Isolate $CD4^+$ T cells from stimulated splenocytes by immunomagnetic separation using negative isolation. After isolation, count $CD4^+$ T cells and resuspend in standard RPMI medium.
5. Culture stimulated $CD4^+$ T cells (**step 2**) overnight at a 1:1 ratio with purified B cells stimulated as described in Subheading 3.2.2. Following overnight culture, collect cells into flow staining tubes and stain with 1 μg of PE-anti-CD4 per million cells for 30 min at 4 °C.
6. Wash cells once with PBS, then once with Annexin V buffer centrifuging for 5 min at 450 × *g*.
7. Prepare FITC-Annexin V and PI solutions in Annexin V buffer using the manufacturer's recommended concentration for FITC-Annexin V, and a 1:500 dilution of PI. Add 50 μl of Annexin V/PI solution to each sample and incubate for 15 min in the dark at room temperature.
8. Dilute samples with 300 μl of Annexin buffer and run immediately on an appropriate flow cytometer.
9. Recent $CD4^+$ T-cell apoptosis is determined on the basis of cells that are $AnnexinV^+$ and PI^{neg}, while cells that are PI^+ are in later stages of apoptosis or are dead.
10. To determine the role of FasL in the apoptotic response, it is recommended that a neutralizing anti-mouse FasL antibody be used or that B cells are purified from mice carrying the *gld* mutation that eliminates FasL function.

4 Notes

1. The required timing for fibroblasts irradiation is solely dependent on the strength of the radiation source. The time to reach 300 Gray is device-specific and should be calculated based on the irradiator being used. Other methods of stopping the proliferation of fibroblasts, such as through incubation with mitomycin C, may work but have not been tested by our laboratory.
2. This protocol is designed for preparation of spleen cells from individual mice and can be adapted for extraction of cells from pools of 5–20 spleens from a group of mice.
3. The timing of ACK lysis may vary and should be tested for each batch of lysis buffer.
4. In our experience, using medium containing 10% FCS to stop the ACK lysis gives more consistent results in terms of cell viability than using medium alone or balanced salt solutions without proteins.
5. Removing most of the solution at this step makes it much easier to chop the lung tissue up into fine pieces and avoid dilution of the dispersal solution.
6. For best results, perform **steps 3–5** of Subheading 3.1.2 on one sample at a time to avoid drying out of the lung tissue.
7. If the lung tissue chunks are too large to go through the needle, it may work better to use the syringe without the needle for the first few pipetting steps and then attach the needle to the full syringe before proceeding.
8. For best results, hold the mouse abdomen up and insert the needle at a 30° angle to a depth of 0.3–0.5 cm in the lower middle of the abdomen.
9. Liquid pressure may force the solution to initially exit in a powerful stream.
10. Repositioning of the needle and massage of the abdomen may be necessary to increase the yield of lavage fluid, which should be 6–8 mL depending on the amount of solution injected initially.
11. The presence of blood in lavage fluid is not expected or desired but is also not uncommon using this procedure. If at the end of the centrifugation the pellet appears red, sign that a significant contamination by red blood cells is present, an ACK lysis step can be performed.
12. If the sort yield is too low, positive selection of $CD19^+$ B cells by magnetic bead separation may be desired. In our experience, the best results were obtained when the $FasL^+$ B cells were sorted by the most rapid and efficient means available.

13. The exosomes should be in a small visible brown pellet that will be difficult to get back into suspension. Since the second ultracentrifugation step is followed by the addition of SDS lysis buffer to the pellet, it is not necessary to completely resuspend this pellet.
14. For functional assays, flow cytometry or imaging applications, resuspend pelleted exosomes in sterile 1× PBS. For Western blot, use SDS lysis buffer while to analyze and quantify exosomes proteins by ELISA, it is best to use 1× RIPA buffer containing protease inhibitors.
15. A lentiviral vector was used to stably transduce NIH3T3 fibroblasts as described in Morita et al. [65]. This mCD40L-Fb line was provided to us as a gift from Dr. David Fox (Univ. of Michigan) with the permission of the creator of the cell line, Dr. Kevin McDonagh (Univ. of Kentucky). Those interested in obtaining this cell line are encouraged to contact Dr. Steven K. Lundy (sklundya2@gmail.com) or Dr. David A. Fox (dfox@umich.edu). Substitution of this stimulation with an agonist anti-CD40 antibody does lead to stimulation of B cells with similar functions but is very inferior in terms of B-cell proliferation and yield.
16. Recommended medium for NIH3T3 contains adult bovine serum that has not been heat-inactivated. Substitution with fetal or newborn calf serum is strongly discouraged. Note that heat-inactivation of adult bovine serum may result in coagulation into a gel.
17. In our experience, seeding a flask with 0.5 million fibroblasts will yield a confluent monolayer in 4–5 days. Amounts can be adjusted if different timing is desired.
18. This concentration of irradiated fibroblasts typically results in a confluent monolayer if the following amounts are used: 50 μL (96-well plate), 200 μL (48 well), 0.5 mL (24 well), or 2 mL (T25cm^2 flask). Adding the B cells and fibroblasts to the wells at the same time is preferred over trying to carefully layer the B cells on top of a preformed monolayer since the fibroblasts have a tendency to lift off of the bottom of the plate in sheets in the latter scenario.
19. Culture supernatants can be stored overnight at 4 °C or for several months at −80 °C prior to performing ELISA. If supernatants are stored in the freezer, then allow to thaw overnight at 4 °C prior to performing ELISA.
20. Examples of combinations commonly used in our laboratory are the following: PE-anti-FasL/FITC-anti-CD1d/APC-anti-CD5/PECy7-anti-CD19, PE-anti-FasL/FITC-anti-CD24/APC-anti-CD19/PECy7-anti-IgM, PE-anti-FasL/FITC-anti-CD19/APC-anti-CD5/PECy7-anti-IgM.

21. To analyze flow cytometry data, we have used FlowJo and CytoBank. Moreover, we recommend using the guidelines for gating live, single, lymphocytes established by Herzenberg et al. [69].
22. Development of the radiographic film for FasL typically takes up to 30 min while the beta actin signal develops in 1–2 min maximum.
23. To do so, incubate membrane with stripping buffer for 30–60 min at 50 °C with gentle agitation. Rinse the membrane with running water for several minutes and wash the membrane three times with 15 mL of wash buffer. For each wash, incubate membranes at room temperature for 15 min with gentle agitation. To re-probe the stripped membrane, repeat **steps 18–24** of Subheading 3.3.2. Membranes were probed first with anti-FasL antibody, then stripped and re-probed with anti-beta actin antibody.
24. Extensive work was done attempting to simultaneously stain B cells for surface or intracellular FasL and intracellular IL-10. However, measurement of IL-10 requires B-cell activation with mitogens in the presence of agents that block cytokine release from the Golgi apparatus, and these treatments consistently lead to shedding of surface FasL and exosome release [59]. Therefore, sorting of $FasL^+$ B cells followed by activation and measurement of intracellular IL-10 is the preferred method of determining the frequency of IL-10^+ B cells among the $FasL^+$ B-cell subset.

References

1. Roths JB, Murphy ED, Eicher EM (1984) A new mutation, gld, that produces lymphoproliferation and autoimmunity in C3H/HeJ mice. J Exp Med 159(1):1–20
2. Sobel ES, Kakkanaiah VN, Cohen PL, Eisenberg RA (1993) Correction of gld autoimmunity by co-infusion of normal bone marrow suggests that gld is a mutation of the Fas ligand gene. Int Immunol 5(10):1275–1278
3. Lynch DH, Watson ML, Alderson MR, Baum PR, Miller RE, Tough T, Gibson M, Davis-Smith T, Smith CA, Hunter K et al (1994) The mouse Fas-ligand gene is mutated in gld mice and is part of a TNF family gene cluster. Immunity 1(2):131–136
4. Takahashi T, Tanaka M, Brannan CI, Jenkins NA, Copeland NG, Suda T, Nagata S (1994) Generalized lymphoproliferative disease in mice, caused by a point mutation in the Fas ligand. Cell 76(6):969–976
5. Hahne M, Peitsch MC, IrmLer M, Schroter M, Lowin B, Rousseau M, Bron C, Renno T, French L, Tschopp J (1995) Characterization of the non-functional Fas ligand of gld mice. Int Immunol 7(9):1381–1386
6. Adachi M, Watanabe-Fukunaga R, Nagata S (1993) Aberrant transcription caused by the insertion of an early transposable element in an intron of the Fas antigen gene of lpr mice. Proc Natl Acad Sci U S A 90(5):1756–1760
7. Wu J, Zhou T, He J, Mountz JD (1993) Autoimmune disease in mice due to integration of an endogenous retrovirus in an apoptosis gene. J Exp Med 178(2):461–468
8. Nagata S, Suda T (1995) Fas and Fas ligand: lpr and gld mutations. Immunol Today 16 (1):39–43
9. Fisher GH, Rosenberg FJ, Straus SE, Dale JK, Middleton LA, Lin AY, Strober W, Lenardo

MJ, Puck JM (1995) Dominant interfering Fas gene mutations impair apoptosis in a human autoimmune lymphoproliferative syndrome. Cell 81(6):935–946

10. Rieux-Laucat F, Le Deist F, Hivroz C, Roberts IA, Debatin KM, Fischer A, de Villartay JP (1995) Mutations in Fas associated with human lymphoproliferative syndrome and autoimmunity. Science 268(5215):1347–1349
11. Bleesing JJ (2005) Sorting out the causes of ALPS. J Pediatr 147(5):571–574. https://doi.org/10.1016/j.jpeds.2005.09.025
12. Infante AJ, Britton HA, DeNapoli T, Middelton LA, Lenardo MJ, Jackson CE, Wang J, Fleisher T, Straus SE, Puck JM (1998) The clinical spectrum in a large kindred with autoimmune lymphoproliferative syndrome caused by a Fas mutation that impairs lymphocyte apoptosis. J Pediatr 133(5):629–633
13. Sneller MC, Straus SE, Jaffe ES, Jaffe JS, Fleisher TA, Stetler-Stevenson M, Strober W (1992) A novel lymphoproliferative/autoimmune syndrome resembling murine lpr/gld disease. J Clin Invest 90(2):334–341. https://doi.org/10.1172/JCI115867
14. Magerus-Chatinet A, Stolzenberg MC, Loffredo MS, Neven B, Schaffner C, Ducrot N, Arkwright PD, Bader-Meunier B, Barbot J, Blanche S, Casanova JL, Debre M, Ferster A, Fieschi C, Florkin B, Galambrun C, Hermine O, Lambotte O, Solary E, Thomas C, Le Deist F, Picard C, Fischer A, Rieux-Laucat F (2009) FAS-L, IL-10, and double-negative CD4- CD8- TCR alpha/beta + T cells are reliable markers of autoimmune lymphoproliferative syndrome (ALPS) associated with FAS loss of function. Blood 113(13):3027–3030. https://doi.org/10.1182/blood-2008-09-179630
15. Stroncek DF, Carter LB, Procter JL, Dale JK, Straus SE (2001) RBC autoantibodies in autoimmune lymphoproliferative syndrome. Transfusion 41(1):18–23
16. Wu J, Wilson J, He J, Xiang L, Schur PH, Mountz JD (1996) Fas ligand mutation in a patient with systemic lupus erythematosus and lymphoproliferative disease. J Clin Invest 98(5):1107–1113
17. Kojima T, Horiuchi T, Nishizaka H, Sawabe T, Higuchi M, Harashima SI, Yoshizawa S, Tsukamoto H, Nagasawa K, Niho Y (2000) Analysis of fas ligand gene mutation in patients with systemic lupus erythematosus. Arthritis Rheum 43(1):135–139
18. Atkinson EA, Bleackley RC (1995) Mechanisms of lysis by cytotoxic T cells. Crit Rev Immunol 15(3–4):359–384
19. Oshimi Y, Oda S, Honda Y, Nagata S, Miyazaki S (1996) Involvement of Fas ligand and Fas-mediated pathway in the cytotoxicity of human natural killer cells. J Immunol 157(7):2909–2915
20. Hahne M, Renno T, Schroeter M, IrmLer M, French L, Bornard T, MacDonald HR, Tschopp J (1996) Activated B cells express functional Fas ligand. Eur J Immunol 26(3):721–724
21. Lundy SK (2009) Killer B lymphocytes: the evidence and the potential. Inflammation Research 58(7):345–357. https://doi.org/10.1007/s00011-009-0014-x
22. Lundy SK, Lerman SP, Boros DL (2001) Soluble egg antigen-stimulated T helper lymphocyte apoptosis and evidence for cell death mediated by FasL(+) T and B cells during murine Schistosoma mansoni infection. Infect Immun 69(1):271–280
23. Lundy SK, Boros DL (2002) Fas ligand-expressing B-1a lymphocytes mediate CD4(+)-T-cell apoptosis during schistosomal infection: induction by interleukin 4 (IL-4) and IL-10. Infect Immun 70(2):812–819
24. Lundy SK, Berlin AA, Martens TF, Lukacs NW (2005) Deficiency of regulatory B cells increases allergic airway inflammation. Inflammation Research 54(12):514–521. https://doi.org/10.1007/s00011-005-1387-0
25. Lundy SK, Fox DA (2009) Reduced Fas ligand-expressing splenic CD5+ B lymphocytes in severe collagen-induced arthritis. Arthritis Res Ther 11(4):R128. https://doi.org/10.1186/ar2795
26. Tian J, Zekzer D, Hanssen L, Lu Y, Olcott A, Kaufman DL (2001) Lipopolysaccharide-activated B cells down-regulate Th1 immunity and prevent autoimmune diabetes in nonobese diabetic mice. J Immunol 167(2):1081–1089
27. Montandon R, Korniotis S, Layseca-Espinosa E, Gras C, Megret J, Ezine S, Dy M, Zavala F (2013) Innate pro-B-cell progenitors protect against type 1 diabetes by regulating autoimmune effector T cells. Proc Natl Acad Sci U S A 110(24):E2199–E2208. https://doi.org/10.1073/pnas.1222446110
28. Bonardelle D, Benihoud K, Kiger N, Bobe P (2005) B lymphocytes mediate Fas-dependent cytotoxicity in MRL/lpr mice. J Leukoc Biol 78(5):1052–1059. https://doi.org/10.1189/jlb.0904536
29. Zuniga E, Motran CC, Montes CL, Yagita H, Gruppi A (2002) Trypanosoma cruzi infection selectively renders parasite-specific IgG+ B lymphocytes susceptible to Fas/Fas ligand-mediated fratricide. J Immunol 168(8):3965–3973
30. Minagawa R, Okano S, Tomita Y, Kishihara K, Yamada H, Nomoto K, Shimada M,

Maehara Y, Sugimachi K, Yoshikai Y, Nomoto K (2004) The critical role of Fas-Fas ligand interaction in donor-specific transfusion-induced tolerance to H-Y antigen. Transplantation 78(6):799–806. https://doi.org/10.1097/01.tp.0000129799.96439.6f

31. Griffith TS, Brunner T, Fletcher SM, Green DR, Ferguson TA (1995) Fas ligand-induced apoptosis as a mechanism of immune privilege. Science 270(5239):1189–1192
32. Mohan RR, Liang Q, Kim WJ, Helena MC, Baerveldt F, Wilson SE (1997) Apoptosis in the cornea: further characterization of Fas/Fas ligand system. Exp Eye Res 65(4):575–589
33. Stuart PM, Griffith TS, Usui N, Pepose J, Yu X, Ferguson TA (1997) CD95 ligand (FasL)-induced apoptosis is necessary for corneal allograft survival. J Clin Invest 99(3):396–402
34. Jorgensen A, Wiencke AK, la Cour M, Kaestel CG, Madsen HO, Hamann S, Lui GM, Scherfig E, Prause JU, Svejgaard A, Odum N, Nissen MH, Ropke C (1998) Human retinal pigment epithelial cell-induced apoptosis in activated T cells. Invest Ophthalmol Vis Sci 39(9):1590–1599
35. Sapi E, Brown WD, Aschkenazi S, Lim C, Munoz A, Kacinski BM, Rutherford T, Mor G (2002) Regulation of Fas ligand expression by estrogen in normal ovary. J Soc Gynecol Investig 9(4):243–250
36. Li H, Ren J, Dhabuwala CB, Shichi H (1997) Immunotolerance induced by intratesticular antigen priming: expression of TGF-beta, Fas and Fas ligand. Ocul Immunol Inflamm 5 (2):75–84
37. Uckan D, Steele A, Cherry WBY, Chamizo W, Koutsonikolis A, Gilbert-Barness E, Good RA (1997) Trophoblasts express Fas ligand: a proposed mechanism for immune privilege in placenta and maternal invasion. Mol Hum Reprod 3(8):655–662. https://doi.org/10.1093/molehr/3.8.655
38. Kauma SW, Huff TF, Hayes N, Nilkaeo A (1999) Placental Fas ligand expression is a mechanism for maternal immune tolerance to the fetus. J Clin Endocrinol Metab 84 (6):2188–2194
39. Silvestris F, Tucci M, Cafforio P, Dammacco F (2001) Fas-L up-regulation by highly malignant myeloma plasma cells: role in the pathogenesis of anemia and disease progression. Blood 97(5):1155–1164
40. Tinhofer I, Marschitz I, Kos M, Henn T, Egle A, Villunger A, Greil R (1998) Differential sensitivity of CD4+ and CD8+ T lymphocytes to the killing efficacy of Fas (Apo-1/CD95) ligand+ tumor cells in B chronic lymphocytic leukemia. Blood 91(11):4273–4281
41. Lettau M, Paulsen M, Kabelitz D, Janssen O (2009) FasL expression and reverse signalling. Results Probl Cell Differ 49:49–61. https://doi.org/10.1007/400_2008_21
42. Kavurma MM, Khachigian LM (2003) Signaling and transcriptional control of Fas ligand gene expression. Cell Death Differ 10 (1):36–44
43. Chow WA, Fang JJ, Yee JK (2000) The IFN regulatory factor family participates in regulation of Fas ligand gene expression in T cells. J Immunol 164(7):3512–3518
44. Sayed D, He M, Hong C, Gao S, Rane S, Yang Z, Abdellatif M (2010) MicroRNA-21 is a downstream effector of AKT that mediates its antiapoptotic effects via suppression of Fas ligand. J Biol Chem 285(26):20281–20290. https://doi.org/10.1074/jbc.M110.109207
45. Li JH, Rosen D, Ronen D, Behrens CK, Krammer PH, Clark WR, Berke G (1998) The regulation of CD95 ligand expression and function in CTL. J Immunol 161(8):3943–3949
46. Zuccato E, Blott EJ, Holt O, Sigismund S, Shaw M, Bossi G, Griffiths GM (2007) Sorting of Fas ligand to secretory lysosomes is regulated by mono-ubiquitylation and phosphorylation. J Cell Sci 120(Pt 1):191–199. https://doi.org/10.1242/jcs.03315
47. Mincheff M, Loukinov D, Zoubak S, Hammett M, Meryman H (1998) Fas and Fas ligand expression on human peripheral blood leukocytes. Vox Sang 74(2):113–121
48. Martinez-Lorenzo MJ, Anel A, Gamen S, Monle NI, Lasierra P, Larrad L, Pineiro A, Alava MA, Naval J (1999) Activated human T cells release bioactive Fas ligand and APO2 ligand in microvesicles. J Immunol 163 (3):1274–1281
49. Jodo S, Xiao S, Hohlbaum A, Strehlow D, Marshak-Rothstein A, Ju ST (2001) Apoptosis-inducing membrane vesicles. A novel agent with unique properties. J Biol Chem 276(43):39938–39944. https://doi.org/10.1074/jbc.M107005200
50. Sabapatha A, Gercel-Taylor C, Taylor DD (2006) Specific isolation of placenta-derived exosomes from the circulation of pregnant women and their immunoregulatory consequences. Am J Reprod Immunol 56 (5–6):345–355. https://doi.org/10.1111/j.1600-0897.2006.00435.x
51. McKechnie NM, King BC, Fletcher E, Braun G (2006) Fas-ligand is stored in secretory lysosomes of ocular barrier epithelia and released with microvesicles. Exp Eye Res 83 (2):304–314. https://doi.org/10.1016/j.exer.2005.11.028

52. Kang SM, Schneider DB, Lin Z, Hanahan D, Dichek DA, Stock PG, Baekkeskov S (1997) Fas ligand expression in islets of Langerhans does not confer immune privilege and instead targets them for rapid destruction. Nat Med 3 (7):738–743
53. Takeuchi T, Ueki T, Nishimatsu H, Kajiwara T, Ishida T, Jishage K, Ueda O, Suzuki H, Li B, Moriyama N, Kitamura T (1999) Accelerated rejection of Fas ligand-expressing heart grafts. J Immunol 162(1):518–522
54. Gregory MS, Repp AC, Holhbaum AM, Saff RR, Marshak-Rothstein A, Ksander BR (2002) Membrane Fas ligand activates innate immunity and terminates ocular immune privilege. J Immunol 169(5):2727–2735
55. Mariani SM, Matiba B, BaumLer C, Krammer PH (1995) Regulation of cell surface APO-1/Fas (CD95) ligand expression by metalloproteases. Eur J Immunol 25(8):2303–2307
56. Powell WC, Fingleton B, Wilson CL, Boothby M, Matrisian LM (1999) The metalloproteinase matrilysin proteolytically generates active soluble Fas ligand and potentiates epithelial cell apoptosis. Curr Biol 9 (24):1441–1447
57. Sano Y, Yamada J, Ishino Y, Adachi W, Kawasaki S, Suzuki T, Kinoshita S, Okuyama T, Azuma N (2002) Non-cleavable mutant Fas ligand transfection of donor cornea abrogates ocular immune privilege. Exp Eye Res 75(4):475–483
58. Lundy SK, Klinker MW, Fox DA (2015) Killer B lymphocytes and their fas ligand positive exosomes as inducers of immune tolerance. Front Immunol 6:122. https://doi.org/10.3389/fimmu.2015.00122
59. Klinker MW, Reed TJ, Fox DA, Lundy SK (2013) Interleukin-5 supports the expansion of Fas ligand-expressing killer B cells that induce antigen-specific apoptosis of CD4(+) T cells and secrete Interleukin-10. PLoS One 8 (8):e70131. https://doi.org/10.1371/journal.pone.0070131
60. Martin F, Kearney JF (2001) B1 cells: similarities and differences with other B cell subsets. Curr Opin Immunol 13(2):195–201
61. Yang Y, Tung JW, Ghosn EE, Herzenberg LA, Herzenberg LA (2007) Division and differentiation of natural antibody-producing cells in mouse spleen. Proc Natl Acad Sci U S A 104 (11):4542–4546. https://doi.org/10.1073/pnas.0700001104
62. Kantor AB, Stall AM, Adams S, Watanabe K, Herzenberg LA (1995) De novo development and self-replenishment of B cells. Int Immunol 7(1):55–68
63. Yoshimoto M, Montecino-Rodriguez E, Ferkowicz MJ, Porayette P, Shelley WC, Conway SJ, Dorshkind K, Yoder MC (2011) Embryonic day 9 yolk sac and intra-embryonic hemogenic endothelium independently generate a B-1 and marginal zone progenitor lacking B-2 potential. Proc Natl Acad Sci U S A 108 (4):1468–1473. https://doi.org/10.1073/pnas.1015841108
64. Klinker MW, Lundy SK (2012) Multiple mechanisms of immune suppression by B lymphocytes. Mol Med 18:123–137. https://doi.org/10.2119/molmed.2011.00333
65. Morita Y, Gupta R, Seidl KM, McDonagh KT, Fox DA (2005) Cytokine production by dendritic cells genetically engineered to express IL-4: induction of Th2 responses and differential regulation of IL-12 and IL-23 synthesis. J Gene Med 7(7):869–877. https://doi.org/10.1002/jgm.730
66. Schultze JL, Michalak S, Seamon MJ, Dranoff G, Jung K, Daley J, Delgado JC, Gribben JG, Nadler LM (1997) CD40-activated human B cells: an alternative source of highly efficient antigen presenting cells to generate autologous antigen-specific T cells for adoptive immunotherapy. J Clin Invest 100 (11):2757–2765. https://doi.org/10.1172/JCI119822
67. Taitano SH, van der Vlugt L, Shea MM, Yang J, Lukacs NW, Lundy SK (2018) Differential influence on regulatory B cells by TH2 cytokines affects protection in allergic airway disease. J Immunol 201(7):1865–1874. https://doi.org/10.4049/jimmunol.1800206
68. Klinker MW, Lizzio V, Reed TJ, Fox DA, Lundy SK (2014) Human B cell-derived Lymphoblastoid cell lines constitutively produce Fas ligand and secrete MHCII(+)FasL(+) killer Exosomes. Front Immunol 5:144. https://doi.org/10.3389/fimmu.2014.00144
69. Herzenberg LA, Tung J, Moore WA, Herzenberg LA, Parks DR (2006) Interpreting flow cytometry data: a guide for the perplexed. Nat Immunol 7(7):681–685. https://doi.org/10.1038/ni0706-681

Chapter 10

Characterization and Activity of TIM-1 and IL-10-Reporter Expressing Regulatory B Cells

Kanishka Mohib, David M. Rothstein, and Qing Ding

Abstract

In addition to their role in humoral immunity, B cells can exhibit regulatory activity. Such B cells have been termed regulatory B cells (Bregs). Bregs have been shown to inhibit inflammatory immune responses in a variety of autoimmune, alloimmune, and infectious settings. Breg activity is frequently IL-10-dependent, although a number of other mechanisms have been identified. However, our understanding of Bregs has been hampered by their rarity, lack of a specific phenotypic marker, and poor insight into their induction and maintenance. A variety of B-cell subsets enriched for IL-10$^+$ Bregs have been identified in multiple murine disease models that can adoptively transfer Breg activity. However, most of these B-cell subsets actually contain only a minority of all IL-10$^+$ B cells. In contrast, TIM-1 identifies over 70% of IL-10-producing B cells, irrespective of other markers. Thus, TIM-1 can be considered a broad marker for IL-10-expressing Bregs. Moreover, TIM-1 signaling plays a direct role in both the maintenance and induction of Bregs under physiological conditions, in response to both TIM-1 ligation and to apoptotic cells. TIM-1 expression has also been reported on IL-10$^+$ human B cells. Together, these findings suggest that TIM-1 may represent a novel therapeutic target for modulating the immune response and provide insight into the signals involved in the generation and induction of Bregs. Here, we provide the methods to analyze and purify the murine TIM-1$^+$ B-cell subset for further in vitro and in vivo experiments. We also provide methods for in vitro analysis and in vivo tracking of Bregs using IL-10-reporter mice.

Key words B cells, TIM-1, Regulatory B cells, Interleukin 10, Intracellular cytokine staining, Islet transplantation

1 Introduction

B cells not only give rise to antibody-secreting cells but also play an important role in regulating immune responses. B-cell deficiency or depletion can worsen autoimmunity and prevent allograft tolerance, while adoptive transfer of certain B-cell subpopulations can inhibit inflammation and allograft rejection, frequently in an IL-10-dependent fashion [1–4]. However, our understanding of such regulatory B cells (Bregs) is hampered because Bregs are rare and lack a specific marker. Moreover, IL-10 production by B cells capable of regulatory activity can generally be detected only after

Francesca Mion and Silvia Tonon (eds.), *Regulatory B Cells: Methods and Protocols*, Methods in Molecular Biology, vol. 2270, https://doi.org/10.1007/978-1-0716-1237-8_10, © Springer Science+Business Media, LLC, part of Springer Nature 2021

brief stimulation ex vivo [3, 5, 6]. Even then, only 1–2% of all B cells in the spleen, and even less in lymph nodes or bone marrow, are IL-10-competent. Various B-cell subsets have been shown to express IL-10 and exhibit regulatory activity, including Marginal Zone, Transitional, $CD1d^{hi}CD5^{+}$ B cells, and plasma cells [5, 7–11]. However, even in these enriched subsets, IL-10-expressing B cells are a minority (e.g., 5–15% of the population), and these subsets only represent a minority of all $IL\text{-}10^{+}$ B cells present (e.g., <20%) [6]. Thus, these subsets appear to contain the highest proportion of $IL\text{-}10^{+}$ B cells and are therefore capable of adoptively transferring regulatory activity rather than representing a true "Breg phenotype." This is further complicated by the fact that, in a growing number of models, Bregs appear to utilize mechanisms of suppression other than IL-10, and our understanding of such Bregs is even more limited [12–14]. A marker that can identify the majority of $IL\text{-}10^{+}$ B cells is critical for improved understanding of Breg biology, including the relationship between Bregs exhibiting different phenotypes, and reliable protocols for phenotypic identification and characterization of Bregs are of great importance to the study of B-cell-mediated immunoregulation.

T-cell (Transmembrane) Immunoglobulin domain and Mucin domain protein-1 (TIM-1) was first identified as a costimulatory molecule that regulates immune responses by modulating $CD4^{+}$ T-cell effector differentiation [15]. We found that, in vivo, murine TIM-1 is expressed at higher levels on B rather than T cells, both constitutively and after activation [3]. Importantly, $TIM\text{-}1^{+}$ B cells are 8- to 20-fold enriched for IL-10 across all major B-cell subpopulations, including transitional, marginal zone, follicular B cells, and B cells with a $CD1d^{hi}CD5^{+}$ phenotype. In fact, $TIM\text{-}1^{+}$ B cells comprise over 70% of all $IL\text{-}10^{+}$ B cells. Moreover, $TIM\text{-}1^{+}$ B cells and not $TIM\text{-}1^{-}$ B cells can transfer long-term acceptance of islet allografts to otherwise-untreated recipients in an IL-10–dependent fashion, and can also inhibit allergic airway disease. Thus, while TIM-1 is still not a specific marker for $IL\text{-}10^{+}$ Bregs (up to 15% of all $TIM\text{-}1^{+}$ B cells express IL-10), it is a broad marker for Bregs.

TIM-1 is also functionally important for Breg generation and induction. A low-affinity anti-TIM-1 antibody (clone RMT1–10) that normally promotes tolerance in mice, actually accelerated T-cell-mediated immune responsiveness in the absence of B cells, suggesting that B cells are the tolerogenic target of anti-TIM-1 [3]. The number of $TIM\text{-}1^{+}$ B cells approximately doubles and B-cell IL-10 expression increases approximately fivefold, following TIM-1 ligation. Thus, TIM-1 is an inclusive marker for IL-10-producing B cells regardless of other phenotypic markers, and TIM-1 ligation induces $IL\text{-}10^{+}$ Bregs. In addition, the role of TIM-1 in Breg homeostasis has been delineated using knock-in mice expressing $TIM1^{\Delta mucin}$ (a mutant version of TIM-1 lacking the mucin domain) [4, 16]. Mice expressing mutant TIM-1 exhibit a deficiency in IL-10$^+$ B cells, which increases with age, and this is associated with splenomegaly and spontaneous autoimmunity. TIM1$^{\Delta mucin}$ mice exhibit more aggressive allograft rejection that can be prevented by transfer of naïve wild-type TIM-1$^+$ B cells. When crossed onto a lupus-prone (mrl/lpr) background, TIM1$^{\Delta mucin}$ mice exhibited markedly accelerated lupus [16]. B-cell IL-10 can be induced by apoptotic cells, and TIM-1 is a known phosphatidylserine receptor [8, 15]. In this regard, B cells expressing TIM1$^{\Delta mucin}$ exhibit decreased phosphatidylserine binding and are unable to produce IL-10 in response to apoptotic cells [4]. While anti-TIM-1 binds TIM1$^{\Delta mucin}$, it fails to induce IL-10 [4]. These data suggest that TIM-1 signaling plays a direct role in Breg maintenance and induction both under physiological conditions (in response to apoptotic cells) and in response to TIM-1 ligation.

Thus, TIM-1 identifies a majority of IL-10$^+$ Bregs comprised of multiple canonical B-cell subsets and has a key functional role in development and induction of IL-10$^+$ B cells. Moreover, unlike intracellular cytokine staining, TIM-1 can be identified on freshly isolated live B cells, making it a very useful marker for Breg studies, including functional and transfer experiments. Thus, protocols for purification of the TIM-1$^+$ B-cell subset are useful for the study on Breg function. TIM-1 may be of even broader utility to the extent that TIM-1 also identifies B cells that utilize mechanisms of action other than IL-10. We have shown that TIM-1$^+$ B cells are enriched for IL-4 expression and may influence Th2 responses [3]. Indeed, it was recently shown that in addition to IL-10, TIM-1 regulates expression of various anti-inflammatory cytokines and co-inhibitory ligands, and that specific deletion of TIM-1 expression on B cells, results in spontaneous systemic autoimmunity (17A) [17]. It should be noted that CD9 is also a broad marker for IL-10$^+$ B cells, but deletion of CD9 results in augmented IL-10$^+$ B cells suggesting that it may repress Breg development [18]. While this may be a useful marker, it will not be further discussed in this chapter.

In the first part of this chapter, we detail procedures for the identification and purification of the murine TIM-1$^+$ B-cell subset for subsequent in vitro or in vivo experiments. We include our protocol to detect TIM-1$^+$ B-cell IL-10 production using intracellular cytokine staining. While this approach will identify TIM-1$^+$ B cells that are enriched for IL-10, as noted above, only a subset of TIM-1$^+$ B cells actually express IL-10. In this regard, we and others have also demonstrated that fluorescent IL-10-reporters can identify IL-10$^+$ B cells even in the absence of in vitro stimulation [19]. We have recently taken advantage of this strategy to sort-purify relatively pure populations of IL-10$^+$ Bregs for in vitro and in vivo studies. Thus, in the second part of this chapter we describe our approach for the isolation of purified IL-10$^+$ (reporter expressing) Bregs. To the extent that IL-10$^+$ B cells are representative of all Bregs, or that IL-10 is involved in Breg activity in a given model, using IL-10$^+$ B cells offers advantages. However, to the extent that TIM-1 identifies Bregs that utilize suppressive mechanisms other than IL-10, the TIM-1 approach also has advantages. Moreover, isolation of TIM-1$^+$ B cells aids study of the role of this molecule in Breg function and differentiation. Until there is a more specific marker than TIM-1, or one that unifies Bregs utilizing different suppressive mechanisms, we believe that these two approaches represent the current state of the art.

2 Materials

2.1 Mice

To perform the procedures described in this chapter, we suggest using 8- to 10-week-old mice.

1. Male inbred B6.129S6-il10^{tm1Flv}/J IL-10GFP reporter mice.
2. C57BL/6 J and congenic B6.SJL-*Ptprc*^{a} *Pepc*^{b}/BoyJ CD45.1 mice.
3. OT-1 C57BL/6-Tg (TCRαTCRβ)1100 Mjb/J mice.
4. OT-2 C57BL/6-Cg-Tg (TCRαTCRβ)425Cbn/J mice.
5. Male inbred BALB/c, C57BL/6, or B-cell-deficient (B6 background) μMT mice (*see* **Note 1**).

2.2 Laboratory Plasticware

1. 15 mL and 50 mL conical tubes.
2. 1.5 mL tubes.
3. Luer lock syringes.
4. Disposable petri dish 100 × 15mm.
5. Cell strainer: 40 μm and 100 μm mesh size.
6. FACS tubes: round-bottom polypropylene tubes for flow cytometry and fluorescence-activated cell sorting (FACS).
7. Unbreakable plastic cover slips.
8. Disposable cryosection base molds.

2.3 Equipment

1. Refrigerated centrifuge.
2. Humidified incubator maintained at 37 °C and 5% CO_2.
3. Vibratome.
4. Imaging chamber with "in and out" flow ports for medium exchange.
5. Peristaltic pump.
6. Air pump for oxygenation of medium.

7. Scissors and forceps.
8. Cryostat.
9. Charged microscope slides.
10. Cover slips.
11. Slide tray.
12. Scalpel.
13. PAP-Pen (hydrophobic marking pen).
14. Liquid nitrogen container.
15. Stopcock.
16. 25-gauge needle.
17. Paper towel.
18. Magnet for immunomagnetic cell separation.
19. Blood glucose meter.
20. Stereomicroscope.
21. Hemocytometer.
22. FACS cell sorter and flow cytometer (equipped with 532 nm green laser [20]).
23. Fluorescent microscope with three channel acquisition filters and motorized stage.
24. Two-photon intravital microscope.
25. 5% CO_2 and 95% O_2 tank.
26. Vetbond tissue adhesive: n-butyl cyanoacrylate adhesive used to bond tissue together in veterinary procedures.

2.4 Buffers, Media, and General Solutions

1. Phenol-free RPMI 1640 medium warmed up to 37 °C.
2. Fetal bovine serum (FBS).
3. Cell culture medium: 10% FBS, 4 mM L-Glutamine and 5×10^{-5} M 2-mercaptoethanol (2-ME) in RPMI 1640. Store at 4 °C.
4. Ca^{2+}- and Mg^{2+}-free Dulbecco's PBS (D-PBS): 0.20 g/l KCl, 0.20 g/l KH_2PO_4, 8.00 g/l NaCl, 1.15 g/l Na_2HPO_4.
5. FACS buffer: 1% heat-inactivated FBS in D-PBS without Mg^{2+} or Ca^{2+}. Adjust to pH 7.4–7.6, filter through a 0.2-μm pore membrane, and store at 4 °C.
6. Red blood cell lysing buffer.
7. Goat serum solution: 5% solution of goat serum diluted in D-PBS. Store at −20 °C and thaw before using.
8. 95% EtOH stored at room temperature.
9. 4% formalin stored at 4 °C.
10. 0.4% Trypan Blue solution.

Table 1
Antibodies used for immunofluorescent staining of IL-10 reporter mouse spleens

Target	Clone
SIGNR-1	22D1
B220	RA3-6B2
IgM	Polyclonal (*see* **Note 2**)
GFP	Polyclonal (*see* **Note 2**)

Table 2
Monoclonal antibodies used to characterize mouse IL-10⁺TIM-1⁺ B cells by flow cytometry

Target	Clone
CD19	1D3
TIM-1	RMT1-4
IL-10	JES5-16E3

2.5 Reagents and Kits

1. Nitrophenyl(20–25)-chicken gamma globulin (NP-CGG): dilute at 0.5 mg/mL with D-PBS. Store at −80 °C and thaw before using.
2. Nitrophenyl(19)-ovalbumin (NP-OVA): dilute at 0.5 mg/mL with D-PBS. Store at −80 °C and thaw before using.
3. Alum Adjuvant.
4. Specific reagents for immunomagnetic isolation of CD4, CD8, CD11c, and CD19 positive cells. According to lab preference, different separation techniques are available.
5. Carboxyfluorescein succinimidyl ester (CFSE).
6. CellTracker Violet (CTV) BMQC.
7. CellTracker Red (CTR) CMPTX.
8. Antibodies for immunofluorescence (*see* Table 1 and **Note 2**).
9. Avidin-Biotin blocking kit (*see* **Note 3**).
10. OCT compound.
11. Glycerol-based liquid mountant.
12. Fluorescence-labeled antibodies for cell isolation or analysis (*see* Table 2). All antibodies should be tittered to identify optimal concentration that gives the highest mean fluorescence intensity (MFI) while maintaining low background staining of negative populations.
13. Dye for the discrimination of viable from nonviable cells in multicolor flow cytometric applications (e.g., LIVE/DEAD Aqua fluorescent reactive dye). Reconstitute the dye according to the manufacturer's instructions.

14. Fc block: purified rat anti-mouse CD16/CD32 (clone 2.4 G2) antibody.
15. Phorbol 12-myristate 13-acetate (PMA): dissolve at 1 mg/mL in dimethyl sulfoxide (DMSO) and store in single-use aliquots (50 μL/tube) at −20 °C.
16. Ionomycin: dissolve at 1 mg/mL in DMSO and store in single-use aliquots (50 μL/tube) at −20 °C.
17. 2 mM monensin solution. This is a 1000× solution that should be stored at 4 °C.
18. LPS (*Escherichia coli* serotype O111:B4): dissolve at 1 mg/mL in sterile PBS and store at −20 °C (*see* **Note 4**).
19. Collagenase V.
20. Streptozocin: dissolve at 25 mg/mL in 0.1 M citrate buffer (pH 4.5).
21. Fixation/permeabilization solution: 2–4% paraformaldehyde (w/w) in PBS.
22. Permeabilization buffer: 0.1% saponin and 1% FBS in PBS (pH 7.4).

3 Methods

3.1 Identification and Characterization of TIM-1⁺ B Cells

The protocol below is used to identify and analyze murine TIM-1$^+$ Bregs. Single-cell suspensions of splenocytes are treated with *LPS, PMA, ionomycin, plus monensin* (LPIM) for 5 hours in vitro to induce IL-10 expression (*see* **Note 5**). The cells are then stained with fluorochrome-conjugated monoclonal antibodies (mAbs) specific for surface CD19, TIM-1, and cytoplasmic IL-10, followed by flow cytometric analysis. It is important to note that TIM-1$^+$IL-10$^+$ B cells are significantly increased in immunized mice compared to naïve mice. IL-10 expression is reliably increased by day 10 post-immunization. IL-10 and TIM-1 expression can be further enhanced by treating mice with three doses of anti-TIM-1 (clone RMT1–10) antibody: 500 μg on day −1, and 300 μg on day 0 and day 5, relative to immunization [3].

3.1.1 Preparation of Splenocytes Suspensions and Cell Stimulation Protocol for IL-10 Induction

1. Collect spleens from C57BL/6 mice and place them in a petri dish with 10 mL of FACS buffer. Gently disaggregate the spleens by pressing with the flat plastic surface on the top of the plunger from a 3-mL syringe against a sterile cell strainer (mesh size, 100 μm). Up to five spleens can be processed in a single petri dish in a total volume of 10 mL FACS buffer.
2. *Transfer the splenocyte suspension to a 15-mL* conical *tube*, centrifuge at 350 × *g* for 5 min at 4 °C and remove the supernatant by aspiration.

3. According to the number of spleens processed, resuspend the cell pellet in the optimal volume of red blood cell lysing buffer (*see* **Note 6**) and incubate for 4 min at room temperature. Stop the lysis reaction by adding an equal volume of FACS buffer and centrifuge immediately at 350 × *g* for 5 min at room temperature. Decant the supernatant and count the cells.
4. Resuspend splenocytes at 2 × 10^6/mL in cell culture medium containing 50 ng/mL PMA, 500 ng/mL ionomycin, 10 μg/mL LPS, and 1× monensin (LPIM). Culture in 24-well culture plates (1 mL/well) at 37 °C in a CO_2 incubator for 5 h.

3.1.2 Cell Staining

1. After the 5 hours stimulation, harvest the cells and place them into 1.5 mL tubes. Centrifuge the tubes at 350 × *g* for 5 min at 4 °C to pellet the cells. Discard all medium from the tube by aspiration and resuspend the cells in 1 mL D-PBS.
2. Add 1 μL of the reconstituted LIVE/DEAD Aqua fluorescent reactive dye to the cells and mix well. Incubate at room temperature or on ice for 30 min, protected from light. Wash the cells once with 1 mL of D-PBS and resuspend the cells in 100 μL of D-PBS.
3. To block nonspecific antibody binding, add 5 μg/mL Fc block and gently vortex the tubes. Incubate for 15 min at 4 ° C and then centrifuge the tubes at 350 × *g* for 5 min at 4 °C to pellet the cells.
4. Proceed with cell surface staining by adding 50 μL of anti-CD19 and anti-TIM-1 antibodies diluted in FACS buffer at the optimal concentration as determined by titration, as noted above. Vortex tubes gently and incubate at 4 °C for 45 min, protected from light (*see* **Note 7**).
5. Wash cells twice with FACS buffer (1 mL per tube) and pellet by centrifugation (350 × *g* for 5 min at 4 °C).
6. Thoroughly resuspend cells and add 250 μL per tube of fixation/permeabilization solution for 20 min at 4 °C (*see* **Note 8**). Centrifuge cells at 500 × *g* for 5 min and discard supernatant.
7. Wash fixed cells twice with 1 mL of permeabilization buffer and by centrifuging at 500 × *g* for 5 min (*see* **Note 9**).
8. Thoroughly resuspend fixed/permeabilized cells in 50 μL of permeabilization buffer containing a pre-determined optimal concentration of anti-mouse IL-10 (*see* **Note 10**) or of the appropriate negative isotype control (*see* **Note 11**). Incubate at 4 °C for 1 h in the dark.
9. Wash cells twice with 1 mL of permeabilization buffer and by centrifuging at 500 × *g* for 5 min. Resuspend in FACS buffer prior to flow cytometric analysis (*see* **Note 12**). Figure 1 shows the result of phenotypic identification of TIM-1 Breg cells using this procedure.

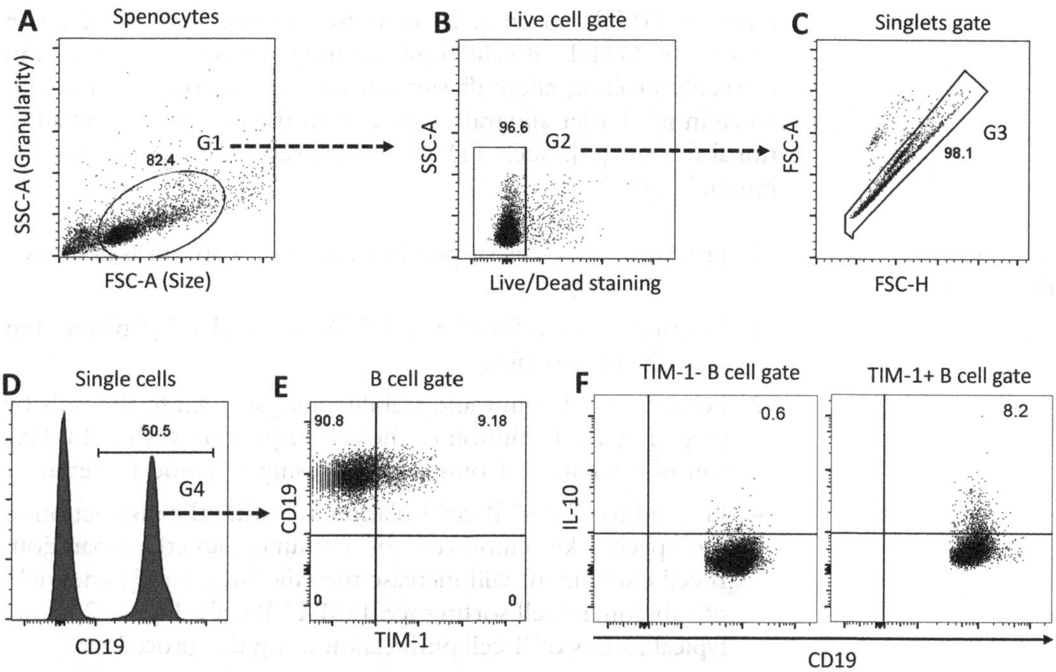

Fig. 1 Representative flow cytometry plots showing the gating strategy for the identification of mouse TIM-1$^+$ Breg cells. This strategy allows B cells to be divided into TIM-1$^+$ and TIM-1$^-$ subsets. (**a**) Forward (FSC-A) versus side scatter (SSC-A) gating is used to identify lymphocytes (G1) based on size and granularity (complexity). (**b**) Using LIVE/DEAD staining, it is possible to identify viable cells (G2). (**c**) G3 defines single cells using a forward scatter area (FSC-A) versus height (FSC-H) plot; cells outside the G3 gate include cell doublets. (**d**) Single cells can be divided according to the expression of the CD19 marker in two regions corresponding to CD19^{pos} (G4) and CD19^{neg} cells. (**e**) From the analysis of the expression of TIM-1 on the CD19^{pos} compartment, TIM-1$^+$ B cells can be discriminated from TIM-1$^-$ B cells. (**f**) From the analysis of the expression of IL-10 on the TIM-1$^+$ or TIM-1$^-$ compartments, the frequencies of IL-10 expressing B cells on TIM-1$^+$ versus TIM-1$^-$ B-cell subsets are assessed

3.2 Isolation of TIM-1$^+$ B Cells

The method described below is for isolating live CD19$^+$TIM-1$^+$ B cells from mouse spleen by cell sorting. A B-cell enrichment step using immunomagnetic separation is performed to reduce the time required for sorting CD19$^+$TIM-1$^+$ and CD19$^+$TIM-1$^-$ subsets by *FACS*. The resultant TIM-1$^+$ B cells, enriched for viable IL-10-producing Bregs, can be used for subsequent functional assays. Importantly, Bregs appear to require activation and/or expansion of antigen-specific cells before they are able to inhibit immune responses. Thus, sort-purified TIM-1$^+$ B cells from spleens of naïve B6 mice are unable to prolong islet allograft survival when transferred into otherwise-untreated B-cell-deficient μMT allograft recipients [3]. However, adoptive transfer of naïve TIM-1$^+$ B cells into μMT mice will prolong islet allograft survival in the setting of anti-TIM-1 treatment, which expands these Bregs during antigen-mediated activation. Allograft prolongation is not observed in anti-TIM-1-treated μMT mice that did not receive B-cell transfer or received TIM-1⁻ B cells. In contrast to naïve B cells, adoptive transfer of TIM-1⁺ B cells from alloantigen-immunized mice can markedly prolong allograft survival and induce long-term acceptance in μMT islet allograft recipients in the absence of any additional therapy [3]. Such TIM-1⁺ Bregs are antigen-specific for the immunizing allospecificity.

3.2.1 Isolation of CD19⁺B Cells

1. Prepare a single-cell suspension from mouse spleen as described in Subheading 3.1.1.
2. Resuspend the cell pellet in FACS buffer (1 mL/spleen) and keep the tube on ice.
3. Perform a cell count and viability analysis. Dilute the cells by preparing a 1:1 dilution of the cell suspension with 0.4% Trypan Blue solution. Count live cells using a hemocytometer.
4. Proceed to CD19⁺ B-cell isolation following the instruction of the specific kit employed for immunomagnetic separation. B-cell enrichment will increase the efficiency, purity, and yield of subsequent cell sorting for TIM-1⁺ B cells. Figure 2 shows typical results of B-cell purification using this procedure.

3.2.2 Cell Sorting of Tim-1⁺ B Cells

1. Resuspend purified B cells at 2×10^8/mL in FACS buffer in sterile 15 mL conical centrifuge tubes with caps.
2. Add optimal amounts of diluted anti-CD19 and anti-TIM-1 mAb and then incubate the cells on ice for 45 min, protected from light, as described in Subheading 3.1.2 (*see* **Note 7**).
3. After incubation, add 5 mL of cold FACS buffer to the tubes and gently mix the cells. Centrifuge at $500 \times g$ for 5 min at 4 °C and remove the supernatant. Repeat twice.

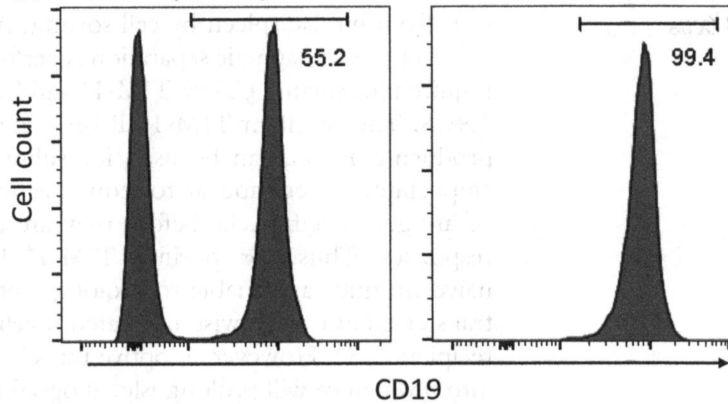

Fig. 2 Analysis of murine splenic B cells. B cells were purified from C57BL/6 splenocytes using immunomagnetic separation. Both splenocytes (**a**) and purified B cells (**b**) were analyzed by flow cytometry to evaluate CD19 expression

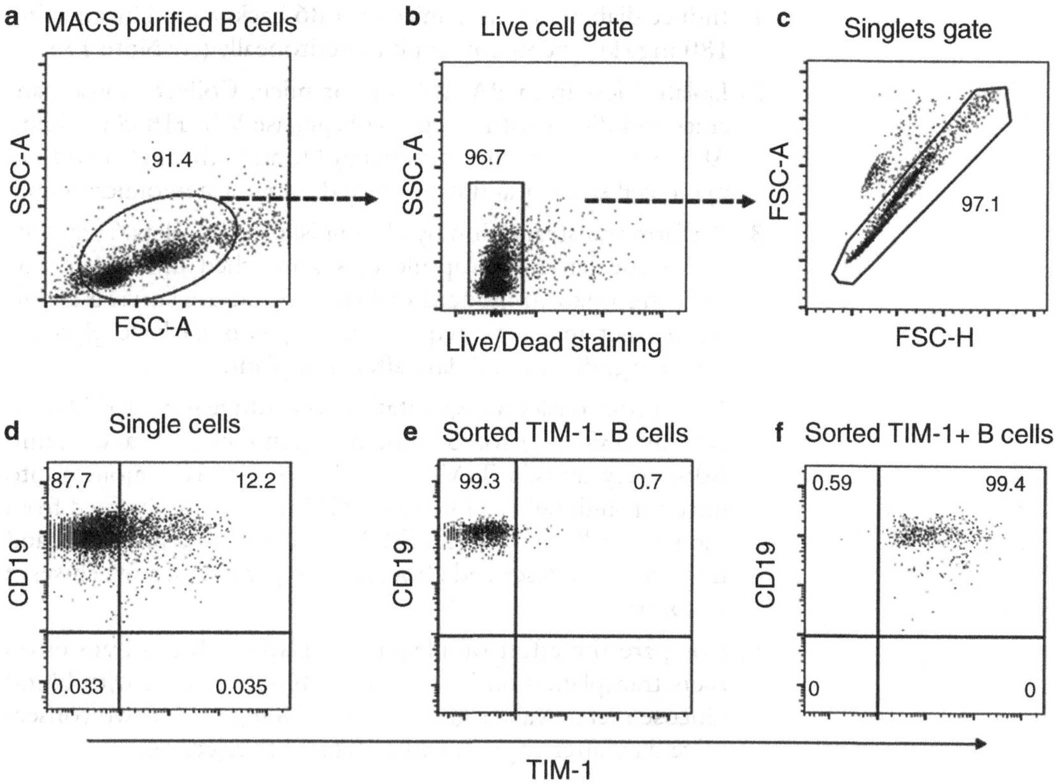

Fig. 3 Representative example of the cell sorting strategy used to purify TIM-1$^+$ B cells from the spleen of adult mice. (**a–c**) The viability of murine splenic B cells was determined by using a dye for the discrimination of viable from nonviable cells in multicolor flow cytometric applications (LIVE/DEAD staining). (**d**) The staining with Alexa-647-conjugated CD19 and PE-conjugated TIM-1 mAbs allows B cells to be subdivided into CD19$^+$TIM-1$^+$ and CD19$^+$TIM-1$^-$ subsets. (**e**, **f**) Dot plot panels show the sorted CD19$^+$TIM-1$^+$ and CD19$^+$TIM-1$^-$ populations

4. Suspend B cells in FACS buffer, generally at a final concentration of 5–8 × 10^7/mL. Filter the cell suspension through a 40-μm sterile cell strainer to remove clumps, before subsequent cell sorting.
5. Prepare sterile 15 mL conical tubes with 500 μL of FBS to collect cells during cell sorting (*see* **Note 13**). Clearly identify each tube with a label corresponding to the single-cell population you are purifying. Figure 3 shows the gating strategy applied to purify the TIM-1$^+$ or TIM-1$^-$ B-cell subsets (*see* **Note 14**).

3.3 Functional Assay for TIM-1$^+$ Breg Cells

The functionality of TIM-1$^+$ Breg cells has been determined in mouse transplantation and in the experimental autoimmune encephalomyelitis (EAE) model. Here we describe a method to test the regulatory properties of TIM-1$^+$ B cells in the context of islet allograft transplantation for the treatment of chemically induced diabetes.

1. Induce diabetes in μMT mice on a B6 background by injecting 180 mg/kg streptozotocin intraperitoneally (*see* **Note 15**).
2. Isolate islets from BALB/c donor mice. Collect mouse pancreas and digest with 1.1 g/l collagenase V in HBSS medium. Allogenic islets are then purified by filtration through a 100-μm nylon cell strainer and hand-picked under a stereomicroscope.
3. Perform transplantation by placing islets (400 islets/recipient) under the left renal capsule of sex-matched μMT recipients with streptozocin-induced diabetes. To ensure survival of sufficient islet mass, we require all recipients to have glycemia $\leq$150 mg/dl within 2 days after transplant.
4. 1 day prior to islet transplantation, centrifuge sorted TIM-1$^+$ B cells at 350 $\times$ g for 5 min, resuspend in PBS and count. Adoptively transfer TIM-1$^+$ B cells ($\geq$ 5 $\times$ 10^6/mouse) into mice through tail veil injection. TIM-1$^-$ B cells obtained from the same cell sort as the TIM-1$^+$ B cells can be processed and transferred as described above, into separate mice which serve as controls.
5. Compare the effect of TIM-1$^+$ or TIM-1$^-$ B-cell transfer on islets transplantation by measuring blood glucose with blood glucose meter. Values greater than 250 mg/dl for two consecutive days after engraftment is defined as rejection.

3.4 Detection of IL-10$^+$ Bregs Utilizing IL-10 Reporter Mice

IL-10 expression by B cells can be detected using GFP reporter mice. Further, immunization of the mice results in expansion of Bregs and a brighter GFP signal. NP-CGG is used for immunization as it is well known for its potent B-cell-stimulating properties (*see* Subheading 3.5). Hence, the detection of IL-10 does not require in vitro stimulation, and this allows for accurate phenotypic analysis, in situ study, and cell transfer of freshly isolated cells. While not required, IL-10 expression by B cells increases even further after in vivo treatment of mice with anti-TIM-1 antibody or in vitro stimulation of B cells with LPIM. This section details the identification of IL-10$^+$ Bregs using IL-10 GFP reporter mice without ex vivo stimulation with mitogens, and provides a protocol for identifying Breg localization in specific splenic niches in situ by immunofluorescence histology, and as well as a protocol for studying Breg function using two-photon microscopy [19].

3.4.1 Direct Identification of IL-10$^+$ Bregs In Vivo from Secondary Lymphoid Organs Using IL-10 Reporter mice by Flow Cytometry

1. Mix 50 μg of NP-CGG/mouse with an equivalent volume of alum adjuvant in a stopcock for 5 min.
2. Immunize IL-10 reporter mice and GFP-negative wild-type controls with a total volume of 200 μL of NP-CGG/alum by intraperitoneal injection using 25-gauge needles (*see* **Note 16**). Inject wild-type B6 mice similarly for staining controls.

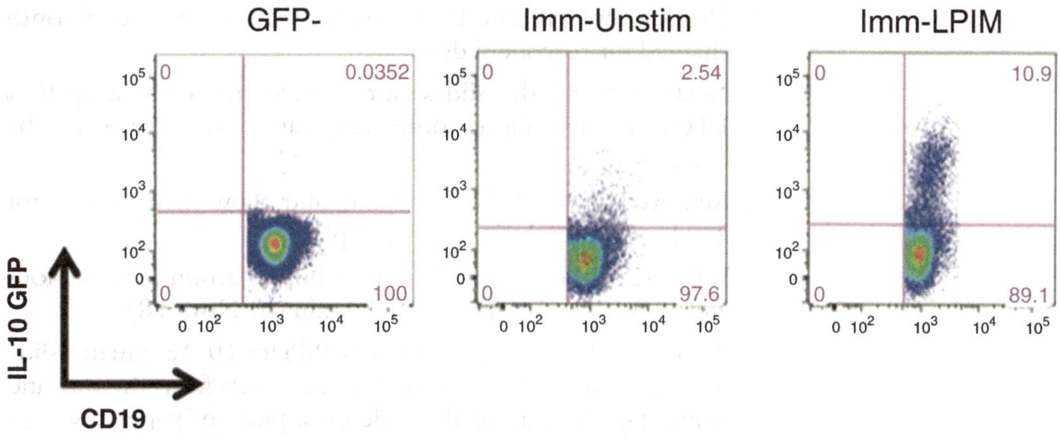

Fig. 4 IL-10-GFP reporter mice or GFP^{neg} littermate controls were immunized with NP-CGG plus Alum, and splenocytes were isolated on day 3. Panels show flow plots of IL-10-GFP expression by CD19^{+} B cells isolated from either GFP^{neg} mice or from immunized IL-10-GFP reporter mice that were unstimulated (Imm-Unstim) or stimulated in vitro with LPS, PMA, ionomycin, and monensin (Imm-LPIM) for 5 h

3. Euthanize mice on days 3–7 and carefully harvest the spleens with forceps and scissors. Process the spleens to obtain a single-cell suspension as described in Subheading 3.1.1.
4. Carry out cell stimulation as described in Subheading 3.1.1 making sure to leave cells unstimulated under the same culture conditions. This will allow you to compare IL-10-GFP expression by stimulated and unstimulated cells (*see* Fig. 4).
5. At the end of the stimulation period, perform staining of the cells as described in Subheading 3.1.2. At this stage, one can include markers that will allow to differentiate individual B-cell subsets such as follicular, marginal zone, and transitional B cells [19]. Make sure not to include a fluorochrome that will have a major overlap with GFP emission.
6. Examine the stained cells by flow cytometry.

3.4.2 In Vivo Detection of IL-10^{+} B Cells in Splenic Cryosections

1. Immunize mice with NP-CGG/alum and harvest spleens as described in **steps 1–3** of Subheading 3.4.1.
2. Cut each spleen into three cross sections to expose the white pulp and embed them in OCT pre-poured into disposable cryosection cartridges. The exposed cross section of the cut side of the spleen should face outwards and vertically when placed into the OCT so that the cryostat cuts parallel to the cross section.
3. Place the cartridges over liquid nitrogen vapor to slowly freeze the OCT (*see* **Note 17**). Once fully frozen, store the cartridges in −80 °C until they are ready to be cryosectioned.

4. Using a cryostat, cut 10 μm spleen sections at −16 °C onto charged microscope slides.
5. Next, immerse the slides into a slide tray containing 95% ETOH for 15 min at room temperature in order to fix the tissue sections.
6. Remove the slides from the tray and allow them to dry for 2–3 h or overnight in a cool dry place.
7. With a PAP-Pen, carefully draw a border around the sections and allow them to dry for 20–30 min (*see* **Note 18**).
8. Rehydrate the tissue sections in D-PBS for 10–15 min in a slide tray (*see* **Note 19**). Then, remove the slides from the tray and gently tap the side of the slide on a piece of paper towel to remove excess D-PBS (repeat this step after every wash to minimized D-PBS diluting reagents).
9. Quickly, pipette 200–500 μL of 5% goat serum solution into the PAP-pen outlined area and allow the slides to rest for 30–45 min at room temperature.
10. Discard the serum block, rinse the slides with D-PBS, and carry out an avidin-biotin block of the section (*see* **Note 20**). Incubate the section in avidin solution for 10 min at room temperature and then wash the section for 5 min in the slide tray containing D-PBS. Subsequently, carry out the biotin block of the sections with the biotin solution for 10 min at room temperature. Again, wash the section for 5 min in the slide tray containing fresh D-PBS.
11. Stain the section with 200 μL of 5% goat serum solution containing anti-GFP (polyclonal, rabbit, 1:200 dilution), anti-SIGNR-1 (monoclonal, hamster, 1:200 dilution), and anti-B220-biotin (monoclonal, rat, 1:200 dilution) antibodies (*see* **Notes 21** and **22**). Incubate for 2 h at room temperature. Wash the section for 15 min in the slide tray containing fresh D-PBS.
12. Stain the slides with 200 μL of 5% goat serum containing anti-IgM-Alexa647 (1:400, *see* **Note 23**), and fluorochrome-conjugated streptavidin (1:1000), anti-rabbit (1:400), and anti-hamster (1:400) secondary reagents to match the primary antibodies listed in **step 11** above. Titrations are provided as a starting point (*see* **Note 22**). Incubate for 45 min and then wash the sections for 15 min in the slide tray containing PBS.
13. Fix the slides with 4% formalin for 10 min.
14. Discard the formalin and quickly mount the slide with mountant and slide cover. Make sure to avoid forming bubbles as this will affect image quality (*see* **Note 24**). Allow the mounted slides to dry in a cool, dry, and dark place overnight.

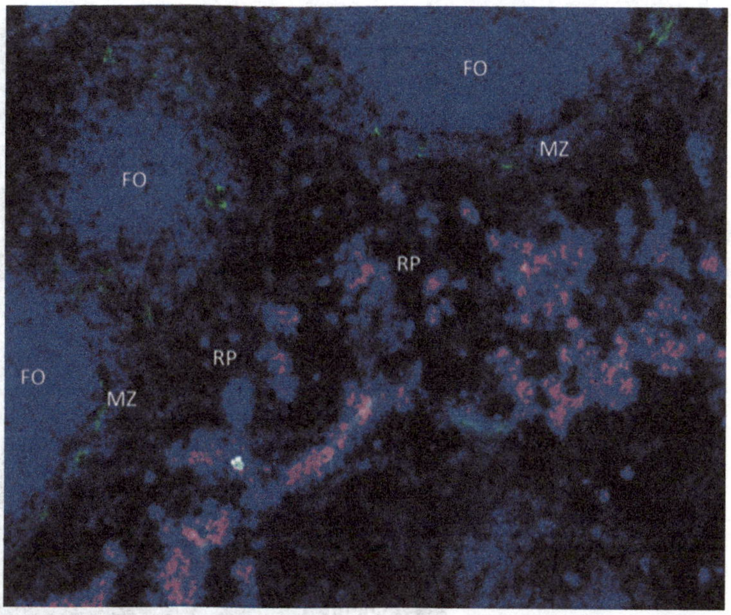

Fig. 5 Representative staining of an IL-10-GFP reporter mouse spleen harvested 72 h after immunization. The cryosection was stained with anti-IgM-Alexa647 (blue), B220-Alexa647 (blue), anti-SIGNR-1-Alexa488 (green), and anti-GFP-Alexa555 (red) in order to distinguish B-cell follicles (FO), marginal zone (MZ), and red pulp (RP) areas of the spleen

15. Acquire large areas of the stained tissue section with a fluorescent microscope equipped with a motorized stage. A representative immunofluorescence staining is shown in Fig. 5.

3.5 Examination of Breg In Vivo Interactions by Two-Photon Intravital Microscopy Using IL-10 GFP Reporter Mice

In vivo interactions between Bregs and other cells may be of paramount importance in understanding Breg function. This can be studied by sorting Bregs from IL-10 GFP reporter mice followed by adoptive transfer into congenic recipients. Here we describe a procedure that allows examination of antigen-specific interactions between Bregs and T cells or DCs using two-photon intravital imaging (*see* Fig. 6). Bregs are generated in response to protein carriers such as chicken gamma globulin (CGG) or ovalbumin (OVA) conjugated to nitrophenyl (NP), a hapten to which there exists a high natural frequency of Ag-specific B cells. In such systems, anti-NP B cells react to the hapten regardless of the carrier. However, the protein carrier is internalized and processed by B cells, and peptide antigens contained therein are bound by MHC molecules and can be presented to T cells. Bregs generated in NP-CGG-immunized mice are pulsed in vitro with fresh antigen (NP) plus the carrier (either CGG or OVA) [21]. When sorted and then pulsed with NP-OVA, Bregs make Ag-specific interactions with OT-1 and OT-2 T cells [19]. In contrast, NP-CGG (taken up by the same NP-reactive B cells) serves as an internal negative

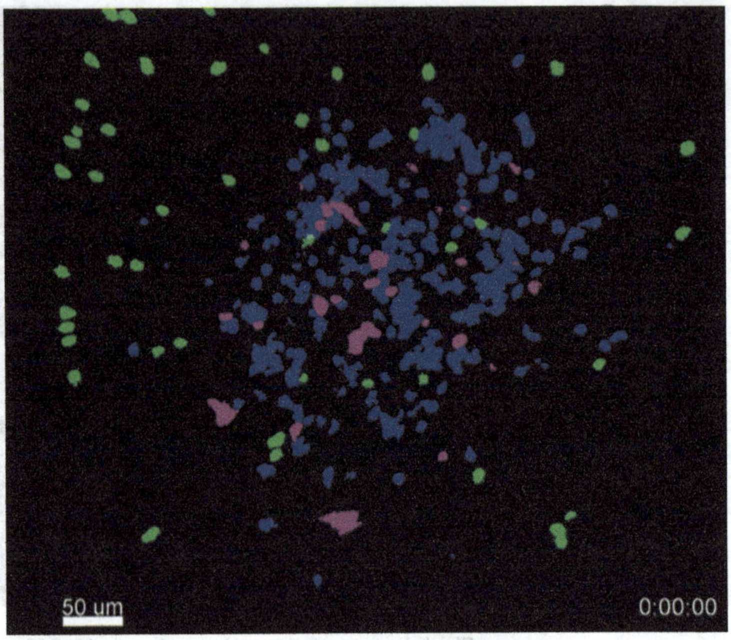

Fig. 6 Snapshot showing two-photon microscopy imaging of a mouse spleen that received bone marrow-derived dendritic cells (pink), OT-1 T cells (blue), and IL-10 GFP$^+$ B cells (green)

control for non-Ag-specific intercellular interactions (*see* Fig. 7 for schematic diagram). Because white pulp is extremely hard to visualize by two-photon microscopy in intact spleen, we visualize cell interactions in situ, in freshly isolated splenic sections.

3.5.1 Intravital Imaging of IL-10$^+$ B Cells in Freshly Cut spleen Sections

1. Mix 50 μg of NP-CGG/mouse with an equivalent volume of alum in a stopcock for 5 min (*see* **Note 25**).
2. Immunize IL-10 reporter mice with a total volume of 200 μL of NP-CGG/alum by intraperitoneal injection using 25-gauge needles (*see* **Note 26**).
3. Harvest spleens on day 7 and prepare cells for sorting as described in Subheading 3.2.3. Omit TIM-1 staining and instead sort for total CD19$^+$GFP$^+$ B cells.
4. Once the sort is finished, resuspend the sorted CD19$^+$GFP$^+$ B cells at 2 × 10^6 cells/mL and pulse them with 10 μg/mL of NP-OVA or NP-CGG for 1 h in RPMI 1640 medium in the incubator at 37 °C.
5. During the last 20 min of incubation, stain the CD19$^+$GFP$^+$ B cells with 1.5 μM CFSE. Wash cells twice with D-PBS.
6. Resuspend the cells at 10 × 10^6 cell/mL in D-PBS and inject 1–2 × 10^6 CD19$^+$GFP$^+$ B cells intravenously into the same congenic B6 CD45.1 mice that received T cells the day before (*see* Subheading 3.5.2 below).

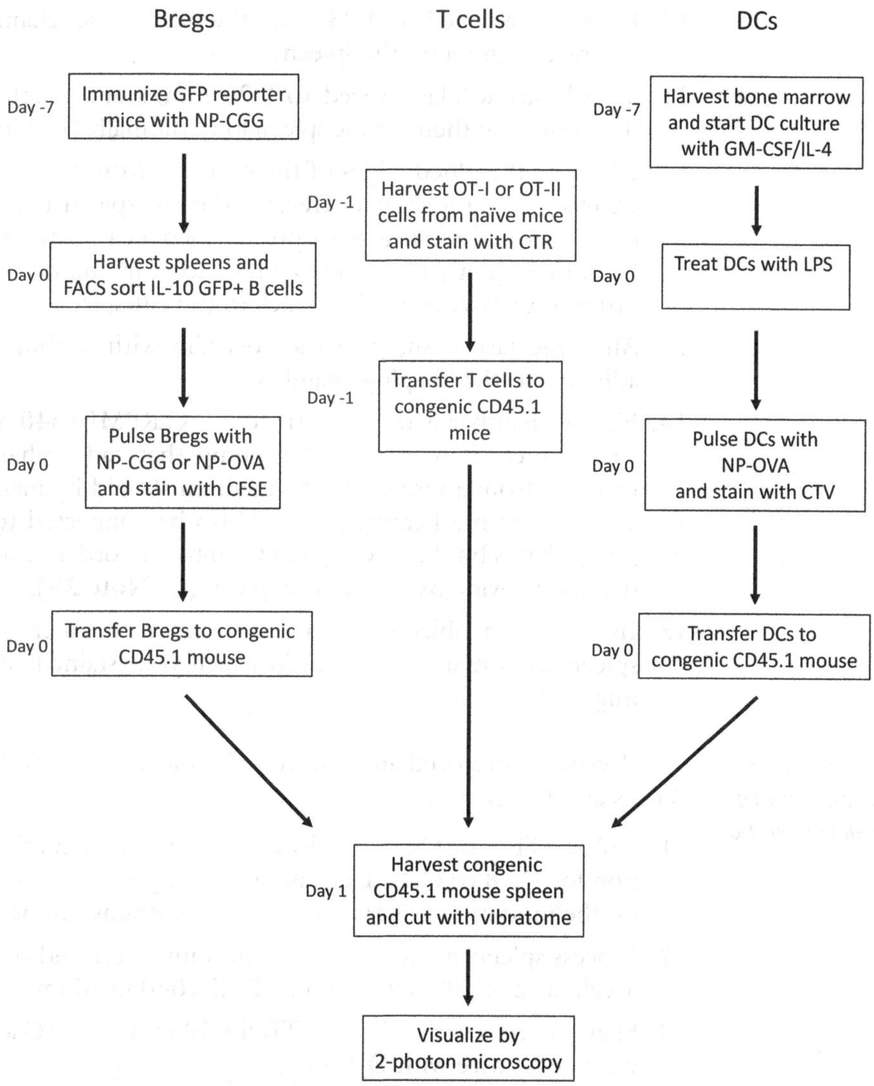

Fig. 7 Schematic diagram showing the approach used to examine Breg interactions with T cells and DCs by two-photon intravital imaging as described in Subheading 3.5

7. Harvest the spleens of recipient mice 15–18 h following cell transfer and quickly glue the smooth side of the spleen to an unbreakable plastic cover slip using the Vetbond tissue adhesive. Gently press on the edges of the spleen to ensure it is glued on well to the coverslip.
8. Transfer the spleen and cover slip to a petri dish containing pre-warmed 37 °C D-PBS (*see* **Note 27**).
9. Move the cover slip and spleen to vibratome chamber and glue the corners of the cover slip to the vibratome stage.

10. Pour pre-warmed D-PBS into the vibratome chamber to completely immerse the spleen.
11. Set vibratome blade speed to 0.20 mm/s and amplitude to 0.55 mm, and then cut the spleen longitudinally (*see* **Note 28**).
12. Dislodge the glued edges of the coverslip from the vibratome chamber using a scalpel. Transfer the cut spleen back to the petri dish and wash it with pre-warmed D-PBS three times. Each time gently pour the D-PBS and swirl the petri dish in order to remove any debris stuck to the cut spleen.
13. After the last wash, glue the coverslip with Vetbond tissue adhesive to the imaging chamber.
14. Fill the chamber with pre-warmed 37 °C RPMI 1640 medium and connect it to a peristaltic pump that can exchange the medium from a reservoir. The medium should be maintained at 37 °C with a heating pad and also be connected to an air pump that is bubbling CO_2 and O_2 into it in order to maintain pH and provide oxygen to the spleen (*see* **Note 29**).
15. Immerse the objective into the imaging chamber over the spleen section and find areas in which your stained cells have migrated.

3.5.2 Preparation of T Cells for Intravital Imaging (Day − 1 from Breg and DC Transfer)

The T cells are prepared and transferred 1 day before $CD19^+GFP^+$ B cells and DC transfer.

1. Isolate OT-1 or OT-2 T cells using immunomagnetic separation for CD8 or CD4 T-cell isolation, respectively. Depending on the model, T cells from other mouse strains can be used.
2. Process spleen as outlined in Subheading 3.1.1 and resuspend T cells at 2×10^6 cells/mL in RPMI 1640 medium.
3. Stain the cells with 2.5 μM CTR for 20 min at 37 °C and then wash cells twice with D-PBS.
4. Resuspend the T cells at 10×10^6 cells/mL in D-PBS and inject 2×10^6 cells intravenously into congenic B6 CD45.1 mice.

3.5.3 Preparation of Dendritic cells for Intravital Imaging (Same Day as $CD19^+GFP^+$ B Cells Transfer)

1. On the day that IL-10 GFP reporter mice are immunized, start generating bone marrow-derived dendritic cells from wild-type B6 mice using the classical method involving culture with GM-CSF and IL-4 which typically requires 7 days [22] (*see* **Note 30**).
2. On the day $CD19^+GFP^+$ B cells are being sorted, treat DCs with 100 ng/mL of LPS for 5–6 h.
3. Harvest the LPS-stimulated DCs, wash them with D-PBS twice and pulse them with 10 μg/mL of NP-OVA for 1 hour, as described above.

4. For the last 20 min of the incubation, stain the DCs with 2.5 μM CTV at 37 °C. Wash the cells twice with D-PBS.
5. Resuspend the cells at 10 × 10^6 cell/mL in D-PBS and inject 1 × 10^6 DCs intravenously into the same congenic B6 CD45.1 mice that will receive Bregs and T cells.

3.5.4 Analysis of In Vivo Breg Interactions

1. Import the two-photon acquired files to the analysis software of your choice. Imaris by Oxford Instruments and Velocity by PerkinElmer are two widely used software application suites that allow two-photon analysis.
2. Start the analysis by subtracting major background signals that appear in every channel.
3. Similarly, subtract signals bleeding from one channel into all others, one by one, in order to clean up false overlapping signals.
4. Next, create surfaces for cells in each individual channel. This will allow you to track single cells and obtain specific parameters such as track length, velocity, displacement, and arrest coefficient (*see* **Note 31**).
5. Examine cell–cell interaction measurements between your channels by either following individual cells manually through each recorded session, or by utilizing built-in algorithms that measure signal overlap duration for a specific tracked cell (*see* **Note 32**). This will allow one to determine whether or not there were differences in Breg interactions with T cells and DCs when the B cells are pulsed with cognate or nonspecific antigen.

4 Notes

1. These mice can be used in a time frame from 6 to 10 weeks of age.
2. Although the choice of the specific antibody supplier depends on the needs of the researcher, we suggest using the rabbit polyclonal antibody to GFP from Abcam (ab6556) since it worked consistently, and the polyclonal goat anti-mouse IgM heavy chain secondary antibody from ThermoFisher Scientific (A-21238), as it gives a very bright signal for IFHC.
3. The avidin-biotin blocking kit is provided by different suppliers. If using the avidin-biotin blocking kit from Vector Laboratories, then prepare the avidin and the biotin solutions by squeezing two droplets from the avidin and biotin bottles into separate tubes containing 10 mL of D-PBS. Shake well before using the solutions to carry out the block.

4. Compared to other *Escherichia coli* serotypes, LPS from the *Escherichia coli* serotype O111:B4 works better for inducing IL-10 expression in vitro.
5. The protein transport inhibitor monensin is recommended in this protocol to inhibit the secretion of IL-10. Empirically, *monensin* works *better* than brefeldin A for detection of IL-10 expression by intracellular staining.
6. If processing one spleen, then use 4 mL of red blood cell lysing buffer. If working with more than 1 but less than 5 spleens, then use a total volume of 7 mL.
7. In our experience, compared to other commercially available conjugates, the PE-conjugated anti-TIM-1 antibody is a better choice for the identification of TIM-1^+ B cells by flow cytometry because it has better resolution. We highly recommend PE-conjugated anti-TIM-1 antibody because it gives the best signal, and we use it in combination with the Alexa Fluor 647-conjugated anti-CD19 mAb. The working concentration of each antibody should be optimized before use. Avoid using excess of fluorescence-labeled antibodies to reduce nonspecific staining.
8. Cell aggregation can be avoided by vortexing prior to the addition of the fixation/permeabilization solution.
9. Permeabilization buffer must be maintained in the washing steps to maintain cell permeabilization.
10. We recommend using a BV-421-labeled anti-IL-10 antibody. BV421 is a polymer-based dye excited by the violet laser (405 nm). Conjugates are typically 10 times brighter than Pacific Blue conjugates and are often as bright as or brighter than PE conjugates.
11. Due to the low MFI of IL-10 expression in B cells, when feasible, B cells from IL-10 KO mice should be used as a superior negative control. Splenocytes from IL-10 KO mice are stimulated with LPIM and stained with BV-421-labeled anti-IL-10 rather than an unrelated isotype control—giving a more accurate gating of IL-10 negative versus IL-10-positive cells.
12. Measurement of the fluorescence emission of PE and PE-tandem dyes is considerably more sensitive when using a green laser (532 nm excitation) as compared with a blue laser (488 nm excitation). In addition, as the absolute number of photoelectrons collected is greater, there is less measurement-error-induced spread into the compensated channels. Moreover, the blue laser produces more cell autofluorescence than the green laser [20].

13. Vortex thoroughly and let FBS in the medium precoat the collection tube wall, to reduce nonspecific adherence of the sticky B cells to collection tube wall.
14. Despite the excellent performance of modern FACS machines, high purity of minor populations is not always easy to obtain, especially when using markers whose expression is low and does not form a distinct peak. Moreover, a certain level of cell death is always expected. Therefore, it is important to check cell purity and viability after cell sorting. Collect 200 μL of each cell population into FACS tubes and reanalyze on the flow cytometer. If the purity of the sorted cells is not satisfactory, spin down the cells at 350 × *g* for 5 min and re-sort the cells. We do not suggest using cells whose post-sort purity does not reach 90–95%.
15. Streptozotocin (STZ) is a broad-spectrum antibiotic that is toxic to the insulin producing β cells of pancreatic islets. We use 0.1 M citrate buffer (pH 4.5) to dissolve the STZ at a concentration of 180 mg/kg in a single intraperitoneal dose after a 20-minute stabilization period at 4 °C. Do not graft within 48 h postinjection to allow the drug to be fully cleared from the mouse's system [23, 24].
16. Any desired immunization can be used instead (i.e., allo-immunization, bacterial or viral).
17. It is important that the sections are frozen slowly over the liquid nitrogen vapor in order to prevent crystal formation and cracking of the tissue. This can be achieved by shaping an aluminum foil basket that can sit in the opening of the nitrogen container so that the nitrogen vapor, but no actual liquid nitrogen, contacts the tissue, allowing for slower cooling.
18. The hydrophobic layer formed by the PAP-pen allows for small volumes of liquid to be retained around the tissue and serves as the means to deliver antibodies for the staining procedure.
19. Once the tissue section is rehydrated with D-PBS, it must not dry out again until the staining is finished, and the slides are mounted.
20. An avidin block is necessary as the tissue may have endogenous biotin sites that may result in nonspecific avidin/streptavidin-fluorochrome binding and background staining. The subsequent biotin block then ensures that all open avidin-binding sites for biotin are blocked before the biotinylated antibody is added.
21. SIGNR-1 is expressed by a specific subset of macrophages called "marginal zone macrophages" that are located within the marginal zone. The marginal zone forms a ring-like

structure around B-cell follicles. The red pulp lies outside of this ring (*see* Fig. 5). Hence, this marker allows to easily distinguish one splenic niche from the other.

22. The suggested antibody types and host species are the most common ones available. Titrating multiple primary and secondary antibodies on tissue sections is quite laborious. Therefore, if the antibody supplier does not provide recommendations for immunohistochemistry, the titers provided in the text are a good starting point. Further titration may be required to optimize the signal.
23. Normally, anti-IgM will mainly stain marginal zone and plasma B cells strongly while follicular B cells stain weakly. In contrast, anti-B220 will strongly stain follicular B cells while weakly staining marginal zone B cells and plasma cells. Hence, if simultaneous visualization of all B-cell zones is desired, we suggest staining the sections with anti-IgM and anti-B220 both labeled with Alexa647, which allows all B cells to be visualized at the same time, saving other colors for other fluorescent markers.
24. Push bubbles out to the edge of the cover slip by gently pressing down near them with a 1-mL pipette tip.
25. NP-CGG is used for the initial immunization in order to avoid any carry over of ovalbumin from mice immunized with NP-OVA, when examining subsequent antigen-specific interactions with OT-1/OT-2 T cells.
26. We recommend immunization of four IL-10 GFP reporter mice to obtain ~2×10^6 Bregs from the sort.
27. It is essential that the spleen is kept warmed at 37 °C at all times. Temperature drops below 37 °C will affect the motility of the cells within the tissue during imaging and skew subsequent results. Therefore, the imaging chamber and media should be maintained at 37 °C as well.
28. You may want to save and cryo-preserve the unattached cut portion of the spleen to carry out immunohistochemistry.
29. For an in-depth review of this procedure, see the work by Zinselmeyer et al. 2009 [25].
30. The GM-CSF and IL-4 culture method will generate an approximately twofold increase in the number of DCs from the starting number of bone marrow cells. Alternatively, DCs may be freshly isolated from B6 mouse spleens by positive selection through immunomagnetic separation. According to lab preference, different separation techniques are available. If you are isolating dendritic cells from a mouse spleen using the EasySep™ mouse CD11c-positive selection kit from Stemcell Tech, you will obtain approximately one million cells/spleen.

31. It is best to start making surfaces on a channel which have relatively bigger objects (cells) and low motility. These properties will allow you to compensate for drift that occurs when imaging live tissue (although with a glued spleen this should be minimal). In this case, it is suggested that you start with the channel that detected your transferred DCs.

32. If you use built-in algorithms, it is recommended you perform some manual tracking yourself in order to verify your results. The software may make mistakes tracking cells when there are a high number of surfaces together in one area. It is necessary at times to manually follow cells and ensure that a given track is properly connected to one cell throughout the entire movie.

Acknowledgments

This work was supported by NIH grant AI114587 (DMR).

References

1. Shen P, Fillatreau S (2015) Antibody-independent functions of B cells: a focus on cytokines. Nat Rev Immunol 15:441–451. https://doi.org/10.1038/nri3857
2. Lund FE, Randall TD (2010) Effector and regulatory B cells: modulators of CD4+ T cell immunity. Nat Rev Immunol 10:236–247. https://doi.org/10.1038/nri2729
3. Ding Q, Yeung M, Camirand G, Zeng Q, Akiba H, Yagita H, Chalasani G, Sayegh MH, Najafian N, Rothstein DM (2011) Regulatory B cells are identified by expression of TIM-1 and can be induced through TIM-1 ligation to promote tolerance in mice. J Clin Invest 121:3645–3656. https://doi.org/10.1172/JCI46274
4. Yeung MY, Ding Q, Brooks CR, Xiao S, Workman CJ, Vignali DA, Ueno T, Padera RF, Kuchroo VK, Najafian N et al (2015) TIM-1 signaling is required for maintenance and induction of regulatory B cells. Am J Transplant 15:942–953. https://doi.org/10.1111/ajt.13087
5. Yanaba K, Bouaziz JD, Haas KM, Poe JC, Fujimoto M, Tedder TF (2008) A regulatory B cell subset with a unique CD1dhiCD5+ phenotype controls T cell-dependent inflammatory responses. Immunity 28:639–650. https://doi.org/10.1016/j.immuni.2008.03.017
6. Mohib K, Cherukuri A, Rothstein DM (2018) Regulatory B cells and transplantation: almost prime time? Curr Opin Organ Transplant 23:524–532. https://doi.org/10.1097/MOT.0000000000000559
7. Brummel R, Lenert P (2005) Activation of marginal zone B cells from lupus mice with type a(D) CpG-oligodeoxynucleotides. J Immunol 174:2429–2434. https://doi.org/10.4049/jimmunol.174.4.2429
8. Gray M, Miles K, Salter D, Gray D, Savill J (2007) Apoptotic cells protect mice from autoimmune inflammation by the induction of regulatory B cells. Proc Natl Acad Sci U S A 104:14080–14085. https://doi.org/10.1073/pnas.0700326104
9. Lenert P, Brummel R, Field EH, Ashman RF (2005) TLR-9 activation of marginal zone B cells in lupus mice regulates immunity through increased IL-10 production. J Clin Immunol 25:29–40. https://doi.org/10.1007/s10875-005-0355-6
10. Flemming A (2018) Natural regulatory plasma cells. Nat Rev Immunol 18:540–541. https://doi.org/10.1038/s41577-018-0057-8
11. Matsumoto M, Baba A, Yokota T, Nishikawa H, Ohkawa Y, Kayama H, Kallies A, Nutt SL, Sakaguchi S, Takeda K et al (2014) Interleukin-10-producing plasmablasts exert regulatory function in autoimmune inflammation. Immunity 41:1040–1051. https://doi.org/10.1016/j.immuni.2014.10.016
12. Rosser EC, Mauri C (2015) Regulatory B cells: origin, phenotype, and function. Immunity

42:607–612. https://doi.org/10.1016/j.immuni.2015.04.005

13. Mauri C, Menon M (2015) The expanding family of regulatory B cells. Int Immunol 27:479–486. https://doi.org/10.1093/intimm/dxv038
14. Alhabbab RY, Nova-Lamperti E, Aravena O, Burton HM, Lechler RI, Dorling A, Lombardi G (2019) Regulatory B cells: development, phenotypes, functions, and role in transplantation. Immunol Rev 292:164–179. https://doi.org/10.1111/imr.12800
15. Kuchroo VK, Dardalhon V, Xiao S, Anderson AC (2008) New roles for TIM family members in immune regulation. Nat Rev Immunol 8:577–580. https://doi.org/10.1038/nri2366
16. Xiao S, Brooks CR, Zhu C, Wu C, Sweere JM, Petecka S, Yeste A, Quintana FJ, Ichimura T, Sobel RA et al (2012) Defect in regulatory B-cell function and development of systemic autoimmunity in T-cell Ig mucin 1 (Tim-1) mucin domain-mutant mice. Proc Natl Acad Sci U S A 109:12105–12110. https://doi.org/10.1073/pnas.1120914109
17. Xiao S, Bod L, Pochet N, Kota SB, Hu D, Madi A, Kilpatrick J, Shi J, Ho A, Zhang H, et al (2020) Checkpoint Receptor TIGIT Expressed on Tim-1(+) B Cells Regulates Tissue Inflammation. Cell Rep 32:107892. https://doi.org/10.1016/j.celrep.2020.107892
18. Sun J, Wang J, Pefanis E, Chao J, Rothschild G, Tachibana I, Chen JK, Ivanov II, Rabadan R, Takeda Y et al (2015) Transcriptomics identify CD9 as a marker of murine IL-10-competent regulatory B cells. Cell Rep 13:1110–1117. https://doi.org/10.1016/j.celrep.2015.09.070
19. Mohib K, Cherukuri A, Zhou Y, Ding Q, Watkins SC, Rothstein DM (2020) Antigen-dependent interactions between regulatory B cells and T cells at the T:B border inhibit subsequent T cell interactions with DCs. Am J Transplant 20:52–63. https://doi.org/10.1111/ajt.15546
20. Perfetto SP, Roederer M (2007) Increased immunofluorescence sensitivity using 532 nm laser excitation. Cytometry A 71:73–79. https://doi.org/10.1002/cyto.a.20358
21. Shulman Z, Gitlin AD, Targ S, Jankovic M, Pasqual G, Nussenzweig MC, Victora GD (2013) T follicular helper cell dynamics in germinal centers. Science 341:673–677. https://doi.org/10.1126/science.1241680
22. Inaba K, Inaba M, Romani N, Aya H, Deguchi M, Ikehara S, Muramatsu S, Steinman RM (1992) Generation of large numbers of dendritic cells from mouse bone marrow cultures supplemented with granulocyte/macrophage colony-stimulating factor. J Exp Med 176:1693–1702. https://doi.org/10.1084/jem.176.6.1693
23. Deeds MC, Anderson JM, Armstrong AS, Gastineau DA, Hiddinga HJ, Jahangir A, Eberhardt NL, Kudva YC (2011) Single dose streptozotocin-induced diabetes: considerations for study design in islet transplantation models. Lab Anim 45:131–140. https://doi.org/10.1258/la.2010.010090
24. de la Garza-Rodea AS, Knaan-Shanzer S, den Hartigh JD, Verhaegen AP, van Bekkum DW (2010) Anomer-equilibrated streptozotocin solution for the induction of experimental diabetes in mice (Mus musculus). J Am Assoc Lab Anim Sci 49: 40–44
25. Zinselmeyer BH, Dempster J, Wokosin DL, Cannon JJ, Pless R, Parker I, Miller MJ (2009) Chapter 16. Two-photon microscopy and multidimensional analysis of cell dynamics. Methods Enzymol 461:349–378. https://doi.org/10.1016/S0076-6879(09)05416-0

Chapter 11

New Method for the Expansion of Highly Purified Human Regulatory Granzyme B-Expressing B Cells

Mélanie Chesneau, Hoa Le Mai, and Sophie Brouard

Abstract

Granzyme B (GZMB)-expressing B cells inhibit CD4$^+$ T-lymphocyte proliferation in a contact- and GZMB-dependent manner, through degradation of TCR zeta or induction of T-cell apoptosis. This regulatory B-cell population is present in human healthy individuals and represents about 1% of circulating B cells. Their small proportion requires the development of expansion methods to enable their study and envision clinical applications. We describe here how to expand GZMB-expressing B cells to obtain more than 90% of highly purified GZMB$^+$ B cells, and the protocol of B/T cells coculture for the evaluation of the suppressive function of the GZMB$^+$ B-cell population.

Key words Breg, Granzyme B, Expansion, Regulation, T/B-cell coculture

1 Introduction

B cells are mainly known for their properties to induce or/and maintain an immune response through their ability to secrete antibodies and their capacity to present antigens [1–3]. However, since several years now, it has been shown that different B-cell subsets can also suppress the pro-inflammatory immune response in rodent models and in human through different mechanisms such as cell contact and the release of various soluble factors [4, 5]. For this reason, these subsets have been described as regulatory B cells. Regulatory B cells are characterized by different phenotypes depending on the immunological context in which they are identified, and on the conditions of activation. Among the different regulatory B cells, a population has been characterized for its ability to secrete the serine protease granzyme B (GZMB) and to play an immunosuppressive and thereby protective role in the early phase of systemic lupus erythematosus [6]. Since then, GZMB-expressing B cells have been described in various immunological contexts such as cancer, autoimmune diseases, viral infection, and transplantation [7–15], with different phenotypes including CD5$^+$, Plasmablast,

Francesca Mion and Silvia Tonon (eds.), *Regulatory B Cells: Methods and Protocols*, Methods in Molecular Biology, vol. 2270, https://doi.org/10.1007/978-1-0716-1237-8_11,

IgD$^-$CD27$^-$, and CD38$^+$CD1d$^+$IgM$^+$CD147$^+$ [6, 7, 10, 16]. Their functional characterization show that GZMB$^+$ B cells inhibit the proliferation of CD4$^+$ T cells in a contact- and GZMB-dependent manner [10], through degradation of TCR zeta [7, 11] or not [10] or induction of T-cell apoptosis [17]. Interestingly, GZMB$^+$ B cells are not only present in pathological situations but also represent about 1% of circulating B cells in healthy individuals, and we report that, in physiological conditions, these cells may potentially be involved in cell homeostasis (Chesneau et al. Submitted). This raises the interest of this population as a tool for cell therapy. Different protocols have already been proposed to expand these cells in vitro. It has been shown that the expression of GZMB by B cells is induced by IL-21, and also by a weak stimulation through CD40 and by BCR stimulation [6, 7, 18]. These protocols allow obtaining about 5–40% of GZMB$^+$ B cells (*see* Table 1). In the present chapter, we describe a protocol that, starting from total purified CD19$^+$ B cells, allows to expand this population and to obtain more than 90% of highly purified GZMB$^+$ B cells after 3 days of expansion with BCR stimulation, CD40L, CpG ODN, IL-21, and IL-2. Moreover, we provide the protocol of B/T cells coculture for the evaluation of the suppressive function of the GZMB$^+$ B-cell population.

2 Materials

2.1 General Equipment

1. Cell incubator maintained at 37 °C and 5% CO_2.
2. Centrifuge equipped with a swinging-bucket rotor.
3. Flow cytometer.
4. 500 mL sterile Vacuum Filtration System (0.22 μm).
5. 50 mL and 15 mL conical tubes.
6. 96-well U-bottom cell culture plates.
7. 96-well V-bottom cell culture plates.
8. 70 μm filters.
9. Eppendorf tube magnet for dynabeads.

2.2 Peripheral Blood Mononuclear Cells (PBMCs) Isolation

1. EDTA tubes for blood collection.
2. Density gradient solution for the isolation of PBMCs (e.g., Ficoll-Paque PREMIUM centrifugation medium).
3. Red blood cell lysis buffer: 17 mM Tris–HCl, 144 mM NH4Cl, pH 7.4.
4. 1× Phosphate-Buffered Saline (PBS): Dulbecco's Phosphate-Buffered Saline (DPBS) powder diluted in sterile water.

Table 1
Protocols for GZMB+ B-cell expansion in vitro

Title of the research paper	Author	Immunological context	Cell type	Stimulation	Duration	% GZMB+
Granzyme B production by activated B cells derived from breast cancer-draining lymph nodes.	Arabpour M [15].	Breast tumor-draining lymph nodes (TDLNs)	B cells from lymph nodes	Anti-BCR / IL-21 / CD40 L	16H	6% in HV
IL-21-dependent Granzyme B production of B cells is decreased in patients with lupus nephritis.	Rabani M [14]	Lupus nephritis	B cells from PBMCs	CPG/ IgG + IgM / IL-21 + BFA	20H	35,1% in HV
Impairment of Granzyme B-producing regulatory B Cells correlates with exacerbated rheumatoid arthritis.	Xu L [19]	Rheumatoid arthritis (RA)	B cells from PBMCs	PMA / iono + BFA	5 h	7,5% in HV
Granzyme B-producing B cells in renal transplant patients.	Zhu J [13]	Renal transplant patient	B cells	IgM/IgG/IL21 + BFA	20 h	18,75% in HV
Increased IL-21 expression induces Granzyme B in peripheral CD5(+) B cells as a potential counter-regulatory effect in primary Sjögren's syndrome.	Papp G [20]	Primary Sjögren's syndrome (pSS)	CD19+ CD5+ from PBMCs	BCR/IL-21 + BFA	18H	5,2% in HV
B-cell-derived circulating Granzyme B is a feature of acute infectious mononucleosis.	Hagn M [12]	Acute infectious mononucleosis	B cells from PBMCS	IL-21/BCR + BFA	16H	29,6% in EBV- 83,3% in EBV+
CD4+ T-cell-derived IL-21 and deprivation of CD40 signaling favor the in vivo development of Granzyme B-expressing regulatory B cells in HIV patients.	Kaltenmeier C [11]	HIV patients	B cells from PBMCs	No		30% in HIV

(continued)

Table 1 (continued)

Title of the research paper	Author	Immunological context	Cell type	Stimulation	Duration	% GZMB+
B-CLL cells acquire APC- and CTL-like phenotypic characteristics after stimulation with CpG ODN and IL-21.	Hagn M [9]	B-cell chronic lymphocytic leukemia (B-CLL)	B cells from PBMCs	IL21/BCR + BFA	16H	25% in HV
Trafficking phenotype and production of Granzyme B by double-negative B cells (IgG + IgD − CD27−) in the elderly	Bulati M [16]	Elderly	IgD − CD27− (DN)	IL-21/α-IgG + BFA	16H	26% in young 30% in elderly donors
Human plasma cells express Granzyme B.	Xu W [8]	Healthy	B cells from PBMCs	IL-15 and IL-21 + BFA	5 days	36,2% in HV
Interleukin 21–induced Granzyme B–expressing B cells infiltrate tumors and regulate T cells	Lindner S [7]	Cancer	B cells from PBMCs	BCR/IL21 + BFA	48 h	31% in Hv
Human B cells differentiate into Granzyme B-secreting cytotoxic B lymphocytes upon incomplete T-cell help	Hagn M [17]	Healthy	B cells	IL-21/BCR + BFA	16H	40% in HV

2.3 B-Cell Enrichment

1. Specific reagents and supports for immunomagnetic isolation of human B cells by negative selection. According to lab preference, different separation techniques are available (*see* **Note 1**).
2. Staining buffer: 0.5% bovine serum albumin (BSA), and 2 mM EDTA in PBS. Sterilize by filtering.

2.4 Reagents for B-Cell Culture

1. Culture medium: 10% fetal calf serum (FCS, hybridoma grade), 0.3 mg/mL L-glutamine, 120 IU/mL penicillin, 120 μg/mL streptomycin in RPMI 1640.
2. Expansion B-cell culture medium: 10 ng/mL IL-21; 50 ng/mL Recombinant Human CD40 Ligand; 1 μg/mL CpG ODN 2006; 5 μg/mL F(ab')2 anti-BCR antibody, and 50 IU/mL IL-2 in culture medium.

2.5 Reagents for GZMB$^+$ B-Cell Staining

1. Brefeldin A.
2. Staining buffer: 0.5% BSA and 2 mM EDTA in PBS. Sterilize by filtering.
3. Fixation and permeabilization solutions for intracellular staining of cytoplasmic proteins (*see* **Note 2**).
4. Dye for the discrimination of viable from nonviable cells in multicolor flow cytometry applications (e.g., LIVE/DEAD Fixable Aqua reactive dye). Reconstitute the dye according to manufacturer's instructions.
5. Anti-human CD19 (clone SJ25C1) and anti-human Granzyme B (clone GB11) antibodies (*see* **Note 3**).

2.6 Evaluation of Suppressive Function of GZMB$^+$ B Cells by B/T-Cell coculture Assays

1. Specific reagents and supports for immunomagnetic isolation of human CD4$^+$ CD25$^-$ T cells by negative selections. According to lab preference, different separation techniques are available (*see* **Note 4**).
2. Staining buffer: 0.5% BSA and 2 mM EDTA in PBS. Sterilize by filtering.
3. Anti-CD3/CD28 beads to stimulate T-cell proliferation (*see* **Note 5**).
4. Fluorescent dye specific for the study of cell proliferation (*see* **Note 6**).
5. Culture medium: 10% fetal calf serum (FCS, hybridoma grade), 0.3 mg/mL L-glutamine, 120 IU/mL penicillin, 120 μg/mL streptomycin in RPMI 1640.
6. Dye for the discrimination of viable from nonviable cells in multicolor flow cytometry applications (e.g., LIVE/DEAD Fixable Aqua reactive dye). Reconstitute the dye according to manufacturer's instructions.

7. Anti-human CD4 (clone SK3) antibody (*see* **Note 7**).
8. GZMB inhibitor (Granzyme B Inhibitor IV).

3 Methods

3.1 PBMCs Isolation

1. Collect human blood samples in EDTA tubes. Dilute 50 mL of blood with 1 volume of PBS in two 50 mL conical tubes and invert 2–3 times to homogenize the blood-PBS solution (*see* **Note 8**).
2. Carefully layer 35 mL of diluted blood over 15 mL of density gradient solution for PBMCs isolation in a 50-mL conical tube and centrifuge at 400 × *g* for 20 min at room temperature (RT) in a swinging-bucket rotor without brake.
3. Aspirate the mononuclear cell layer (lymphocytes, monocytes, and thrombocytes) at the interphase and transfer to a new 50-mL conical tube.
4. Fill the tube up to 50 mL with PBS and remove platelets by centrifuging at 200 × *g* for 10 min at RT. Carefully remove supernatant completely.
5. If following the density separation of PBMCs, there is still a lot of red cells than proceed to their removal by resuspending the cell pellet in 5 mL of red blood cell lysis buffer for 5 min at RT (*see* **Note 9**).
6. Fill the tube up to 50 mL with PBS and centrifuge at 350 × *g* for 10 min at RT.
7. Discard the supernatant and resuspend the cell pellet in 5 mL of staining buffer. Count the number of cells. The expected yield of PBMCs from 50 mL of blood is usually between 75 and 100 million.
8. Divide the obtained PBMC population into two fractions. Half the population is used for B-cell isolation (*see* Subheading 3.2), while the other half should be resuspended at 2×10^6 cells/mL in culture medium, and kept overnight in a 50-mL conical tube at 4 °C for subsequent isolation of $CD4^+$ T cells (*see* Subheading 3.4).

3.2 B-Cell Enrichment by Immunomagnetic Separation

1. Centrifuge the PBMC suspension at 350 × *g* for 10 min at 4 °C and aspirate supernatant completely.
2. Resuspend the cell pellet in 40 μL of staining buffer per 10^7 total cells and proceed to immunomagnetic isolation of B cells by negative selection. Follow the instructions provided by the manufacturer of the employed kit (*see* **Notes 1** and **10**).
3. Collect the unlabeled cell fraction and determine the number of enriched B cells obtained by magnetic separation. 40 million of PBMCs usually give two million of B cells.

3.3 GZMB+ B-Cell Expansion and Staining

1. In order to expand GZMB+ B cells, culture the enriched B-cell fraction in a 96-well round-bottom cell culture plate (10^6 cells/mL) with 200 μL of expansion B-cell culture medium for 1–3 days in a cell incubator at 37 °C and 5% CO_2 (*see* **Note 11**). As a control, culture the enriched B-cell fraction in culture medium, which is free of stimuli (resting B cells).
2. For GZMB detection, add 10 μg/mL Brefeldin A solution into the culture medium of both expanded and resting B cells 4 h before the end of the 3 days culture.
3. Collect cells from the 96-well cell culture plate and resuspend 10^6 cells in 100 μL of PBS in a 96-well plate V-bottom (*see* **Note 12**).
4. Add the optimal dose of the chosen dye for the discrimination of viable from nonviable cells and incubate 20 min at 4 °C protected from light. After incubation, wash by adding 100 μL of PBS and centrifuge cells 600 × *g* for 2 min at 4 °C. Discard the supernatant.
5. Resuspend cells in staining buffer and add the optimal dose of anti-CD19 mAb (*see* **Note 13**). Incubate 20 min at 4 °C protected from light.
6. Wash twice by adding 100 μL of staining buffer and centrifuge 600 × *g* for 2 min at 4 °C. Discard the supernatant.
7. Resuspend cells in Intracellular Fixation & Permeabilization Buffer and incubate 30 min at 4 °C protected from light. Wash by adding 100 μL of Permeabilization Buffer and centrifuge 600 × *g* for 2 min at 4 °C (*see* **Note 14**). Discard the supernatant.
8. Resuspend cells in 100 μL of Permeabilization Buffer and add the optimal dose of anti-GZMB mAb and incubate 30 min at 4 °C protected from light (*see* **Notes 13** and **15**). After incubation, wash twice by adding 100 μL of Permeabilization Buffer and centrifuge 600 × *g* for 2 min at 4 °C. Discard the supernatant.
9. Resuspend stained cells in an appropriate volume of staining buffer and analyze samples by flow cytometry. Figure 1 shows a representative analysis of GZMB+ B cells among expanded and resting B cells after 3 days of culture.

3.4 Evaluation of the Suppressive Function of GZMB+ B Cells by B/T-Cell coculture Assays

The evaluation of the suppressive function of GZMB+ B cells can be performed 18–24 h after GZMB+ B-cell expansion through the analysis of their capacity to suppress CD3/CD28-induced T-cell proliferation (*see* **Note 16**).

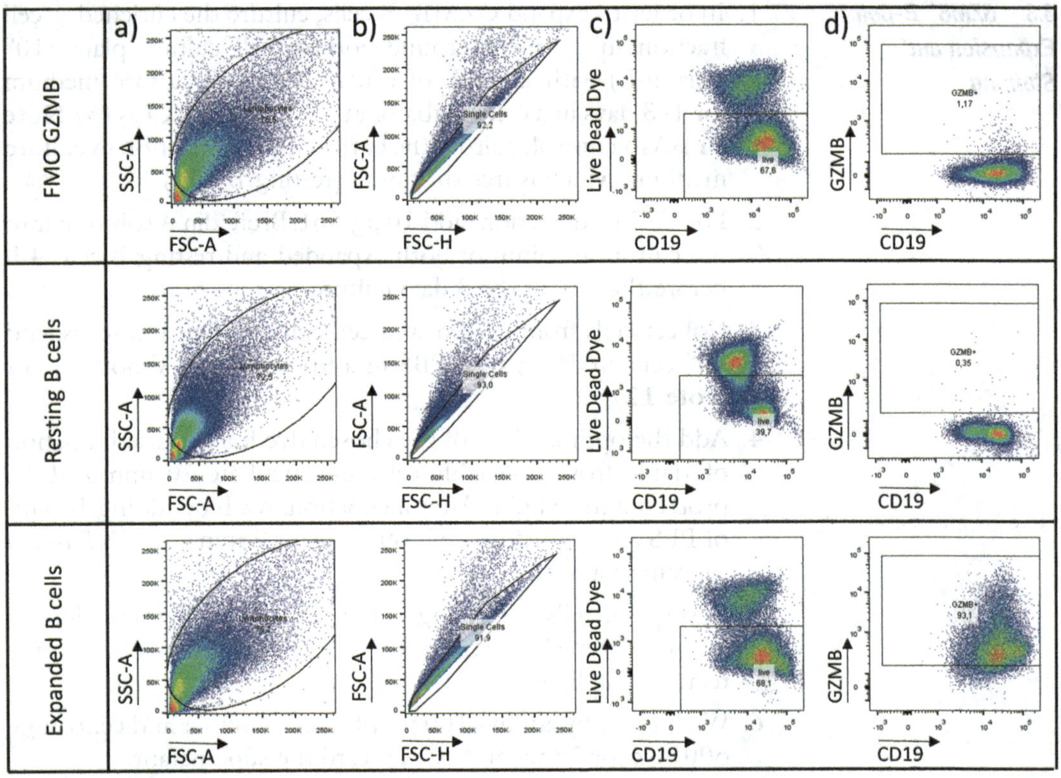

Fig. 1 Expressions of GZMB in resting and expanded B cells after 3 days of culture. Dot plots show the gating strategy to identify GZMB$^+$ B cells by intracellular staining. Start by gating on lymphocytes on the basis of their size and granularity (**a**), and on singlet cells to exclude doublets of sticky cells (**b**). Then, select alive lymphocytes which are negative for the Live/Dead dye (**c**), and finally identify GZMB$^+$CD19$^+$ GZMB-producing B cells (**d**). The first row of dot plots shows the FMO control, while the middle and bottom rows display GZMB expression in resting and expanded B cells, respectively.

3.4.1 T-Cell Preparation

1. Isolate CD4$^+$ T cells from PBMCs kept overnight at 4 °C (*see* Subheading 3.1, **step 8**). Filter the cell suspension on a 70-μm filter and proceed to the immunomagnetic isolation of CD4$^+$ T cells by negative selection. Follow the instructions provided by the manufacturer of the employed kit (*see* **Notes 4** and **10**).
2. Collect the unlabeled cell fraction and determine the number of enriched CD4$^+$ T cells obtained by magnetic separation. 40 million of PBMCs usually give ten million of CD4$^+$ T cells.
3. Resuspend CD4$^+$ T cells in 80 μL of sorting buffer per 10^7 total cells and proceed to immunomagnetic isolation of CD25$^-$ cells by negative selection. Follow the instructions provided by the manufacturer of the employed kit (*see* **Notes 4** and **10**).
4. Collect the unlabeled cell fraction and determine the number of enriched CD4$^+$CD25$^-$ T cells obtained by magnetic separation. ten million of CD4$^+$ T cells usually give around four million of CD4$^+$CD25$^-$ T cells.

5. Resuspend $CD4^+CD25^-$ in PBS and add the selected fluorescent dye specific for the study of cell proliferation. Follow the instructions provided by the manufacturer of the employed kit (*see* **Note 6**).
6. Resuspend the stained $CD4^+CD25^-$ cells in culture medium at 10^6 cells/mL and keep them out of the light and on ice.

3.4.2 Set up of the B/T-Cell Coculture

1. Recover the B cells which were put in culture in normal or expansion B-cell culture medium the previous day (*see* Subheading 3.3, **step 1**) and wash them by adding warm culture medium. Centrifuge the cell suspensions at 350 × *g* for 10 min at RT and resuspend $GZMB^+$ expanded and resting B cells at 10^6 cells/mL in culture medium. Keep cells on ice.
2. At the same time prepare the anti-CD3/CD28 beads, following the instructions provided by the manufacturer of the employed kit (*see* **Note 17**).
3. Plate 10^5 $GZMB^+$ expanded or resting B cells, 5×10^4 $CD4^+CD25^-$ effector T cells and 5×10^4 anti-CD3/CD28 beads (*see* **Notes 5** and **17**) in a U-bottom 96-well plate. Coculture B and T cells in a final volume of 200 μL of culture medium for 3 days in a cell incubator at 37 °C and 5% CO_2. Determine the GZMB-dependent regulatory function of expanded B cells by adding a GZMB inhibitor (10 μg/mL) to the B/T-cell coculture (*see* **Note 18**).

3.4.3 Evaluation of the Suppression of T-Cell Proliferation by Flow Cytometry

1. Following the 3 days of coculture (*see* Subheading 3.4, **step 9**), collect the cells from the U-bottom 96-well cell culture plate and transfer them to a V-bottom 96-well plate (*see* **Note 12**), centrifuge 600 × *g* for 2 min at 4 °C, discard the culture medium, and resuspend cells in 100 μL PBS.
2. Add the optimal dose of the chosen dye for the discrimination of viable from nonviable cells and incubate 20 min at 4 °C protected from light. After incubation, wash cells by adding 100 μL of PBS and centrifuge cells 600 × *g* for 2 min at 4 °C. Discard the supernatant.
3. Resuspend cells in staining buffer and add the optimal dose of anti-CD4 mAb (*see* **Note 13**). Incubate 20 min at 4 °C protected from light.
4. Wash twice by adding 100 μL of staining buffer and centrifuge 600 × *g* for 2 min at 4 °C. Discard the supernatant.
5. Resuspend stained cells in an appropriate volume of staining buffer and analyze samples by flow cytometry. Figure 2 shows a representative analysis of how T-cell proliferation changes when cultured in the presence of $GZMB^+$ expanded or resting B cells.

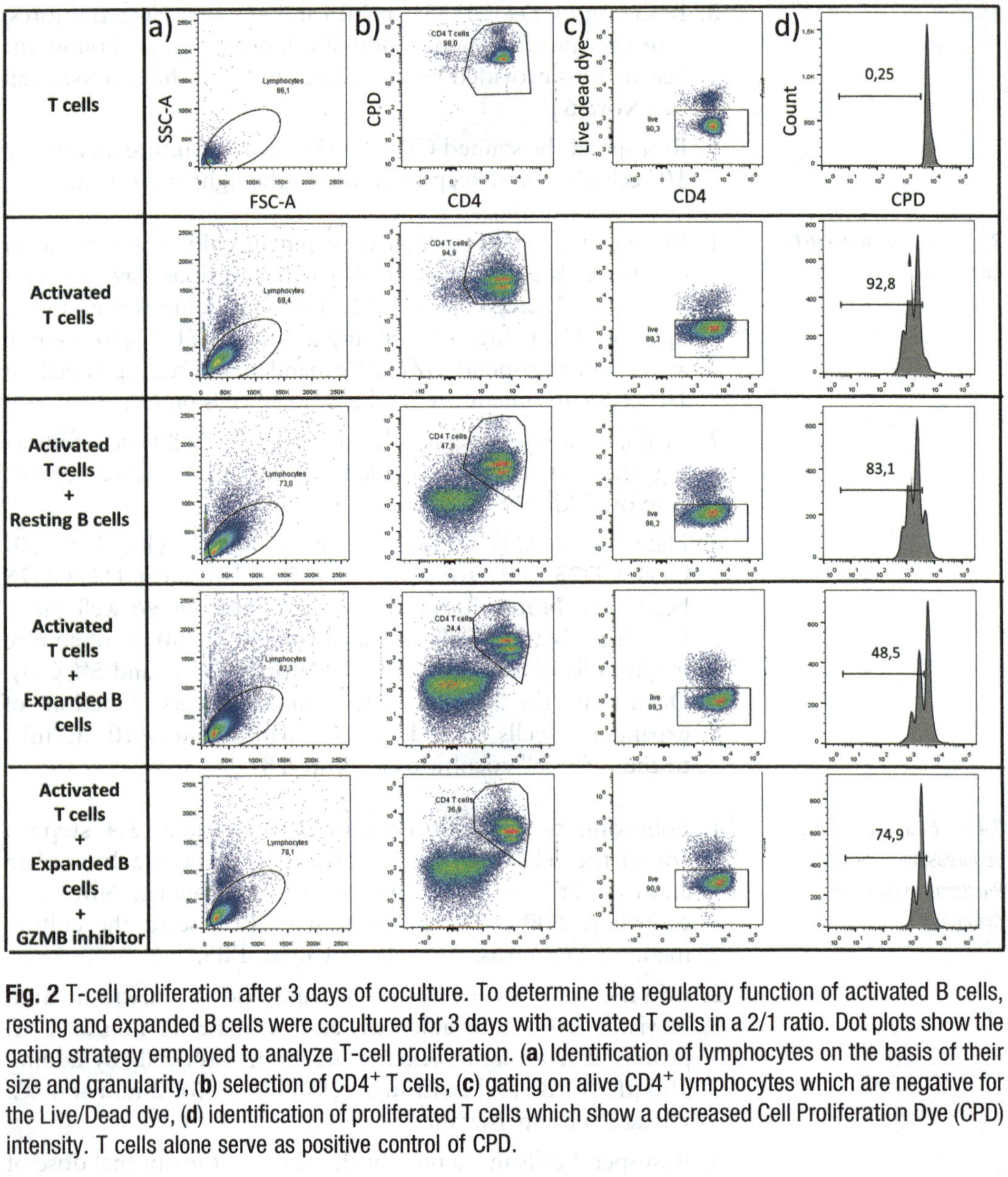

Fig. 2 T-cell proliferation after 3 days of coculture. To determine the regulatory function of activated B cells, resting and expanded B cells were cocultured for 3 days with activated T cells in a 2/1 ratio. Dot plots show the gating strategy employed to analyze T-cell proliferation. (**a**) Identification of lymphocytes on the basis of their size and granularity, (**b**) selection of $CD4^+$ T cells, (**c**) gating on alive $CD4^+$ lymphocytes which are negative for the Live/Dead dye, (**d**) identification of proliferated T cells which show a decreased Cell Proliferation Dye (CPD) intensity. T cells alone serve as positive control of CPD.

4 Notes

1. B cells can be positively selected based on the binding of cell surface markers, such as CD19 or CD20. However, we prefer adopting negative selection due to possible activation of B cells by CD19 and as it makes easier a subsequent staining with an anti-CD19 mAb. We routinely use the B-cell isolation kit II, human, from Miltenyi Biotec. When using the Miltenyi technology, magnetic cell separation can be performed either

manually using MS or LS columns, or with the autoMACS Pro Separator following the manufacturer's instruction, depending on the number of cells.

2. We suggest using commercially available kits and, in particular, the Intracellular Fixation & Permeabilization Buffer Set (eBioscience). According to manufacturer's instructions, 1× Permeabilization Buffer was prepared by mixing one part of 10× Permeabilization Buffer with nine parts of distilled water. However, the staining of GZMB can also be performed using in-house-made reagents for fixation and permeabilization.
3. The anti-human CD19 and anti-GZMB antibodies routinely used in our laboratory to follow $GZMB^+$ B cells are conjugated to BV786 and BV421, respectively. These fluorochromes are part of the BD Horizon™ Brilliant Violet™ family of dyes. Use of more common dyes is quite possible for this staining.
4. There are several human $CD4^+$ T-lymphocyte isolation kits commercially available. We suggest using a kit that employs a negative selection method for $CD4^+$ T-cell enrichment (e.g., $CD4^+$ T Cell Isolation Kit, human, Miltenyi) as a second isolation step with CD25 microbeads (e.g., CD25 MicroBeads II, human Miltenyi) should be performed to purify effectors $CD25^-$ cells.
5. For T-cell activation, we routinely use Dynabeads Human T-activator CD3/CD28. Anti-CD3/CD28 beads should be carefully titrated before use. Alternatively, one could choose to coat the wells of the culture plate with anti-CD3 and anti-CD28 mAb.
6. We routinely use the CellTrace Cell proliferation kit which allows to trace multiple generations using dye dilution by flow cytometry. We use the CellTrace Violet, but other dyes are available and could also be used.
7. The anti-human CD4 antibody used in this study is conjugated to PE-C7. Use of other dyes is quite possible for this staining, according to the choice of the specific cell proliferation dye.
8. For this protocol, blood samples can be stored for up to 24 h at room temperature after collection.
9. The quantity of red cell lysis solution should be adapted according to the initial quantity of blood, and according to the grade of red cell contamination after Ficoll. If the cell pellet still has red cells, it is preferable to perform two successive lyses. Exceeding 5 min of red cell lysis may increase lymphocyte mortality.
10. All buffers should be sterile and kept cold until use.
11. The percentage of $GZMB^+$ B cells increases until the third day of culture, then it decreases while lymphocyte mortality

increases. Depending on the applications, the duration of culture can be reduced. To test GZMB$^+$ B-cell suppressive effect, an 18- to 24-h stimulation is recommended to avoid a too high mortality of lymphocytes at the end of the coculture.

12. The transfer of cells to a V-bottom 96-well plate avoids cell loss during staining for flow cytometry. Multichannel pipette can be used. For cell staining, the cells and buffers should be always kept cold to avoid background staining.
13. The working concentration of each antibody should be optimized before use. Avoid using excess of fluorescence-labeled antibodies to reduce nonspecific staining.
14. The Perm/Wash solution must be maintained in washing steps to keep cells permeabilized.
15. Simultaneous to the GZMB staining, it is necessary to do the fluorescence minus one (FMO) of GZMB as a control of the GZMB staining.
16. To test the suppressive function of the GZMB$^+$ B cells, a coculture is carried out between CD4$^+$CD25$^-$ effectors T cells and B cells expanded for 18–24 h. The choice of this shorter time frame for GZMB$^+$ B-cell expansion is due to the fact that, after 3 days of culture, expanded B cells become more sensitive to apoptosis. As a consequence, after 3 more days in coculture we observed a higher cell mortality and a regulatory function that is not increased.
17. Wash Dynabeads Human T-activator CD3/CD28 to obtain a bead-to-cell ratio of 1:1. Staining buffer can be used for the Dynabeads washing procedure.
18. As a negative control of effector CD4$^+$ T-cell proliferation, we prepare a well with CD4$^+$CD25$^-$ T cells without CD3/CD28 stimulation. The positive control is a well with CD4$^+$CD25$^-$ T cells with CD3/CD28 stimulation. We determine the regulatory function of expanded B cells on T-cell proliferation by comparing the wells in which expanded and resting B cells are cultured with CD4$^+$CD25$^-$ T cells in the presence of CD3/CD28 stimulation.

Acknowledgments

This work was supported by a grant from the ANR project BIKET (ANR-17-CE17-0008). French National Research Agency (ANR-11-JSV1-0008-01) and supported in part by the RTRS Fondation de Coopération Scientifique CENTAURE, which supports a French transplantation research network. This work was performed as a part of the IHU-Cesti project, which received French government financial support managed by the Agence

Nationale de la Recherche via the "Investment into the Future" program ANR-10-IBHU-005. The IHU-Cesti project is also supported by Nantes Metropole and the Pays de la Loire Region. This work was also supported by the FP7 VISICORT project, which has received funding from the European Union's Seventh Framework Programme for research, technological development, and demonstration under grant agreement 602470. This work was performed as a part of the LabEX IGO program supported by the National Research Agency via the Investment into the Future program ANR-11-LABX-0016-01 and in the context of the ANR project PRELUD (ANR-18-CE17-0019).

References

1. Parker Harp CR, Archambault AS, Sim J, Ferris ST, Mikesell RJ, Koni PA, Shimoda M, Linington C, Russell JH, Wu GF (2015) B cell antigen presentation is sufficient to drive neuroinflammation in an animal model of multiple sclerosis. J Immunol 194:5077–5084. https://doi.org/10.4049/jimmunol.1402236
2. Liu S (2018) Release of antibodies and cytokines from B cells. Methods Mol Biol 1868:201–207. https://doi.org/10.1007/978-1-4939-8802-0_20
3. Matsushita T (2019) Regulatory and effector B cells: friends or foes? J Dermatol Sci 93:2–7. https://doi.org/10.1016/j.jdermsci.2018.11.008
4. Floudas A, Amu S, Fallon PG (2016) New insights into IL-10 dependent and IL-10 independent mechanisms of regulatory B cell immune suppression. J Clin Immunol 36 (Suppl 1):25–33. https://doi.org/10.1007/s10875-016-0263-8
5. Wąsik M, Nazimek K, Bryniarski K (2018) Regulatory B cell phenotype and mechanism of action: the impact of stimulating conditions. Microbiol Immunol 62:485–496. https://doi.org/10.1111/1348-0421.12636
6. Hagn M, Ebel V, Sontheimer K, Schwesinger E, Lunov O, Beyer T, Fabricius D, Barth TFE, Viardot A, Stilgenbauer S, Hepp J, Scharffetter-Kochanek K, Simmet T, Jahrsdörfer B (2010) CD5+ B cells from individuals with systemic lupus erythematosus express granzyme B. Eur J Immunol 40:2060–2069. https://doi.org/10.1002/eji.200940113
7. Lindner S, Dahlke K, Sontheimer K, Hagn M, Kaltenmeier C, Barth TFE, Beyer T, Reister F, Fabricius D, Lotfi R, Lunov O, Nienhaus GU, Simmet T, Kreienberg R, Möller P, Schrezenmeier H, Jahrsdorfer B (2013) Interleukin 21-induced granzyme B-expressing B cells infiltrate tumors and regulate T cells. Cancer res 73:2468. https://doi.org/10.1158/0008-5472.CAN-12-3450
8. Xu W, Narayanan P, Kang N, Clayton S, Ohne Y, Shi P, Herve M-C, Balderas R, Picard C, Casanova J-L, Gorvel J-P, Oh S, Pascual V, Banchereau J (2014) Human plasma cells express granzyme B. Eur J Immunol 44:275–284. https://doi.org/10.1002/eji.201343711
9. Hagn M, Blackwell SE, Beyer T, Ebel V, Fabricius D, Lindner S, Stilgenbauer S, Simmet T, Tam C, Neeson P, Trapani JA, Schrezenmeier H, Weiner GJ, Jahrsdörfer B (2014) B-CLL cells acquire APC- and CTL-like phenotypic characteristics after stimulation with CpG ODN and IL-21. Int Immunol 26:383–395. https://doi.org/10.1093/intimm/dxu001
10. Chesneau M, Michel L, Dugast E, Chenouard A, Baron D, Pallier A, Durand J, Braza F, Guerif P, Laplaud D-A, Soulillou J-P, Giral M, Degauque N, Chiffoleau E, Brouard S (2015) Tolerant kidney transplant patients produce B cells with regulatory properties. J Am Soc Nephrol 26:2588. https://doi.org/10.1681/ASN.2014040404
11. Kaltenmeier C, Gawanbacht A, Beyer T, Lindner S, Trzaska T, van der Merwe JA, Härter G, Grüner B, Fabricius D, Lotfi R, Schwarz K, Schütz C, Hönig M, Schulz A, Kern P, Bommer M, Schrezenmeier H, Kirchhoff F, Jahrsdörfer B (2015) CD4+ T Cell-Derived IL-21 and Deprivation of CD40 Signaling Favor the In Vivo Development of Granzyme B-Expressing Regulatory B Cells in HIV Patients. J Immunol. https://doi.org/10.4049/jimmunol.1402568
12. Hagn M, Panikkar A, Smith C, Balfour HH, Khanna R, Voskoboinik I, Trapani JA (2015) B

cell-derived circulating granzyme B is a feature of acute infectious mononucleosis. Clin Transl Immunology 4:e38. https://doi.org/10.1038/cti.2015.10

13. Zhu J, Zeng Y, Dolff S, Bienholz A, Lindemann M, Brinkhoff A, Schedlowski M, Xu S, Sun M, Guberina H, Kirchhof J, Kribben A, Witzke O, Wilde B (2017) Granzyme B producing B-cells in renal transplant patients. Clin Immunol 184:48–53. https://doi.org/10.1016/j.clim.2017.04.016
14. Rabani M, Wilde B, Hübbers K, Xu S, Kribben A, Witzke O, Dolff S (2018) IL-21 dependent Granzyme B production of B-cells is decreased in patients with lupus nephritis. Clin Immunol 188:45–51. https://doi.org/10.1016/j.clim.2017.12.005
15. Arabpour M, Rasolmali R, Talei A-R, Mehdipour F, Ghaderi A (2019) Granzyme B production by activated B cells derived from breast cancer-draining lymph nodes. Mol Immunol 114:172–178. https://doi.org/10.1016/j.molimm.2019.07.019
16. Bulati M, Buffa S, Martorana A, Candore G, Lio D, Caruso C, Colonna-Romano G (2014) Trafficking phenotype and production of granzyme B by double negative B cells (IgG(+)IgD(−)CD27(−)) in the elderly. Exp Gerontol 54:123–129. https://doi.org/10.1016/j.exger.2013.12.011
17. Hagn M, Sontheimer K, Dahlke K, Brueggemann S, Kaltenmeier C, Beyer T, Hofmann S, Lunov O, Barth TFE, Fabricius D, Tron K, Nienhaus GU, Simmet T, Schrezenmeier H, Jahrsdörfer B (2012) Human B cells differentiate into granzyme B-secreting cytotoxic B lymphocytes upon incomplete T-cell help. Immunol Cell Biol 90:457–467. https://doi.org/10.1038/icb.2011.64
18. Hagn M, Jahrsdörfer B (2012) Why do human B cells secrete granzyme B? Insights into a novel B-cell differentiation pathway. Onco Targets Ther 1:1368–1375. https://doi.org/10.4161/onci.22354
19. Xu L, Liu X, Liu H, Zhu L, Zhu H, Zhang J, Ren L, Wang P, Hu F, Su Y (2017) Impairment of Granzyme B-producing regulatory B cells correlates with exacerbated rheumatoid arthritis. Front Immunol 8:768. https://doi.org/10.3389/fimmu.2017.00768
20. Papp G, bor, Gyimesi E, Szab, Krisztina, Z, Ld, va, Zeher M (2016) Increased IL-21 expression induces granzyme B in peripheral CD5. Mediators of inflammation 2016. https://doi.org/10.1155/2016/4328372

Chapter 12

Characterization of the Cell Surface Phenotype and Regulatory Activity of B-Cell IgD Low (BD_L) Regulatory B Cells

Mohamed Khalil, Avijit Ray, and Bonnie N. Dittel

Abstract

B-cell IgD Low (BD_L) B cells have been shown to promote immunological tolerance by inducing proliferation of $CD4^+Foxp3^+$ T-regulatory cells (Treg) in a glucocorticoid-induced tumor necrosis factor receptor-related protein ligand (GITRL, *Tnfsf18*)-dependent manner. BD_L cells constitute a small subset of splenic B lymphocytes that, in mice, are characterized by the $B220^+IgM^{int}CD21^{int}CD23^+CD93^-IgD^{low/-}$ cell surface expression profile. In this chapter, we show the flow cytometry gating strategy developed to identify and purify BD_L. In addition, we describe an in vitro assay and two in vivo assays to assess BD_L regulatory activity by quantitating Treg expansion/proliferation and indicate how they can be used in mouse models of disease. Collectively, these methods are useful to track and quantitate BD_L and Treg numbers and assess their regulatory activity in inflammatory disease models.

Key words B-cell IgD low (BD_L), $CD4^+Foxp3^+$ T-regulatory cells (Treg), B-cell-deficient mice (μMT), Flow cytometry, Fluorescence activated cell sorting (FACS), Proliferation

1 Introduction

A regulatory role for B cells was first described in autoimmunity utilizing the experimental autoimmune encephalomyelitis (EAE) mouse model of multiple sclerosis, where it was shown that mice deficient in B cells (μMT) did not recover from the signs of disease [1]. This seminal study demonstrated that B cells play a critical role in negatively regulating the extent of inflammation and initiated the search for regulatory B-cell phenotypes and their mechanism of action [2–4]. To that end, we identified a novel B-cell subset, which we termed B-cell IgD low (BD_L) because they are separated from conventional follicular (FO) B cells by low/negative IgD expression [5]. When we investigated their mechanism of action, we found that mice deficient in B cells due to genetic disruption or B-cell depletion with anti-CD20 antibody had a significant reduction in the absolute number of $CD4^+Foxp3^+$ T-regulatory cells

Francesca Mion and Silvia Tonon (eds.), *Regulatory B Cells: Methods and Protocols*, Methods in Molecular Biology, vol. 2270, https://doi.org/10.1007/978-1-0716-1237-8_12,

(Treg) [5, 6]. This result was of importance because Treg are an essential tolerance mechanism preventing autoimmune responses [7]. To study the mechanism whereby BD_L maintain Treg homeostasis, we developed both in vitro and in vivo assays [5, 6]. We found that adoptive transfer of BD_L into μMT mice induced Treg proliferation and that only BD_L, but not FO IgD^{hi} or marginal zone (MZ) B cells, induced Treg expansion [5]. We also demonstrated that the in vitro co-culture of total B cells or BD_L with labeled Treg or their cotransfer into μMT mice induced proliferation of the labeled Treg [5, 6]. These data indicated that BD_L:Treg interactions likely occur leading to Treg proliferation. When we investigated the mechanism, we found that BD_L expression of glucocorticoid-induced tumor necrosis factor receptor-related protein ligand (GITRL, *Tnfsf18*) was required to induce Treg proliferation [5, 6]. These findings are consistent with its receptor GITR being highly expressed by Treg and a known inducer of Treg proliferation [8, 9]. We have also shown that BD_L adoptive transfer prior to induction of EAE or contact hypersensitivity leads to increased Treg cell numbers and attenuated disease severity [5].

Here, we provide detailed flow cytometry-based methods for the identification and purification of BD_L for their subsequent tracking and utilization in BD_L activity assays. In addition, we provide methods to assess the ability of BD_L to induce Treg proliferation both in vitro and in vivo. These methods can be adapted to study whether BD_L play a role in specific diseases and to further identify BD_L and Treg mechanisms resulting in the attenuation of inflammation using animal models of disease.

2 Materials

2.1 Equipment

1. 24-well polystyrene tissue culture plates.
2. 15-mL polypropylene conical tubes.
3. 45-μm cell strainers.
4. Staining tubes or microtiter plates.
5. Magnets for immunomagnetic sorting.
6. Flow cytometer (*see* **Note 1**).
7. Flow cytometry analysis software (*see* **Note 2**).
8. Cell sorter (*see* **Note 3**).

2.2 General Reagents

1. 1× Phosphate-buffered saline (PBS).
2. Cell staining buffer: 2% Fetal Bovine Serum (FBS) and 0.1% sodium azide in 1× PBS.
3. FACS staining buffer: 5% FBS in 1× PBS.

4. Cell sorting collection solution: 1 mL FBS and 25 mM HEPES.
5. Culture medium: RPMI 1640 medium containing 10% FBS, 2 mM L-glutamine, 0.05 mM 2-mercaptoethanol and 100 U/mL penicillin and streptomycin.
6. 2% paraformaldehyde.

2.3 Mice

For all of our studies, we utilized μMT mice deficient in B cells due to disruption of the IgM heavy chain, on the B10.PL or C57BL/6 background [10]. However, other B-cell-deficient mouse models can be employed. Both male and female mice can be utilized at 6–10 weeks of age (*see* **Note 4**).

1. C57BL/6 mice.
2. B10.PL mice.
3. Foxp3^{EGFP} mice.
4. B-cell-deficient (μMT) mice.

2.4 Assessing BD_L and Treg Cell Surface Phenotype by Flow Cytometry

1. Single cell suspension of mouse splenocytes (*see* **Note 5**).
2. Fluorescent-conjugated mAb for the detection of Treg cells (*see* **Note 6**) and of cell surface molecules of BD_L and other B-cell subsets (*see* Table 1). Every antibody needs to be titrated starting from manufacturer's instructions.

2.5 Fluorescence Activated Cell Sorting (FACS) and Magnetic Bead Enrichment

1. Single cell suspension of mouse splenocytes (*see* **Note 5**).
2. Streptavidin-coated beads and anti-mouse thy1-biotin and anti-mouse CD11b-biotin antibodies for immunomagnetic enrichment of B cells through positive selection of T cells and myeloid cells (*see* **Notes** 7 and **8**).
3. Streptavidin-coated beads and anti-mouse B220-biotin, anti-CD8-biotin, and anti-mouse CD11b-biotin antibodies for immunomagnetic enrichment of $CD4^+$ T cells through positive selection of B cells, $CD8^+$ T cells, and myeloid cells (*see* **Notes 7** and **8**).
4. Sterile fluorochrome-conjugated mAbs for detection of BD_L and Treg cell surface molecules (*see* Table 1).

2.6 Reagents for In Vitro Treg Proliferation Assay

1. Functional-grade anti-mouse-CD3 and anti-mouse-CD28 antibodies purified locally or purchased from a commercial source (*see* **Note 9**).
2. Cell proliferation dye (*see* **Note 10**).
3. Anti-mouse CD4 antibody conjugated to a fluorochrome of choice.
4. 7-Aminoactinomycin D (7AAD).

Table 1
List of fluorochrome-conjugated mAb for the detection and FACS purification of BD_L and Treg cells

Fluorochrome	Antigen	Clone
PE/dazzle 594	IgM	RMM-1
Efluor 450	CD21/CD35	4E3
PE/Cy7	CD23	B3B4
PE-CF594	CD45R (B220)	RA3-6B2
PE	CD93	AA4.1
APC	IgM	II/41
FITC	IgD	11-26c
PE	IgD	11-26c.2a
FITC	CD4	GK1.5
PE	FoxP3	FJK-16 s
AF700	CD45R (B220)	RA3-6B2

2.7 Reagents for the In Vivo Treg Expansion and Maintenance Assays

1. Optional-fixation and permeabilization buffers optimized for the staining of transcription factors and nuclear proteins (*see* **Note 6**).
2. Optional- reagents to detect cell proliferation: cell proliferation dye, anti-Ki-67 or BrdU (*see* **Note 11**).

3 Methods

3.1 Detecting the BD_L Cell Surface Phenotype by Flow Cytometry

BD_L are a rare population of B cells that are identified by low expression of IgD along with additional cell surface markers that are differentially expressed on other B-cell subsets [5]. The lack of unique identifying markers makes it difficult to identify BD_L within tissues. Because of the ability to measure protein expression levels on millions of cells, flow cytometry is an optimal method to identify, quantitate, and track BD_L.

1. Euthanize mice and collect the spleen. Isolate mouse splenocytes by mashing the spleen between the frosted ends of microscope slides. Centrifuge, aspirate the supernatant and then loosen the cell pellet by flicking the bottom of the tube. Proceed to red blood cell lysis.
2. Wash total splenocytes twice with 1× PBS and then determine the absolute cell number. Resuspend total splenocytes at $10–20 \times 10^6$ cells/mL and stain with a cocktail of anti-B220, -CD21, -IgM, -CD23, -CD93, and -IgD antibodies (*see* Table 1) diluted in cell staining buffer. Antibodies should be titrated before use.

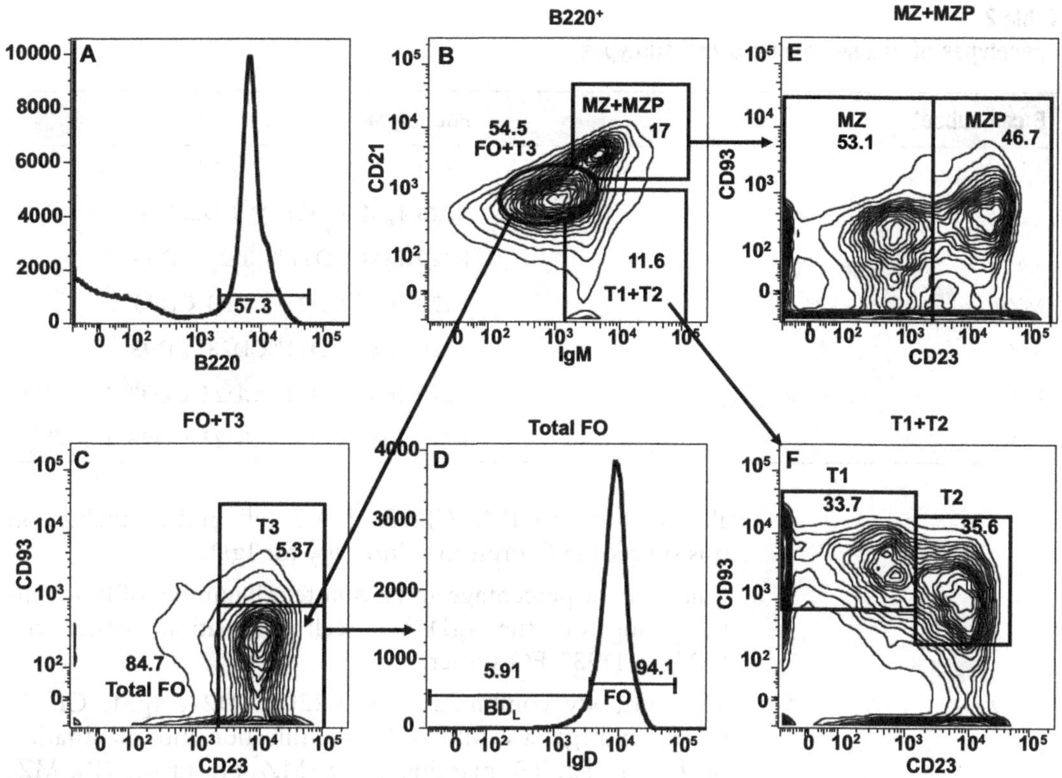

Fig. 1 Flow cytometry gating strategy for the identification of different B-cell subsets in the spleen of mice. Splenocytes were surface stained with anti-B220, -CD21, -IgM, -CD23, -CD93, and -IgD antibodies and analyzed by flow cytometry. Cells were first gated based on the size and granularity using FSC and SSC to exclude debris (not shown) and then gated as $B220^+$ B cells (**a**). $B220^+$ B cells were subsequently analyzed for CD21 and IgM expression and $IgM^{int}CD21^{int}$ cells, that contain follicular (FO) and transitional (T) 3 cells, were selected (**b**). The differential expression of CD23 and CD93 between FO and T3 cells allows the selection of the $CD23^+CD93^-$ FO B-cell population (**c**) and to subsequently gate on $IgD^{low/-}$ BD_L (**d**). The antibody combination of B220, CD21, IgM, CD23, CD93, and IgD also allows the identification and quantitation of transitional (T) subsets and mature marginal zone (MZ) B cells. The $B220^+IgM^+CD21^{hi}$ subset (**b**) can be subdivided into $CD23^-$ MZ B cells and $CD23^+$ T2-MZP (**e**). The $IgM^{hi}CD21^-$ subset (**b**) can be subdivided into the $CD23^-CD93^+$ T1 and $CD23^+CD93^+$ T2 subsets (**f**)

3. Incubate for 15 min in the dark at 4 °C and then wash twice with staining buffer by centrifuging at 300 × *g* for 5 min. Discard the supernatant and resuspend the cell pellet at 1–2 × 10^6 cells/mL in staining buffer or fix with 2% paraformaldehyde.

4. Acquire samples on the flow cytometer and analyze data (*see* **Notes 1** and **2**). Figure 1 outlines the gating strategy used to identify BD_L cells based on their peculiar phenotype. Gate on $B220^+$ B cells and then subsequently gate on $IgM^{int}CD21^{int}$ cells that contain follicular (FO) and transitional (T) 3 cells. The differential expression of the CD23 and CD93 markers

Table 2
Phenotypes of mouse splenic B-cell subtypes

B cell subset	Phenotype
T1	$B220^+IgM^{hi}CD21^{low/-}CD23^-CD93^+$
T2	$B220^+IgM^{hi}CD21^{low/-}CD23^+CD93^+$
T3	$B220^+IgM^+CD21^{int}CD23^+CD93^+$
MZP	$B220^+IgM^{hi}CD21^{hi}CD23^+CD93^{int}$
MZ	$B220^+IgM^{hi}CD21^{hi}CD23^-CD93^-$
FO	$B220^+IgM^{hi}CD21^{int}CD23^+CD93^-IgD^{hi}$
BD_L	$B220^+IgM^{hi}CD21^{int}CD23^+CD93^-IgD^{low/-}$

allows to select $CD23^+CD93^-$ FO B cells and to analyze on this subset the fluorescence intensity for IgD.

5. Calculate the percentage and absolute cell number of BD_L cells by gating on the $IgD^{low/-}$ cell population within the $CD23^+CD93^-$ FO subset.
6. The antibody combination of B220, CD21, IgM, CD23, CD93, and IgD also allows the identification and quantitation of the T1, T2, T3, marginal zone (MZ) precursors (P), MZ, total FO, and FO IgD^{hi} B-cell subsets (*see* Table 2).

3.2 Detection of Treg by Flow Cytometry

Treg are a rare T-cell subset that can be tracked by the expression of CD4 in combination with Foxp3. Although intranuclear staining of Foxp3 can be utilized to follow Treg, this staining procedure results in the death of the cells, which cannot be utilized in functional assays. An alternative that allows to bypass this problem is the employment of $Foxp3^{EGFP}$ reporter mice using flow cytometry which permits the identification and quantitation of the small numbers of Treg [5].

1. Isolate mouse splenocytes and quantitate the absolute cell number as in Subheading 3.1.
2. Stain total splenocytes at 10–20 × 10^6 cells/mL with the anti-mouse CD4 antibody (*see* Table 1) diluted in cell staining buffer (*see* **Note 6**). Incubate for 15 min in the dark at 4 °C.
3. At the end of incubation, wash twice with staining buffer by centrifuging at 300 × *g* for 5 min. Discard the supernatant and resuspend the cell pellet at 1–2 × 10^6 cells/mL in staining buffer or fix with 2% paraformaldehyde.
4. Acquire samples on the flow cytometer and analyze flow cytometry data (*see* **Notes 1** and **2**). Analyze the Treg population as $CD4^+FoxP3/EGFP^+$ (*see* **Note 6**). To obtain the absolute

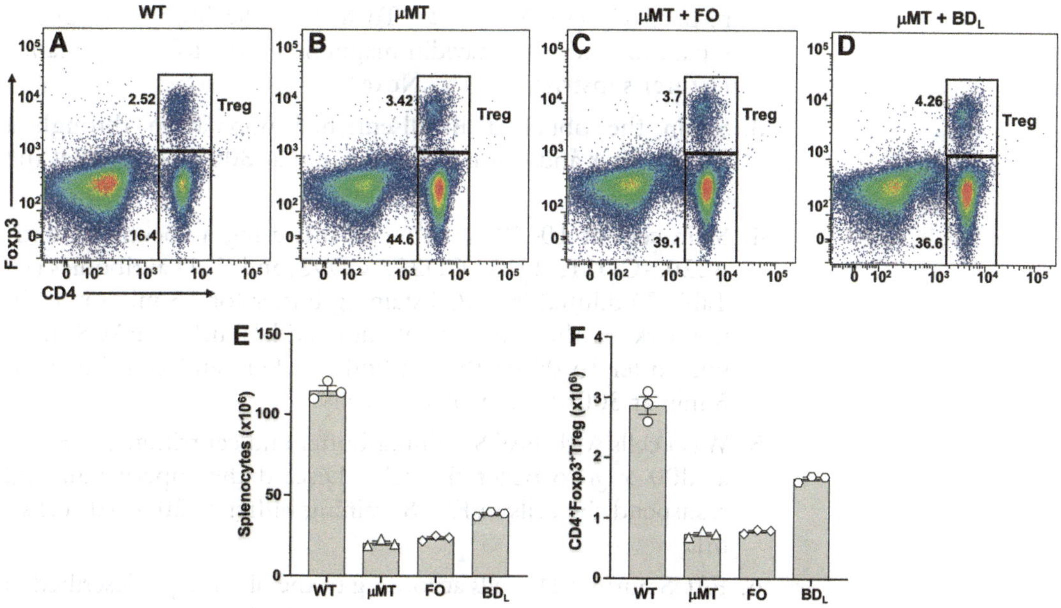

Fig. 2 Flow cytometry gating strategy for Treg identification and quantification in the spleen of mice. To detect $CD4^+Foxp3^+$ Treg, gate on lymphocytes using forward and light scatter and then generate a two-color flow plot with CD4 and EGFP (Foxp3) (**a–d**). Shown are representative flow cytometry plots of Treg in WT (**a**) and μMT (**b**) mice, and in μMT mice adoptively transferred with FO (**c**) or BD_L (**d**) B cells 7 days prior Treg analysis. For Treg quantification, first determine the absolute number of total splenocytes from each mouse (**e**) and then multiply with the percentage of Treg obtained in the flow cytometry plots (**f**)

number of Treg from the starting mononuclear cell number, gate on $CD4^+$ T cells and then calculate the percentage of Treg within the $CD4^+$ gate (*see* Fig. 2).

3.3 FACS Purification of BD_L

Because BD_L do not express a unique cell surface identifier and share markers with other B-cell subsets, magnetic bead positive selection cannot be used for their purification. Thus, FACS needs to be utilized. Since BD_L are rare, we suggest to couple immunomagnetic separation, necessary to enrich the starting population in B cells, to the following sorting of BD_L. This will reduce the time required for their purification by FACS. Moreover, FACS has the added advantage of providing a very high cell purity, which is fundamental for BD_L functional assays [11]. All steps of this method should be performed under sterile conditions.

1. Isolate mouse splenocytes and quantitate the absolute cell number as in Subheading 3.1.
2. Enrich the splenocyte population for B cells by positive selection of T cells and myeloid cells. To do so, first add anti-thy1-biotin and anti-CD11b biotin antibodies according to manufacturer's instructions for T-cell and myeloid-cell depletion,

respectively (*see* **Note 12**). To finalize the immunomagnetic separation, add streptavidin magnetic beads, following manufacturer's instructions (*see* **Note** 7).

3. Strain the obtained B-cell-enriched population through a 45-μm filter and centrifuge for 5 min at 300 × *g* to pellet the cells.
4. Stain cells at 10–20 × 10^6 cells/mL using a cocktail of anti-B220, -CD21, -IgM, -CD23, -CD93, and -IgD antibodies (*see* Table 1) diluted in FACS staining buffer for 15 min on ice in the dark. At the end of incubation, add 10 mL of FACS staining buffer to dilute the antibody cocktail and centrifuge for 5 min at 300 × *g* to pellet the cells.
5. Wash cells with FACS staining buffer and centrifuge for 5 min at 300 × *g* to pellet the cells. Discard the supernatant and resuspend the cells in FACS staining buffer at 20 × 10^6 cells/mL.
6. FACS purify BD_L cells according to the phenotype described in Table 2 and Fig. 1. Collect the cells in 15 mL polypropylene conical tubes containing 1 mL of cell sorting collection solution.
7. Once all the samples are sorted, centrifuge the collection tubes, combine cells, and perform a cell count. 1.5–2 × 10^6 BD_L can be obtained from one spleen.

3.4 $CD4^+Foxp3^{EGFP}$ Treg FACS Purification

The unique identifier for Treg is Foxp3. Since this is an intranuclear protein, antibody detection cannot be used for their purification. Thus, we utilized the $Foxp3^{EGFP}$ reporter and the staining of the cell surface marker CD4 to identify Treg. Since Treg are a rare T-cell subset, we suggest using magnetic beads to enrich for $CD4^+$ T cells prior to proceed with cell sorting, to reduce the time required for their purification. All steps of this method should be performed under sterile conditions.

1. Isolate mouse splenocytes and quantitate the absolute cell number as in Subheading 3.1.
2. Deplete B cells, $CD8^+$ T cells and myeloid cells by adding anti-B220-biotin or anti-CD19-biotin, anti-CD8-biotin, and anti-CD11b-biotin, respectively, according to manufacturer's instructions (*see* **Note 12**). To finalize the immunomagnetic separation, add streptavidin magnetic beads, following the manufacturer's instructions (*see* **Note** 7).
3. Strain the enriched T-cell population through a 45-μm filter and centrifuge for 5 min at 300 × *g* to pellet the cells.
4. Stain cells with the anti-mouse CD4 antibody (*see* Table 1) for 15 min in FACS staining buffer. At the end of the incubation,

add 10 mL of FACS staining buffer to dilute the anti-CD4 antibody and centrifuge for 5 min at 300 × *g* to pellet the cells. Repeat the wash.

5. Wash cells with FACS staining buffer and centrifuge for 5 min at 300 × *g* to pellet the cells. Discard the supernatant and resuspend the cells in FACS staining buffer at 20 × 10^6 cells/mL.
6. FACS purify Treg according to their $CD4^+Foxp3^+$ phenotype as shown in Fig. 2. Collect the cells in 15 mL polypropylene conical tubes containing 1 mL of cell sorting collection solution.
7. Centrifuge the collection tubes, combine cells, and perform a cell count.

3.5 In Vitro Treg Proliferation Assay

The assessment of BD_L-induced Treg proliferation in vitro allows for the quick screening of BD_L effector mechanisms using antibodies, inhibitors, and knockout mice without the requirement of B-cell-deficient mice. Although the protocol is written using mouse splenocytes, the in vitro assay can be easily modified to any species including human. In addition, alternative sources of BD_L and Treg could be obtained from such as human peripheral blood [5]. All steps of this method should be performed under sterile conditions.

1. Coat 24-well plates with 1–10 μg/mL anti-CD3 and 1–10 μg/mL anti-CD28 antibody diluted in 250 μL PBS for 12–24 h at 4 °C (*see* **Note 9**).
2. FACS purify BD_L cells as described in Subheading 3.3.
3. FACS purify $CD4^+EGFP^+$ Treg cells as described in Subheading 3.4 and label the cells using 3 μM cell proliferation dye eFluor 670, following manufacturer's instructions (*see* **Note 10**).
4. Aspirate the antibody solution from the wells of the 24-well plate and wash one time with culture medium.
5. Mix 5 × 10^4 labeled Treg with or without 1 × 10^5 BD_L in culture medium and co-culture on the Ab-coated 24-well plates in a final volume of 0.5 mL. As a control of BD_L cell function, FACS-purified FO IgD^{hi} or MZ B cells (obtained as described in Fig. 1) can be included in the assay since they will not induce Treg proliferation [5].
6. After 4 days, collect the cellular contents from each well and transfer samples to staining tubes. Wash one time with cell staining buffer, and stain for CD4 detection by adding the anti-mouse CD4 antibody diluted in cell staining buffer (*see* Subheading 3.2).
7. Prior to proceeding with the flow cytometry analysis, add 5 μg/mL 7AAD to exclude dead cells from the analysis.

8. Assess $CD4^+$ Treg cell proliferation by flow cytometry based on cell proliferation dye eFluor 670 dilution.
9. To quantitate the absolute cell number of $CD4^+$ Treg, run the entire content of the sample tube through the flow cytometer. For the analysis, gate on $CD4^+Foxp3^+$ T cells and determine the event count and then gate on Treg that had undergone dye dilution to determine the number of Treg that had undergone proliferation.

3.6 In Vivo Treg Expansion Assay

The in vivo Treg expansion assay was designed to identify BD_L effector mechanisms. After the transfer of BD_L into μMT mice, they are the only B-cell subset present, thus any increase in Treg absolute cell numbers can be attributed to their presence and activity. BD_L effector functions can be assessed using antibody blocking or gene knockout mice. As an example of antibody blocking, we treated FACS-purified BD_L with anti-GITRL blocking antibody prior to adoptive transfer into μMT mice. When we assessed Treg expansion/proliferation, we found that GITRL blocking of BD_L resulted in a significantly lower number of Treg as compared to mice that were transferred unblocked BD_L [5]. By using knockout mice deficient in MHC class II (C2ta) or CD80/CD86 molecules, we determined that BD_L:Treg cognate interactions are not required for Treg expansion [5, 6].

1. FACS purify BD_L cells as described in Subheading 3.3.
2. Adoptively transfer 3–5 × 10^6 BD_L cells per mouse in 200 μL of sterile PBS by intravenous (i.v.) injection into μMT mice (*see* **Note 13**). Intravenously inject 200 μL of PBS to wild-type and μMT control mice. As a B-cell negative control, FACS purify FO IgD^{hi} or MZ B cells (obtained as in Fig. 1) and adoptively transfer in mice in place of BD_L cells. This B-cell-negative control will not induce Treg proliferation.
3. Seven to 10 days later, sacrifice mice and harvest the spleen. Isolate mouse splenocytes and determine cell number.
4. Transfer up to 1 × 10^6 splenocytes to a cell staining tube, wash with cell staining buffer by centrifuging for 5 min at 300 × *g* and cell surface stain the splenocytes with an anti-mouse CD4 antibody (*see* **Note 6**). If the interest is not only the detection of Treg but also their proliferative state, stain for Ki-67 or BrdU using fixation and permeabilization buffers optimized for the staining of transcription factors and nuclear proteins (*see* **Note 11**).
5. Analyze by flow cytometry and determine the absolute cell number of Treg and those that are proliferating, if measuring.

6. Optional- to verify the presence of BD_L, first stain for BD_L and then analyze by flow cytometry and quantitate their absolute cell number.

3.7 In Vivo Treg Maintenance Assay

The in vivo Treg maintenance assay was designed to specifically monitor the fate of a marked population of Treg. In our published studies, we monitored Treg proliferation following adoptive transfer into μMT mice alone or in combination with BD_L. We found that cotransfer with BD_L, but not FO (IgD^{hi}) or MZ B cells increased Treg expansion beyond mice receiving Treg alone. By examining Treg-cell surface markers, this assay can be used to track the expansion and survival of specific Treg subsets in the context of BD_L effector function.

1. FACS purify BD_L cells as described in Subheading 3.3 and $CD4^+Foxp3/EGFP^+$ Treg cells as described in Subheading 3.4.
2. In the case in which Treg proliferation will be monitored, label Treg with a cell proliferation dye (*see* **Note 10** and **14**).
3. Adoptive transfer 2×10^5 Treg with or without $2–5 \times 10^6$ BD_L in 200 μL of sterile PBS by i.v. injection into μMT mice. Intravenously inject 200 μL of PBS to wild-type and μMT control mice.
4. As a B-cell-negative control, FACS purify FO IgD^{hi} or MZ B cells (obtained as in Fig. 1) and adoptive transfer in mice in place of BD_L cells. This B-cell-negative control will not induce Treg proliferation.
5. Seven days later sacrifice mice and harvest the spleen. Isolate mouse splenocytes and determine cell count.
6. Cell surface stain the splenocytes with an anti-mouse CD4 antibody (*see* **Note 6**). If the intent is to monitor Treg proliferation, stain for Ki-67 or label with BrdU (*see* **Note 11**).
7. Analyze by flow cytometry and determine the absolute cell number of Treg and those that are proliferating, if measuring.
8. Optional- to verify the presence of BD_L, first stain for BD_L and then analyze by flow cytometry and quantitate their absolute cell number.

3.8 Assess BD_L Activity in Mouse Models of Disease

In our studies, we utilized EAE as a model system in which to monitor BD_L effector function. EAE was a good disease model for this analysis because μMT mice deficient in B cells on the B10. PL background do not recover from the signs of EAE [1, 12]. In addition, the adoptive transfer of B cells into μMT mice restored EAE recovery [6]. EAE recovery is also enhanced by increasing Treg numbers by adoptive transfer [13]. By transferring BD_L into μMT mice, we were able to demonstrate that the increase in the absolute number of Treg was directly correlated with EAE recovery [5]. We utilized EAE to confirm the role for BD_L GITRL expression in their effector function [6]. We have also utilized the mouse model of allergic contact dermatitis, contact hypersensitivity to confirm our findings in EAE [5]. Thus, our protocol for assessing BD_L activity can be modified for use in other disease models of interest. Here below, the passive induction of EAE will be detailed as an example of how to assess BD_L activity in mouse models of disease.

1. Generate encephalitogenic T cell lines from myelin basic protein (MBP)-TCR transgenic mice as previously described [12, 14].
2. On day −4, sublethally irradiate B10.PL WT control and B10. PL μMT mice.
3. On day −3, adoptively transfer 3–5 × 10^6 BD_L and control B cells by i.v. injection (*see* Subheading 3.6, **steps 1**–**2**).
4. On day 0, induce EAE by adoptive transfer of 1 × 10^6 MBP-TCR encephalitogenic T cells by i.v. injection.
5. On day 7, start scoring mice for EAE using a 5-point scale: 0, no disease; 1, limp tail; 1.5, hind limb ataxia; 2, hind limb paresis; 2.5, partial hind limb paralysis; 3, total hind limb paralysis; 4, hind and fore limb paralysis; and 5, death [12, 14].
6. At various timepoints along the disease course, track and quantitate Treg and BD_L by flow cytometry as described in Subheadings 3.1 and 3.2, respectively.

4 Notes

1. For our studies, we utilized a LSRII flow cytometer from BD Biosciences equipped with four lasers: 488 nm, 532 nm, 640 nm, and 405 nm. However, any equivalent flow cytometer can be utilized. The antibody fluorochrome combinations outlined in Table 1 will need to be adjusted according to the laser configuration of the flow cytometer utilized.
2. For our studies, we utilized the FlowJo analysis software (Tree Star Inc., Ashland, OR, USA). However, any comparable flow cytometry analysis software can be utilized.
3. For FACS, we utilized the FACSAriaII cell sorter from BD Biosciences with four lasers: 488 nm, 561 nm, 633 nm, and 405 nm. However, any equivalent cell sorter can be utilized. The antibody fluorochrome combinations outlined in Table 1 will need to be adjusted according to the laser configuration of the cell sorter utilized.

4. While both BD_L and Treg can be purified from any strain of mice, we have only analyzed their phenotype and function in B10.PL and C57BL/6 mice purchased from The Jackson Laboratory (Bar Harbor, ME). BD_L and Treg are utilized in a syngeneic manner. In our studies we utilized $Foxp3^{EGFP}$ reporters, on both the B10.PL and C57BL/6 background, generated by Chatila and Williams [15]; however, other Foxp3 reporter mice could be utilized.
5. Always quantitate the absolute number of the starting population of splenocytes so that the absolute number of specific cell subsets can be quantitated from the flow cytometry analysis.
6. Although for our studies we have primarily utilized a $Foxp3^{EGFP}$ reporter mouse [15], we have also identified $CD4^+$ Treg by intranuclear staining of Foxp3 with or without $CD25^{hi}$ cell surface expression [5, 6]. Indeed, in the absence of a Foxp3 reporter, the positive expression of CD4 and FoxP3 can be combined with a high expression of CD25 to identify and purify by FACS the Treg cell population. If not using a $Foxp3^{EGFP}$ mice, detect intranuclear Foxp3 using fixation and permeabilization buffers optimized for the staining of transcription factors and nuclear proteins, following manufacturer's instruction.
7. We utilized STEMCELL magnetic beads. However, they can be substituted with any equivalent product.
8. This is an optional reagent. Indeed, negative selection is not required, but greatly shortens the timing of subsequent FACS isolation of the rare BD_L and Treg subsets.
9. The final concentration of the anti-CD3 and anti-CD28 antibodies used in the assay should be titrated because antibody affinity and plate absorption will differ depending upon the source of the antibodies and microtiter plates, respectively.
10. We used eFluor 670 (eBioscience), but there are a number of cell proliferation dyes that could substitute this reagent according to the laser configuration of the flow cytometry utilized.
11. We have detected Treg proliferation in μMT mice using cell proliferation dyes, Ki-67 staining, and BrdU labeling with equivalent results [5, 6].
12. In the case you are not using a commercial kit, experimentally determine antibody concentrations.
13. Four mice are required to obtain a sufficient number of BD_L for one recipient mouse.
14. If Foxp3 reporter mice are not available, there are a number of options that can be utilized to track Treg cells after adoptive transfer: [1] Treg can be labeled with cell proliferation dye prior to be transferred in mice. This method has the advantage

of allowing the quantitation of the absolute number of transferred Treg cells that have undergone proliferation [2]. Utilize donor and recipient mice that differ in CD45 isoforms. For instance, Treg can be obtained from CD45.1 mice and transferred into CD45.2 μMT mice [16, 17] [3]. Utilize donor and recipient mice that differ in Thy1 isoforms. For instance, Treg can be obtained from Thy1.1 mice and transferred into Thy1.2 μMT mice. Antibodies that allow to distinguish between the different isoforms of both CD45 and Thy1 are commercially available.

Acknowledgments

This work was supported by NIH grants R01 AI069358, 1R56AI122655-01A1, and 1R56AI129348-01A1, National Multiple Sclerosis Society grants RG 3299-A-2 and RG 1501-03034 and the Versiti Blood Research Institute Foundation.

References

1. Wolf SD, Dittel BN, Hardardottir F, Janeway CA Jr (1996) Experimental autoimmune encephalomyelitis induction in genetically B cell-deficient mice. J Exp Med 184:2271–2278
2. Ray A, Mann MK, Basu S, Dittel BN (2010) A case for regulatory B cells in controlling the severity of autoimmune-mediated inflammation in experimental autoimmune encephalomyelitis and multiple sclerosis. J Neuroimmunol 230:1–9
3. Ray A, Wang L, Dittel BN (2015) IL-10-independent regulatory B-cell subsets and mechanisms of action. Int Immunol 27:531–536
4. Ray A, Dittel BN (2017) Mechanisms of regulatory B cell function in autoimmune and inflammatory diseases beyond IL-10. J Clin Med 6
5. Ray A, Khalil MI, Pulakanti KL, Burns RT, Gurski CJ, Basu S, Wang D, Rao S, Dittel BN (2019) Mature IgD(low/−) B cells maintain tolerance by promoting regulatory T cell homeostasis. Nat Commun 10:190
6. Ray A, Basu S, Williams CB, Salzman NH, Dittel BN (2012) A novel IL-10-independent regulatory role for B cells in suppressing autoimmunity by maintenance of regulatory T cells via GITR ligand. J Immunol 188:3188–3198
7. Rudensky AY (2011) Regulatory T cells and Foxp3. Immunol Rev 241:260–268
8. Liao G, Nayak S, Regueiro JR, Berger SB, Detre C, Romero X, de Waal Malefyt R, Chatila TA, Herzog RW, Terhorst C (2010) GITR engagement preferentially enhances proliferation of functionally competent CD4+CD25+FoxP3+ regulatory T cells. Int Immunol 22:259–270
9. Liao G, O'Keeffe MS, Wang G, van Driel B, de Waal Malefyt R, Reinecker HC, Herzog RW, Terhorst C (2014) Glucocorticoid-induced TNF receptor family-related protein ligand is requisite for optimal functioning of regulatory CD4(+) T cells. Front Immunol 5:35
10. Kitamura D, Roes J, Kuhn R, Rajewsky K (1991) A B cell-deficient mouse by targeted disruption of the membrane exon of the immunoglobulin mu chain gene. Nature 350:423–426
11. Basu S, Campbell HM, Dittel BN, Ray A (2010) Purification of specific cell population by fluorescence activated cell sorting (FACS). J Vis Exp 10(41):1546
12. Dittel BN, Merchant RM, Janeway CA Jr (1999) Evidence for Fas-dependent and Fas-independent mechanisms in the pathogenesis of experimental autoimmune encephalomyelitis. J Immunol 162:6392–6400
13. Kohm AP, Carpentier PA, Anger HA, Miller SD (2002) Cutting edge: CD4+CD25+ regulatory T cells suppress antigen-specific autoreactive immune responses and central nervous system inflammation during active experimental autoimmune encephalomyelitis. J Immunol 169:4712–4716

14. Mann MK, Maresz K, Shriver LP, Tan Y, Dittel BN (2007) B cell regulation of $CD4^+CD25^+$ T regulatory cells and IL-10 via B7 is essential for recovery from experimental autoimmune encephalomyelitis. J Immunol 178:3447–3456
15. Haribhai D, Lin W, Relland LM, Truong N, Williams CB, Chatila TA (2007) Regulatory T cells dynamically control the primary immune response to foreign antigen. J Immunol 178:2961–2972
16. Basu S, Ray A, Dittel BN (2011) Cannabinoid receptor 2 is critical for the homing and retention of marginal zone B lineage cells and for efficient T-independent immune responses. J Immunol 187:5720–5732
17. Basu S, Ray A, Dittel BN (2013) Differential representation of B cell subsets in mixed bone marrow chimera mice due to expression of allelic variants of CD45 (CD45.1/CD45.2). J Immunol Methods 396:163–167

Part III

Methods for the Ex Vivo Expansion and Molecular Characterization of IL-10 Producing B Cells

Chapter 13

Use of Toll-Like Receptor (TLR) Ligation to Characterize Human Regulatory B-Cells Subsets

Mathilde A. M. Chayé, Chiara Tontini, Arifa Ozir-Fazalalikhan, Astrid L. Voskamp, and Hermelijn H. Smits

Abstract

Toll-like receptors (TLRs) are pattern recognition receptors (PRRs), which constitute key components in the recognition of pathogens, thereby initiating innate immune responses and promoting adaptive immune responses. In B cells, TLR ligation is important for their activation and, together with CD40, for their differentiation. TLR ligands are also strong promoters of regulatory B (Breg)-cell development, by enhancing the production of IL-10 and their capacity to induce tolerance. In inflammatory diseases, such as autoimmunity or allergies, Breg-cell function is often impaired, while in chronic infections, such as with helminths, or cancer, Breg-cell function is boosted. Following pathogen exposure, B cells can respond directly by producing cytokines and/or IgM (innate response) and develop into various memory B (Bmem)-cell subsets with class-switched immunoglobulin receptors. Depending on the disease state or chronic infection conditions, various Breg subsets can be recognized as well. Currently, a large array of surface markers is known to distinguish between these large range of B-cell subsets. In recent years, the development of mass cytometers and spectral flow cytometry has allowed for high-dimensional detection of up to 48 markers, including both surface and intracellular/intranuclear markers. Therefore, this novel technology is highly suitable to provide a comprehensive overview of Bmem/Breg-cell subsets in different disease states and/or in clinical intervention trials. Here, we provide detailed instructions of the steps necessary to obtain high-quality data for high-dimensional analysis of multiple human Breg-cell subsets using various TLR ligands.

Key words Regulatory B cells, IL-10, Human, TLR ligands, Flow cytometry, Mass cytometry, Subset, Validation

1 Introduction

Toll-like receptors (TLRs) are pattern recognition receptors (PRRs) that are key components of the innate immune response to pathogens. TLRs are expressed on a variety of immune cells, such as dendritic cells, macrophages, neutrophils, and B cells. Such receptors recognize pathogen-associated molecular patterns (PAMPs) of viruses, bacteria, or parasites, and endogenous damage-associated molecular patterns (DAMPs) associated with

Francesca Mion and Silvia Tonon (eds.), *Regulatory B Cells: Methods and Protocols*, Methods in Molecular Biology, vol. 2270, https://doi.org/10.1007/978-1-0716-1237-8_13,

cell stress, apoptosis, necrosis, or tissue damage. In B cells, TLR ligation enhances the effector function by increasing antigen presentation, immunoglobulin class-switch recombination, as well as chemokine and cytokine production. However, TLR ligands are also strong promoters of regulatory B (Breg)-cell activation and development, by enhancing the production of IL-10 and increasing their capacity to induce tolerance. For example, during *Salmonella typhimurium* or *Helicobacter felis* infection, MyD88-signaling in B cells suppresses infection-induced pathology and/or protective immunity via IL-10, suggesting roles for TLR2 and/or TLR4 in direct microbial sensing by B cells [1–3]. TLR7 ligand uridine-containing ssRNA and TLR9 ligand CpG oligonucleotides (ODN) were also described as strong inducers of IL-10 expression in murine and human B cells [4–8]. In addition to bacterial-derived TLR ligands, TLR2, and/or TLR4 ligands present in parasites, such as *Echinococcus granulosus protoscoleces*, *Leishmania major*, *Brugia malayi* and *Schistosoma mansoni*, also induced IL-10-producing B cells [9–12]. These studies show an important role for TLR2, TLR4, TLR7, and TLR9 ligation in the development of Breg cells and highlight their potential use in studying Breg cell development in homeostasis, as well as in conditions where Breg cells are lacking, their function is impaired (as in chronic inflammatory diseases and transplant rejection) or where they are over-active (such as chronic infections or cancer).

Breg cells are heterogenous and their features depend on environmental triggers and on their maturation status [13]. In both mice and men, distinct Breg subsets have been described, with similar cell phenotypes across species [13]. Here we will focus on the characterization of human Breg cell subsets and their link with human disease, i.e., inflammatory disorders, transplantation, chronic infections, and cancer. In patients affected by the systemic lupus erythematosus (SLE) autoimmune disorder, a population of transitional $CD19^{+}CD24^{high}CD38^{high}$ Breg cells was impaired [14], while $CD19^{+}CD24^{high}CD27^{+}$ Breg cells were reported to produce less IL-10 in patients with allergic rhinitis, asthma, and autoimmune diseases [15–17]. In addition, other subsets such as $CD19^{+}CD25^{high}CD71^{high}CD73^{low}$ Brl cells and $CD19^{+}CD5^{+}$ Breg cells, that were also impaired in allergic subjects [18, 19], expanded in patients undergoing allergen-specific immunotherapy [20, 21, 18]. In regard to Breg-cell subsets in transplantation, $CD19^{+}CD27^{+}IgM^{+}$ memory B cells were impaired in chronic graft-versus-host disease (cGVHD) patients [22], while cytokine production of $CD24^{hi}CD38^{hi}$ transitional Breg cells was altered in patients with graft dysfunctions [23]. In contrast, chronic infections are associated with increased development and activity of $CD19^{+}CD1d^{high}CD5^{+}$ Breg cells, as shown in patients with chronic infection with hepatitis B virus [24], *Mycobacterium tuberculosis* [7], or *Schistosoma haematobium* [25, 26]. In cancer, the

Breg-cell population expands and contributes to the tumor immunosuppressive microenvironment. The presence of Breg cells was linked to disease progression via IL-10-mediated immune regulation and/or Treg-cell induction [27–29]. The aforementioned Breg-cell subsets have also been detected in numerous types of cancer [29, 30], with an additional PD-1^{hi}CD5^{hi}CD$24^{-/+}$CD$27^{hi/+}$CD38^{dim} subset identified in hepatocellular carcinoma [27]. In healthy subjects, IL-10-producing CD$27^{hi/int}$CD38^{+} regulatory plasmablasts were also described [31]. Furthermore, several non-IL-10-producing Breg cell subsets were also identified, including TGF-β-producing CD19^{+}CD5^{+} [32] and CD19^{+}CD25^{high} CD27^{high}CD86^{high}CD1d^{high} B cells, granzyme (GrB)-producing CD19^{+}CD38^{+}CD1d^{+}IgM^{+}CD147^{+} B cells [33], adenosine-producing CD39^{+}CD73^{+} B cells [34], PD-L1^{high}CD19^{+} CD21^{+}CD27^{-} B cells [35], and Tim-1^{+}CD5^{hi}CD$24^{-/+}$CD$27^{-/+}$ CD$38^{+/hi}$ [36]. The multiplicity of Breg-cell phenotypes may suggest that various B-cell subsets can acquire different regulatory mechanisms over time depending on the environmental conditions, and may indicate a certain plasticity of these cells [13]. Most studies investigating the presence and function of Breg cells restrict to IL-10 as the major cytokine, potentially overlooking the role of other anti-inflammatory cytokines such as TGF-β or GrB, or the co-production of counteracting pro-inflammatory cytokines. In fact, TLR ligation can promote and contribute to the development of both anti- and pro-inflammatory responses simultaneously [5, 25]. For instance, CpG, LPS, and the TLR2/6 agonist Pam3Cys, which are all inducers of IL-10 production in B cells, also increase to variable degrees the pro-inflammatory cytokines IL-1α, IL-1β, IL-6, IL-8, and TNF-α [3, 5, 6, 37–39]. Studies in mice and humans have partially deciphered the downstream signaling cascade of TLR ligation leading to enhanced IL-10 transcription, and several key signaling molecules have been identified [40]. TLRs are transmembrane receptors that can be expressed on the cell surface (TLR1, 2, 4, 5, and 6) or located in intracellular compartments such as the endoplasmic reticulum (ER), endosomes, lysosomes, or endolysosomes (TLR3, 7, 8, 9) [41]. TLR-mediated IL-10 expression in B cells is mainly dependent on the activity of three key transcription factors, namely STAT3, NF-κB, and NFAT. STAT3 signaling can be induced by TLR ligation through the activation of Bruton Tyrosine Kinase (BTK) by the signaling adaptor B-cell linker protein (BLNK) [42–44]. TLR ligation associated with A Proliferation Inducing Ligand (APRIL) binding to Transmembrane Activator and CAML Interactor (TACI) signals through NF-κB to induce IL-10 expression [45]. TLR4 ligation specifically signals through NF-κB, Hypoxia-Inducible Factor 1 α (HIF1α) and STAT3 to induce IL-10 expression [46, 47]. Furthermore, a role for Fas Ligand (FasL) in TLR4 signaling was reported, involving both

NF-κB and NFAT. Thus, for in-depth analysis of Breg-cell activation and development in clinical patient cohorts, intracellular analysis of STAT3, NFAT, and NF-κB should be considered as key signaling molecules leading to IL-10 expression following TLR ligation. Importantly, Breg-cell development does not only rely on TLR stimulation but also result from triggering the B-cell receptor (BCR) [48, 49], cross-linking of CD40-CD40L [14, 50], activation through CD86/CD80 [51], and/or innate cytokines [52, 53]. However, the activation of these pathways may also induce a broader B-cell activation profile and the development of memory B-cell formation/germinal center reactions. Therefore, TLR ligation is a relatively homogenous and efficient way to induce Breg-cell development and study their presence and activity in different contexts. Thorough investigation of Breg-cell subsets and of their activity requires simultaneous analysis of a considerable number of surface markers, immunoglobulins, cytokines, and/or other anti-inflammatory molecules, as well as signaling and transcription factors. The recent development of mass cytometry and new generations of spectral flow cytometers allows for high-dimensional analysis of up to 48 different markers, throughout multiple cell regions (i.e., surface, intracellular, or intranuclear molecules) [54]. These novel technologies are ultimately designed for a more comprehensive and detailed characterization of human Breg-cell subsets and can be applied to different diseases or clinical intervention trials. Although these techniques have a far-reaching potential, their complexity also requires thorough preparation and validation steps to guarantee harmonized and reproducible data with a low signal-to-noise ratio. To this aim, the steps required for validation and optimization are discussed in the figures and notes of this chapter, and the use of reference samples and barcoding are described in order to reduce batch effects. A table that summarizes the differences in B-cell recovery using different methods for single-cell analysis is also provided (*see* Table 1). Altogether, in this chapter, we provide information and detailed instructions on how to validate and harmonize high-dimensional experiments for the analysis of multiple human Breg-cell subsets by using various TLR ligands.

2 Materials

All materials and solutions listed should be sterile and handled at room temperature, unless otherwise specified.

2.1 General Equipment

1. 50 mL, 15 mL, and 5 mL tubes.
2. 50 mL and 25 mL serological pipettes.
3. 3 mL Pasteur pipettes.

Table 1
Differences in B-cell recovery using different methods for single-cell analysis

Technique	Sample type	# cells/subject (average)	Viability % (average)	# Absolute number of recovered B cells (average)	B-cell yield % (average)
Flow cytometry	PBMCs (n = 18)	0.5×10^6	41–83.4 (68.1)	1571–18,677 (7357.7)	2.15–14.8 (6.7)
	Isolated B cells (n = 10)	0.5×10^6	78.5–90.9 (86.8)	10,630–108,863 (68592)	2.1–21.8 (13.7)
Mass cytometry with barcoding	PBMCs (n = 8)	2×10^6	94.3–96.7 (95.4)	36,999–50,050 (41827)	1.8–2.5 (2.1)
	Isolated B cells (n = 34)	$0.32–4.36 \times 10^6$ (1.33×10^6)	51–98.7 (86)	10,800–690,104 (205341)	3.8–33.5 (16.1)

The recovery of live B cells is subject to both donor-to-donor variation and differences in the type of sample analyzed (PBMC versus isolated B cells). Additional factors that may affect recovery are the number of processing steps required for both flow and mass cytometry and the viability of samples after stimulation. When analyzing B cells, isolation of B cells allows better visualization of small cell subsets, ensuring sufficient events per subset during acquisition and analysis. However, if isolation of B cells cannot be performed (e.g., limited number of cells available and limited resources) or the aim of the study is to analyze different cell types simultaneously or to assess cell–cell interactions, analysis of total PBMCs is a possible solution, taking into account that the measurement of small subsets may be less precise compared to isolated B cells. n: number of healthy donors analyzed

4. 2–20 μL and 20–200 μL multichannel pipettes.
5. 96-Well round-bottom plates and 96-well conical bottom plates.
6. Heparin collection tubes.
7. 1.4 mL polystyrene fluorescence-activated cell sorting (FACS) tubes.
8. Counting chamber.
9. Optical microscope.
10. Mr. Frosty® freezing container.
11. 1.8 mL cryovials.
12. Water bath at 37 °C.
13. Plate sealing foil.
14. Flow cytometer.
15. Devices for immunomagnetic separation (separator system and columns).

2.2 Buffers and Media

1. Culture medium: RPMI 1640 supplemented with 10% Heat-Inactivated Fetal Calf Serum (HI-FCS), 1 mM pyruvate, 2 mM L-glutamine, 100 U/mL penicillin, and 100 μg/mL streptomycin.
2. Freezing medium: RPMI 1640 supplemented with 20% HI-FCS, 1 mM pyruvate and 2 mM L-glutamine, 100 U/mL penicillin, and 100 μg/mL streptomycin.
3. D-Methyl-Sulfoxide (DMSO) freezing medium: RPMI 1640 supplemented with 20% DMSO, 20% HI-FCS, 1 mM pyruvate and 2 mM L-glutamine, 100 U/mL penicillin, and 100 μg/mL streptomycin.
4. Thawing medium: RPMI 1640 supplemented with 50% HI-FCS, 1 mM pyruvate and 2 mM L-glutamine, 100 U/mL penicillin, and 100 μg/mL streptomycin.
5. Hank's Balanced Salt Solution: resuspend in ultrapure water 140 mg/l Calcium Chloride ($CaCl_2$), 100 mg/l Magnesium Chloride ($MgCl_2$-$6H_2O$), 100 mg/l Magnesium Sulfate ($MgSO_4$-$7H_2O$), 400 mg/l Potassium Chloride (KCl), 60 mg/l Potassium Phosphate monobasic (KH_2PO_4), 350 mg/l Sodium Bicarbonate ($NaHCO_3$), 8 g/l Sodium Chloride (NaCl), 48 mg/l Sodium Phosphate dibasic (Na_2HPO_4), 1 gr/l D-Glucose (Dextrose).
6. Phosphate-buffered saline (PBS): resuspend in ultrapure water 8 gr/l NaCl, 200 mg/l KCl, 1.15 gr/l Na_2HPO_4, 200 mg/l KH_2PO_4, pH 7.2.
7. 10× FACS buffer: 5% Bovine Serum Albumin (BSA), 20 mM Ethylenediamine tetraacetic acid (EDTA) in PBS. Non-sterile.

8. 1× FACS buffer: dilute the 10× FACS buffer 1:10 in non-sterile PBS.
9. MACS buffer: 0.5% BSA, 0,09% azide and 2 mM EDTA in PBS. Sterile.
10. Non-sterile ultrapure water.
11. 37% Paraformaldehyde (PFA).
12. 1× permeabilization buffer: dilute a commercial 10× permeabilization buffer stock 1:10 with ultrapure water.

2.3 Antibodies, Cytokines, and Other Reagents

1. Human TLR ligands: CpG ODN 2006, Ultrapure LPS, and Pam3-Cys.
2. Phorbol 12-myristate 13-acetate (PMA).
3. Ionomycin.
4. Brefeldin A.
5. Density gradient centrifugation medium for the separation of mononuclear cells from human blood (e.g., 1.077 g/mL Ficoll Paque).
6. Türk stain: 10 mg gentian violet plus 1 mL acetic acid in 100 mL of demineralized water or PBS.
7. 0.4% Trypan blue solution in PBS.
8. B-cell isolation kit (*see* **Note 1**).
9. Live-dead fixable Aqua dead cell staining kit (Invitrogen) or equivalent by another supplier.
10. Flow cytometry anti-human CD3 PerCP-eF710 (clone SK7), CD14 BV450 (clone MφP9), CD19 PerCP-eFluor 710 (clone SJ25C1), CD20 FITC (clone 2H7), CD23 PE (clone EBVCS2), CD24 BV711 (clone ML5), CD25 BB515 (clone 2A3), CD27 BV650 (clone O323), CD38 BV605 (clone HB7), IL-10 APC (clone JES3-19F1) and TNF-α eFluor 450 (clone MAb11) antibodies. Antibodies must be titrated starting from manufacturer's instructions.
11. FcγR-binding inhibitor.
12. Cytometric Bead Array (CBA) Human Soluble Protein Master Buffer Kit and Human Flex sets (BD Biosciences) for the following cytokines: IL-6 (bead position A7), GM-CSF (C9), IL-10 (B7), TNF-alpha (C4) (*see* **Note 2**).

2.4 Software

1. Flow data acquisition and analysis software such as FACSDiva, BD Biosciences, or FlowJo, Tree Star Inc.
2. Excel and GraphPad spreadsheets for calculation of standard curves and results.

3 Methods

3.1 Isolation of Human Peripheral Blood Mononuclear Cells (PBMCs) by Density Centrifugation and Cryopreservation

Peripheral blood is collected from healthy donors, after informed consent, by venipuncture. PBMCs should be isolated within 1–2 hours of collection, to preserve cell viability.

3.1.1 Isolation of PBMCs Via Density Gradient Centrifugation

1. Transfer 20 mL of blood to a 50-mL tube, dilute 1:1 with HBSS and mix gently by inversion. Aliquot 20 mL of blood-HBSS in an additional 50 mL tube.
2. Layer 13 mL of 1.077 g/mL Ficoll Paque underneath the blood-HBSS suspension. Avoid shaking or mixing the layered fluids. Centrifuge tubes for 25 min at room temperature at 400 × *g*, with no brake or low brake.
3. Remove the top layer carefully with a 10-mL serological pipette until 1 cm above the white ring, then collect the PBMCs white ring from the interface using a 3-mL sterile-Pasteur pipette. Transfer and pool PBMCs of the same donor into a new sterile 50-mL tube and add HBSS until 50 mL volume is reached.
4. Centrifuge the tube(s) for 10 min at 500 × *g*, room temperature. Pour off the liquid and resuspend the pellet in 10 mL of HBSS. Centrifuge again for 10 min at 500 × *g* at room temperature and resuspend the pellet in 2 mL of culture medium.
5. Transfer 10 μL of cell suspension to a non-sterile conical bottom plate and add 10 μL Türk stain. Count manually using a counting chamber and optical microscope (*see* **Note 3**).

3.1.2 Cryopreservation of Isolated PBMCs

The decision to perform cryopreservation of cells depends on several factors, not only related to the specific research question but also to the practical issues related to sample collection, logistics, and processing as often observed in the context of multicentral clinical trials. Typically, to ensure consistency in the processing of samples and analysis of the data, most trials require experiments to be performed in a central laboratory as opposed to multiple testing sites. The logistics of shipping biological specimens is daunting, especially when dealing with live cells: mishandling, difficulty in reaching test site locations, and delays during shipment may lead to variable sample quality and unreliable results. Furthermore, same-day shipping of fresh samples in a controlled environment is expensive and infeasible in certain geographical areas. To circumvent this, PBMCs can be cryopreserved and shipped in bulk on dry ice or in liquid nitrogen. As cryopreservation may affect the expression of markers and cytokine production, extensive testing should be included to assess the impact of cryopreservation on the cell subsets of interest when designing the experiments.

1. Cool down the Mr. Frosty freezing container to 4 °C in the fridge for at least 20 min before loading the cryovials.

2. Centrifuge PBMCs at 500 × *g*, at room temperature, pour off the supernatant and resuspend cells in ice-cold freezing medium at a concentration of 2 × 10^7 cells/mL. Keep PBMCs on ice.
3. Prepare DMSO freezing medium and put on ice (*see* **Note 4**). Label cryovials with pencil or alcohol resistant marker and put on ice.
4. Use a 3-mL sterile Pasteur pipette to add 1:1 DMSO freezing medium to the cells. Always add drop-by-drop to the suspension, while gently shaking the tube. The final number of frozen cells will be 10^7 cells/cryovial.
5. Aliquot 1 mL of cell suspension to each cryovial on ice. Put cryovials in ice-cold Mr. Frosty and transfer to a − 80 °C freezer for at least 4 h. Then transfer the vials to liquid nitrogen for long-term storage.

3.2 Thawing and Count of Cryopreserved PBMCs

The thawing step is crucial to ensure the optimal recovery and viability of frozen cells and should therefore be performed quickly and carefully in sterile conditions, using warm medium and centrifuges at room temperature to reduce cell loss, where required.

1. Warm up water bath to 37 °C and label a 15-mL tube for each donor. Add to each tube a quantity of thawing medium twice the volume of a single cryovial. If multiple cryovials from the same donor are thawed, they can be pooled in the same tube. If the total volume exceeds 15 mL, use a 50-mL tube. Move tubes with thawing medium to the water bath.
2. Take the cryovials from cold storage. If stored in liquid nitrogen, open the cryovials under a flow hood for few seconds to let liquid nitrogen evaporate before thawing. Thaw cells quickly in the 37 °C water bath, until a small ice clump is still visible. Disinfect tubes with 70% ethanol and move cryovials and tubes with thawing medium into a sterile hood.
3. Using a sterile Pasteur pipette collect around 200 μL of thawing medium from tubes and add to the cryovial. Resuspend cells and transfer around 200 μL of PBMCs to the tube with thawing medium, adding drop-by-drop while shaking the tube gently. Repeat the steps for five times until all the cryovial contents are transferred to the 15 mL tube.
4. Centrifuge the cells at 500 × *g* for 10 min at room temperature. Discard the supernatant and resuspend the cells with 2–5 mL of culture medium. Repeat the previous washing step and resuspend cells in 1 mL of culture medium.
5. Count cells by diluting 1:1 in 0.4% Trypan blue and using a counting chamber (or automated counter).

6. Centrifuge the cells at 500 × *g*, for 10 min at room temperature. Carefully remove all the supernatant above the cell pellet using a 1000-μL pipette. Resuspend cells to a final concentration of 10^7 cells/mL in culture medium.
7. Transfer 10^6 PBMCs to a sterile 96-well round-bottom culture plate and add 50 μL of culture medium to each well (*see* **Note 5**).
8. Proceed either with cell resting or cell stimulation.

3.3 Human B-Cell Isolation

Depending on the research question, B-cell analysis can be performed either on total PBMCs or on purified B cells (*see* **Note 6**). Isolation of B cells can be performed either directly after PBMCs isolation or after thawing, by positive or negative selection (*see* **Notes 1**, **7**, and **8**).

1. Perform isolation of B cells from PBMCs as described by the manufacturer and collect isolated cells in 5 mL tubes.
2. Transfer 10 μL of the purified B-cell suspension to a non-sterile conical bottom plate and add 10 μL of the 0.4% Trypan blue solution. Count manually using a counting chamber and optical microscope, or using a cell counting slide and an automatic cell counter.
3. Add 5 mL culture medium to cells, and centrifuge at 500 × *g* for 5 min at room temperature.
4. Discard supernatant and resuspend cells to a final concentration of 10^7 cells/mL in culture medium.
5. Transfer 10^6 B cells into a sterile 96-well round-bottom culture plate and add 50 μL of culture medium to the wells (*see* **Note 9**). For culture of more than 10^6 cells, culture cells in 250 μL medium per million cells in 5 mL tubes.
6. Check B-cell purity by flow cytometry using anti-CD20, anti-CD3, and anti-CD14 antibodies (*see* Fig. 1). Negative selection typically results in an enrichment of 80–85% CD19$^+$ B cells.

3.4 Cell Resting and Cell Stimulation through TLR Ligands

Whether the scientific focus is total PBMCs or purified B cells (*see* **Note 10**), the researcher can choose to directly proceed with the stimulation step or, alternatively, introduce a resting step before incubation with activating stimuli. The resting step consists in leaving cells at 37 °C in culture medium overnight, with no stimuli added, right after being thawed. This extra process is not mandatory but might significantly affect cytokine production and marker expression by some cell subsets. Therefore, the choice to include an overnight resting step needs to be carefully examined and tested, according to the research question.

In our experience, overnight resting has a positive impact on the ability of B cells to produce cytokines as documented by both

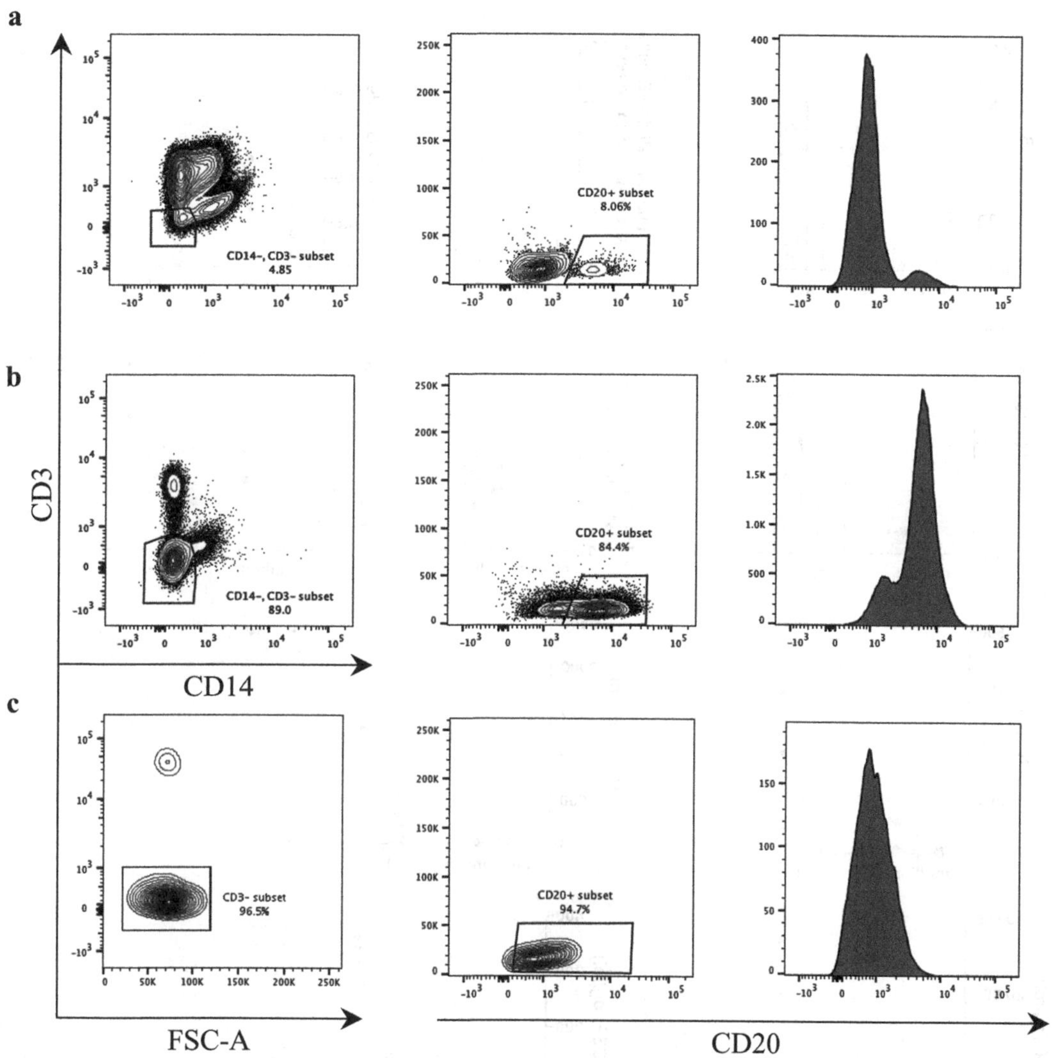

Fig. 1 Comparison of positive and negative selection for human B-cell isolation from cryopreserved PBMCs. Directly after thawing, B cells were isolated using a negative selection-based B-cell isolation kit. Purity was determined by flow cytometry by analyzing the expression of the CD20, CD3, and CD14 markers before (**a**) and after (**b**) negative selection. (**c**) Positive B-cell selection was performed using CD20 beads immediately after thawing. Purity was assessed by flow cytometry following the expression of the CD20 and CD3 markers after selection.

intracellular flow cytometry (*see* Fig. 2a-b) and cytometric bead array (CBA) performed on cell culture supernatants of isolated B cells (*see* Fig. 2c) (*see* **Note 11**).

1. For the resting step, cells must be incubated overnight in an incubator set at 37 °C with 5% CO_2.
2. Whether the stimulation is done immediately or following the resting phase, add 50 μL of stimuli-containing medium to the

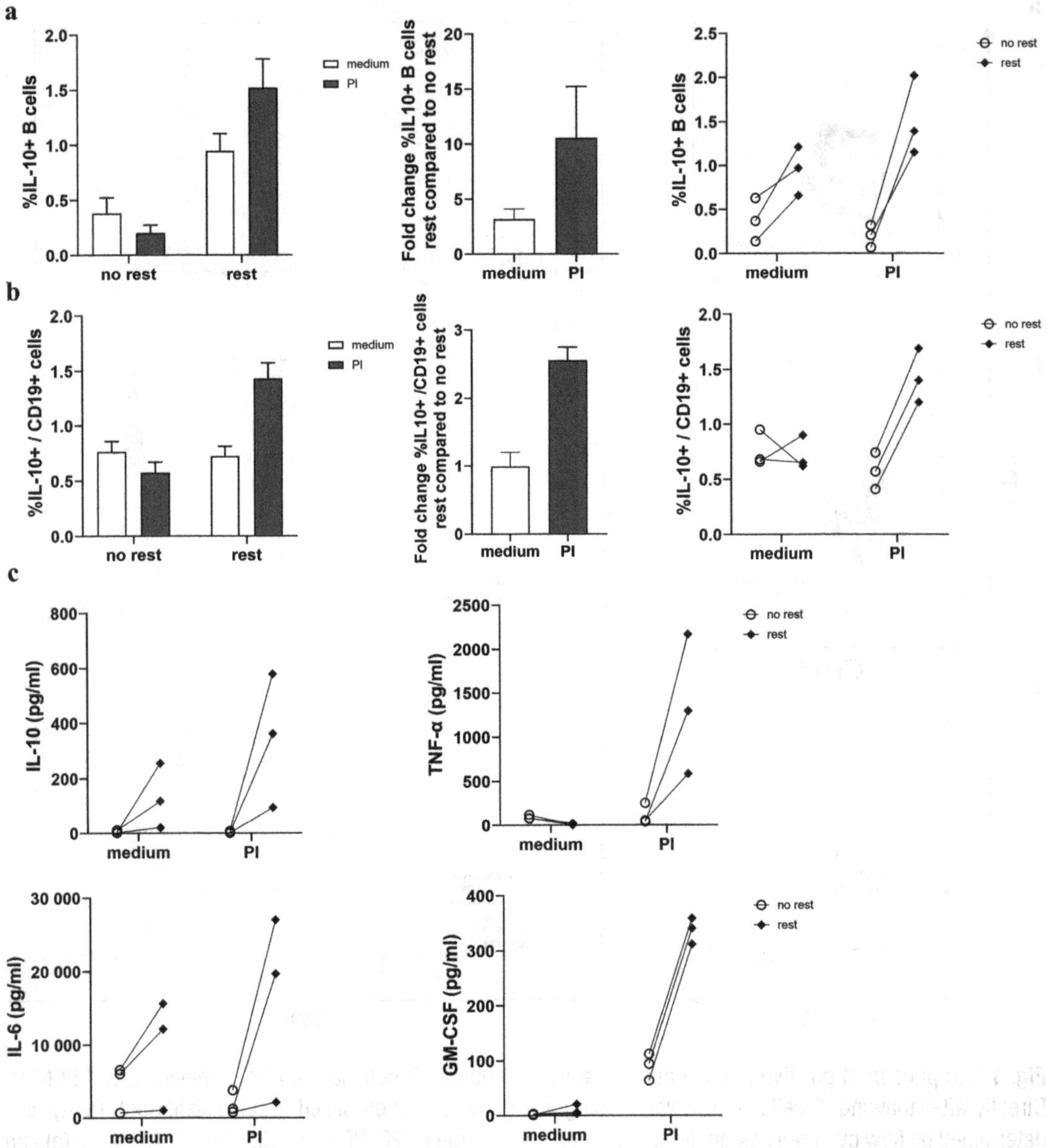

Fig. 2 Effect of overnight resting on the ability of cryopreserved human B cells to produce cytokines. (**a-b**) Analysis of intracellular IL-10 in isolated B cells (**a**) and PBMCs (**b**). 5×10^5 purified B cells or PBMCs collected from healthy adult donors were either stimulated immediately after thawing and/or isolation (no rest), or after overnight resting at 37 °C in culture medium (rest). Cells were stimulated with either 100 ng/mL PMA, 1 μg/mL ionomycin and 10 μg/mL Brefeldin A (PI) or medium and 10 μg/mL Brefeldin A (medium) for 6 h (B cells) or 5 h (PBMCs). IL-10 production was measured by flow cytometry. Data are expressed as mean ± SEM (n = 3). (**c**) Secretion of IL-10, GM-CSF, IL-6, and TNF-α by cryopreserved isolated B cells. 5×10^5 B cells were either stimulated immediately after thawing and isolation, or after resting overnight, and stimulated with either PMA/ionomycin or medium alone for 6 h. Cytokine content was analyzed in cell culture supernatants using CBA (n = 3)

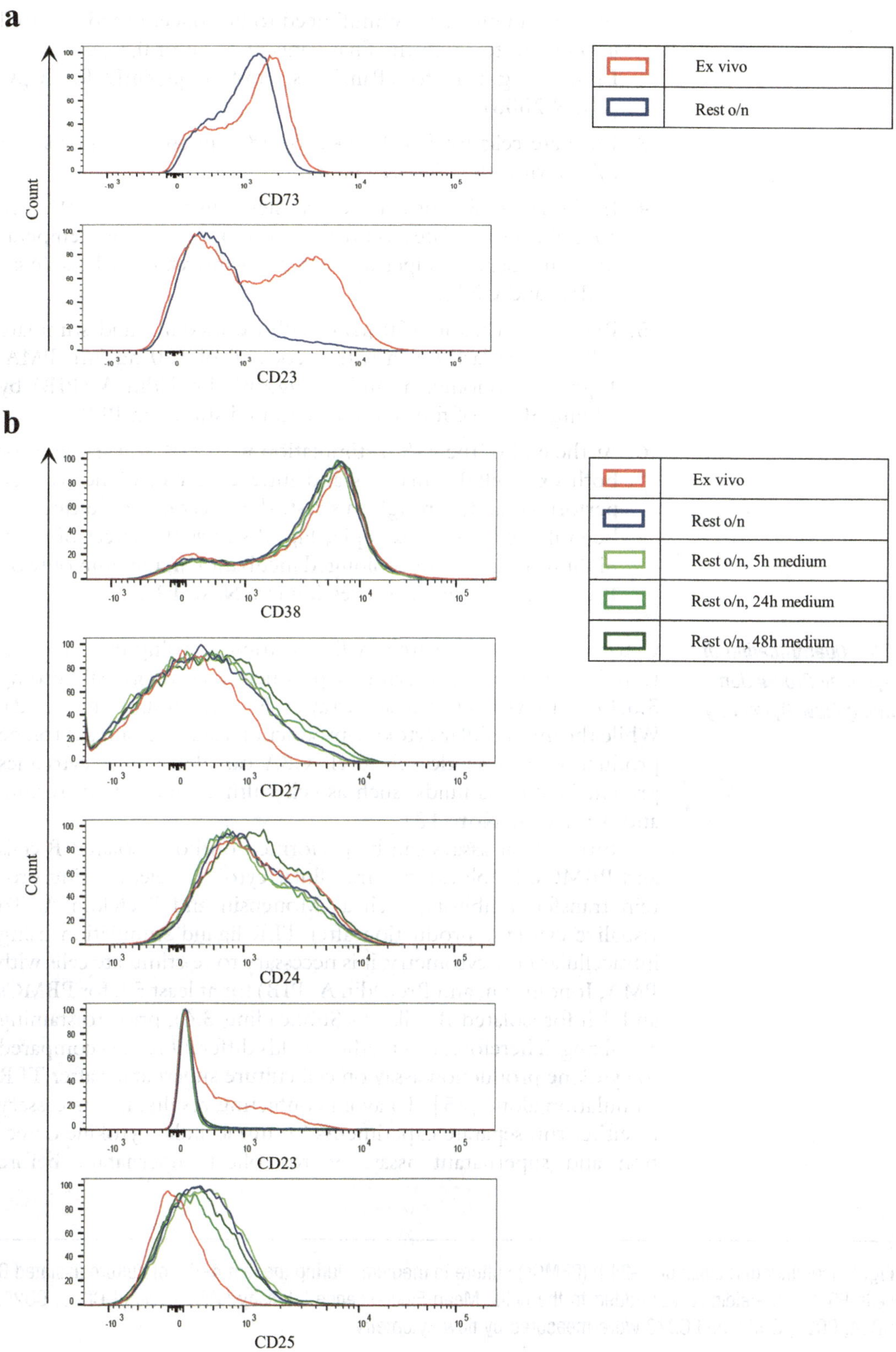

Fig. 3 Effect of overnight resting and/or prolonged incubation in medium only on B-cell surface markers expression. Expression of various surface markers was measured on isolated B cells (**a**) and PBMCs (**b**) directly after isolation or thawing (ex vivo) and after overnight resting (rest o/n) with or without 5–24 h (isolated

corresponding wells. Stimuli need to be concentrated fourfold in medium to reach the final concentration of 0.1 μg/mL for LPS, 5 μg/mL for Pam3Cys, and 1 μg/mL for CpG (ODN 2006).

3. Incubate cells for 5–6 h, 24 h or 48 h in an incubator set at 37 °C with 5% CO_2 (*see* Fig. 3).
4. In the last 4–5 h of culture, transfer cells into sterile 96-well conical bottom plates, centrifuge at 400 × *g* at room temperature and harvest supernatant for downstream analysis (e.g., ELISA and CBA).
5. Resuspend cells in 150 μL of culture medium and stimulate cells for the last 4–5 h with a cocktail of 100 ng/mL PMA, 1 μg/mL ionomycin, and 10 μg/mL brefeldin A (PIB) by adding 50 μL of fourfold concentrated stimuli in PBS.
6. At the end of the 4–5 h stimulation with PIB, the staining for both extracellular markers and intracellular cytokines can be performed and, through this test, the effect of cell resting can be evaluated. As an example, Fig. 3 shows the effect of overnight resting and/or prolonged incubation in medium only on B-cell surface markers expression (*see* **Note 12**).

3.5 Quantification of Cytokine Production Using Flow Cytometry

Cytokines can be measured by flow cytometry using two different techniques: intracellular cytokine production assay (*see* Subheading 3.5.1) and Cytometric Bead Array (CBA, *see* Subheading 3.5.2). While the intracellular cytokine production assay measures cytokine production at a single cell level, CBA can detect free cytokines present in various fluids, such as cell culture supernatant, serum, and plasma (*see* **Note 13**).

Intracellular assays can be performed on both isolated B cells and PBMCs, by blocking extracellular cytokine release using protein transfer inhibitors, such as Monensin and Brefeldin A. To visualize cytokine production after TLR ligand stimulation using intracellular flow cytometry, it is necessary to re-stimulate cells with PMA, Ionomycin, and Brefeldin A (PIB) for at least 5 h for PBMCs and 4 h for isolated B cells (*see* Subheading 3.4), prior to staining and fixing. Therefore, this method yields different results compared to cytokine production assay on cell culture supernatant after TLR stimulation alone [55]. To avoid conflicting results, it is necessary to either run separate experiments for intracellular cytokine detection and supernatant assay, or to collect supernatant before

Fig. 3 (continued) B cells) or 6–24 h (PBMCs) culture in medium. During the last 4–5 h of culture (isolated B cells-PBMC), Brefeldin A was added to the cells. Mean Fluorescence Intensity (MFI) levels of CD23, CD25, CD24, CD27, CD38, and CD73 were measured by flow cytometry

re-stimulation with PIB. Furthermore, the use of Brefeldin A hinders cytokine detection in the supernatant, especially relevant for stimulations of short duration. It is therefore advisable to run duplicate experiments to include non-Brefeldin A-treated cells for short stimulations, or to collect supernatant prior to adding Brefeldin A for longer stimulations.

CBA is a fluorescence-based capture assay that can be run on any flow cytometer equipped with red (633 nm) and green (488 nm) lasers. The advantage of using CBA compared to other capture-based methods is the possibility of customizing and multiplexing up to 30 cytokines/proteins using a small sample volume (5–50 μL) (*see* **Notes 14** and **15**). The quantitative results obtained by CBA and other cytokine quantification assays (i.e., ELISA) from the same sample may differ and can therefore not be used interchangeably.

3.5.1 B-Cell Phenotyping and Quantification of Intracellular Cytokine Production by Flow Cytometry

1. Stimulate cells as in Subheading 3.4. Transfer the cells from 96-well round-bottom plates into sterile 96-well conical bottom plates. Centrifuge plates 3 min at 400 × *g* at room temperature, discard or collect supernatant depending on downstream analysis, and resuspend cells in 200 μL PBS per well. Wash again and flick off supernatant. Add 50 μL of live/dead fixable Aqua stain diluted 1:500 with non-sterile PBS to the cells and incubate for 15–20 min at room temperature.
2. In the meantime, prepare the antibody staining mix for the extracellular markers of interest by adding the appropriate amount of each antibody (e.g., anti-CD24, -CD27, and -CD38 for B-cell phenotyping) and 0.01 mg/l FcγR-binding inhibitor to 1× FACS buffer (*see* **Notes 16**, **17**, and **18**). Keep the mix at 4 °C and protected from light.
3. Wash cells with 150 μL PBS, add 50 μL of staining mix, and incubate for 30 min at 4 °C. Wash cells again with 100 μL 1× FACS buffer, resuspend in 200 μL per well of 1.9% PFA diluted in PBS, and incubate for 15 min at room temperature.
4. Prepare the antibody staining mix for the intracellular markers of interest, such as the IL-10 and TNF-α cytokines, by adding the appropriate amount of each antibody and 0.01 mg/l FcγR-binding inhibitor to 1× permeabilization buffer. Keep the mix at 4 °C and protected from light.
5. Wash cells and resuspend in 200 μL of 1× permeabilization buffer per well. Wash cells again, then add 50 μL of intracellular antibody staining mix and incubate for 30 min at 4 °C.
6. Wash cells with 150 μL 1× permeabilization buffer, resuspend cells with 100 μL FACS Buffer, transfer cells to polystyrene FACS tubes and acquire samples on a flow cytometer.

Table 2
Gating strategy for analysis of single, live B cells by flow cytometry

Step n°	Y Axis	X Axis	Gate name	Meaning
1	SSC-A	FSC-A	Lymphocytes	By gating the acquired events based on side scatter (SSC) and forward scatter (FSC) area (A), the lymphocyte population ($SSC\text{-}A^{+}FSC\text{-}A^{+}$) can be selected and debris ($SSC\text{-}A^{-/low}$ $FSC\text{-}A^{-/low}$) removed from the analysis
2	FSC-A	FSC-W	Singlets	Doublet exclusion by plotting FSC-A and FSC-width (W) and selecting cells with equal area and width. $FSC\text{-}W^{+}FSC\text{-}A^{-}$ events should be removed. Doublets are the result of dead cells clumping together and being recorded as a single event by the cytometer. Therefore, removing doublets improves the quality of the sample analyzed.
3	SSC-A	Live/dead marker	Live cells	It is crucial to actively remove dead cells from the analysis for better result quality. Several fluorescent dyes are commercially available and can be adapted for any cytometry panel. Cells that are positive for the dead cell marker should be excluded from the analysis.
4	–	–	"AND population"	Create a Boolean intersect gate of "lymphocytes," "Singlets," and "live cells." Boolean gating is a feature available in most cytometry data analysis softwares, which merges two or more subpopulations of interest, by including events that express all of the pre-selected markers ("AND" gate), or any of them ("OR" gate). Select events included only in the "AND population" gate and move to step 5.
5	SSC-A	CD19	Live B cells	Select $CD19^{+}$ events to gate on the live B-cell population. Perform marker analysis from the "live B cells" gate only.

7. Before acquiring the cells, plot and gate in the flow cytometry acquisition software the gates listed in Table 2. First, draw the lymphocyte gate on the forward scatter area (FSC-A) versus (vs.) side scatter area (SSC-A) plot and then exclude doublets by gating on singlets on the FSC-A vs. FSC-W plot. Viable cells are selected by gating on the population that is negatively stained by a live/dead dye (SSC-A vs. live/dead marker). Create a Boolean intersect gate of the three gates ("AND" population), then plot SSC-A vs. CD19 and gate out the $CD19^{+}$ population ("Live B cells").
8. Acquire a minimum of 350.000 total events per donor, and/or 2000 live B-cell events or, when measuring IL-10 production, a minimum of 100 events in $IL\text{-}10^{+}$ B-cell gates (precision ±10%) (*see* **Note 19**).

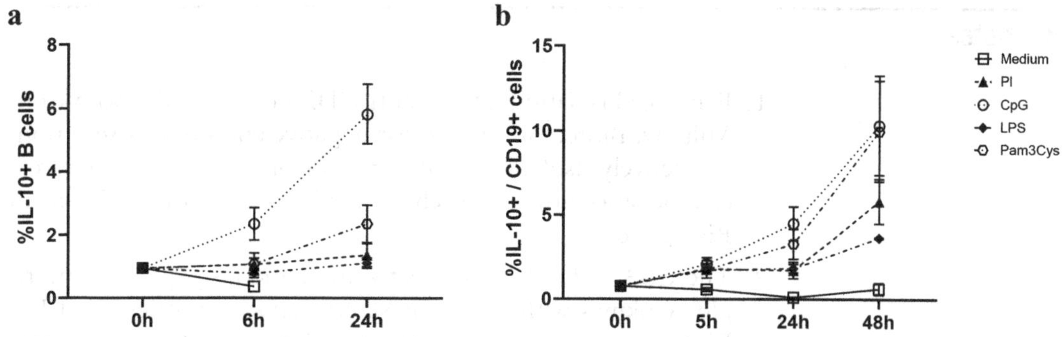

Fig. 4 Kinetics of IL-10 expression after stimulation of B cells and PBMCs with TLR ligands. 5×10^5 cryopreserved purified B cells (**a**) and PBMCs (**b**) collected from healthy adult donors were thawed and rested in culture medium overnight, followed by incubation with either medium, PMA and ionomycin (PI), 1 ug/mL CpG, 0.1 ug/mL LPS, or 5 ug/mL Pam3Cys for 5–6 h, 24 h, and 48 h. Cells were re-stimulated with either PMA, ionomycin and Brefeldin A or Brefeldin A only for the last 4 (B cells) or 5 (PBMC) h of culture. IL-10 production was analyzed by intracellular flow cytometry (n = 2)

9. Analyze data using FlowJo, and identify the main Breg-cell subsets of interest according to the phenotype described in detail in the introduction, for instance: immature transitional B cells ($CD19^+CD24^{high}CD38^{high}$), $CD19^+CD24^{high}CD27^+$ B cells, and IL-10-producing B cells ($CD19^+IL\text{-}10^+$) (*see* **Note 20**).
10. As an example, Fig. 4 shows the kinetics of IL-10 expression after stimulation of B cells and PBMCs with TLR ligands, detected by intracellular cytokine staining and flow cytometry analysis (*see* **Note 21**).

3.5.2 Quantification of Cytokine Production by Cytometric Bead Array (CBA)

1. Stimulate cells as in Subheading 3.4. and harvest supernatants before PIB addition. To perform cytokine quantification by CBA, reconstitute standards for each cytokine (*see* **Note 22**) and perform all other steps required as detailed in the manufacturer's instructions.
2. Setup the flow cytometer using the setup beads and instructions provided by the manufacturer. Acquire a minimum of 100 beads per cytokine.
3. Analyze the data using a flow cytometry analysis software (i.e., FlowJo), gate individual beads in the APC-Cy7 vs. APC scatter plot, and identify the position of each bead/cytokine according to manufacturer's instructions. Calculate the geometric median of the PE channel to obtain the MFI data of individual cytokines.
4. Using a calculation spreadsheet (i.e., Excel and GraphPad), convert the MFI of the standard curves to a logarithmic scale, check the R^2 value for each standard curve, which should be higher than 0.98, and convert the result to pg/mL using the serial dilution concentrations of the standard.

4 Notes

1. Pan B-cell isolation kit and anti-CD20 microbeads (both from Miltenyi Biotec) were used for negative and positive selection, respectively. Isolation beads or kits from other manufacturers can be also utilized, such as MojoSort isolation kits from Biolegend.
2. The CBA technology allows to simultaneously quantify multiple cytokines within a single sample and is proprietary of BD Bioscience. An alternative could be Luminex Multiplex Assays which technology enables simultaneous detection and quantitation of multiple secreted proteins or expressed genes. Basically, the principle is the same, but the methods and instrumentation required differ between the two.
3. Two different solutions can be used to manually count cells, namely Türk stain and Trypan blue. While both discriminate nonviable cells by coloring dead cells in purple and blue, respectively, Türk stain contains acetic acid that lyses both erythrocytes and platelets, hence facilitating the manual counting using an optical microscope. We recommend using Türk stain, if available, for the counting step after PBMC isolation, where erythrocytes and platelets are present if no extra washing or lysing steps have been performed to actively remove these cells. On the other hand, the freezing and thawing steps contribute to the natural lysis and removal of erythrocytes and platelets, therefore there is no added benefit in using Türk stain for manual counting after thawing PBMCs and Trypan blue can be used as an alternative.
4. Always use freshly prepared freezing medium and add DMSO as the final component. Do not let DMSO come into contact with the plastic side of the tube and avoid exposure to direct light sources.
5. If total PBMCs are used for analysis, it is important to obtain sufficient B-cell numbers for subset analysis and/or assessment of IL-10 production. In our experience of studying B-cell subsets within PBMCs, the number of cells required for optimal live B-cell recovery is at least 10^6 PBMCs per well cultured in 96-well plates. This estimation is made on the basis of several factors that may influence B-cell recovery, which should be considered during experimental design and optimization: (1) The percentage of B cells in healthy subjects varies according to ethnic origin, sex, and age, ranging from 2 to 20% of total lymphocytes measured by flow cytometry [56]; (2) Cryopreservation, thawing, and stimulation of PBMCs significantly affect the yield and viability of B cells (*see* Table 1); (3) The frequency of IL-10-positive B cells after TLR ligand

stimulation measured in flow cytometry will be in the range of 0.5–10% of recovered live B cells, depending on the stimuli used and donor-to-donor variation; (4) When studying low frequency subsets by flow cytometry, a higher number of events should be acquired to obtain enough cell numbers for reliable analysis of the population of interest. An estimate of the standard deviation of a measured subset can be calculated as $n^{-1/2}$, n being the number of events acquired per gate [57]. This calculation provides an estimate of the precision of measurement for subpopulations within a specific gate, hence serving as an empirical guide to ensure having enough cell numbers.

6. The decision to use isolated B cells or total PBMCs may also depend on the research question. B-cell responses will most likely differ if cultured as isolated cells or within total PBMCs, due to possible interactions with neighboring immune cells. For instance, cytokine secretion by isolated B cells stimulated using either PI or different TLR ligands tends to be lower than that of B cells within total PBMCs (*see* Figs. 2 and 3). This could be explained by the presence of other immune cells within PBMCs, such as T cells or monocytes, which may support B-cell expression of cytokines through co-stimulatory molecules, CD40 ligation, or expression of cytokines.
7. Isolation of B cells through negative selection by Miltenyi Biotec beads is less efficient in terms of purity and recovery compared to positive selection isolation. Despite the lower purity, the main reasons to use negative selection are as follows: (1) to not induce activation or blocking of function of B cells, which may interfere with future measurements, (2) to substantially reduce the number of irrelevant cells included in the analysis, to save time and reduce the number of cells to be acquired by flow cytometer or mass cytometer, which are usually costly procedures (*see* Fig. 1); (3) to ensure that traces of antibodies or beads used for isolation will not hamper further labeling of B cells with pan-B marker antibodies also used in positive isolation kits such as CD19 or CD20 [58]. Indeed, the staining of CD20 is substantially lower after positive selection by anti-CD20 microbeads (*see* Fig. 1c).
8. To increase isolated B-cell purity after negative selection, it is essential to remove all supernatant after centrifugation, before adding the antibody cocktail. Leaving supernatant on top of the cell pellet will dilute the antibody concentration and greatly decrease the purity of selected cells (in our hands from >80% B cells to <60%). 15 mL tubes allow for a denser and smaller cell pellet in the bottom of the tube upon centrifugation, making complete removal of supernatant more achievable. As stated in the manufacturer's protocol, it is necessary to scale up reagent

volumes if more than 10^7 PBMCs are stained, but the volumes should not be scaled down below the recommended amount, if less than 10^7 cells are to be stained.

9. In our experience, the optimal concentration of isolated B cells is 0.5×10^6 cells/well in 200 μL (96-well plates), or 10^6 cells/250 μL medium (5 mL tubes) for cultures of more than 10^6 cells (*see* Table 1).
10. There are two main differences between stimulation and culture conditions of PBMC and that of isolated B cells. For optimal cell survival, PBMCs are plated at 1×10^6 cells/well in 200 μL of 96 wells plates, while 0.5×10^6 cells/well is optimal for isolated B-cell culture (200 μL per well in 96-well plate). We routinely stimulate PBMC for 5, 24, or 48 h, with addition of PMA, Ionomycin, and Brefeldin A in the last 5 h of culture, while isolated B cells are stimulated for 6, 24, or 48 h and re-stimulated with PMA, Ionomycin, and Brefeldin A during the last 4 h.
11. A resting period of 16–20 h increases the production of IL-10 by stimulated B cells and PBMCs and allows for better detection and measure when stimulating for 5–6 h (*see* Fig. 2). Resting also increases production of TNF-α, IL-6, and GM-CSF by stimulated B cells cultured for 6 h. The necessity of resting might depend on the stimuli and readout, hence we recommend testing and compare the effect of stimulation with and without resting.
12. The expression of CD23 and CD73 by B cells is reduced during overnight resting compared to both ex vivo isolated B cells and PBMC, while CD24 and CD27 expression in PBMC increases over time in medium (unstimulated PBMC control). Changes in the expression of certain surface markers are observed upon thawing or culture in medium, unrelated to stimulation. Therefore, any surface marker for Breg phenotyping must be tested according to the research question and experiment design.
13. Note that any cytokine detection method performed on supernatants of PBMC cultures cannot discriminate the source of cytokine production, particularly when using pleiotropic stimuli such as TLR ligands. Depending on the research question, cytokine production of cell subsets can be measured from PBMC culture supernatants by CBA/ELISA; however, for some cytokines (e.g., IL-10, IL-6, and TNF-α), interference from other cell subsets (e.g., monocytes) is likely, unless cell-specific stimuli are used. To assess B-cell-specific cytokine production after pleiotropic stimulation, it is recommended to use supernatants of cultured isolated B cells rather than PBMCs.

However, the purity of the isolated B-cell population is crucial when measuring cytokines in supernatant as contaminating cells may influence cytokine levels.

14. When performing CBA, always confirm the cytokine/protein of choice is in a unique bead position to allow for multiplexed analysis. Different assay sensitivities can be combined according to the research needs. Certain cytokines, such as the abundantly expressed IL-6, may require increased dilution of the samples to be measured, making it difficult to multiplex with lowly expressed cytokines.
15. The volumes of CBA reagents and cell supernatants can be reduced after extensive testing of the limits of cytokine detection. After validation, we routinely use 5 μL of culture supernatant and diluted standards and 0.1 μL of capture beads per cytokine in 5 μL of capture/detection diluent volume per sample.
16. All antibodies used for flow cytometry should be titrated according to the cell subset studied and the amount of PBMCs per well to reach an optimal staining index [59].
17. When acquiring flow cytometry samples, always add appropriate controls (e.g., unstimulated samples as negative control and stimuli and/or conditions used as positive control). When performing experiments on separate days, it is advisable to add a reference sample (i.e., aliquots of PBMCs or isolated B cells from a single donor along with the test samples) to track any batch effect [59]. Analysis of B-cell subsets should be performed after gating on lymphocytes and removing doublets using side and forward scatter parameters, and excluding dead cells and nonrelevant cell populations from the analysis (i.e., $CD14^+$, $CD3^+$, $CD56^+$ cells) [59]. In order to set accurate gates, the use of Fluorescence-minus-one (FMO) controls is highly recommended [59].
18. Manufacturers recommend adding FcγR-binding inhibitor to the cells 10 min prior to antibody staining. In our experience, FcγR-binding inhibitor can be added to the antibody mix for ease and convenience but should be tested first.
19. A substantial number of cells can be lost during cell culture, processing, and measurement. To minimize this, several actions can be taken. Addition of survival factors, such as IL-2, IL-4, or IL-21 [60], will decrease cell loss during culture, but may also skew B-cell responses. For mass cytometry, sample barcoding can be very efficient in reducing cell loss during staining and measurement (*see* Table 1). Barcoding is a technique extensively used in high-throughput cytometry and genomics, which allows labeling of individual cells, DNA, or RNA fragments with unique tracers (e.g., metals, proteins, and

fluorescent labels) used to retain information on the sample source when pooling (i.e., subject identification and cell lineage). Several barcoding techniques exist and can be applied to either live or fixed cells [61–63]. Lastly, cell loss during staining and/or measurement can be reduced by adding extra cells to the samples, such as nonrelevant unstained carrier cells (e.g., PBMCs) after cell staining, or by including a barcoded reference sample with other barcoded samples. Reference samples are cells of a healthy donor, usually PBMCs derived from a single blood draw, the presence of which assists in identifying and correcting potentially inconsistent antibody staining and batch effects [64].

20. In addition to the identification of IL-10 production, the functionality of IL-10-producing B cells should be validated before being termed "regulatory B cells." Further investigations should be performed to confirm Breg cell's ability to drive regulatory T-cell development, or their capacity to reduce cytokine expression or T-cell proliferation [26, 65].
21. B-cell production of IL-10 varies depending on the TLR ligand used to stimulate the cells and the duration of stimulation. In human B cells, the most effective TLR ligand to induce IL-10 production is CpG, with the optimal stimulation duration of 24 h for isolated B cells, and 48 h for PBMC. Prolonged culture of isolated B cells (i.e., beyond 24 h), without any additional survival factors, severely decreases B cell's viability in medium, thus hindering possible comparisons with PBMCs measured at later time points (data not shown). Furthermore, 48 h cultures of PBMCs allows interactions between different cell types and B cells to be studied, which would not be possible using isolated B cells only.
22. For better results, we recommend using fresh standards for each experiment. Frozen standards should be avoided as freezing reduces the stability/activity of cytokines, ultimately affecting the reliability of the standard curves.

References

1. Neves P, Lampropoulou V, Calderon-Gomez-E, Roch T, Stervbo U, Shen P, Kuhl AA, Loddenkemper C, Haury M, Nedospasov SA, Kaufmann SH, Steinhoff U, Calado DP, Fillatreau S (2010) Signaling via the MyD88 adaptor protein in B cells suppresses protective immunity during Salmonella typhimurium infection. Immunity 33(5):777–790. https://doi.org/10.1016/j.immuni.2010.10.016
2. Sayi A, Kohler E, Toller IM, Flavell RA, Muller W, Roers A, Muller A (2011) TLR-2-activated B cells suppress Helicobacter-induced preneoplastic gastric immunopathology by inducing T regulatory-1 cells. J Immunol 186 (2):878–890. https://doi.org/10.4049/jimmunol.1002269
3. Jagannathan M, Hasturk H, Liang Y, Shin H, Hetzel JT, Kantarci A, Rubin D, McDonnell ME, Van Dyke TE, Ganley-Leal LM, Nikolajczyk BS (2009) TLR cross-talk specifically regulates cytokine production by B cells from chronic inflammatory disease patients. Journal

of immunology (Baltimore, Md: 1950) 183 (11):7461-7470. doi:https://doi.org/10.4049/jimmunol.0901517

4. Khan AR, Amu S, Saunders SP, Hams E, Blackshields G, Leonard MO, Weaver CT, Sparwasser T, Sheils O, Fallon PG (2015) Ligation of TLR7 on CD19(+) CD1d(hi) B cells suppresses allergic lung inflammation via regulatory T cells. Eur J Immunol 45 (6):1842–1854. https://doi.org/10.1002/eji.201445211
5. Barr TA, Brown S, Ryan G, Zhao J, Gray D (2007) TLR-mediated stimulation of APC: Distinct cytokine responses of B cells and dendritic cells. 37(11):3040–3053. https://doi.org/10.1002/eji.200636483
6. Jiang W, Lederman MM, Harding CV, Rodriguez B, Mohner RJ, Sieg SF (2007) TLR9 stimulation drives naïve B cells to proliferate and to attain enhanced antigen presenting function. 37(8):2205–2213. https://doi.org/10.1002/eji.200636984
7. Agrawal S, Gupta SJJCI (2011) TLR1/2, TLR7, and TLR9 Signals Directly Activate Human Peripheral Blood Naive and Memory B Cell Subsets to Produce Cytokines, Chemokines, and Hematopoietic Growth Factors. 31 (1):89–98. https://doi.org/10.1007/s10875-010-9456-8
8. Karlsen M, Jonsson R, Brun JG, Appel S, Hansen T (2015) TLR-7 and -9 Stimulation of Peripheral Blood B Cells Indicate Altered TLR Signalling in Primary Sjögren's Syndrome Patients by Increased Secretion of Cytokines. 82(6):523–531. https://doi.org/10.1111/sji.12368
9. Pan W, Xu HW, Hao WT, Sun FF, Qin YF, Hao SS, Liu H, Cao JP, Shen YJ, Zheng KY (2018) The excretory-secretory products of Echinococcus granulosus protoscoleces stimulated IL-10 production in B cells via TLR-2 signaling. BMC immunology 19(1):29. https://doi.org/10.1186/s12865-018-0267-7
10. Velupillai P, Harn DA (1994) Oligosaccharide-specific induction of interleukin 10 production by B220+ cells from schistosome-infected mice: a mechanism for regulation of CD4+ T-cell subsets. Proc Natl Acad Sci U S A 91 (1):18–22. https://doi.org/10.1073/pnas.91.1.18
11. Ronet C, Hauyon-La Torre Y, Revaz-Breton-M, Mastelic B, Tacchini-Cottier F, Louis J, Launois P (2010) Regulatory B cells shape the development of Th2 immune responses in BALB/c mice infected with Leishmania major through IL-10 production. J Immunol 184 (2):886–894. https://doi.org/10.4049/jimmunol.0901114
12. Palanivel V, Posey C, Horauf AM, Solbach W, Piessens WF, Harn DA (1996) B-cell outgrowth and ligand-specific production of IL-10 correlate with Th2 dominance in certain parasitic diseases. Exp Parasitol 84 (2):168–177. https://doi.org/10.1006/expr.1996.0102
13. Baba Y, Saito Y, Kotetsu Y (2019) Heterogeneous subsets of B-lineage regulatory cells (Breg cells). Int Immunol. https://doi.org/10.1093/intimm/dxz068
14. Blair PA, Norena LY, Flores-Borja F, Rawlings DJ, Isenberg DA, Ehrenstein MR, Mauri C (2010) CD19(+)CD24(hi)CD38(hi) B cells exhibit regulatory capacity in healthy individuals but are functionally impaired in systemic Lupus Erythematosus patients. Immunity 32 (1):129–140. https://doi.org/10.1016/j.immuni.2009.11.009
15. Iwata Y, Matsushita T, Horikawa M, DiLillo DJ, Yanaba K, Venturi GM, Szabolcs PM, Bernstein SH, Magro CM, Williams AD, Hall RP, St Clair EW, Tedder TF (2011) Characterization of a rare IL-10–competent B-cell subset in humans that parallels mouse regulatory B10 cells. Blood 117 (2):530-541. doi:10.1182/blood-2010-07-294249 %J
16. Kamekura R, Shigehara K, Miyajima S, Jitsukawa S, Kawata K, Yamashita K, Nagaya T, Kumagai A, Sato A, Matsumiya H, Ogasawara N, Seki N, Takano K, Kokai Y, Takahashi H, Himi T, Ichimiya S (2015) Alteration of circulating type 2 follicular helper T cells and regulatory B cells underlies the comorbid association of allergic rhinitis with bronchial asthma. Clinical Immunology 158 (2):204–211. https://doi.org/10.1016/j.clim.2015.02.016
17. van der Vlugt LE, Mlejnek E, Ozir-Fazalalikhan A, Janssen Bonas M, Dijksman TR, Labuda LA, Schot R, Guigas B, Möller GM, Hiemstra PS, Yazdanbakhsh M, Smits HH (2014) CD24(hi)CD27(+) B cells from patients with allergic asthma have impaired regulatory activity in response to lipopolysaccharide. Clin Exp Allergy 44(4):517–528. https://doi.org/10.1111/cea.12238
18. van de Veen W, Stanic B, Yaman G, Wawrzyniak M, Sollner S, Akdis DG, Ruckert B, Akdis CA, Akdis M (2013) IgG4 production is confined to human IL-10-producing regulatory B cells that suppress antigen-specific immune responses. J Allergy Clin Immunol 131(4):1204–1212. https://doi.org/10.1016/j.jaci.2013.01.014
19. Noh J, Lee JH, Noh G, Bang SY, Kim HS, Choi WS, Cho S, Lee SS (2010) Characterisation of allergen-specific responses of IL-10-

producing regulatory B cells (Br1) in cow Milk allergy. Cell Immunol 264(2):143–149. https://doi.org/10.1016/j.cellimm.2010.05.013

20. Noh J, Noh G, Kim HS, Kim AR, Choi WS (2012) Allergen-specific responses of CD19(+) CD5(+)Foxp3(+) regulatory B cells (Bregs) and CD4(+)Foxp3(+) regulatory T cell (Tregs) in immune tolerance of cow milk allergy of late eczematous reactions. Cell Immunol 274(1):109–114. https://doi.org/10.1016/j.cellimm.2012.01.005
21. Oliveria J-P, El-Gammal AI, Yee M, Obminski CD, Scime TX, Watson RM, Howie K, O'Byrne PM, Sehmi R, Gauvreau GM (2018) Changes in regulatory B-cell levels in bone marrow, blood, and sputum of patients with asthma following inhaled allergen challenge. Journal of Allergy and Clinical Immunology 141(4):1495–1498.e1499. https://doi.org/10.1016/j.jaci.2017.11.013
22. Khoder A, Sarvaria A, Alsuliman A, Chew C, Sekine T, Cooper N, Mielke S, de Lavallade H, Muftuoglu M, Fernandez Curbelo I, Liu E, Muraro PA, Alousi A, Stringaris K, Parmar S, Shah N, Shaim H, Yvon E, Molldrem J, Rouce R, Champlin R, McNiece I, Mauri C, Shpall EJ, Rezvani K (2014) Regulatory B cells are enriched within the IgM memory and transitional subsets in healthy donors but are deficient in chronic GVHD. Blood 124 (13):2034–2045. doi:https://doi.org/10.1182/blood-2014-04-571125%JBlood
23. Cherukuri A, Rothstein DM, Clark B, Carter CR, Davison A, Hernandez-Fuentes M, Hewitt E, Salama AD, Baker RJ (2014) Immunologic human renal allograft injury associates with an altered IL-10/TNF-<em>α</em> expression ratio in regulatory B cells. Journal of the American Society of Nephrology. 25 (7):1575-1585. Doi:https://doi.org/10.1681/ASN.2013080837%J
24. Zhang M, Zheng X, Zhang J, Zhu Y, Zhu X, Liu H, Zeng M, Graner MW, Zhou B, Chen X (2012) CD19+CD1d+CD5+ B cell frequencies are increased in patients with tuberculosis and suppress Th17 responses. Cell Immunol 274(1):89–97. https://doi.org/10.1016/j.cellimm.2012.01.007
25. Correale J, Farez M (2009) Helminth Antigens Modulate Immune Responses in Cells from Multiple Sclerosis Patients through TLR2-Dependent Mechanisms. The Journal of Immunology. 183 (9):5999–6012. doi: https://doi.org/10.4049/jimmunol.0900897%J
26. van der Vlugt LE, Labuda LA, Ozir-Fazalalikhan A, Lievers E, Gloudemans AK, Liu KY, Barr TA, Sparwasser T, Boon L, Ngoa UA, Feugap EN, Adegnika AA, Kremsner PG, Gray D, Yazdanbakhsh M, Smits HH (2012) Schistosomes induce regulatory features in human and mouse CD1d(hi) B cells: inhibition of allergic inflammation by IL-10 and regulatory T cells. PLoS One 7(2): e30883. https://doi.org/10.1371/journal.pone.0030883
27. Xiao X, Lao X-M, Chen M-M, Liu R-X, Wei Y, Ouyang F-Z, Chen D-P, Zhao X-Y, Zhao Q, Li X-F, Liu C-L, Zheng L, Kuang D-M (2016) PD-1^{hi} Identifies a Novel Regulatory B-cell Population in Human Hepatoma That Promotes Disease Progression. Cancer Discovery. 6 (5):546–559. doi:https://doi.org/10.1158/2159-8290.CD-15-1408%J
28. Ishigami E, Sakakibara M, Sakakibara J, Masuda T, Fujimoto H, Hayama S, Nagashima T, Sangai T, Nakagawa A, Nakatani Y, Otsuka M (2019) Coexistence of regulatory B cells and regulatory T cells in tumor-infiltrating lymphocyte aggregates is a prognostic factor in patients with breast cancer. Breast Cancer 26(2):180–189. https://doi.org/10.1007/s12282-018-0910-4
29. Lechner A, Schlößer HA, Thelen M, Wennhold K, Rothschild SI, Gilles R, Quaas A, Siefer OG, Huebbers CU, Cukuroglu E, Göke J, Hillmer A, Gathof B, Meyer MF, Klussmann JP, Shimabukuro-Vornhagen A, Theurich S, Beutner D, von Bergwelt-Baildon M (2019) Tumor-associated B cells and humoral immune response in head and neck squamous cell carcinoma. Onco Targets Ther 8(3):1535293–1535293. https://doi.org/10.1080/2162402X.2018.1535293
30. Zhou X, Su Y-X, Lao X-M, Liang Y-J, Liao G-Q (2016) CD19+IL-10+ regulatory B cells affect survival of tongue squamous cell carcinoma patients and induce resting CD4+ T cells to CD4+Foxp3+ regulatory T cells. Oral Oncol 53:27–35. https://doi.org/10.1016/j.oraloncology.2015.11.003
31. Matsumoto M, Baba A, Yokota T, Nishikawa H, Ohkawa Y, Kayama H, Kallies A, Nutt Stephen L, Sakaguchi S, Takeda K, Kurosaki T, Baba Y (2014) Interleukin-10-producing Plasmablasts exert regulatory function in autoimmune inflammation. Immunity 41(6):1040–1051. https://doi.org/10.1016/j.immuni.2014.10.016
32. Lee JH, Noh J, Noh G, Choi WS, Cho S, Lee SS (2011) Allergen-specific transforming growth factor-beta-producing CD19+CD5+ regulatory B-cell (Br3) responses in human late eczematous allergic reactions to cow's milk. J Interf Cytokine Res 31(5):441–449. https://doi.org/10.1089/jir.2010.0020

33. Lindner S, Dahlke K, Sontheimer K, Hagn M, Kaltenmeier C, Barth TFE, Beyer T, Reister F, Fabricius D, Lotfi R, Lunov O, Nienhaus GU, Simmet T, Kreienberg R, Möller P, Schrezenmeier H, Jahrsdörfer B (2013) Interleukin 21–Induced Granzyme B–Expressing B Cells Infiltrate Tumors and Regulate T Cells. Cancer Research. 73 (8):2468–2479. doi: https://doi.org/10.1158/0008-5472.CAN-12-3450%J
34. Saze Z, Schuler PJ, Hong C-S, Cheng D, Jackson EK, Whiteside TL (2013) Adenosine production by human B cells and B cell–mediated suppression of activated T cells. Blood 122 (1):9–18. doi:10.1182/blood-2013-02-482406 %J
35. Khan AR, Hams E, Floudas A, Sparwasser T, Weaver CT, Fallon PG (2015) PD-L1hi B cells are critical regulators of humoral immunity. Nat Commun 6(1):5997. https://doi.org/10.1038/ncomms6997
36. Ye L, Zhang Q, Cheng Y, Chen X, Wang G, Shi M, Zhang T, Cao Y, Pan H, Zhang L, Wang G, Deng Y, Yang Y, Chen G (2018) Tumor-derived exosomal HMGB1 fosters hepatocellular carcinoma immune evasion by promoting TIM-1(+) regulatory B cell expansion. J Immunother Cancer 6(1):145–145. https://doi.org/10.1186/s40425-018-0451-6
37. Ganley-Leal LM, Liu X, Wetzler LM (2006) Toll-like receptor 2-mediated human B cell differentiation. Clin Immunol 120 (3):272–284. https://doi.org/10.1016/j.clim.2006.04.571
38. Molnarfi N, Bjarnadottir K, Benkhoucha M, Juillard C, Lalive PH (2017) Activation of human B cells negatively regulates TGF-beta1 production. J Neuroinflammation 14(1):13. https://doi.org/10.1186/s12974-017-0798-5
39. Shin H, Zhang Y, Jagannathan M, Hasturk H, Kantarci A, Liu H, Van Dyke TE, Ganley-Leal LM, Nikolajczyk BS (2009) B cells from periodontal disease patients express surface toll-like receptor 4. J Leukoc Biol 85(4):648–655. https://doi.org/10.1189/jlb.0708428
40. Cerqueira C, Manfroi B, Fillatreau S (2019) IL-10-producing regulatory B cells and plasmocytes: Molecular mechanisms and disease relevance. Seminars in Immunology:101323. doi:https://doi.org/10.1016/j.smim.2019.101323
41. Kawasaki T, Kawai T (2014) Toll-like receptor signaling pathways. Front Immunol 5:461. https://doi.org/10.3389/fimmu.2014.00461
42. Jin G, Hamaguchi Y, Matsushita T, Hasegawa M, Le Huu D, Ishiura N, Naka K, Hirao A, Takehara K, Fujimoto M (2013) B-cell linker protein expression contributes to controlling allergic and autoimmune diseases by mediating IL-10 production in regulatory B cells. Journal of Allergy and Clinical Immunology 131 (6):1674–1682.e1679. doi: https://doi.org/10.1016/j.jaci.2013.01.044
43. Wang D, Feng J, Wen R, Marine J-C, Sangster MY, Parganas E, Hoffmeyer A, Jackson CW, Cleveland JL, Murray PJ, Ihle JN (2000) Phospholipase Cγ2 is essential in the functions of B cell and several fc receptors. Immunity 13 (1):25–35. https://doi.org/10.1016/S1074-7613(00)00005-4
44. Khan WN, Alt FW, Gerstein RM, Malynn BA, Larsson I, Rathbun G, Davidson L, Müller S, Kantor AB, Herzenberg LA, Rosen FS, Sideras P (1995) Defective B cell development and function in Btk-deficient mice. Immunity 3 (3):283–299. https://doi.org/10.1016/1074-7613(95)90114-0
45. Fehres CM, van Uden NO, Yeremenko NG, Fernandez L, Franco Salinas G, van Duivenvoorde LM, Huard B, Morel J, Spits H, Hahne M, Baeten DLP (2019) APRIL induces a novel subset of IgA(+) regulatory B cells that suppress inflammation via expression of IL-10 and PD-L1. Front Immunol 10:1368. https://doi.org/10.3389/fimmu.2019.01368
46. Meng X, Grötsch B, Luo Y, Knaup KX, Wiesener MS, Chen X-X, Jantsch J, Fillatreau S, Schett G, Bozec A (2018) Hypoxia-inducible factor-1α is a critical transcription factor for IL-10-producing B cells in autoimmune disease. Nat Commun 9(1):251. https://doi.org/10.1038/s41467-017-02683-x
47. Frede S, Stockmann C, Freitag P, Fandrey J (2006) Bacterial lipopolysaccharide induces HIF-1 activation in human monocytes via p44/42 MAPK and NF-κB. Biochem J 396 (3):517–527. doi:10.1042/BJ20051839%J
48. Bouaziz JD, Calbo S, Maho-Vaillant M, Saussine A, Bagot M, Bensussan A, Musette P (2010) IL-10 produced by activated human B cells regulates CD4(+) T-cell activation in vitro. Eur J Immunol 40(10):2686–2691. https://doi.org/10.1002/eji.201040673
49. Matsumoto M, Fujii Y, Baba A, Hikida M, Kurosaki T, Baba Y (2011) The calcium sensors STIM1 and STIM2 control B cell regulatory function through Interleukin-10 production. Immunity 34(5):703–714. https://doi.org/10.1016/j.immuni.2011.03.016

50. Haeberlein S, Obieglo K, Ozir-Fazalalikhan A, Chaye MAM, Veninga H, van der Vlugt L, Voskamp A, Boon L, den Haan JMM, Westerhof LB, Wilbers RHP, Schots A, Schramm G, Hokke CH, Smits HH (2017) Schistosome egg antigens, including the glycoprotein IPSE/alpha-1, trigger the development of regulatory B cells. PLoS Pathog 13(7):e1006539. https://doi.org/10.1371/journal.ppat.1006539
51. Lemoine S, Morva A, Youinou P, Jamin C (2011) Human T cells induce their own regulation through activation of B cells. J Autoimmun 36(3):228–238. https://doi.org/10.1016/j.jaut.2011.01.005
52. Menon M, Blair PA, Isenberg DA, Mauri C (2016) A regulatory feedback between Plasmacytoid dendritic cells and regulatory B cells is aberrant in systemic lupus Erythematosus. Immunity 44(3):683–697. https://doi.org/10.1016/j.immuni.2016.02.012
53. Obieglo K, Costain A, Webb LM, Ozir-Fazalalikhan A, Brown SL, MacDonald AS, Smits HH (2019) Type I interferons provide additive signals for murine regulatory B cell induction by Schistosoma mansoni eggs. Eur J Immunol 49(8):1226–1234. https://doi.org/10.1002/eji.201847858
54. Han G, Spitzer MH, Bendall SC, Fantl WJ, Nolan GP (2018) Metal-isotope-tagged monoclonal antibodies for high-dimensional mass cytometry. Nat Protoc 13 (10):2121–2148. https://doi.org/10.1038/s41596-018-0016-7
55. van der Vlugt LEPM, Mlejnek E, Ozir-Fazalalikhan A, Janssen Bonas M, Dijksman TR, Labuda LA, Schot R, Guigas B, Möller GM, Hiemstra PS, Yazdanbakhsh M, Smits HH (2014) CD24hiCD27+ B cells from patients with allergic asthma have impaired regulatory activity in response to lipopolysaccharide. 44(4):517–528. https://doi.org/10.1111/cea.12238
56. Zalocusky KA, Kan MJ, Hu Z, Dunn P, Thomson E, Wiser J, Bhattacharya S, Butte AJ (2018) The 10,000 Immunomes Project: Building a Resource for Human Immunology. Cell reports 25 (2):513–522.e513. doi: https://doi.org/10.1016/j.celrep.2018.09.021
57. Roederer M (2008) How many events is enough? Are you positive? Cytometry A 73A (5):384–385. https://doi.org/10.1002/cyto.a.20549
58. Wang K, Wei G, Liu D (2012) CD19: a biomarker for B cell development, lymphoma diagnosis and therapy. Exp Hematol Oncol 1 (1):36. https://doi.org/10.1186/2162-3619-1-36
59. Cossarizza A, Chang H-D, Radbruch A, Acs A, Adam D, Adam-Klages S, Agace WW, Aghaeepour N, Akdis M, Allez M, Almeida LN, Alvisi G, Anderson G, Andrä I, Annunziato F, Anselmo A, Bacher P, Baldari CT, Bari S, Barnaba V, Barros-Martins J, Battistini L, Bauer W, Baumgart S, Baumgarth N, Baumjohann D, Baying B, Bebawy M, Becher B, Beisker W, Benes V, Beyaert R, Blanco A, Boardman DA, Bogdan C, Borger JG, Borsellino G, Boulais PE, Bradford JA, Brenner D, Brinkman RR, Brooks AES, Busch DH, Büscher M, Bushnell TP, Calzetti F, Cameron G, Cammarata I, Cao X, Cardell SL, Casola S, Cassatella MA, Cavani A, Celada A, Chatenoud L, Chattopadhyay PK, Chow S, Christakou E, Čičin-Šain L, Clerici M, Colombo FS, Cook L, Cooke A, Cooper AM, Corbett AJ, Cosma A, Cosmi L, Coulie PG, Cumano A, Cvetkovic L, Dang VD, Dang-Heine C, Davey MS, Davies D, De Biasi S, Del Zotto G, Dela Cruz GV, Delacher M, Della Bella S, Dellabona P, Deniz G, Dessing M, Di Santo JP, Diefenbach A, Dieli F, Dolf A, Dörner T, Dress RJ, Dudziak D, Dustin M, Dutertre C-A, Ebner F, Eckle SBG, Edinger M, Eede P, Ehrhardt GRA, Eich M, Engel P, Engelhardt B, Erdei A, Esser C, Everts B, Evrard M, Falk CS, Fehniger TA, Felipo-Benavent M, Ferry H, Feuerer M, Filby A, Filkor K, Fillatreau S, Follo M, Förster I, Foster J, Foulds GA, Frehse B, Frenette PS, Frischbutter S, Fritzsche W, Galbraith DW, Gangaev A, Garbi N, Gaudilliere B, Gazzinelli RT, Geginat J, Gerner W, Gherardin NA, Ghoreschi K, Gibellini L, Ginhoux F, Goda K, Godfrey DI, Goettlinger C, González-Navajas JM, Goodyear CS, Gori A, Grogan JL, Grummitt D, Grützkau A, Haftmann C, Hahn J, Hammad H, Hämmerling G, Hansmann L, Hansson G, Harpur CM, Hartmann S, Hauser A, Hauser AE, Haviland DL, Hedley D, Hernández DC, Herrera G, Herrmann M, Hess C, Höfer T, Hoffmann P, Hogquist K, Holland T, Höllt T, Holmdahl R, Hombrink P, Houston JP, Hoyer BF, Huang B, Huang F-P, Huber JE, Huehn J, Hundemer M, Hunter CA, Hwang WYK, Iannone A, Ingelfinger F, Ivison SM, Jäck H-M, Jani PK, Jávega B, Jonjic S, Kaiser T, Kalina T, Kamradt T, Kaufmann SHE, Keller B, Ketelaars SLC, Khalilnezhad A, Khan S, Kisielow J, Klenerman P, Knopf J, Koay H-F, Kobow K, Kolls JK, Kong WT, Kopf M, Korn T, Kriegsmann K,

Kristyanto H, Kroneis T, Krueger A, Kühne J, Kukat C, Kunkel D, Kunze-Schumacher H, Kurosaki T, Kurts C, Kvistborg P, Kwok I, Landry J, Lantz O, Lanuti P, LaRosa F, Lehuen A, LeibundGut-Landmann S, Leipold MD, Leung LYT, Levings MK, Lino AC, Liotta F, Litwin V, Liu Y, Ljunggren H-G, Lohoff M, Lombardi G, Lopez L, López-Botet M, Lovett-Racke AE, Lubberts E, Luche H, Ludewig B, Lugli E, Lunemann S, Maecker HT, Maggi L, Maguire O, Mair F, Mair KH, Mantovani A, Manz RA, Marshall AJ, Martínez-Romero A, Martrus G, Marventano I, Maslinski W, Matarese G, Mattioli AV, Maueröder C, Mazzoni A, McCluskey J, McGrath M, McGuire HM, McInnes IB, Mei HE, Melchers F, Melzer S, Mielenz D, Miller SD, Mills KHG, Minderman H, Mjösberg J, Moore J, Moran B, Moretta L, Mosmann TR, Müller S, Multhoff G, Muñoz LE, Münz C, Nakayama T, Nasi M, Neumann K, Ng LG, Niedobitek A, Nourshargh S, Núñez G, O'Connor J-E, Ochel A, Oja A, Ordonez D, Orfao A, Orlowski-Oliver E, Ouyang W, Oxenius A, Palankar R, Panse I, Pattanapanyasat K, Paulsen M, Pavlinic D, Penter L, Peterson P, Peth C, Petriz J, Piancone F, Pickl WF, Piconese S, Pinti M, Pockley AG, Podolska MJ, Poon Z, Pracht K, Prinz I, Pucillo CEM, Quataert SA, Quatrini L, Quinn KM, Radbruch H, Radstake TRDJ, Rahmig S, Rahn H-P, Rajwa B, Ravichandran G, Raz Y, Rebhahn JA, Recktenwald D, Reimer D, Reis e Sousa C, EBM R, Richter L, Rico LG, Riddell A, Rieger AM, Robinson JP, Romagnani C, Rubartelli A, Ruland J, Saalmüller A, Saeys Y, Saito T, Sakaguchi S, Sala-de-Oyanguren F, Samstag Y, Sanderson S, Sandrock I, Santoni A, Sanz RB, Saresella M, Sautes-Fridman C, Sawitzki B, Schadt L, Scheffold A, Scherer HU, Schiemann M, Schildberg FA, Schimisky E, Schlitzer A, Schlosser J, Schmid S, Schmitt S, Schober K, Schraivogel D, Schuh W, Schüler T, Schulte R, Schulz AR, Schulz SR, Scottá C, Scott-Algara D, Sester DP, Shankey TV, Silva-Santos B, Simon AK, Sitnik KM, Sozzani S, Speiser DE, Spidlen J, Stahlberg A, Stall AM, Stanley N, Stark R, Stehle C, Steinmetz T, Stockinger H, Takahama Y, Takeda K, Tan L, Tárnok A, Tiegs G, Toldi G, Tornack J, Traggiai E, Trebak M, TIM T, Trotter J, Trowsdale J, Tsoumakidou M, Ulrich H, Urbanczyk S, van de Veen W, van den Broek M, van der Pol E, Van Gassen S, Van Isterdael G, van Lier RAW, Veldhoen M, Vento-Asturias S, Vieira P, Voehringer D, Volk H-D, von Borstel A, von Volkmann K, Waisman A, Walker RV, Wallace PK, Wang SA, Wang XM, Ward MD, Ward-Hartstonge KA, Warnatz K, Warnes G, Warth S, Waskow C, Watson JV, Watzl C, Wegener L, Weisenburger T, Wiedemann A, Wienands J, Wilharm A, Wilkinson RJ, Willimsky G, Wing JB, Winkelmann R, Winkler TH, Wirz OF, Wong A, Wurst P, JHM Y, Yang J, Yazdanbakhsh M, Yu L, Yue A, Zhang H, Zhao Y, Ziegler SM, Zielinski C, Zimmermann J, Zychlinsky A (2019) Guidelines for the use of flow cytometry and cell sorting in immunological studies (second edition). European Journal of Immunology 49 (10):1457–1973. https://doi.org/10.1002/eji.201970107

60. Su K-Y, Watanabe A, Yeh C-H, Kelsoe G, Kuraoka M (2016) Efficient culture of human naive and memory B cells for use as APCs. J Immunol 197(10):4163–4176. https://doi.org/10.4049/jimmunol.1502193

61. Hartmann FJ, Simonds EF, Bendall SC (2018) A universal live cell barcoding-platform for multiplexed human single cell analysis. Sci Rep 8(1):10770. https://doi.org/10.1038/s41598-018-28791-2

62. Mei HE, Leipold MD, Schulz AR, Chester C, Maecker HT (2015) Barcoding of live human peripheral blood mononuclear cells for multiplexed mass cytometry. J Immunol 194 (4):2022–2031. https://doi.org/10.4049/jimmunol.1402661

63. Schulz AR, Mei HE (2019) Surface Barcoding of Live PBMC for Multiplexed Mass Cytometry. Methods in molecular biology (Clifton, NJ) 1989:93–108. doi:https://doi.org/10.1007/978-1-4939-9454-0_7

64. Kleinsteuber K, Corleis B, Rashidi N, Nchinda N, Lisanti A, Cho JL, Medoff BD, Kwon D, Walker BD (2016) Standardization and quality control for high-dimensional mass cytometry studies of human samples. 89 (10):903–913. https://doi.org/10.1002/cyto.a.22935

65. Flores-Borja F, Bosma A, Ng D, Reddy V, Ehrenstein MR, Isenberg DA, Mauri C (2013) CD19+CD24hiCD38hi B cells maintain regulatory T cells while limiting TH1 and TH17 differentiation. Sci Transl Med 5 (173):173ra123. https://doi.org/10.1126/scitranslmed.3005407

Chapter 14

Use of Cocultures for the Study of Cellular Interactions Influencing B-Cell Regulatory Functions

Giada Pace and Viviana Valeri

Abstract

Although IL-10-producing B cells have been shown to play key roles in regulating immune responses involved in autoimmunity, inflammation, and cancer, the mechanisms at the base of the generation and maintenance of the pool of regulatory B cells are still poorly characterized. Several evidences show that the cross talk between B cells and other immune cell types promotes IL-10 production by B lymphocytes. Soluble mediators released into the microenvironment, together with direct cell–cell contact, are key signals in the process of regulatory B-cell development and differentiation. Here we describe the methods required to follow IL-10-producing B cells in MC- and MDSC-B-cell cocultures as examples of in vitro systems that induce the expansion of the regulatory B-cell population. These protocols can be also adapted for the study of other immune cell systems.

Key words B cells, IL-10, MCs, MDSCs, Coculture, Soluble mediators, Interaction mechanisms

1 Introduction

The immune response is orchestrated by a well-organized balance between immune activation and suppression that depends on the co-working between effector and regulatory cells of the immune system [1]. While the relevant role played by B cells in the humoral response has been deeply studied, the regulatory function of this immune cell type has been explored only in the last two decades. In 2002, Fillatreau and colleagues revealed a key role of B cells with regulatory functions in controlling autoimmunity. They showed the presence of a population of IL-10-producing B cells in mice with experimental autoimmune encephalomyelitis (EAE) and demonstrated the ability of these B cells to expand during the inflammatory phase that was correlated with the reduction of disease severity [2]. Since then, it has been a succession of studies that have supported the suppressive role of B cells and have led to coining the term regulatory B cells (Bregs) [3, 4]. Subsequent studies established the ability of IL-10^{+} B cells to target many

Francesca Mion and Silvia Tonon (eds.), *Regulatory B Cells: Methods and Protocols*, Methods in Molecular Biology, vol. 2270, https://doi.org/10.1007/978-1-0716-1237-8_14, © Springer Science+Business Media, LLC, part of Springer Nature 2021

immune cell types such as DCs [5], macrophages [6], and Th cells [7], confirming their function in the maintenance of immune tolerance. Although B cells are able to inhibit T-cell proliferation and cytokine production through the release of regulatory antibodies and cytokines such as TGF-β or IL-35, immunosuppression occurs mainly through the release of the anti-inflammatory cytokine IL-10 [3]. Moreover, the Breg immunosuppressive activity can also be mediated by cell contact-dependent mechanisms in which the CD40/CD40L axis and the co-stimulatory molecules CD80 and CD86 are involved [8]. Beyond the attention put in determining the functional involvement of Bregs in precise pathological settings, identifying the specific stimuli and mechanisms involved in the induction of a regulatory phenotype in B cells is of great interest. Soluble or membrane-mediated signals provided by the gut microbiota [9] or by different immune cell types such as dendritic cells (DCs) [10, 11], mast cells (MCs) [12], invariant natural killer T cells (iNKT) [13], myeloid-derived suppressor cells (MDSC) [14], and follicular regulatory helper T cells (T_{FR}) [15] are shown to be able to induce Bregs. DCs are antigen-presenting cells originating from bone marrow precursors and responsible of immune-surveillance and activation of T cells. Although DCs give rise to immunological responses, a tolerogenic role has also been demonstrated for this immune cell type. Several works underlined the ability of DCs to induce splenic B cells to differentiate into a Breg subset with immunosuppressive functions [10] and to amplify IL-10 production in TLR4-activated B cells in a contact-dependent mechanism [11].

MCs are hematopoietic cells that populate almost all vascularized tissues after having completed their differentiation in peripheral tissues. In mice, mucosal MCs and connective tissue MCs are classically identified based on their anatomical localization and granular content even if, in the last years, a remarkable phenotypical heterogeneity and functional plasticity emerged with regard to these cells [16, 17]. The interaction between MCs and B cells is well established, and it has been demonstrated that, besides providing supporting effect in terms of B-cell survival, proliferation, and antibody production, MCs are able to differentiate and expand IL-10-competent B cells [12]. The CD40/CD40L axis was shown to play a key role in this process.

MDSCs originate from a block of the myeloid maturation process during myelopoiesis that impedes immature myeloid cells to differentiate into mature myeloid cells, leading to the generation of a population with immunosuppressive functions [18]. MDSCs have been characterized in two main subsets: the granulocytic or polymorphonuclear MDSCs (G-MDSCs or PMN-MDSCs) and the monocytic MDSCs (M-MDSCs) that differ for the phenotype ($CD11b^{+}Ly6G^{+}Ly6C^{low}$ and $CD11b^{+}Ly6G^{-}Ly6C^{high}$, respectively) and the immunosuppressive mechanisms exerted [19]. The accumulation of MDSCs has been associated with cancer progression and correlated with poor prognosis and survival in cancer patients [20, 21]. Additionally, an increasing amount of data demonstrated the correlation between the large accumulation of MDSCs and the modulation of B-cell differentiation and function [22]. A recent study showed that MDSCs can transform normal B cells to a subtype of Bregs, characterized by a PD-1^{-}PD-L1^{+}CD19^{+} phenotype, which inhibits T-cell response [14].

In this chapter, we present the methods that are necessary to investigate the ability of a partner cell type to promote the expansion of IL-10-competent B cells and/or to induce IL-10 transcription and production by B lymphocytes. We also provide the description of techniques that permit to discriminate between the contribution of soluble versus membrane-bound factors in the induction of Bregs. As examples, the B cell/MCs and B cells/MDSCs coculture systems are described, and detailed protocols to isolate, purify, and coculture B cells with MCs and MDSCs are provided. However, the described procedures can be easily adapted for the study of other different cell types.

2 Materials

2.1 Equipment

1. Surgical instruments (tweezers, scissors, blades).
2. 5 and 10 mL syringes and 26G needles.
3. 1.5 mL microcentrifuge tubes, 15 and 50 mL conical tubes.
4. FACS tubes: round-bottom polypropylene tubes for flow cytometry cell analysis.
5. 70 μm nylon cell strainers.
6. T25 and T75 sterile flasks for suspension cell culture, petri dishes and 24 multi-well flat-bottom culture plates.
7. Transwell-24 well permeable inserts with 0.4 μm pore size and 6.5-mm diameter.
8. Columns and separators for immunomagnetic isolation of specific cell types.
9. Centrifuge.
10. Cell incubator, maintained at 37 °C and 5% CO_2.
11. Flow cytometer and flow cytometry software for data analysis such as the Flowjo Software, or similar.
12. Spectrophotometer.
13. Real-time PCR detection system.
14. ELISA plate reader.

2.2 Mice

1. 6- to 12-week-old female C57BL/6 mice (*see* **Note 1**).

2.3 Buffers, Solutions and Media

1. Phosphate-buffered saline (PBS), pH 7.4: 137 mM NaCl; 2.68 mM KCl; 8.1 mM Na_2HPO_4; 1.47 mM KH_2PO_4.
2. 70% ethanol in water.
3. 0.192 M sodium citrate in PBS. Freshly prepare 20 mL per each spleen. Filter-sterilize. This stock solution should be diluted 10× in the final medium.
4. Red blood cell (RBC) lysis buffer.
5. Peritoneal lavage solution: 3% fetal bovine serum (FBS), 100 U/mL penicillin, and 100 μg/mL streptomycin in PBS. Store at +4 °C.
6. Wash medium: 10% FBS; 20 mM Hepes; 2 mM L-glutamine; 100 U/mL penicillin and 100 μg/mL streptomycin in RPMI 1640. Store at +4 °C.
7. B-cell complete culture medium: 10% FBS; 20 mM Hepes; 2 mM L-glutamine; 1 mM sodium pyruvate; 1× nonessential amino acids (from 100× mix); 100 U/mL penicillin and 100 μg/mL streptomycin; 50 mM β-mercaptoethanol in RPMI 1640. Store at +4 °C.
8. BMMC complete culture medium: 20% FBS; 20 mM Hepes; 2 mM L-glutamine; 1 mM sodium pyruvate; 1× non-essential amino acids (from 100× mix); 100 U/mL penicillin and 100 μg/mL streptomycin; 50 mM β-mercaptoethanol; 20 ng/mL IL-3 in RPMI 1640. Store at +4 °C.
9. PDMC complete culture medium: 20% FBS; 20 mM Hepes; 2 mM L-glutamine; 1 mM sodium pyruvate; 1× non-essential amino acids (from 100× mix); 100 U/mL penicillin and 100 μg/mL streptomycin; 50 mM β-mercaptoethanol; 20 ng/mL IL-3; 20 ng/mL SCF in RPMI 1640. Store at +4 °C.
10. MACS buffer: 2 mM EDTA; 0.5% Bovine serum albumin (BSA) in PBS. Filter-sterilize and store at +4 °C.
11. Fixation/permeabilization solution and permeabilization buffer for intracellular cytokine staining (*see* **Note 2**).
12. 1.5% paraformaldehyde (PFA) in PBS.

2.4 Reagents and Antibodies

1. Specific reagents for immunomagnetic isolation of B cells by negative selection. According to lab preference, different separation techniques are available.
2. Specific reagents for immunomagnetic isolation of MDSC. According to lab preference, different separation techniques are available.

Table 1
Fluorochrome-conjugated antibodies used for immunophenotyping

Specificity of antibody	Clone
CD11b	M1/70
Gr-1	RB6-8C5
Ly6C	HK1.4
Ly6G	1A8
CD19	6D5
CD4	RM4–5
IL-10	JES5-16E3
FcεRIa	Mar-01
CD117 (c-kit)	ACK2

3. Dinitrophenol (DNP): reconstitute at 20 μg/mL in sterile PBS. Store at +4 °C.
4. DNP-specific IgE. Store at −20 °C.
5. Lipopolysaccharide (LPS from *Escherichia coli* O55:B5): reconstitute at 1 mg/mL in sterile PBS. Aliquot and store at −20 °C.
6. Phorbol 12-myristate 13-acetate (PMA): 1 mg/mL in dimethyl sulfoxide (DMSO). Store at −20 °C (*see* **Note 3**).
7. Ionomycin: 1 mg/mL in DMSO. Store at −20 °C (*see* **Note 3**).
8. Monensin.
9. Dye for the discrimination of viable from nonviable cells in multicolor flow cytometric applications (e.g., LIVE/DEAD Fixable Green reactive dye). Reconstitute the dye according to manufacturer's instructions.
10. FcBlock reagent: unconjugated anti-CD16/CD32 (clone 2.4G2) monoclonal antibody diluted in cell staining buffer according to manufacturer's instructions.
11. Fluorescent-conjugated antibodies for flow cytometry analysis (*see* Table 1).

2.5 Other

1. RNA extraction reagent for cells and tissues (kit or phenol and guanidine isothiocyanate based solution).
2. Kit for complementary DNA (cDNA) synthesis.
3. DNA intercalant dye for real-time quantitative PCR.
4. Primers for real-time PCR reaction. Sequences are reported in Table 2.
5. Mouse IL-10 ELISA kit.

Table 2
Primers used for real-time PCR

Target gene	Forward primer	Reverse primer
Murine *il10*	5′-TGTGAAAATAAGAGCAAGGCAGTG-3′	5′-CATTCATGGCCTTGTAGACACC-3′
Murine *g3pdh*	5′-TCAACAGCAACTCCCACTCTTCCA-3′	5′-ACCCTGTTGCTGTAGCCGTATTCA-3′

3 Methods

3.1 Cell Preparation

Depending on the anatomic distribution and abundancy, the immune cell types used in the coculture experiments can either be in vitro differentiated or freshly isolated. Moreover, depending on the purpose of the study, the B cell type used in the assay can derive from different mouse compartments. Here below we provide the protocols for the in vitro differentiation of MCs and for MDSC and B-cell isolation from mouse spleen.

3.1.1 Mouse B-Cell Purification

Although B cells used for the coculture experiments can be purified from different organs, we describe here the protocol of splenic B-cell purification since the spleen is the organ with the higher number of B cells at several differentiation stages. In spite of the fact that several procedures can be used to isolate splenic B cells, we routinely use a B-cell isolation kit based on negative selection, that is fast and allows obtaining high levels of purity (*see* **Note 4**). The B-cell isolation kit uses the immunomagnetic column technology: columns are made of an optimized matrix which generates a strong magnetic field between the beads bound to cells and the magnet when the columns are in contact with the magnet. As shown in Fig. 1, the grade of B-cell purity obtained with this methodology is around 95–99%. All the following steps should be performed under sterile conditions.

1. Euthanize mice by cervical dislocation and spray them with 70% ethanol. Collect the spleen in a small volume of wash medium supplemented with 0.0192 M sodium citrate.
2. Place the spleen in a petri dish and dissociate the tissue by gently scratching the spleen with a scalpel in sterile PBS supplemented with 0.0192 M sodium citrate. Collect the splenocyte suspension and filter through a cell strainer placed on the top of a 50-mL tube.
3. Centrifuge at 300 × *g* for 5 min and discard the supernatant.
4. Resuspend the cell pellet in 2 mL of RBC lysing buffer and incubate for 2 min at room temperature (RT). Mix gently. At

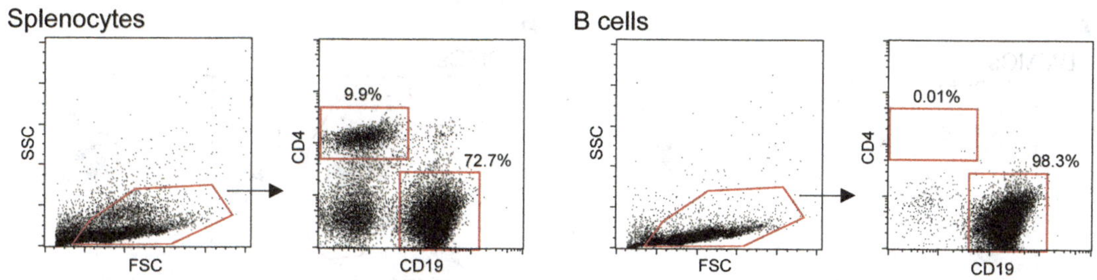

Fig. 1 Percentages of B cells (and of $CD4^+$ T cells as a control) among total splenocytes and following B-cell purification. Cells were labeled using anti-CD19-APC and anti-CD4-FITC mAbs. The CD4 and CD19 plots are selected on FSC versus SSC gate

the end of incubation, dilute the buffer with 50 mL of wash medium supplemented with 0.0192 M sodium citrate and centrifuge at 300 × *g* for 7 min. Discard the supernatant and determine cell number.

5. For every 10^7 cells, add 40 μL of MACS buffer and proceed to B-cell isolation following manufacturer's instructions (*see* **Note 4**).
6. Collect the purified B cells in a 15-mL conical tube. Wash the cells with PBS and resuspend them in B-cell complete medium at the final concentration of 2 × 10^6 cell/mL. Cells are now ready to be used for coculture experiments.

3.1.2 BMMC Differentiation

As described in the introduction, mature MCs are tissue resident cells. In spite of that, primary cultures of mouse MCs can be obtained by in vitro differentiation of bone marrow progenitors, the so-called bone marrow-derived MCs (BMMCs). This procedure allows to generate large numbers of MCs that can be cocultured with B cells. IL-3 is added to the culture medium of BMMCs to mediate MC differentiation into a phenotype similar to that of mucosal MCs.

1. Euthanize 5- to 8-week-old mice and spray them with 70% ethanol (*see* **Note 5**).
2. Peel the skin off from the extremities to expose femurs and tibiae, clean the bones by removing the muscles and the connective tissue with the help of scissors. Excise the femur from the hip join and the tibia from the ankle keeping them together.
3. Rinse the bones with PBS, then put them into 15-mL conical tubes containing wash medium.
4. Under sterile conditions, divide femurs from tibiae. Process one bone at the time. Cut both ends in order to expose the bone marrow, hold it with a nipper and insert in one extremity a 26G needle settled in a 5-mL syringe filled with wash

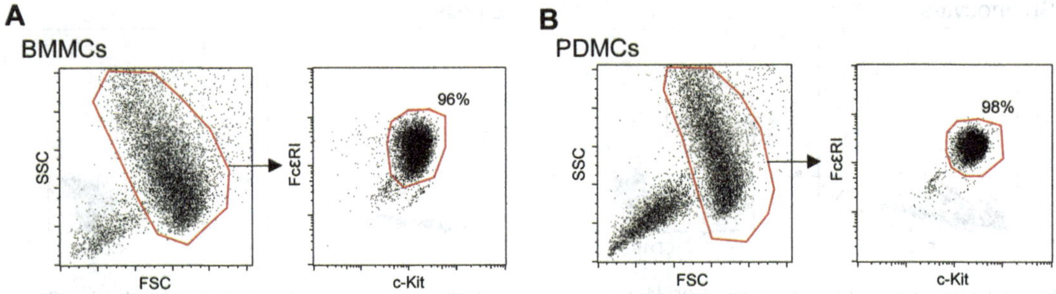

Fig. 2 Flow cytometry analysis of differentiated BMMCs and expanded PDMCs. Cells were labeled using anti-FcεRIa-PE and -CD117 (c-kit)-PE-Cy7 mAbs. BMMCs (**a**) and PDMCs (**b**) are selected on FSC versus SSC plot, and their double positivity for FcεRIa and c-Kit is shown in the corresponding gates

medium. Press half of the liquid down until the marrow comes out, then repeat by inserting the needle in the opposite extremity. Collect in a 50-mL conical tube.

5. Once all the marrow is collected, centrifuge for 5 min at 300 × *g*. Discard supernatant.
6. Resuspend cell pellet in 25 mL per 1 mouse bone marrow (flushed from both femurs and tibiae) of BMMCs complete medium and transfer the cell suspension to a T75 flasks for suspension cell. Adjust medium volumes by maintaining cells at a concentration between 1 and 2 × 10^6/mL and change completely the medium once a week. Culture the cells at 37 °C, 5% CO_2 for 5 weeks before confirming MC differentiation by flow cytometry. Use anti-FcεRIa and anti-c-Kit conjugated antibodies to assess BMMCs purity. As shown in Fig. 2a, the c-Kit$^+$ and FcεRIa$^+$ cells are usually ≥96%.

3.1.3 PDMC Isolation and Expansion

Mature MCs existing in the mouse peritoneal cavity can alternatively be expanded in vitro to obtain peritoneal-derived MCs (PDMCs). The combination of IL-3 and SCF is used in the PDMC culture medium to favor both the differentiation and the expansion of preexisting mature connective-type MCs.

1. Euthanize mice and spray them with 70% ethanol.
2. Inject about 6–8 mL of ice-cold peritoneal lavage solution into the peritoneal cavity.
3. Gently massage the peritoneum to dislodge any attached cell into the peritoneal lavage solution and collect the fluid into sterile tubes. Repeat twice **steps 2–3** to ensure maximal peritoneal cell collection.
4. Centrifuge cell suspension at 300 × *g* for 10 min at +4 °C. Suspend the pelleted cells in 6 mL of PDMCs complete culture medium and culture cells in a T25 flask for suspension cell at 37 °C in 5% CO_2 atmosphere.

5. At day 3 discard nonadherent cells and add fresh medium to the flask.
7. At day 10 check suspension cells by flow cytometry. Use anti-FcεRIa and anti-c-Kit conjugated antibodies to assess PDMCs purity. As shown in Fig. 2b, the c-Kit^{+} and FcεRIa^{+} cells are usually ≥96% (*see* **Note 6**).

3.1.4 Purification of MDSCs

The protocol here below refers to the isolation of MDSCs from the spleen of MC38-tumor-bearing mice that were obtained by subcutaneous injection of 0.2 × 10^{6} MC38 colon carcinoma cells into the left flank of 9-week-old female wild-type mice. Mice were scarified, and the spleen was recovered when the tumor reached the correct dimensions. MDSCs were isolated using a kit that is based on the column technology (*see* Subheading 3.1.1) and that allows the isolation of polymorphonuclear Gr1^{high}Ly6G^{+} and mononuclear Gr-1^{dim}Ly6G^{-}. The obtained purity of the recovered cell fractions using this protocol might be variable depending on the specific source organ. During the MDSC isolation procedure, all steps should be performed under sterile conditions and keeping cells cold.

1. After spleen collection and splenocytes isolation (*see* Subheading 3.1.1, **steps 1–4**), transfer 1 × 10^{8} viable cells into a 50-mL tube and add fresh MACS buffer in order to perform centrifugation with at least 15 mL. Centrifuge the suspension 10 min at 300 × *g* and discard the supernatant.
2. Hereafter, the adopted procedure for the MDSC isolation is in accordance with the manufacturer's instructions.
3. Put the Gr-1^{high}Ly6G^{+} and the Gr-1^{dim}Ly6G^{-} recovered cell fractions on ice. Perform cell count and check MDSC purity by flow cytometry. As shown in Fig. 3, the expected purity is around 90–95% for PMN-MDSCs and about 80% for M-MDSCs (*see* **Note** 7).
4. Wash the cells and resuspend them at a final concentration of 2 × 10^{6} cell/mL in complete culture medium. Cells are now ready to be used for coculture experiments.

3.2 Cocultures

The aim of this subheading is to describe the essential steps necessary to set up a B/MC or B/MDSC coculture. This is preliminary for the study of the role of the partner cell type on the induction of Bregs. An important aspect is that in the coculture panel the outcomes derived from each single cell types should be distinguished. Moreover, the addition of stimulatory factors in the coculture medium can impact the behavior of both cell types cultured in the same well plate. Therefore, single cell type cultures are mandatory controls in this setting. Indeed, MCs and MDSCs could produce and release IL-10 as well as B cells do [23, 24].

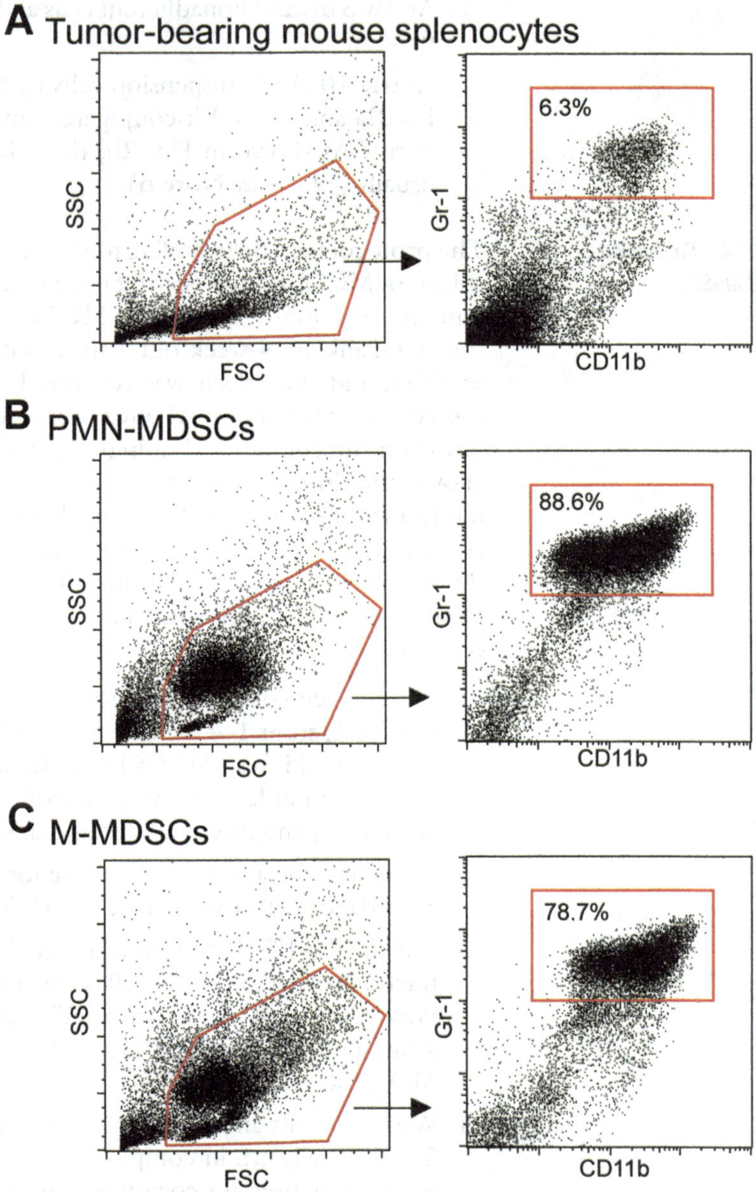

Fig. 3 Flow cytometry analysis of MDSCs from tumor-bearing mice. Cells were labeled using anti-CD11b-FITC and anti Gr-1-PE-Cy7 mAbs. (**a**) The flow cytometry plots show the frequency of MDSC among total splenocytes before immunomagnetic separation. The percentages of PMN-MDSCs (**b**) and M-MDSCs (**c**) are highly increased following immunomagnetic separation. MDSC plots are selected on FSC versus SSC in the left side, and their double positivity for CD11b and Gr-1 is shown in the right panels

3.2.1 B/MC Coculture

The procedure described below can be applied for the study of the interaction between B cells and both BMMCs or PDMCs.

1. Count MCs and wash the required number of cells twice with wash medium. Starve MCs for 3 h in B-cell complete culture medium, IL-3- and SCF-free (*see* **Note 8**). Resuspend cells at 1×10^6 cells/mL. Cells can be either starved in resting condition or sensitized with 1 μg/mL DNP-specific IgE for IgE-dependent activation.
2. After 3 h, wash the cells twice and resuspend them at 2×10^6 cells/mL in fresh B-cell complete culture medium alone (for resting MCs) or supplemented with 200 ng/mL DNP to challenge IgE-stimulated MCs. Cells are now ready to be seeded in a 1:1 ratio culture with B cells.
3. In the meantime, prepare the B cells by resuspending them at a concentration of 2×10^6 cells/mL in B-cell complete culture medium. Plate 300 μL of the cell suspension in each corresponding well of a 24-multi-well plate.
4. Add 300 μL of resting or IgE/DNP triggered MCs in each well. B cells and MCs will have a final concentration of 1×10^6/mL and an equivalent of 0.6×10^6 cells per condition. Gently pipette the wells to allow cell redistribution in the whole volume. Single cell type controls (B cells and MCs only) should be maintained under the same culture conditions. An example of the minimal conditions to include in the coculture plate is shown in Fig. 4a.
5. Incubate the plate in a sterile incubator at 37 °C, 5% CO_2, in a humidified atmosphere. Timing of cell culture will be adjusted to the specific downstream assay (*see* Subheading 3.3).

3.2.2 B/MDSC Coculture

1. Freshly purified B cells (*see* Subheading 3.1.1) are resuspended at a concentration of 2×10^6 cells/mL in B-cell complete culture medium. Plate 300 μL of the cell suspension in each corresponding well of a 24-multi-well plate.
2. Add 300 μL of resting or LPS (10 μg/mL) triggered PMN-MDSCs or M-MDSCs in each well. B cells and MDSCs will have a final concentration of 1×10^6/mL and an equivalent of 0.6×10^6 cells per condition. Gently pipette the wells to allow cell redistribution in the whole volume. Single cell type controls (only B, only PMN-MDSCs and only M-MDSCs) should be maintained under the same culture conditions. An example of the coculture plate for the B/MDSC coculture is shown in Fig. 4b.
3. Incubate the plate in a sterile incubator at 37 °C, 5% CO_2, in a humidified atmosphere for 48 h.

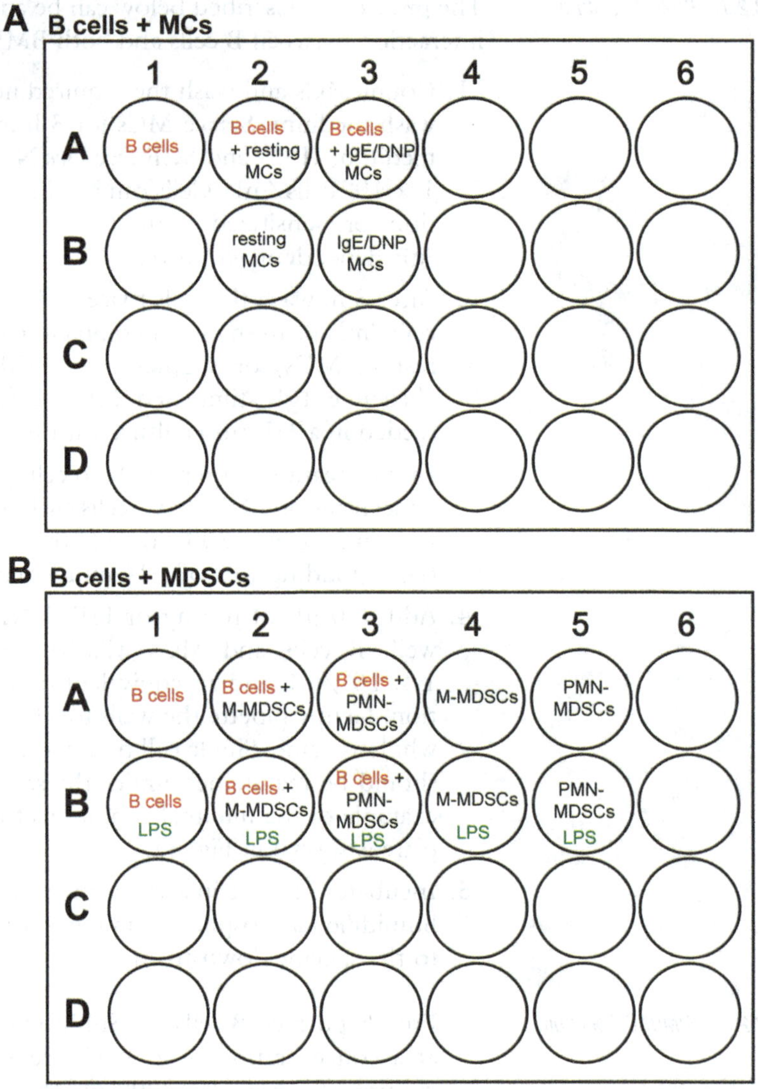

Fig. 4 Basic experimental setup for the coculture experiment between B cells and MCs (**a**) and B cells and MDSCs (**b**). If other stimuli are included in the scheme (here is shown the case of LPS stimulation in the B/MDCS cross talk), corresponding single cell control conditions must be included

3.3 Evaluation of MC and MDSC Ability to Induce IL-10 Production in B Cells

Hereafter we show three different methods to assess the production of IL-10 by B cells after coculture with the partner cell type. These techniques can be applied to both the coculture systems described so far.

3.3.1 Real-Time qPCR for Il-10 Gene Expression

Cytokine IL-10 production and release can be predicted by the study of the expression of *il10* gene transcripts. Prior to RNA extraction, the two cell types in coculture must be separated.

1. Set up coculture as described in Subheading 3.2 (*see* **Note 9**).
2. After 5 h of coculture, collect cells by pipetting up and down. Centrifuge for 5 min at 300 × *g* and discard the supernatant.
3. Proceed to cell separation. Depending on lab availability, positive selection of B cells can be performed through immunomagnetic separation or FACS.
4. Once B cells have been isolated, centrifuge at 300 × *g* for 5 min and proceed with total RNA isolation. Extract total RNA with phenol–chloroform protocol or using a specific kit according to manufacturer's instructions.
5. Assess RNA concentration and purity by using a spectrophotometer and reverse transcribe 1 μg of RNA with an appropriate kit for complementary DNA (cDNA) synthesis, following manufacturer's instructions.
6. Perform RT-qPCR analyses with the SYBR Green chemistry using a real-time PCR detection system. Quantify *il10* gene expression by using glyceraldehyde 3-phosphate dehydrogenase (*g3pdh*) as normalizer gene and perform each reaction in triplicate.

3.3.2 ELISA for IL-10

1. Set up coculture as described in Subheading 3.2 (*see* **Note 10**).
2. After 48 h, collect the cell suspension from each well and transfer to 1.5 mL microcentrifuge tubes. Centrifuge for 5 min at 500 × *g* to pellet viable cells and cell debris.
3. Collect the supernatants in clean microcentrifuge tubes and discard cell pellets. Samples can be immediately tested to assess IL-10 concentration or stored at −80 °C until detection.
4. Test secreted IL-10 by ELISA. Each condition should be tested at least in duplicate. Here we used a commercial mouse IL-10 ELISA kit, and manufacturer's instructions were followed.

3.3.3 Intracellular Staining (ICS) for IL-10

The intracellular IL-10 staining technique is a very reliable tool to assess the ability of the partner cell type to induce the expansion of the IL-10-producing B-cell population already present in the pool of B cells in analysis. Since the majority of these cells do not produce detectable cytoplasmic IL-10, a 5-h in vitro stimulation with LPS, PMA, and ionomycin is required to follow these B cells that are competent for IL-10 production. A protein transport inhibitor such as monensin should be added to the stimulation mix to block IL-10 secretion.

1. Set up coculture as described in Subheading 3.2 (*see* **Note 11**).
2. During the last 5 h of coculture, add 70 μL/well of B-cell complete culture medium containing 50 ng/mL PMA,

500 ng/mL ionomycin, 10 μg/mL LPS, and 2 μM monensin (LPIM). The concentration of PMA, ionomycin, LPS, and monensin are referred to the final volume present in the cell culture well (670 μL) which includes the coculture medium (600 μL) and the medium added with the stimulation mix (70 μL). Culture for 5 h at 37 °C and 5% CO_2.

3. At the end of the 5 h of stimulation, collect the cells in FACS tubes by gently pipetting and add 2 mL of PBS. Centrifuge for 5 min at 300 × *g* and discard the supernatant (*see* **Note 12**).
4. Resuspend the cells in 50 μL of the dye for the discrimination of viable from nonviable cells diluted in PBS according to manufacturer's instructions.
5. Vortex and, immediately after, add 50 μL of anti-CD16/CD32 mAb diluted in PBS according to manufacturer's instructions. Incubate for 15 min and then wash by adding 2 mL of PBS and perform a 5-min centrifugation at 300 × *g*.
6. Perform B-cell staining by incubating cells for 30 min with 50 μL of anti-CD19 mAb diluted in PBS (*see* **Note 13**).
7. After surface staining, fix the cells with 250 μL of fixation buffer and incubate for 20 min. Wash twice the cells with 1 mL of permeabilization buffer which helps to maintain cells in a permeabilized state. Centrifuge 5 min at 300 × *g* and discard supernatant.
8. Resuspend the cells in permeabilization buffer containing anti-IL-10 mAb and incubate for 30 min (*see* **Note 13**).
9. Wash cells twice with 1 mL of permeabilization buffer and resuspend in 250 μL of 1.5% PFA in PBS.
10. Analyze cells by flow cytometry. Figure 5 shows a representative analysis performed to assess $CD19^+IL\text{-}10^+$ cells in the B/MDSC coculture system.

3.4 Contact-Dependent Mechanisms and the Role of Soluble Mediators

The IL-10 inductive signals provided by the partner cell type can either be cell contact or soluble-mediated. The methods described henceforth are meant to help to understand which is the mechanism responsible for the induction of IL-10 production by B cells.

3.4.1 Transwell Assay

The reason for using coculture inserts, such as transwells, consists in impeding surface contact between two cell types of interest by placing a physical barrier in the coculture system. The inserts are equipped with variable pores that allow bi-directional exchange of soluble mediators between the two separated cell populations. The procedure described below outlines the coculture between splenic B cells and BMMCs but can be adapted to MDSCs or other cell types (*see* **Note 14**).

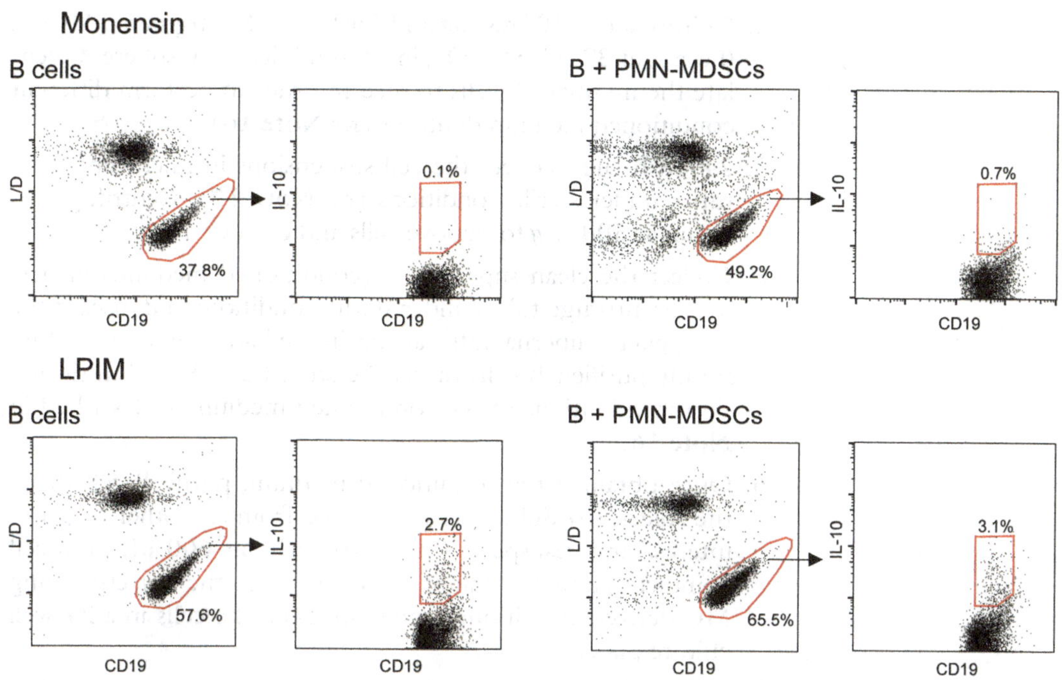

Fig. 5 Gating strategy adopted to analyze IL-10 intracellular staining in B cells cultured alone or cocultured with PMN-MDSCs. Viable B cells are first selected based on the dual staining with the anti-CD19 mAb and the green Live/Dead probe. IL-10$^+$ B cells are then identified by comparing monensin and LPIM-treated cells

1. Seed 0.6×10^6 freshly purified B cells in the bottom chamber of the 24-well culture plate in 0.6 mL of B-cell complete culture medium.
2. Add a transwell insert in each well and then place 0.2×10^6 resting or IgE/DNP-stimulated BMMCs in a volume of 0.2 mL (*see* **Note 15**).
3. Incubate cells for 48 h in a sterile incubator at 37 °C, 5% CO_2.
4. If the downstream assay consists in soluble IL-10 measurements, remove the transwell and proceed as in Subheading 3.3.2. If the experiment involves an ICS for IL-10, add LPIM during the last 5 h and then proceed as indicated in Subheading 3.3.3.

3.4.2 Conditioned Media

To investigate the possible involvement of soluble mediators in the IL-10 inductive capacity of the partner cell type, the conditioned medium obtained by the partner cell type culture can be used. Indeed, resting or stimulated immune cells release factors that can be responsible for inducing IL-10 in B cells. B cells are cultured in this cell-free medium, and the downstream assays described in Subheading 3.3 are then performed.

1. Prepare MCs as in Subheading 3.1.2 or 3.1.3.

2. Culture 0.6 × 10^6 resting and/or IgE/DNP-triggered MCs in 0.6 mL at 37 °C, 5% CO_2, in a humidified atmosphere. Calculate the number of wells to seed in order to perform different conditioned medium dilutions (*see* **Note 16**).
3. 24–48 h later, collect the cell suspensions in microcentrifuge tubes under sterile conditions (*see* **Note 17**). Centrifuge for 5 min at 500 × *g* to remove cells and cell debris.
5. Collect the clean supernatant (conditioned medium) in new microcentrifuge tubes under sterile conditions and discard the cell pellet. Supernatants can be immediately used to culture freshly purified B cells or can be stored at −80 °C until use. Perform dilutions of the conditioned medium as described in **Note 16**.
6. Once obtained the conditioned medium, purify B cells from the spleen (*see* Subheading 3.1.1) or from any other organ of interest and resuspend 0.6 × 10^6 cells in 600 μL of B-cell complete culture medium (control) or of the corresponding MC-derived conditioned medium. Seed the cells in a 24-well culture plate.
7. Incubate for 48 h in a sterile incubator at 37 °C, 5% CO_2 before performing the downstream assay (*see* Subheading 3.3).

3.4.3 Blocking Antibodies

The techniques described above might give an indication concerning the mechanism responsible for the induction of IL-10 in B cells by the partner cell type. In order to determine the contribution of a specific soluble or membrane-bound factor, we suggest the strategy of testing neutralizing Abs for a target molecule. As an example, here below we describe the usage of the anti-CD40L blocking Ab to evaluate the role of the CD40L/CD40 axis in the coculture between B cells and MCs.

1. Prepare B/MC cocultures as described in Subheading 3.2.1. Three wells for each condition (B cells only, MCs only, and B cells plus MCs) should be seed in the plate: the first well is the experimental control in which no Ab is added, the second well is for testing the blocking Ab (e.g., 50 μg/mL anti-CD40L blocking Ab), and the third one is the negative control condition, in which a primary Ab of the same isotype, without any B cell or BMMC specificity, is added (*see* **Note 18**). An example of the plate is shown in Fig. 6.
2. Incubate for 48 h in a sterile incubator at 37 °C, 5% CO_2, then perform the downstream assay (*see* Subheading 3.3).

3.4.4 Use of Genetically Deficient Mice

When feasible, this approach is useful to confirm the result obtained through the usage of blocking Abs. Indeed, if the addition of a specific blocking Ab to the coculture system suggests the involvement of a specific axis, MCs and MDSCs can be obtained by

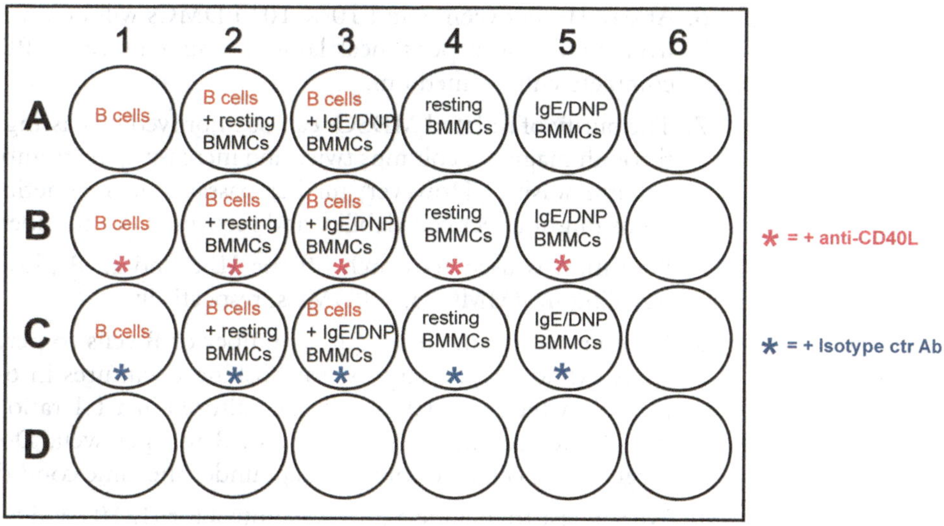

Fig. 6 Coculture scheme between B cells and resting or IgE/DNP-activated BMMCs to determine the role of CD40L, expressed by MCs, in the induction of regulatory B cells. The blocking antibody (anti-CD40L) and its control (Isotype control Ab) are added for each cell condition

knockout mice in which this axis is impaired and can be used to establish cocultures with B cells for the evaluation of downstream assays (*see* **Note 19**).

4 Notes

1. The age of mice depends on the specific immune cell type one wants to work with. For B-cell isolation from mouse spleen, we suggest using 8- to 12-week-old mice while younger mice (4- to 6-week-old mice) are needed for the differentiation of BMMCs from bone marrow precursors.
2. Depending on the availability of the laboratory, either commercially available kits or in-house-made reagents for fixation and permeabilization can be used. Fixation buffer is made of a 4% paraformaldehyde solution in PBS while the recipe for our permeabilization buffer is made of 1% fetal calf serum and 0.1% saponin in PBS.
3. Once reconstituted, prepare small, single-use aliquots to avoid the freeze-thaw. Use fresh aliquots for each experiment.
4. If B cells are isolated from the peritoneum, we recommend proceeding with a positive selection method such as the one obtained by using mouse CD19 microbeads.
5. Pulling femurs and tibiae of two mice will allow to obtain a culture of up to 100×10^6 BMMCs after 5 weeks of cell culture in BMMC complete culture medium.

6. At day 10, between 5 and 10×10^6 PDMCs will be obtained from two mouse peritoneal lavages after culture in PDMC complete culture medium.
7. The purity of isolated MDSCs can be improved by passing cells through magnetic columns twice and increasing the number of column washes. However, further passages in magnetic columns might affect cell viability and recovered cell numbers.
8. Starvation is used to switch off the IL-3 and IL-3 plus SCF signaling in BMMCs and PDMCs, respectively.
9. In order to obtain an adequate number of B cells to perform RNA extraction, we suggest establishing cocultures in 6-well plates in which 3×10^6 B cells are cultured in a 1:1 ratio with the partner cell in a final volume of 3 mL per well. Do not forget single cell type controls, kept under the same conditions.
10. We suggest to include a positive control for IL-10 production. Here we used 10 μg/mL LPS-stimulated B cells as a positive control.
11. We suggest performing the intracellular cytokine staining for IL-10 using at least 10^6 cells per condition. In the absence of a specific immunological signal triggering IL-10 production, $CD19^+IL\text{-}10^+$ cells are present at very low frequencies. Based on our experience, working with 10^6 cells will allow to perform a reliable flow cytometry analysis of IL-10-producing B cells also in the condition in which B cells are cultured alone.
12. Hereafter use precooled solutions and work at +4 °C. Protect samples from light.
13. The working concentration of each antibody should be optimized before use by performing a titration assay.
14. The presented methodology is based on experiments performed in the B/MC coculture. When working with other partner cell types, preliminary tests should be performed to establish the amounts of cells to add in the plate well and in the transwell insert.
15. The 0.4-μm pore size of transwells must be preferred since it allows the passage of cytokines, but not of cells, from the upper to the lower compartment and vice versa. The number of BMMCs seeded in the upper chamber was chosen on the basis of titration experiments. When working with partner cell types different from BMMCs, it is recommended to test different cell ratios and to not exceed the 0.2 mL volume in the bottom chamber.
16. Since the cell metabolism and the amount of released mediators are peculiar of each cell type, pilot experiments should be performed to determine working dilution of the conditioned

medium in fresh culture medium (e.g., 100%, 75%, 50%, 25% of the pure conditioned medium in fresh medium) to use for B-cell culture.

17. The timing for the collection of conditioned medium depends on the functional characteristics of the partner cell type employed in the study. However, it is recommended not to go over a 48-h culture to avoid medium consumption.
18. We recommend titrating neutralizing/blocking Abs to determine their optimal working concentration.
19. Be aware that other molecular alterations may be present when utilizing knockout animals-derived cells.

References

1. Pelanda R, Piccirillo CA (2008) Tolerance, immune regulation, and autoimmunity: cells and cytokines that make a difference. Curr Opin Immunol 20:629–631
2. Fillatreau S, Sweenie CH, McGeachy MJ et al (2002) B cells regulate autoimmunity by provision of IL-10. Nat Immunol 3:944–950
3. Mauri C, Bosma A (2012) Immune regulatory function of B cells. Annu Rev Immunol 30:221–241
4. Vitale G, Mion F, Pucillo C (2010) Regulatory B cells: evidence, developmental origin and population diversity. Mol Immunol 48:1–8
5. Matsushita T, Horikawa M, Iwata Y et al (2010) Regulatory B cells (B10 cells) and regulatory T cells have independent roles in controlling experimental autoimmune encephalomyelitis initiation and late-phase Immunopathogenesis. J Immunol 185:2240–2252
6. Wong S-C, Puaux A-L, Chittezhath M et al (2010) Macrophage polarization to a unique phenotype driven by B cells. Eur J Immunol 40:2296–2307
7. Tian J, Zekzer D, Hanssen L et al (2001) Lipopolysaccharide-activated B cells Down-regulate Th1 immunity and prevent autoimmune diabetes in nonobese diabetic mice. J Immunol 167:1081–1089
8. Sattler S, Vlugt LEPM van der, Hussaarts L, et al (2012) Regulatory B Cells - Implications in Autoimmune and Allergic Disorders, In: Recent Advances in Immunology to Target Cancer, Inflammation and Infections, pp. 177–200 InTech
9. Rosser EC, Oleinika K, Tonon S et al (2014) Regulatory B cells are induced by gut microbiota–driven interleukin-1β and interleukin-6 production. Nat Med 20:1334–1339
10. Qian L, Qian C, Chen Y et al (2012) Regulatory dendritic cells program B cells to differentiate into CD19hiFcγIIbhi regulatory B cells through IFN-β and CD40L. Blood 120:581–591
11. Boldison J, Rosa LC, Da Davies J et al (2019) Dendritic cells license regulatory B cells to produce IL-10 and mediate suppression of antigen-specific CD8 T cells. Cell Mol Immunol:1–13
12. Mion F, D'Incà F, Danelli L et al (2014) Mast cells control the expansion and differentiation of IL-10–competent B cells. J Immunol 193:4568–4579
13. Vomhof-DeKrey EE, Yates J, Hägglöf T et al (2015) Cognate interaction with iNKT cells expands IL-10–producing B regulatory cells. Proc Natl Acad Sci 112:12474–12479
14. Shen M, Wang J, Yu W et al (2018) A novel MDSC-induced PD-1- PD-L1+ B-cell subset in breast tumor microenvironment possesses immuno-suppressive properties. Oncoimmunology Ther 7:e1413520
15. Burger F, Miteva K, Baptista D, et al (2020) Follicular regulatory helper T cells control the response of regulatory B cells to a high-cholesterol diet, In: Cardiovascular Research
16. Cildir G, Pant H, Lopez AF et al (2017) The transcriptional program, functional heterogeneity, and clinical targeting of mast cells. J Exp Med 214:2491–2506
17. Frossi B, Mion F, Sibilano R et al (2018) Is it time for a new classification of mast cells? What do we know about mast cell heterogeneity? Immunol Rev 282:35–46
18. Alicea-Torres K, Gabrilovich DI (2018) Biology of myeloid-derived suppressor cells. Oncoimmunology Ther:181–197

19. Youn J-I, Nagaraj S, Collazo M et al (2008) Subsets of myeloid-derived suppressor cells in tumor-bearing mice. J Immunol 181:5791–5802
20. Gabrilovich DI, Nagaraj S (2009) Myeloid-derived suppressor cells as regulators of the immune system. Nat Rev Immunol 9:162–174
21. Solito S, Marigo I, Pinton L et al (2014) Myeloid-derived suppressor cell heterogeneity in human cancers. Ann N Y Acad Sci 1319:47–65
22. Xu X, Meng Q, Erben U et al (2017) Myeloid-derived suppressor cells promote B-cell production of IgA in a TNFR2-dependent manner. Cell Mol Immunol 14:597–606
23. Galli SJ, Grimbaldeston M, Tsai M (2008) Immunomodulatory mast cells: negative, as well as positive, regulators of immunity. Nat Rev Immunol 8:478–486
24. Park M-J, Lee S-H, Kim E-K et al (2018) Interleukin-10 produced by myeloid-derived suppressor cells is critical for the induction of Tregs and attenuation of rheumatoid inflammation in mice. Sci Rep 8:3753

Chapter 15

Use of Inhibitory Compounds to Dissect the Molecular Pathways Involved in Regulatory B-Cell Differentiation

Maik Luu and Alexander Visekruna

Abstract

Regulatory B cells (Bregs) are IL-10-producing lymphocytes able to suppress inflammatory and autoimmune responses. Pharmacological inhibition of key enzymes within metabolic or signaling pathways enables the identification of factors involved in the differentiation and function of Bregs. Isolation and treatment of splenic B cells derived from IL-10 reporter mice allow fast screening for modulatory compounds influencing IL-10 secretion via flow cytometry. In this chapter, we outline the protocol for the induction of highly potent and metabolically active Bregs using the short-chain fatty acid pentanoate. Moreover, we show how the utilization of inhibitory compounds facilitates the dissection of the engaged pathways in Bregs.

Key words Regulatory B cells, IL-10, Short-chain fatty acids, Pentanoate, Inhibitory compounds

1 Introduction

IL-10 is one of the most important regulatory cytokines dampening inflammatory responses and thereby protecting the host from damage. Due to their strong IL-10-producing capacities, regulatory B cells (Bregs) have become a major research subject in order to find novel therapeutic approaches for inflammatory or autoimmune diseases [1]. Therefore, understanding the underlying molecular mechanisms of IL-10 induction in Bregs may offer new opportunities for developing targeted therapies.

While various Breg subsets have been described and characterized within pathological and autoimmune environments by the expression of their surface markers, such as $CD19^{+}CD21^{hi}CD23^{+}CD24^{hi}$ or $CD5^{+}CD1d^{hi}$ [2, 3], much less is known about the molecular prerequisites necessary for their suppressive phenotype. Different research groups have agreed on in vitro generation of Bregs by agonistic CD40 stimulation [4]. Furthermore, both B-cell receptor (BCR) and Toll-like receptor (TLR) signaling were shown to induce IL-10 production in B cells. TLR ligands activate numerous signaling cascades, of which the MAPK

Francesca Mion and Silvia Tonon (eds.), *Regulatory B Cells: Methods and Protocols*, Methods in Molecular Biology, vol. 2270, https://doi.org/10.1007/978-1-0716-1237-8_15,

signaling through p38 and ERK1/2 plays a crucial role in inducing IL-10 expression in B cells [5, 6]. For instance, the activation with TLR ligands promotes the Blimp1-dependent generation of IL-10-producing IgM^{+}CD138^{hi} plasma cells [7]. Moreover, a recent study has revealed that the induction of Bregs by microbiota via the TLR2-MyD88-PI3K axis contributes to the maintenance of colonic homeostasis [8].

Previous research by our group has shown that not only microbiota-derived TLR agonists but also bacterial metabolites can strongly increase the suppressive capacity of Bregs. Short-chain fatty acids (SCFAs) are a major class of bacteria-derived small molecules generated by the fermentation of dietary fibers modulating cellular metabolism and epigenetic features [9]. Upon activation with the TLR9 agonist CpG, splenic B cells treated with the SCFA pentanoate enhanced both their glycolytic activity and oxidative phosphorylation in a mTOR-dependent manner, in cooperation with p38 signaling. Of note, transfer of pentanoate-treated Bregs was sufficient to suppress pathogenic Th17 response in the central nervous system, in contrast to their untreated counterparts [10].

In this chapter, we describe the detailed methods needed for the in vitro expansion of SCFA-triggered CD19^{+}IL-10^{hi} murine B cells for the screening of inhibitory compounds to identify new pathways involved in IL-10 production and Breg differentiation.

2 Materials

Prepare all solutions under a sterile hood and perform sterile filtration of cell culture buffers. Unless otherwise stated, store all reagents at 4 °C.

2.1 Mice

1. C57BL/6 or IL-10 reporter mice such as tiger mice (Jackson laboratory, strain 008379, B6.129S6-*Il10*^{tm1Flv}/J) (*see* **Note 1**).

2.2 Magnetic-Activated Cell Sorting (MACS)

1. 30 μm cell strainer.
2. 1 mL syringe.
3. 2 mL, 15 mL, and 50 mL tubes.
4. Polypropylene fluorescence activated cell sorting (FACS) tubes.
5. Balanced Salt Solution (BSS): 9.7 g Hanks' Balanced Salts with phenol red ($NaHCO_3$-free), 1.425 g $NaHCO_3$, 2.83 g HEPES, add 1 l H_2O, pH 7.2.
6. Phosphate Buffered Saline (PBS, 1×): 9.6 g PBS powder (Ca^{2+}- and Mg^{2+}-free) in 1 l H_2O, pH 7.2.

7. Ethanol.
8. Sodium borate.
9. Sodium phosphate.
10. Borate Buffered Saline (BBS, 10 x): 0.2 M phosphate, 0.5 M borate, pH 8.0.
11. Red blood cell lysis buffer: 0.17 M NH_4Cl, 20 mM HEPES at room temperature.
12. Trypan Blue for cell counts.
13. MACS Buffer: 1× PBS, 0.5% bovine serum albumin (BSA), 2 mM EDTA.
14. B-cell antibody mix: FITC-conjugated anti-mouse CD8 (53–6.7), CD4 (GK1.5), CD11b (M1/70), CD11c (N418), TER-119 (Ter-119), CD49b (DX5), combine 5 μg each (*see* **Note 2**).
15. Anti-FITC-biotin (0.5 mg/mL).
16. Streptavidin.
17. PerCP-conjugated anti-mouse CD19 (clone 1D3, 0.5 mg/mL).
18. Magnetic beads: NH2-cross-linked magnetic dextran nanoparticles with a 300 nm diameter.
19. (+)-Biotin N-hydroxysuccinimide ester.
20. Magnetic tube stand.
21. FACS Buffer: 1% fetal calf serum (FCS) in 1× PBS.
22. Tube rotator.
23. Storage buffer: 0.1% PEG6000 in 1× PBS, pH 7.0.
24. 1 mM biotin-NHS solution: mix 1 mL ethanol and 1 mL H_2O and then add 30 μL of 300 mM biotin-NHS in DMSO and 8 mL of H_2O.

2.3 Cell Culture and Treatment

1. Fully supplemented RPMI: 2 mM L-Glutamine, 1× MEM non-essential amino acids, 10% FCS, 0.01% penicillin-streptomycin, 50 μM 2-mercaptoethanol in RPMI-1640 medium.
2. CpG-2395 (*see* **Notes 3** and **4**).
3. 100 mM sodium pentanoate.
4. Cell culture plates.
5. 10 mM SB203580.
6. 100 μM Rapamycin.
7. 1 mM GSK23370.
8. 10 mM AKT Inhibitor IV.
9. 10 mM Wortmannin.

10. Annexin V buffer: 9.7 g Hanks' Balanced Salts (phenol red- and $NaHCO_3$-free), 0.35 g $NaHCO_3$, add 1 l H_2O, pH 7.4.
11. 50 μg/mL Alexa Fluor 647-conjugated Annexin V.

2.4 Intracellular Phospho-Staining

1. Wash buffer: 2% FCS, 0.2% Tween-20 in 1× PBS.
2. Fixation buffer: 2% formaldehyde in 1× PBS.
3. Permeabilization buffer: 98% methanol at −20 °C.
4. PE-conjugated anti-phospho-Akt1 (Ser473).

3 Methods

3.1 Isolation of Splenic B Cells by Negative Selection

In this section, we describe the basic protocols needed for efficient isolation of murine splenic B cells by negative selection.

3.1.1 Biotinylation of Magnetic Beads

1. Wash the magnetic beads in 2 mL tubes on the magnetic stand with storage buffer. Repeat this step four times.
2. Before conjugation, bring 100 mg of magnetic beads in storage buffer to room temperature (RT).
3. Combine 10 mL of 1 mM biotin-NHS with 10 mL of magnetic beads in storage buffer and mix well for 1–2 min.
4. Add 2 mL of 10× BBS and mix well.
5. Incubate the reaction for 1 h at RT.
6. Distribute the magnetic bead suspension in 1.5 mL tubes on the magnet and wash with storage buffer. Repeat this step 15 times.
7. Resuspend beads in 1 mL of storage buffer at 4 °C (*see* **Note 5**).

3.1.2 Preparation of Anti-FITC-Streptavidin

1. Suspend 1 mg streptavidin in 20 μL of PBS with 0.5% BSA and centrifuge for 10 min at 10.000 × *g*.
2. Add 10 μL anti-FITC-biotin and mix well. Repeat this step five times.
3. Centrifuge for 10 min at 10.000 × *g* and incubate for 24 h or longer at 4 °C.
4. Use 3 μL per 10^8 total cells.

3.1.3 Isolation of Murine Splenocytes

1. Sacrifice IL-10 reporter mice by CO_2 inhalation, cervical dislocation, or any other approved method.
2. Isolate spleen from mice and put in 2 mL tubes with cold BSS on ice.
3. In a sterile flow hood, gently mash the spleens through a 30-μm cell strainer into either 15 or 50 mL tubes using the

flat end of the plunger from a 1 mL syringe. Wash filter with BSS and centrifuge the single cell suspension for 5 min, 4 °C, 450 × *g*.

4. Discard the supernatant and resuspend the pellet in 3 mL of red blood cell lysis buffer per spleen. Incubate the cell suspension for 7 min at RT to perform erythrocyte lysis with vortexing in between. Fill the tube to the top with MACS buffer. Centrifuge for 5 min, 4 °C, 450 × *g*.
5. Resuspend cells in 5–10 mL MACS buffer and count cells with a hemocytometer. Subsequently, pelletize the cells. Centrifuge for 5 min, 4 °C, 450 × *g* (*see* **Note 6**).

3.1.4 MACS Negative Selection of Splenic B Cells

1. Resuspend pellet in 250 μL MACS buffer per 10^8 cells and add 2.5 μL of B-cell antibody mix. Incubate for 10 min at 4 °C in the dark.
2. Wash the cells by filling the tube to the top with MACS buffer and by subsequent centrifugation for 5 min, 4 °C, 450 × *g* (*see* **Note 7**).
3. Discard supernatant and resuspend the pellet in 100 μL of MACS buffer per 10^8 cells before addition of 3 μL (45 μg) of anti-FITC-biotin/streptavidin.
4. Incubate for 15 min at 4 °C in the dark.
5. Wash twice as described in **step 2** and adjust the volume to 1.5 mL per 10^8 cells.
6. Add 50 μL (5 mg) biotinylated beads per 10^8 cells and distribute 1.5 mL of cell suspension in 2 mL tubes.
7. Put 2 mL tubes on tube rotator at 4 °C. Open tube lids and place the 2 mL tubes in the magnetic stand for 15–20 min (*see* **Note 8**).
8. Collect and pool the supernatants carefully with a pipette and wash the cells in fully supplemented RPMI.
9. Count cells using a hemocytometer.
10. Determine B-cell purity by transferring 2 × 10^5 cells into a 5-mL flow cytometry tube and resuspending them in 100 μL of PBS with 0.125 μg of anti-CD19-PerCP antibody. Incubate the suspension for 5 min at 4 °C, wash the cells in FACS buffer (fill the tube to the top and centrifuge for 5 min, 4 °C, 450 × *g*) and finally analyze the purity of the cell population using a flow cytometer and an analysis software. A purity of >90% should be achieved for the following experiments (*see* **Note 9**).

3.2 Induction of IL-10 Production in Splenic B Cells by SCFAs and Use of Inhibitors

In this section, we describe the use of sodium pentanoate as metabolic enhancer and inducer of IL-10 production in B cells. By application of pharmacological inhibitors, we show an example of how we identified pentanoate-mediated mTOR and p38 pathway induction as underlying mechanism. Inhibition of mTOR by rapamycin or selective blockade of the upstream molecules PI3K/PDKI/AKT acts synergistically with p38 inhibitors to reduce pentanoate-mediated IL-10 production in B cells [10].

3.2.1 Induction of Bregs by pentanoate and CpG-2395

1. Adjust cell number to 1 × 10^6 B cells per 1 mL in fully supplemented RPMI.
2. Add the TLR9 agonist CpG-2395 to the final concentration of 4 μg/mL.
3. Plate 2 × 10^5 cells in 200 μL per well of a 96-well plate (*see* **Note 10**).
4. Incubate the cells for 24 h at 37 °C and 5% CO_2 saturation.
5. Treat the cells with 5 mM pentanoate 24 h post B-cell activation with CpG-2395 for 72 h (*see* **Note 11**).

3.2.2 Determination of Optimal Working Concentration of Inhibitory Compounds

In order to identify molecules involved in the induction of IL-10 production by CpG-2395 and pentanoate, incubate the cells with pharmacological inhibitors of the mTOR and p38 pathways 2 h prior to pentanoate treatment (*see* Fig. 1).

1. Treat the B cells as described in **steps 1–4** of Subheading 3.2.1.
2. Solve the inhibitory compounds in the appropriate solvent according to manufacturer's instructions (*see* Table 1).
3. 2 h prior the administration of pentanoate, incubate the B cells with increasing concentrations of mTOR and p38 pathway inhibitors. As a control sample, treat B cells with the same volume of the respective solvent or, when commercially available, with the inactive analogue of the specific inhibitor in analysis.
4. Collect the supernatants after 72 h of pentanoate treatment for IL-10 detection through ELISA. Supernatants can be stored at −80 °C until processed.
5. Harvest the cells in 5 mL flow cytometry tubes and wash the samples with Annexin V buffer by centrifugation for 5 min, 4 °C, 500 × *g*.
6. Resuspend the pellet in 100 μL Annexin V buffer containing 250 ng Annexin V-Alexa Fluor 647 and incubate the suspension for 30 min at 4 °C in the dark.
7. Add additional 200 μL Annexin V buffer and immediately analyze apoptotic Annexin V^+ cells via flow cytometry (*see* **Note 12**).
8. For each inhibitory compound, determine the optimal concentration that is the one with the lowest toxicity and strongest capacity to reduce IL-10 production.

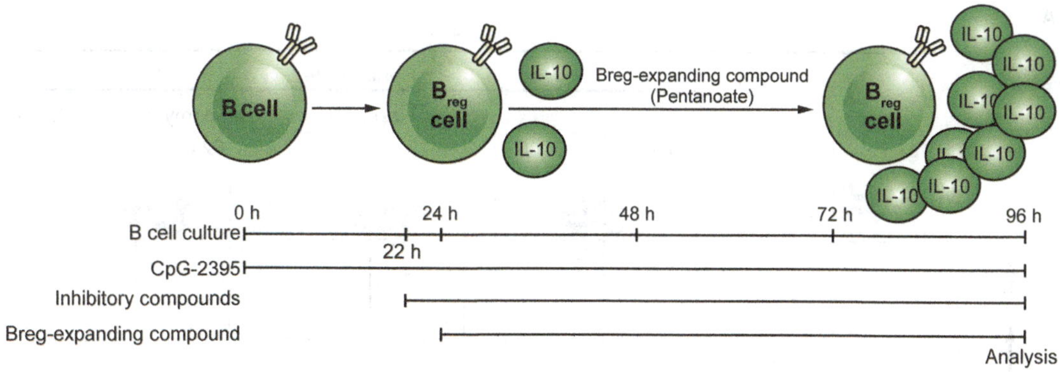

Fig. 1 Experimental design for pentanoate-mediated IL-10 production in Bregs and usage of inhibitory compounds. B cells are activated with CpG-2395 for 24 h. Inhibitory compounds should be added 2 h prior to pentanoate administration. After 72 h of pentanoate treatment, cells can be analyzed for IL-10 production via flow cytometry or ELISA

Table 1
Inhibitory compounds used to dissect the molecular pathways for IL-10 production in Bregs.

Target	Inhibitory compound (Solvent)	Working concentration	Subtoxic concentration
PI3K	Wortmannin (DMSO)	350 nM	1 μM
PDK1	GSK2334470 (DMSO)	150 nM	750 nM
AKT	AKT inhibitor IV (DMSO)	75 nM	100 nM
mTOR	Rapamycin (DMSO)	100 nM	250 nM
p38	SB203580 (DMSO)	5 μM	15 μM

3.2.3 IL-10 Detection

1. 96 h after CpG-2395 administration, collect cultured cells and their supernatants and centrifuge for 5 min, 4 °C, 500 × *g*. Cells can be used to either follow IL-10 production by flow cytometry (*see* Fig. 2a and **Note 13**) or to assess *Il10* gene expression by qPCR (*see* Fig. 2c). Supernatants can be stored at −80 °C for detection of IL-10 release by ELISA (*see* Fig. 2b).
2. In order to follow IL-10 production by flow cytometry, harvest the cells in 5 mL flow cytometry tubes and wash the samples with 4 mL FACS buffer by centrifugation for 5 min, 4 °C, 500 × *g*.
3. If the experiment is performed with the IL-10 reporter mouse, then cells can be directly prepared for analysis via flow cytometry. Instead, if C57BL/6 mice are used, a re-stimulation step is required in order to detect IL-10 by flow cytometry (*see* **Note 14**).

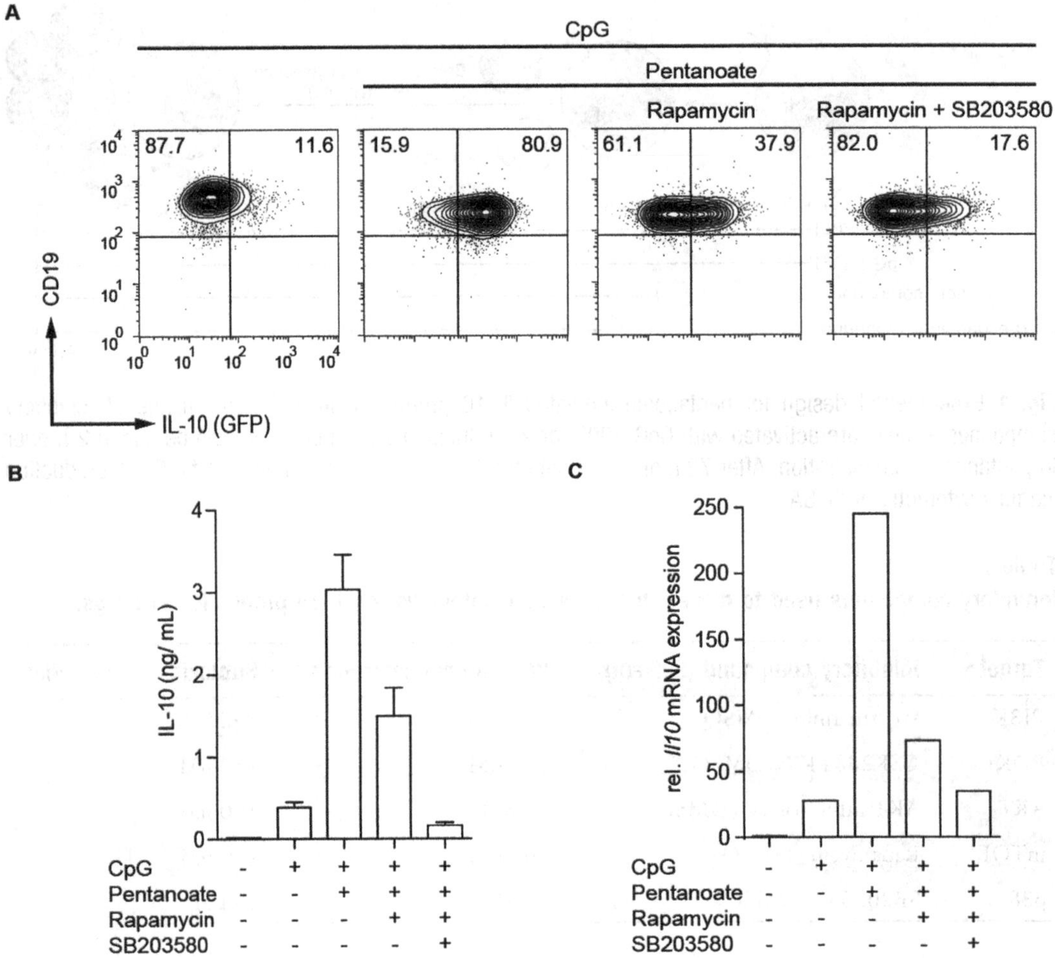

Fig. 2 Analysis of IL-10-producing B cells. Isolated splenic B cells derived from an IL-10 (GFP)-reporter mouse were activated with CpG-2395. Bregs were treated with pharmacological inhibitors of the mTOR (rapamycin) or p38 MAPK (SB203580) pathway, and subsequently incubated for three days in the presence of pentanoate. (**a**) Representative contour plots of IL-10-producing B cells treated with inhibitory compounds. (**b**) IL-10 secretion was determined in B cell supernatants by ELISA. (**c**) Representative RT-qPCR analysis of *Il10* expression in pentanoate-induced Bregs

4. Resuspend the pellet in 100 μL PBS with 0.125 μg of anti-CD19-PerCP antibody and incubate the suspension for 15 min at 4 °C.
5. Wash the cells by addition of 4 mL FACS buffer and centrifuge for 5 min, 4 °C, 450 × *g*.
6. If the IL-10 reporter mouse is used, then directly analyze cells for reporter expression via flow cytometry. Instead, if C57BL/6 mice are used, proceed with the IL-10 intracellular cytokine staining before sample acquisition (*see* **Note 15**).

3.3 Staining for Intracellular Phospho-Proteins

In this section, the staining protocol for the detection of phosphorylated proteins involved in the engaged molecular pathways, such as phospho-AKT1 (Ser473), will be described (*see* **Note 16**).

1. Generate Bregs as Described in Subheading 3.2.1 and Harvest Cells in 5 MmL FACS Tubes
2. Add 2 mL of cold PBS on ice and centrifuge the cells for 5 min at 4 °C, 450 × *g*.
3. Discard the supernatant and resuspend cell pellet in 400 μL of fixation buffer. Incubate for 10 min at 37 °C.
4. Put the samples on ice and permeabilize by slow addition of 3.6 mL permeabilization buffer (*see* **Note 17**). Centrifuge for 4 min, 4 °C, 450 × *g*.
5. Discard the supernatant and resuspend cell pellet in 1 mL of wash buffer. Centrifuge for 4 min, 4 °C, 625 × *g* (*see* **Note 18**).
6. Discard the supernatant and resuspend cell pellet in 100 μL of wash buffer. Add 0.5 μg of PE-conjugated phospho-AKT1 antibody per sample.
7. Incubate at RT for 45–60 min in the dark.
8. Add 1 mL of wash buffer and continue incubation for another 10 min at RT. Centrifuge the samples for 4 min at 625 × *g*.
9. Discard the supernatants and resuspend cell pellet in 200 μL of PBS. Proceed with the flow cytometry analysis.

4 Notes

1. The experiments can be performed with any mouse strain, sex, or age. The protocol provided in Subheading 3.2.1 allows the in vitro generation of a sufficient number of Bregs for adoptive transfer experiments or molecular analysis and screening approaches. However, in order to keep the background on in vivo induced Bregs low, we recommend the use of 8- to 12-weeks-old mice. Moreover, using IL-10 reporter mouse models such as the tiger mouse enables also in vivo identification of IL-10 producers without the need of re-stimulation.
2. The negative-selection process using FITC-conjugate antibodies enables the isolation of untouched B cells. By rearrangement of the antibody composition, the enrichment of other cell types, such as CD4 or CD8 T cells, is possible.
3. CpG-2395 (Type C): 5′-tcgtcgttttcggcgcgcgccg-3′ (22-mer).
4. Other TLR agonists such as LPS have been shown to induce Bregs, as well as the signaling through the BCR or through co-stimulatory molecules (e.g., CD40L-CD40 interaction). However, compared to other stimuli, CpG-2395

administration showed the highest survival rate and IL-10 production of B cells in combination with pentanoate treatment.

5. The biotinylated beads can be stored for up to 12 months at 4 °C.
6. During the cell count, dead cells should also be considered in the total cell number since they contribute to the amount of available antibody epitopes. We recommend to consider a higher cell number to increase the purity by an excess amount of antibodies.
7. During the washing process, accumulation of leftover tissue and fat can occur. These aggregates should be removed in order to avoid loss of antibodies and a consequent decrease in the level of purity.
8. After mixing beads and cell suspension, the beads become separated on the magnetic stand. Open the lid of the tubes before placing them in the stand. Avoid vibrations or movements of the stand to keep the beads fixed to the magnet. For an increase in isolated cells, another cycle of washing the beads in MACS buffer and magnetic separation can be performed.
9. Due to the magnetic separation of FITC-positive cells, the purity has to be determined using a different fluorochrome conjugate. A high number of FITC-positive cells hints toward an inefficient coupling with anti-FITC-biotin/streptavidin or biotinylated beads, whereas the detection of a FITC-negative population can be caused by insufficient administration of primary surface marker-FITC conjugate antibody. Repeating the purification protocol steps can further increase the purity.
10. Design the experiment including an unstained sample and cells for single stainings since these controls are needed to set the gating strategies or compensation.
11. B cells reach the peak of IL-10 production 72 h after pentanoate administration. At this time point, the cells can also be used for adoptive transfer to test their suppressive capacity in vivo.
12. Importantly, it has to be considered that many pharmacological compounds modulate essential factors involved in gene transcription or cellular metabolism, thereby interfering with regulatory processes within the cells and influencing both proliferation and survival. Cell survival can be determined by a viability assay that requires cell staining with compounds such as Annexin V and Zombie Aqua. Additionally, the impact on proliferation can be investigated by CFSE staining.
13. IL-10-producing B cells can also be analyzed using fluorescence microscopy which, unlike flow cytometry, allows the measurement of cell size and surface receptor expression.

14. If non-reporter mice are used for the experiments, the cells have to be re-stimulated with LPS, phorbol myristate acetate (PMA), and ionomycin in the presence of a protein transport inhibitor (e.g., monensin and BD *GolgiStop*) for 4 h at 37 °C and 5% CO_2 saturation.
15. For intracellular cytokine staining, after re-stimulation and optional surface staining, the cells should be fixed with fixation buffer for 20 min at RT prior to washing with permeabilization buffer (e. g. saponin buffer). Permeabilized cells can be further stained intracellularly with anti-IL-10 specific antibodies.
16. Phosphorylation of proteins is a sensitive modification which suffers from signal loss due to cellular phosphatase activity. Therefore, all the reagents should be prepared freshly and pre-tempered as described (PBS on ice, methanol at −20 °C). For kinetic experiments, schedule efficiently the processing of the samples at different time points and work fast.
17. The final concentration of methanol is 90%.
18. To synchronize the antibody staining, samples generated by experimental kinetics can be stored on ice at this step. Depending on the specific factor and cell type, the kinetics can be induced starting with the longest incubation time point and ending with the shortest induction periods which allows a synchronized fixation of all samples.

Acknowledgments

We would like to thank the Studienstiftung des deutschen Volkes and the Von Behring-Röntgen-Stiftung for funding Maik Luu. Alexander Visekruna is funded by the German Research Foundation (startup grant from DFG-KFO325).

References

1. Peng B, Ming Y, Yang C (2018) Regulatory B cells: the cutting edge of immune tolerance in kidney transplantation. Cell Death Dis 9 (2):109. https://doi.org/10.1038/s41419-017-0152-y
2. Evans JG, Chavez-Rueda KA, Eddaoudi A et al (2007) Novel suppressive function of transitional 2 B cells in experimental arthritis. J Immunol 178(12):7868–7878. https://doi.org/10.4049/jimmunol.178.12.7868
3. Yanaba K, Bouaziz J-D, Haas KM et al (2008) A regulatory B cell subset with a unique CD1dhiCD5+ phenotype controls T cell-dependent inflammatory responses. Immunity 28(5):639–650. https://doi.org/10.1016/j.immuni.2008.03.017
4. Yoshizaki A, Miyagaki T, DiLillo DJ et al (2012) Regulatory B cells control T-cell autoimmunity through IL-21-dependent cognate interactions. Nature 491(7423):264–268. https://doi.org/10.1038/nature11501
5. Bankó Z, Pozsgay J, Szili D et al (2017) Induction and Differentiation of IL-10-Producing Regulatory B Cells from Healthy Blood Donors and Rheumatoid Arthritis Patients. J Immunol 198(4):1512–1520. https://doi.org/10.4049/jimmunol.1600218

6. Mion F, Tonon S, Toffoletto B, Cesselli D, Pucillo CE, Vitale G (2014) IL-10 production by B cells is differentially regulated by immune-mediated and infectious stimuli and requires p38 activation. Mol Immunol 62 (2):266–276. https://doi.org/10.1016/j.molimm.2014.05.018
7. Suzuki-Yamazaki N, Yanobu-Takanashi R, Okamura T et al (2017) IL-10 production in murine IgM+ CD138hi cells is driven by Blimp-1 and downregulated in class-switched cells. Eur J Immunol 47(3):493–503. https://doi.org/10.1002/eji.201646549
8. Mishima Y, Oka A, Liu B et al (2019) Microbiota maintain colonic homeostasis by activating TLR2/MyD88/PI3K signaling in IL-10-producing regulatory B cells. J Clin Invest 130. https://doi.org/10.1172/JCI93820
9. Luu M, Visekruna A (2019) Short-chain fatty acids: Bacterial messengers modulating the immunometabolism of T cells. Eur J Immunol 49(6):842–848. https://doi.org/10.1002/eji.201848009
10. Luu M, Pautz S, Kohl V et al (2019) The short-chain fatty acid pentanoate suppresses autoimmunity by modulating the metabolic-epigenetic crosstalk in lymphocytes. Nat Commun 10(1):760. https://doi.org/10.1038/s41467-019-08711-2

Chapter 16

Methods to Study the Transcriptome of Regulatory B Cells

Maud Maho-Vaillant and Sebastien Calbo

Abstract

Regulatory B cells do not constitute a distinct cell lineage because no unique marker or set of markers can exclusively identify neither murine nor human regulatory B cells, and efficient IL-10 production is their only known distinguishing feature. After purification of IL-10-secreting B cells, one may want to characterize them by analyzing their gene expression profile. This goal can be achieved by using different technologies: RT-qPCR, microarrays, Nanostring's nCounter technology, Biomark HD are techniques that will allow you to analyze their gene expression, whether in a targeted (RT-qPCR), extended but targeted (Nanostring's nCounter technology, Biomark HD) or exhaustive (Microarray) way. Aim of this chapter is the description of these techniques in the view of their application to the study and characterization of regulatory B cells.

Key words B Cells, Gene expression profiling, RT-qPCR, Microarrays, mRNA

1 Introduction

The immune system comprises a network of cells, tissues, and organs that mediate host defense against pathogens. By using flow cytometry, immune cells can be readily classified into distinct types based on the differential expression of specific surface markers. However, not all immune cell types can be fully resolved by the sole analysis of phenotypic markers since many of these are expressed by multiple cell lineages or are differentially regulated under non-homeostatic conditions, such as during inflammation [1]. This concept is particularly true when it comes to regulatory B cells (Bregs). Bregs represent a small population of B cells that was shown to modulate the immune response against autoimmune and infectious diseases, and tumors [2]. Similarly to regulatory T cells, B cells employ a wide array of immunosuppressive mechanisms which include the production of IL-10, IL-35, and TGF-β, secondary antigen presentation, and interaction with other immune cells. If on one hand, the B-cell research community agrees on the existence of a B-cell population that exhibits immunomodulatory

Francesca Mion and Silvia Tonon (eds.), *Regulatory B Cells: Methods and Protocols*, Methods in Molecular Biology, vol. 2270, https://doi.org/10.1007/978-1-0716-1237-8_16,

functions, an accurate identification of these regulatory B cells is still challenging more than 20 years after their discovery. Indeed, the functional properties of regulatory B cells have been associated to several different phenotypes among which are transitional two marginal-zone precursor (T2-MZP) cells, CD1d^{hi}CD5^{+} B10 cells, marginal-zone (MZ) B cells, Tim-1^{+} B cells, CD138^{+} plasma cells, and plasmablasts [3]. Given the different results obtained from the study of B-cell surface marker expression, the researcher's intent of finding a specific Breg marker has moved to the analysis of the expressed mRNA, thanks to different techniques. Until recently, gene expression studies were performed on bulk populations of purified B cells in attempt to better understand their transcriptomes. During this process, new and unique population markers have been identified. Nonetheless, this type of analysis does not consider variability, especially if you want to distinguish the factors that govern a B cell to differentiate into pro- or anti-inflammatory B cell. Bulk approaches to the analysis of cells that exist in a continuum of differentiation and activation states lead to averaging of their distinct characteristics. Advances in transcriptome technologies have recently made possible to analyze B cells at the level of individual cells, whether you are targeting the analysis of specific genes or whether your analysis is exhaustive [1]. RNA-sequencing (RNA-seq) at the single cell level is now widely employed in immunological studies seeking to resolve cellular heterogeneity [4] and understanding the gene regulatory networks that predict immune function [5]. A targeted analysis can be considered if the involvement of a gene or of a set of genes in the differentiation of a sub-population needs to be tested. Moreover, other techniques that are easier to implement, quicker to master, and less expensive are available. In this chapter, we provide different methods useful to analyze mRNA expressed by B-cell subpopulations of interest, among which is Bregs. A comparison of different key aspects of qPCR, microarrays, Nanostring's nCounter technology, Biomark HD, and bulk RNA-seq techniques (not described in this chapter) is summarized in Table 1.

Table 1
Key cues of different transcriptomic technologies

	Methods				
	qPCR	**BioMark HD system**	**Microarray**	**Nanostring**	**RNA-seq**
RNA quantity	1 ng	10 ng	100 ng	50 ng	10 ng
RT amplification	Yes	Yes	Yes	No	Yes
Throughput	Low	High	High	High	Low
Labor intensity	High	Low	Low	Low	High

2 Materials

2.1 General Equipment

1. 2100 Bioanalyzer (Agilent Technologies).
2. Individual thin-walled 200 μL PCR tubes or 96-well plates for PCR.
3. Sealing films for 96-well plates.
4. RNAse-free 1.5 mL microcentrifuge tubes.

2.2 RNA Isolation

1. RNAse removal product (*see* **Note 1**).
2. RNA extraction kit specific for RNA isolation from a low number of cells (*see* **Note 2**).
3. RNase-free water (DEPC-treated H_2O).

2.3 cDNA Reverse Transcription

1. Kit for the synthesis of first-strand cDNA (*see* **Note 3**).
2. Random primers, oligo (dT) and deoxynucleotide (dNTP) solution mix (if not provided with the kit).
3. Tris-EDTA (TE) buffer: 10 mM Tris-HCl, 1 mM disodium EDTA, pH 8.0. Prepared with high-quality reagents and 0.2 μm filtered.

2.4 Gene Quantification by RT-qPCR

1. Ready-to-use qPCR kit containing DNA Polymerase, reaction buffer, dNTPs, SYBR Green dye (*see* **Note 4**).
2. 10 μM forward and reverse primers. A list of useful primers for the study of regulatory B cells is reported in Table 2.
3. Real-time PCR detection system.

2.5 Gene Quantification by BioMark HD System

1. BioMark HD System.
2. BioMark dynamic array nanofluidic chip (Fluidigm): 48.48 Dynamic Array™ IFC.
3. 20× GE Sample Loading Reagent (Fluidigm).
4. 2× Assay Loading Reagent (Fluidigm).
5. Low EDTA TE buffer: 10 mM Tris-HCl, 0.1 mM EDTA.
6. TaqMan Fast Universal PCR Master Mix, primer pairs and probes (*see* **Note 5**).

2.6 Gene Quantification by Nanostring nCounter

1. nCounter GX CodeSet (NanoString Technologies).
2. nCounter Master Kit (NanoString Technologies).

2.7 Gene Quantification by Microarrays

1. DNA Microarray Scanner GB and Feature Extraction Software 10.5.1.1 (Agilent Technologies).
2. 4 × 44 K Whole Human or Mouse Genome microarray kit (Agilent Technologies).

Table 2
List of primers for RT-qPCR

Human		Mouse	
IL-10	5′-TGCAAAACCAAACCACAAGA 5′-TCTCGGAGATCTCGAAGCAT	IL-10	5′-AGCCGGGAAGACAATAACTG 5′-CATTTCCGATAAGGCTTGG
CD27	5′-CAGAGAGGCACTACTGGGCT 5′-CGGTATGCAAGGATCACACTG	CD1d	5′-CTGTCTGCGGGCTGTGAAAT 5′-TCCCCAGAATCTCACGACATATT
CD38	5′-AGACTGCCAAAGTGTATGGGA 5′-GCAAGGTACGGTCTGAGTTCC	CD5	5′-CTCACCGTCATCTGCTCTGAT 5′-CTCCCGACATAGCTCTTCCC
CD24	5′-CTCCTACCCACGCAGATTTATTC 5′-AGAGTGAGACCACGAAGAGAC	CD138	5′-ACTTCACCTTTGAAACATCTGGG 5′-CATCCGGTACAGCATGAAAGC
β2microglobulin	5′-GAGGCTATCCAGCGTACTCCA 5′-CGGCAGGCATACTCATCTTTT	TIM-1	5′-AGCAGTCGGTACAACTTAAAGG 5′-ACTCGACAACAATACAGACCAC
HPRT1	5″-ACCAGTCAACAGGGGACATAA 5′-CTTCGTGGGGTCCTTTTCACC	LAG3	5′-CCTCGATGATTGCTAGTCCCT 5′-GTAGACAGGCACTCGGTTCTG
GAPDH	5′-ACAACTTTGGTATCGTGGAAGG 5′-GCCATCACGCCACAGTTTC	βactin	5′-TGGAATCCTGTGGCATCCATGAAAC 5-TAAAACGCAGCTCAGTAACAGTCC
		β2microglobulin	5′-TTCTGGTGCTTGTCTCACTGA 5′-CAGTATGTTCGGCTTCCCATTC
		HPRT	5′-TCAGTCAACGGGGGACATAAA 5′-GGGGCTGTACTGCTTAACCAG
		GAPDH	5′-AGGTCGGTGTGAACGGATTTG 5′-TGTAGACCATGTAGTTGAGGTCA

3. Gene Expression Microarrays Hybridization kit (Agilent Technologies).
4. Low Input QuickAmp Labeling Kit (Agilent Technologies).

3 Methods

The methods described here are kept general, with no reference to the cell type. However, these techniques can be performed either on murine or human purified B cells, isolated by different anatomical sites. When possible, tips related to the analysis of Bregs are provided.

3.1 RNA Isolation from B Cells and cDNA Synthesis

B cells with regulatory functions are usually rare, and, as a consequence, experiments aimed at characterizing this functional subset might consider the limitation of working with very small numbers of cells. We recommend using the PicoPure RNA isolation kit if you have less than 100 cells (*see* **Note 2 and 6**).

1. Prior to perform RNA extraction, it is safer to clean all pipettes and bench with RNAse removal product (*see* **Note 1**). Wear disposable gloves and change them frequently to prevent the introduction of RNAses from skin surfaces and use only plastic ware that is certified nucleic acid-free.
2. Collect from 100 to 100,000 B cells of interest in RNAse-free 1.5 mL microcentrifuge tubes and pellet through centrifugation at 400 × *g* for 5 min at room temperature (RT). Discard the supernatant.
3. Proceed to RNA isolation with the chosen kit, following manufacturer's instructions.
4. Quantify RNA using the 2100 Bioanalyzer which is able to detect up to a minimum of 50 pg of RNA (expect a yield of 20 pg of RNA per cell). Nucleic acid analysis is done on a chip and is based on the traditional gel electrophoresis assay. The chip format dramatically reduces separation time as well as sample and reagent consumption. The system provides automated sizing and quantification in a digital format. The Agilent 2100 Expert Software also provides the RNA Integrity Number (RIN) tool. Only RNA samples exhibiting an RNA Integrity Number $\geq$ 8.5 should be employed for downstream assays.
5. Reverse-transcribe RNA to cDNA using a high-performing cDNA synthesis kit (*see* **Note 3**). Proceed following manufacturer's instructions. Depending on the selected downstream analysis, reverse-transcribe the appropriate quantity of RNA (*see* Table 1).
6. The obtained cDNA can be store at −20 °C and used for downstream applications.

3.2 Fluorescence-Based Quantitative Real-Time PCR (qRT-PCR)

qRT-PCR is the gold standard for quantitatively determining concentrations of target mRNAs. Although well established and reliable, this method is low throughput, costly, and time-consuming. Furthermore, only a limited number of transcripts can be studied (*see* **Note 7**).

1. Prepare a different master mix for each primer pair (*see* Table 2) to be run. Prepare sufficient mix for the samples, standard curve reactions, and no-template controls (all in duplicate, plus calculate an extra 10% to allow for pipetting error). The cDNA to be used as template can be diluted 1:2 for low expressed genes and from 1:10 to 1:100 for medium to high expressed genes (*see* **Note 4** and **8**).
2. An example of reaction master mix for SYBR Green detection can be the following: for a 20-μL single reaction, add 1 μL forward primers, 1 μL reverse primers (*see* **Note 8**), 3 μL RNase-free water, 10 μL qPCR Master mix (2×) (*see* **Note 4**).
3. Add 5 μL of appropriate template serial dilution (standard curve), sample test cDNA or water to the defined tubes or wells.
4. Add 15 μL of master mix to each tube or well. Cap tubes or seal the PCR plate.
5. A typical cycling condition could be as follows: denaturation 95 °C, 30 sec plus (95 °C, 5 sec; 60 °C, 30 sec) × 40 cycles. Remember to determine the optimal annealing temperature of primers before performing RT-qPCR on your samples (*see* **Note 8**).
6. Analyze your data.

3.3 BioMark HD System

Recent technology has automated PCR reactions in nanoliter volumes in a single microfluidic device, consequently using less sample and reagents. The BioMark HD system is a technique that allows a large number of results to be obtained in a very short time. By using 48 × 48 Fluidigm Dynamic Arrays (48 samples and 48 different primers) (*see* **Note 5**), the BioMark HD System gives a total of 2304 reactions per plate which allows to test 48 genes per sample [6, 7]. The amount of cDNA needed for the BioMark HD System is about 40- to 50-fold less than for regular qPCR, and unlike qPCR, triplicates are not needed.

1. Depending on the quantity of starting material, dilute each cDNA sample in low EDTA TE buffer (*see* **Note 9**). Then, divide the diluted cDNA into 48 separate reactions that will be employed to perform qPCR using the BioMark 48.48 dynamic array nanofluidic chip.

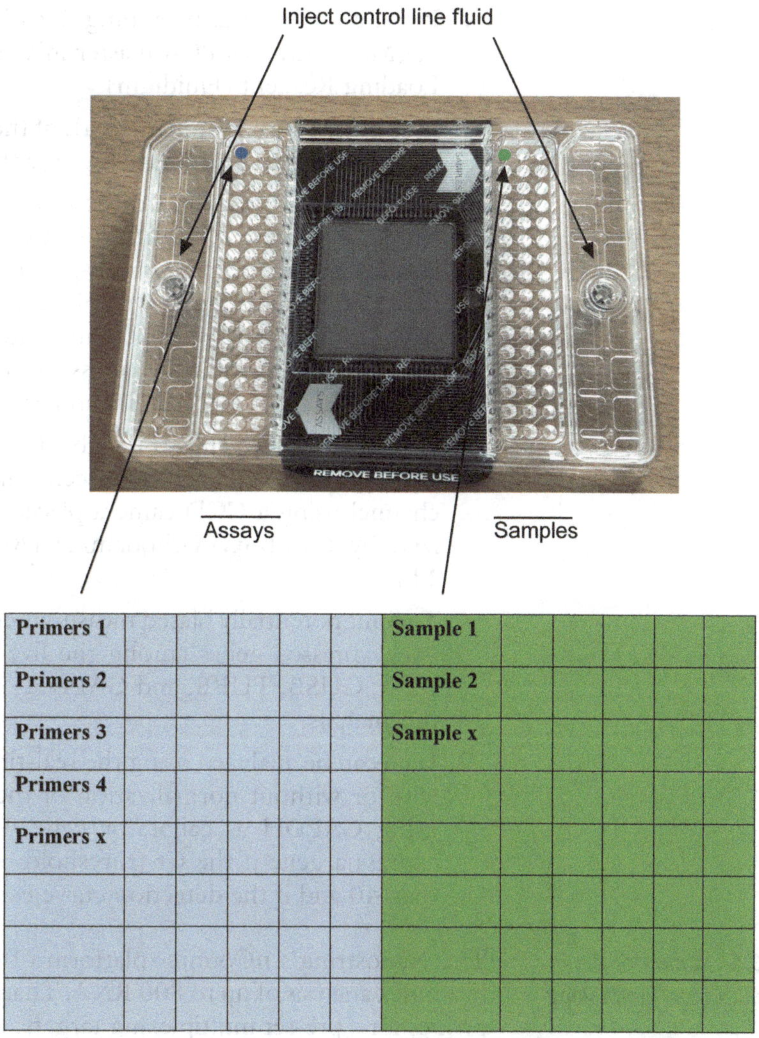

Fig. 1 Photo of 48 × 48 chip Biomark HD. Holes to inject control line fluid are shown by arrows. Assay solutions containing primers (assay) are loaded on the left side of the plate, while the samples mix on the right side. Prepare the scheme of assays and samples mix on a 96-well plate and note their position. Use the 96-well plate to load assays and samples mix on the chip. Position for primer 1 is shown by a blue dot and for sample 1 by a green dot

2. Perform hydraulic chip priming using the NanoFlex integrated fluidic circuit controller which pressurizes the control lines and closes the interface valves to prevent sample mixing.
3. Take a 96-well PCR plate and prepare the scheme of the 96-well plate that will be equivalent to the chip and note the future position of each sample (*see* Fig. 1, lower panel). A well containing the equivalent quantity of cDNA of one hundred cells and a well without any cell should be prepared as positive and negative controls, respectively.

4. Prepare sample mix by adding 2.7 μL of cDNA with 3 μL of TaqMan Universal PCR master mix and 0.3 μL of GE Sample Loading Reagent (Fluidigm).
5. Prepare the assay by mixing 3 μL of the Assay Loading Reagent (Fluidigm) with 3 μL of each primer pair.
6. Cover with a cover-film, vortex and centrifuge the 96-well PCR plate. By using an 8-channel pipette, transfer samples mix and assays (specific Taqman primer-probes for individual transcripts of interest) from the 96-well plates into the 48.48 nanofluidic chip. Transfer 6 μL of sample mix into wells on the right-hand side of the chip and 6 μL of assays into wells on the left-hand side of the chip (*see* **Note 10** and Fig.1).
7. Thermocycle the chip through 40 cycles using the BioMark HD System and detect fluorescence in the Fluorescein (FAM) channel using a CCD camera placed above the chip, normalized by 6-carboxy-X-rhodamine (ROX) intensity (*see* **Note 11**).
8. To limit potentially biased measurement, samples with less than two expressed genes among the five control genes (HPRT1, B2M, GUSB, TUBB, and GAPDH) should be excluded from the analysis.
9. Data can be analyzed using the real-time PCR analysis software with or without normalization of the Ct value for each gene using GAPDH as calibrator gene. We considered that cells express a gene if the Ct (threshold of detection) value is less than 40 and if the detection curve is a sigmoid.

3.4 Nanostring's nCounter Technology

The Nanostring's nCounter platform offers a simple solution for multiplex analysis of up to 800 RNA. Thanks to molecular barcodes probes for a pre-set multiplexing targets, the Nanostring's nCounter technology provides an easy to use, fully automated system. The Nanostring's nCounter system hybridizes two probes to each target transcript: a biotin-labeled capture probe and a fluorescent barcode-labeled reporter probe. Reporter probes hybridize with specific RNAs in a sample while capture probes lock them via avidin onto a static surface. The Nanostring's nCounter analysis system counts the immobilized RNAs using their barcodes. Like other hybridization-based systems, the Nanostring's nCounter platform is not for discovery.

1. Choose the nCounter immunology panel more suitable with the aim of the study. The nCounter immunology panel can perform multiplex gene expression analysis of more than 500 genes related to the immune response, and the user can choose between human and mouse systems.

2. Remove aliquots of both Reporter CodeSet and Capture ProbeSet reagents from the freezer and thaw on ice. Invert several times to mix well and spin down reagents. For each tube, prepare a mix with 10 μL of Reporter CodeSet reagent and 10 μL of hybridization buffer.
3. Add the RNA sample (maximum volume 5 μL) for a total of 100 ng to each tube. Complete by adding RNAse-free water to bring the final volume of each hybridization assay to 25 μL.
4. Add 5 μL of Capture ProbeSet reagent to each tube and incubate tubes for at least 12 h at 65 °C until ready for processing. Maximum hybridization time should not exceed 30 h.
5. Once removed from 65 °C, proceed immediately to post-hybridization processing with the nCounter Prep-station. Do not store hybridizations at 4 °C.
6. Since the system is automated, please follow the manufacturer's instruction.

3.5 Microarrays

Microarrays that detect nucleic acids in a sample by hybridization to probes on microchips are particularly useful for analyzing large mammalian transcriptomes. Microarrays measure the abundances of a defined set of transcripts via their hybridization to an array of complementary probes (*see* **Note 12**). Therefore, microarrays detect only known sequences, so they cannot be used for discovery. However, microarray technology allows the assay of thousands of transcripts simultaneously at a greatly reduced cost per gene and labor saving. Here we describe the method to perform one-colored gene expression profiling using 4 × 44 K Whole Human Genome from Agilent Technologies [8, 9].

1. In order to perform one-colored human gene expression profiling with microarray, 4 × 44 K Whole Human Genome from Agilent Technologies can be used. Collect 100 ng of RNA for each sample from different donors (3–5 different donors) and using the Low Input QuickAmp Labeling Kit, label them with Cyanine-3 according to the manufacturer's instructions.
2. Perform hybridization at 65 °C for 17 h using the hybridization kit.
3. After wash steps, microarrays must be scanned with a 5-μm pixel size using the DNA Microarray Scanner GB. Image analysis and extraction of raw data are performed with the Feature Extraction Software. Data can be normalized using 75 percentile shift and baseline transformed by median of all samples. Only spots that passed these quality controls on 100% of arrays in at least one of two conditions (e.g., condition can be positivity/negativity for a selection marker) can be selected for further analysis.

4 Notes

1. We usually employ RNase AWAY from ThermoFisher Scientific™.
2. The PicoPure RNA isolation Kit (Arcturus) and the RNeasy mini kit (Qiagen) are based on a spin column system and are very efficient to extract good-quality RNA out of few cells. Other kits may be of equivalent quality, but we have not tested them.
3. We routinely use SuperScript III reverse transcriptase (ThermoFisher Scientific™). The enzyme is supplied with a vial of 5× first-strand buffer and a vial of 100 mM DTT. Store at −20 °C. cDNA can be generated using random priming or oligo-dT method.
4. Use the appropriate SYBR Green qPCR ReadyMix compatible with your instrument. An interesting option when working with rare populations is the CellsDirect qRT-PCR kit (ThermoFisher Scientific™).
5. Primers are not provided with the chips. The user can choose between Taq Man probes which are designed and validated by ABI Applied Biosystems, or can design its own primers and probes. Although, Biomark HD system can also be used with regular primers using Sybr green technology, we routinely use and recommend TaqMan probes.
6. The technic employed by the PicoPure RNA isolation kit works well also with a larger number of cells (up to 100,000 cells), but, in this case, it is safer to remove genomic DNA by DNAse treatment.
7. Since the number of isolated Bregs is often very low, we suggest using the Cells Direct qRT-PCR kit which allows to perform real-time qPCR analysis directly from cells, without the need for an RNA purification step. In addition to the advantage of eliminating costly and time-consuming RNA purification procedures, it allows to test with less than 10,000 cells per reaction to as low as 1 cell.
8. cDNA dilution, forward and reverse primers concentration usage and temperature have to be optimized prior to run on samples.
9. The quantity of starting material depends of the number of cells you have purified and on the results obtained from the validation of your primers. Usually, it is diluted four times, but it could be less if you have low quantities of starting RNA and cannot amplify the gene.

10. The BioMark HD system is robust and reliable, but you have absolutely to avoid making bubbles when pipetting reagents on the microfluidic cartridge, otherwise reactions will not run properly. Air bubbles can be removed by gently tapping the side of the tips until the bubbles surface, by centrifuging the cartridge or by dislodging them with a clean pipette tip.
11. The Biomark HD system comes with excitation sources and emission filters for FAM, VIC, and ROX.
12. If the aim of the researcher is to qualitatively and quantitatively analyze any RNA type including mRNAs, microRNAs, small interfering RNAs, and long noncoding RNAs as well as RNA isoforms, then RNA-seq is a more suitable technique.

References

1. Chattopadhyay PK, Gierahn TM, Roederer M, Love JC (2014) Single-cell technologies for monitoring immune systems. Nat Immunol 15 (2):128–135. https://doi.org/10.1038/ni.2796
2. Rincon-Arevalo H, Sanchez-Parra CC, Castano D, Yassin L, Vasquez G (2016) Regulatory B cells and mechanisms. Int Rev Immunol 35(2):156–176. https://doi.org/10.3109/08830185.2015.1015719
3. Rosser EC, Mauri C (2015) Regulatory B cells: origin, phenotype, and function. Immunity 42 (4):607–612. https://doi.org/10.1016/j.immuni.2015.04.005
4. Zheng GX, Terry JM, Belgrader P, Ryvkin P, Bent ZW, Wilson R, Ziraldo SB, Wheeler TD, McDermott GP, Zhu J, Gregory MT, Shuga J, Montesclaros L, Underwood JG, Masquelier DA, Nishimura SY, Schnall-Levin M, Wyatt PW, Hindson CM, Bharadwaj R, Wong A, Ness KD, Beppu LW, Deeg HJ, McFarland C, Loeb KR, Valente WJ, Ericson NG, Stevens EA, Radich JP, Mikkelsen TS, Hindson BJ, Bielas JH (2017) Massively parallel digital transcriptional profiling of single cells. Nat Commun 8:14049. https://doi.org/10.1038/ncomms14049
5. Shalek AK, Satija R, Adiconis X, Gertner RS, Gaublomme JT, Raychowdhury R, Schwartz S, Yosef N, Malboeuf C, Lu D, Trombetta JJ, Gennert D, Gnirke A, Goren A, Hacohen N, Levin JZ, Park H, Regev A (2013) Single-cell transcriptomics reveals bimodality in expression and splicing in immune cells. Nature 498 (7453):236–240. https://doi.org/10.1038/nature12172
6. Berkani N, Joly P, Golinski ML, Colliou N, Lim A, Larbi A, Riou G, Caillot F, Bernard P, Bedane C, Delaporte E, Chaby G, Dompmartin A, Hertl M, Calbo S, Musette P (2019) B-cell depletion induces a shift in self antigen specific B-cell repertoire and cytokine pattern in patients with bullous pemphigoid. Sci Rep 9(1):3525. https://doi.org/10.1038/s41598-019-40203-7
7. Hebert V, Petit M, Maho-Vaillant M, Golinski ML, Riou G, Derambure C, Boyer O, Joly P, Calbo S (2019) Modifications of the Transcriptomic profile of autoreactive B cells from pemphigus patients after treatment with rituximab or a standard corticosteroid regimen. Front Immunol 10:1794. https://doi.org/10.3389/fimmu.2019.01794
8. Golinski ML, Demeules M, Derambure C, Riou G, Maho-Vaillant M, Boyer O, Joly P, Calbo S (2020) CD11c(+) B cells are mainly memory cells, precursors of antibody secreting cells in healthy donors. Front Immunol 11:32. https://doi.org/10.3389/fimmu.2020.00032
9. Lin W, Cerny D, Chua E, Duan K, Yi JT, Shadan NB, Lum J, Maho-Vaillant M, Zolezzi F, Wong SC, Larbi A, Fink K, Musette P, Poidinger M, Calbo S (2014) Human regulatory B cells combine phenotypic and genetic hallmarks with a distinct differentiation fate. J Immunol 193 (5):2258–2266. https://doi.org/10.4049/jimmunol.1303214

Chapter 17

Purification of Murine IL-10$^+$ B Cells for Analyses of Biological Functions and Transcriptomics

Jianbo Sun and Uttiya Basu

Abstract

B10 cells are the most frequently investigated subset of Breg cells, capable of suppressing immunity through the expression of the immunosuppressive cytokine IL-10. B10 cells are enriched in phenotypically diverse B-cell subsets. Recently, CD9 was identified as a marker of B10 cells in mice (human B10 cells have a separate set of markers that do not overlap with murine B10 cells). Together with a combination of other B10 markers, CD9 can be used to distinguish both mature and immature B10 cells from nonregulatory B cells and support selective purification of B10 cells. Here we provide five methods for the characterization and activity evaluation of CD9$^+$ B cells. The first method is used for the preparation of leukocytes, the second and third are used for the characterization of CD9$^+$ B cells, while the last two methods serve to evaluate CD9$^+$ B-cell activities. Finally, we detail the purification of RNA from B10 cells and the performance of transcriptomic assays.

Key words Regulatory B cells, B10 cell, CD9, IL-10, Transcriptome

1 Introduction

B cells play important roles in both promoting and suppressing immune responses [1]. B cells are capable of antigen presentation, antibody production, proinflammatory cytokine production, and acting as co-stimulators for immune promotion. Moreover, B cells can produce immune-suppressive cytokines such as IL-10, IL-35, and TGF-b1, induce regulatory T cells (Treg), and eliminate autoantigens for immune suppression [2]. Regulatory B cells (Breg) are B cells with immune suppressive functions. Bregs have been shown to be involved in various autoimmune- and inflammation-induced diseases [3], including systemic lupus erythematosus [4] and allergies [5], both in patients and in mouse models.

Bregs are found to be enriched in phenotypically diverse B-cell subsets [6]. Mice and humans possess distinct sets of Breg markers, and there is a scarcity of unique markers in either organism that can exclusively and exhaustively identify Breg cells. B10 cells constitute

Francesca Mion and Silvia Tonon (eds.), *Regulatory B Cells: Methods and Protocols*, Methods in Molecular Biology, vol. 2270, https://doi.org/10.1007/978-1-0716-1237-8_17,

one of the most studied Breg subsets, capable of secreting IL-10 and thereby of suppressing immunity. In a search of unique markers that could allow B10 purification and biochemical characterization—important since the lack of unique surface markers has foiled detailed investigations into the origin, development, and immunological roles of B10 cells—B10 cell surface markers have been updated regularly from the original $CD19^{+}CD1d^{hi}CD5^{+}$ phenotype [3, 7]. The identification of B10 cells requires stimulation with specific reagents such as LPS plus PMA, ionomycin, and monensin for cytokine secretion, with this stimulation possibly masking the real differences between B10 cells and other kinds of B cells, especially in terms of expression profiles.

We and others have identified CD9, a tetraspanin family transmembrane protein, as a marker of B10 cells in mice [6]. CD9 can distinguish both mature and immature B10 cells from nonregulatory B cells. Thus, it provides a system to study unperturbed gene expression profiles of Breg progenitors and Bregs without the stimulation required in the past to prompt the IL-10 secretion necessary for Breg identification. With the designation of CD9 as a marker of B10 cells, the identification of physiologically relevant transcription factors driving B10 differentiation becomes a real possibility. Furthermore, as $CD9^{+}$ B cells possess immune suppressive function(s) and can be enriched easily, another application is their adoptive transfer into murine autoimmune disease models to study their immunoregulatory function in vivo. The elimination of immunosuppressive IL-10-expressing plasma cells could allow cytotoxic T-cell-dependent eradication of therapy-resistant tumors [8]. In this light, the possibility that $CD9^{+}$ B-cell depletion could be an effective alternative to specific depletion of B10 cells for tumor immunotherapy should be investigated. Finally, transcriptomics of B10 cells can be performed on B10 cells that have been purified based on their positive expression of CD9. In this chapter we provide five methods for the characterization and functional evaluation of $CD9^{+}$ B cells.

2 Materials

2.1 Equipment

1. 5 mL (12 × 75 mm) and 14 mL (17 × 100 mm) polystyrene round-bottom tubes with snap caps.
2. 50 mL (33 × 115 mm) conical centrifuge tubes.
3. 35 mm dish or 6-well plate.
4. Cell culture plates: sterile 6-well, 24-well, or 48-well flat-bottom culture plates.
5. Pipettes, sterile pipette tips and disposable transfer pipettes.

6. Scissors, sterile cell strainers (40 μm) and sterile 1–10 mL syringes.
7. Device for immunomagnetic isolation of the cell type of interest (e.g., columns, magnets, and stand).
8. Refrigerated centrifuge with swinging-bucket rotor suitable for 5 mL, 14 mL, and 50 mL tubes.
9. BSL-2 cabinet/hood for cell culture, and cell culture supplies.
10. Vortexer.
11. CO_2 incubator, 37 °C, 5% CO_2.
12. Flow cytometer and sorter with multiparameter cytometry capability.
13. Bioanalyzer (Agilent Technologies).
14. Wet ice, to keep cells and reagents at 4 °C.

2.2 Mice

1. Female or male C57BL/6 J mice.
2. Female or male, 6–8 weeks old CD19 KO mice.

2.3 Cell Preparation, Culture, and Stimulation

1. Commercially available sterile Dulbecco's phosphate-buffered saline (D-PBS) without Ca^{2+} and Mg^{2+}. Store at 4 °C or on ice.
2. Ammonium-Chloride-Potassium (ACK) lysing buffer for the lysis of red blood cells.
3. MACS buffer: 0.5% bovine serum albumin (BSA) and 2 mM EDTA in D-PBS. Sterilize by filtration and keep sterile. Store at 4 °C or on ice.
4. Lymphocytes culture medium (LCM): 10% fetal bovine serum (FBS), 100 IU/mL penicillin, 100 μg/mL streptomycin, 2 mM L-Glutamine, 2 mM sodium pyruvate, 2 mM MEM NEAA, 4 mM HEPES buffer, and 55 μM 2-mercaptoethanol in sterile RPMI 1640.
5. Staining buffer: 2% FBS in D-PBS. Store at 4 °C.
6. Mouse CD19 beads for immunomagnetic isolation of B cells.
7. Purified anti-mouse CD40 antibody (Clone HM40–3).
8. Lipopolysaccharides (LPS) from *Escherichia coli* O111:B4: dissolve at 5 mg/mL in sterile D-PBS. Sterilize with a 0.2-μm pore size filter and store in 200 μL aliquots at −20 °C. The thawed aliquots should be kept at 4 °C.
9. Phorbol 12-myristate 13-acetate (PMA): dissolve at 100 ng/μ L in dimethyl sulfoxide (DMSO) and store in 20 μL aliquots at −20 °C.
10. Ionomycin: dissolve at 1 μg/μL in DMSO and store in 20 μL aliquots at −20 °C.

Table 1
List of antibodies

Staining	Target	Clone	Fluorophore
B cells	CD19	6D5	APC
	CD9	MZ3	FITC
	IL-10	JES5-16E3	PE
T cells	CD4	GK1.5	PE/Cy7
	CD25	PC61	FITC
	Rat IgG2b	RTK4530	PE

11. Monensin: the final working concentration is 2 μM. Store at 4 °C.
12. Dye for the discrimination of viable from nonviable cells in multicolor flow cytometric applications (e.g., LIVE/DEAD™ Fixable Near IR Dead Cell Stain Kit, LIVE/DEAD™ Fixable Blue Dead Cell Stain Kit, for UV excitation from Thermo Fisher). Reconstitute the dye according to the manufacturer's instructions.
13. Violet fluorescent cell proliferation dye such as VPD450 (Becton Dickinson) or eFluor 450 (Thermo Fisher).

2.4 Cell Immunofluorescence Staining, Sorting, and Enrichment

1. Purified anti-mouse CD16/CD32 (Clone 2.4G2) mAb.
2. Fluorochrome-conjugated antibodies (*see* Table 1). All antibodies should be tittered to identify optimal concentration starting from specific manufacturer's indications.
3. Cell fixation/permeabilization solution and permeabilization buffer.
4. 1.5% formaldehyde fixing solution: dilute 36% formalin 24-fold in D-PBS, and store at room temperature for up to 1 month.
5. Mouse IL-10 secretion assay (Miltenyi Biotec).
6. Mouse CD90.2 beads.
7. FITC-microbeads.
8. DNase I: diluted at the final concentration of 20 mg/mL in buffer containing 20 mM Tris-HCl, 1 mM $MgCl_2$, 50% (w/v) glycerol, pH 7.5. Store this solution at −15 to −25 °C for up to 18 months.

2.5 RNA Profiling of B10 Cells

1. Guanidine thiocyanate and phenol reagent for phenol–chloroform-based RNA extraction (e.g., Trizol by Thermo Fisher, Tri-Reagent by Sigma).
2. rRNA removal kit.
3. Illumina TruSeq and TruSeq Stranded.
4. Ingenuity Pathway Analysis (IPA) software program (Qiagen).

2.6 Ex Vivo Function of CD9+ B Cells

1. Transwell for 96-well plates, with a 0.4-μm membrane pore size.
2. 96-well, cell culture-treated, U-shaped-bottom microplate.
3. Purified anti-mouse CD28 (Clone 37.51) antibody.
4. Purified anti-mouse CD3e (Clone 145-2C11) antibody.
5. Purified anti-mouse CD9 (Clone MZ3) antibody and its isotype control. Customized without sodium azide.

2.7 Reconstitution of B-Cell-Deficient Mice and Contact Hypersensitivity (CHS) Assay

1. 4-Ethoxymethylene-2-phenyl-2-oxazolin-5-one (oxazolone): reconstitute the powder at 100 mg/mL in acetone/olive oil (4:1 v/v).
2. Oxazolone solution: 10 mg/mL oxazolone in acetone/olive oil (4:1 v/v).
3. A constant force, calibrated digital thickness gauge.
4. Isoflurane and anesthesia ventilators (*see* **Note 1**).
5. 0.5% proparacaine hydrochloride ophthalmic solution (*see* **Note 1**).

3 Methods

3.1 B-Cell Preparation and Culture

For cell culture or further application in vivo, all media, solutions, tips, and tubes should be sterile, and all operations should be performed in a biosafety cabinet (tissue culture hood).

3.1.1 Isolation of B Cells from the Spleen

1. Collect the spleens from C57BL/6 J mice and homogenize with the plunger of a 10-mL syringe on a 40-μm cell strainer in a 35-mm dish or 6-well plate containing 3 mL ice-cold D-PBS (*see* **Note 2**).
2. Transfer the homogenized solution to a 14-mL round-bottom tube and wash the 35-mm dish or 6-well plate with 2-mL D-PBS. Combine the suspensions and pipet several times for further disassociation of cells from the tissue, then spin at 500 × *g* for 8 min at 4 °C.
3. Discard the supernatant and resuspend the cell pellet in 5 mL of ACK lysing buffer by gentle brief vortex, and keep at room temperature (RT) for 5 min with occasional shaking, then spin at 300 × *g* for 5 min at 4 °C (*see* **Note 3**).
4. Discard the supernatant, resuspend the pellet in 5 mL of MACS buffer and then spin at 300 × *g* for 5 min to remove residual ACK lysis buffer. The obtained pellet consists of spleen mononuclear cells that can be either stained with fluorescence antibodies for analysis or cell sorting (*see* Subheading 3.4) or used to purify CD19+ B cells (**step 5**).

5. Purify CD19$^+$ cells by immunomagnetic isolation. Use magnetic microbeads following the instructions outlined in the kit.

3.1.2 Isolation of Peritoneal B Cells

1. Isolate leukocytes from the peritoneal cavity by injecting 10 mL of ice-cold MACS buffer with a syringe into the peritoneal cavity, followed by careful aspiration of the fluid back into the syringe after a gentle palpitation of the abdomen. Use the appropriate number of mice which allows to obtain a leukocyte population sufficient to meet the needs of downstream analyses.
2. Wash collected cells once with MACS buffer and then proceed to perform the CD19$^+$ B-cell isolation, employing the same protocol used in **Step 5** of Subheading 3.1.1.

3.1.3 B-Cell Stimulation for B10 and B10pro Cell Analysis

The primary B cells enriched from splenocytes contain both B10 cells and B10pro cells which are capable of differentiating into B10 cells after culture with the anti-CD40 antibody for 48 h. For intracellular staining of IL-10, cells should be cultured for 5 h with 10 mg/mL LPS, 50 ng/mL PMA, 500 ng/mL ionomycin, and 2 mM monensin (LPI + M), which increase the accumulation of IL-10 by blocking the IL-10 transport process. For the cell sorting of alive IL-10$^+$ B cells, cells should be stimulated with LPI rather than LPI + M for 4 h: taking advantage of the IL-10 secretion assay developed by Miltenyi Biotec, secreted IL-10 is captured by the catch reagent on the cell surface and cells can be stained for the cytokine without the need of permeabilization.

1. To induce B10pro cell differentiation into B10 cells, culture single-cell CD19$^+$ B cells at 2×10^6 cells/mL in LCM containing 1 μg/mL purified anti-mouse CD40 antibody for 48 h at 37 °C in a tissue culture incubator with a 5% CO_2 atmosphere.
2. For B10 cell analysis, culture single-cell primary CD19$^+$ B cells at 2×10^6 cells/mL in LCM containing LPI + M at 37 °C in a tissue culture incubator with a 5% CO_2 atmosphere for 5 h to induce IL-10 production (*see* **Note 4**).
3. For B10 and B10pro cell analysis, culture single-cell CD19$^+$ B cells at 2×10^6 cells/mL in LCM containing 1 μg/mL purified anti-mouse CD40 antibody for 48 h plus LPI + M for the terminal 5 h at 37 °C in a tissue culture incubator with a 5% CO_2 atmosphere.

3.1.4 Differentiation of B10 cells from CD9$^+$ B Cells

1. Stain the purified B cells obtained from Subheadings 3.1.1 and 3.1.2 with anti-CD19 and -CD9 antibodies, following the method of cell surface staining outlined in Subheading 3.2, **steps 1–5**). Resuspend the cells in D-PBS at 0.5–1 $\times 10^7$ cells/mL and proceed to fluorescence-activated cell sorting (FACS) of viable CD19$^+$CD9$^+$ and CD19$^+$CD9$^-$ cells (*see* **Note 5**).

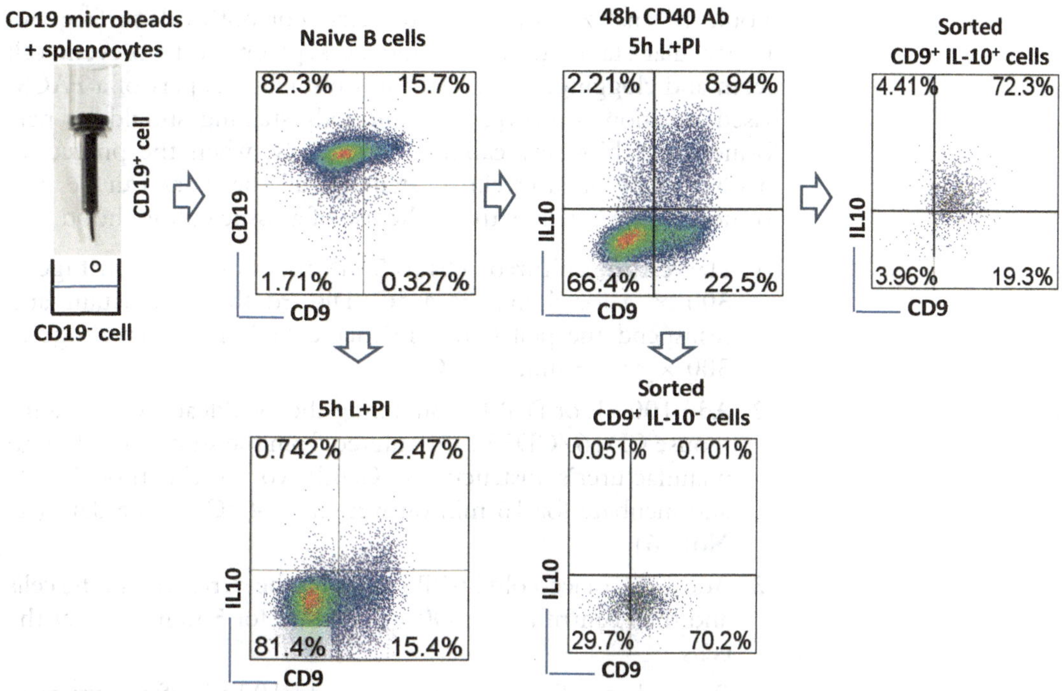

Fig. 1 Cell sorting. Splenocytes are incubated with CD19 microbeads and then naïve $CD19^+$ B cells are enriched through immunomagnetic separation. The frequency of $CD19^+CD9^+$ B cells is shown in the plot. Dot plots also show the expression of CD9 and IL-10 in $CD19^+$ B cells which are treated either with LPI for 5 h or with an anti-CD40 antibody for 48 h plus LPI for the last 5 h, after staining with an IL-10 secretion assay kit as described in Subheading 3.1.4. The purity of $CD9^+IL\text{-}10^+$ and $CD9^+IL\text{-}10^-$ B cells sorted from the cells cultured for 48 h is shown. After sorting, the fluorescence of the sorted cells demonstrates obvious attenuation

2. Culture purified B cells at 2×10^6 cells/mL in 6-well plates with LCM containing LPI for 4 h to induce IL-10 secretion. Stain responding cells, in terms of IL-10 secretion, using the IL-10 secretion assay kit following manufacturer's instructions and then stain the cells with CD19 and CD9 antibodies as previously described. Isolate viable $CD9^-IL10^-$, $CD9^+IL10^-$, and $CD9^+IL10^+$ B cells through FACS (*see* Fig.1 and **Note 5**).
3. Culture the sorted $CD9^+$, $CD9^-$, $CD9^-IL10^-$, $CD9^+IL10^-$, and $CD9^+IL10^+$ B cells in 96-well plates with LCM containing 1 μg/mL purified anti-mouse CD40 antibody for 48 h at 37 °C plus LPI + M for the terminal 5 h.
4. At the end of the stimulation step, collect the cells for flow cytometry analysis of $CD9^+$ Breg cells (*see* Subheading 3.2).

3.2 Flow Cytometry Analysis of $CD9^+$ Breg Cells

The protocol outlined below allows the user to follow the expression of IL-10, CD9, and other reported Breg markers on B cells stimulated with either LPI + M for 5 h or with anti-CD40 antibody for 48 h plus LPI + M for the terminal 5 h. After staining, B cells should be analyzed by flow cytometry. For both cell surface and intracellular staining, cells should be kept on ice to prevent cell death and clogging. When cell surface staining is part of a FACS-based isolation protocol, then antibody staining should be performed in a biosafety cabinet. Conversely, when the procedure involves steps of intracellular staining, all the work can be performed on the bench without the use of a tissue culture hood.

1. Harvest the cultured cells to 5 mL tubes on ice, centrifuge at 300 × *g* for 5 min at 4 °C. Discard the supernatant and resuspend the pellet in 1 mL ice-cold D-PBS, centrifuge at 300 × *g* for 5 min at 4 °C.
2. Add 100 μL of D-PBS containing the live/dead dye and anti-mouse CD16/CD32 mAb diluted from the stock according to manufacturer's instructions. Gently vortex the tube briefly and incubate for 15 min on wet ice (~ 4 °C) in the dark (*see* **Note 6**).
3. Add 1 mL of ice-cold D-PBS to each tube to resuspend the cells and then centrifuge at 300 × *g* at 4 °C for 5 min to pellet the cells.
4. Proceed to cell surface staining. Add 100 μL of a mixture of anti-CD19 and anti-CD9 antibodies (*see* Table 1) diluted in staining buffer according to manufacturer's instructions. A titration of antibody can be performed. Vortex briefly and then incubate for 20–30 min on wet ice in the dark (*see* **Notes 6** and **7**).
5. Add 1 mL of ice-cold D-PBS, centrifuge at 300 × *g* at 4 °C for 5 min to pellet the cells and discard the supernatant. Repeat once.
6. Thoroughly resuspend the cell pellet in fixation/permeabilization solution following manufacturer's instructions. Incubate on wet ice in the dark for 20 min.
7. Add 1 mL of perm/wash buffer and centrifuge at 500 × *g* at 4 °C for 5 min. Discard the supernatant. Repeat once.
8. Thoroughly resuspend the permeabilized cells in 100 μL of ice-cold perm/wash buffer containing the PE anti-mouse IL-10 antibody, diluted according to manufacturer's instructions. A titration of antibody can be performed. Incubate the cell mixture on wet ice for 30 min in the dark.
9. Wash the cells twice with ice-cold perm/wash buffer and resuspend the cell pellet in 250 μL of ice-cold 1.5% formaldehyde fixative. Mix the samples thoroughly by vortexing.
10. Keep the cells on ice or refrigerated at 4 °C before analyzing the stained cells by flow cytometry (*see* Fig. 1).

3.3 RNA Profiling of CD9⁺ B10 cells for the Analysis of the Transcriptome

3.3.1 Induction and Isolation of CD9⁺IL-10⁺ B Cells

1. Induce B10pro cell differentiation as in **step 1** of Subheading 3.1.3. During the last 4 h of B-cell stimulation through the anti-CD40 mAb, add LPI to induce IL-10 secretion.
2. Stain and isolate the CD40-responding cells based on their secretion of IL-10 using the IL-10 secretion assay kit and following manufacturer's instructions, as described previously [9]. Briefly, collect and wash the cells, incubate the cells with the IL-10 catch reagent, and culture the cells with LCM containing LPI for one additional hour to let the reagent on the cells catch the secreted IL-10. Stain the cells with the IL-10 detection antibody provided by the kit.
3. Collect the B cells and stain for dead cells and for the CD9 surface marker (*see* Subheading 3.2).
4. Isolate viable CD9⁺IL10⁻ and CD9⁺IL10⁺ B cells through FACS. Collect cells in LCM (*see* **Note 5**).

3.3.2 RNA Preparation

1. Transfer the FACS-sorted CD9⁺IL10⁻ and CD9⁺IL10⁺ populations to 50 mL tubes and add an equal volume of D-PBS. Centrifuge the cells at 500 × *g* at 4 °C for 10 min.
2. Discard the supernatant and resuspend the cell pellet in 1 mL of a guanidine thiocyanate and phenol reagent, such as Trizol™. Total RNA is prepared following manufacturer's instructions. Resuspend the RNA in 30 μL of the indicated buffer.
3. Deplete the rRNA via a rRNA removal kit, following manufacturer's instructions. Quantify the RNA amount by a device such as a Bioanalyzer (*see* **Note 8**).
4. Send the rRNA-depleted total RNA to an internal or external facility for RNA sequencing.

3.3.3 RNA Profiling

1. Libraries are prepared with Illumina TruSeq and TruSeq Stranded total RNA sample prep kits, and then sequenced with 50–60 million of 2 × 100 bp paired raw passing filter reads on an Illumina HiSeq 2000 V3 instrument.
2. All reads of total RNAs are first mapped to the mouse reference genome (mm9) with TopHat (v. 1.3.2). Cufflinks (v. 1.2.1) is subsequently applied to assemble the whole transcriptome and to identify all possible transcripts.
3. To obtain short RNAs, set the overlap radius as 1 and merge repeated samples. All resulting transcripts can be further annotated using a comprehensive collection of RNA databases including mRNA, snoRNA, long intergenic noncoding RNA (lincRNA), microRNA, and other annotated noncoding RNAs.
4. Once the transcriptome has been generated, the individual transcripts can be annotated. Specifically, all assembled

transcripts can be overlapped with known RNAs in the collected database (information for source of coordinates of various RNAs can be accessed from [6]), and the transcripts can be annotated by their adjacent known RNAs. Biological replicates indicate that each RNA-seq data set should be generated from B cells isolated from separate mice.

5. The generated list of differentially expressed factors can be analyzed through the "Core Analysis" option in the IPA software program [10]. Rank change (RC) and fold change (FC) levels of various noncoding RNAs, including long noncoding RNA (lnRNA), as well as mRNAs compared between $B10^+$ and $B10^-$ cells can be analyzed.

3.4 Ex Vivo Activity of $CD9^+$ B Cells

The protocol outlined here below allows the evaluation of the immune suppressive activity of $CD9^+$ B cells through a T-cell proliferation assay. $CD4^+CD25^-$ T cells are sorted from the $CD19^-$ non-B cell fraction, stained with a violet fluorescent cell proliferation dye such as VPD450, and then seeded in 96-well round-bottom plates coated with the anti-CD3e antibody at an appropriate density. $CD9^+$ and $CD9^-$ B cells are sorted from the $CD19^+$ B-cell fraction and then cocultured with VPD450-stained $CD4^+CD25^-$ T cells. The coculture is treated with or without 10 μg/mL of anti-CD9 blocking antibody or of its isotype control to check whether CD9 is involved in the suppressive activity of $CD9^+$ B cells.

3.4.1 T-Cell Proliferation Assay

1. Pretreat each well of a 96-well round-bottom plate with 100 μL of 5 μg/mL anti-CD3e antibody and then incubate overnight at 4 °C. Wash twice with 200 μL D-PBS per well before seeding cells for the T/B-cell coculture.
2. Isolate splenocytes and collect both the $CD19^+$ B-cell and $CD19^-$ non-B-cell fractions using CD19 microbeads, following the instruction of the kit.
3. Prepare the T-cell fraction for the T/B-cell coculture. Stain unstimulated $CD19^-$ cells with anti-CD4 and anti-CD25 antibodies (*see* Table 1) for 30 min at 4 °C and then purify $CD4^+CD25^-$ T cells through FACS. Finally, stain $CD4^+CD25^-$ T cells with VPD450 following manufacturer's instructions.
4. Prepare the $CD19^+CD9^-$ and $CD19^+CD9^+$ B-cell fractions for the T/B-cell coculture. Subsets are sorted from $CD19^+$ cells which were first stimulated for 48 h with anti-CD40 antibody and LPS for the last 5 h to prime the suppressive activity (*see* **Note 9**), and then stained with the anti-CD19 and anti-CD9 antibodies.

5. Seed both T and B cells on the 96-well round-bottom plate pretreated with the anti-CD3e antibody. Coculture 1–2 × 10^5 VPD450-stained CD4$^+$CD25$^-$ T cells with different numbers of autologous CD19$^+$CD9$^+$ B cells or CD19$^+$CD9$^-$ B cells, in the presence or absence of 10 μg/mL anti-CD9 blocking antibody or of its isotype control. Incubate the coculture for 72 h, but change the medium after 48 h to avoid nutrients exhaustion. If one of the final outcomes of the T/B-cell coculture is the detection of B10 cells by flow cytometry, then cells should be stimulated with PMA, ionomycin, and monensin for the terminal 5 h of culture.
6. At the end of the incubation, the cocultured cells should be collected, washed once with PBS, and then stained with the anti-CD9, -CD4, and -CD19 antibodies to check the final frequencies of the T-cell, B-cell, and B10-cell subsets by flow cytometry (*see* **Note 10**).
7. Finally, analyze the changes in T-cell proliferation by following the dilution of the VPD450 dye by flow cytometry.

3.4.2 Evaluation of Cell Contact Contribution on the T-Cell Proliferation Assay

A transwell system can be used to check whether cell–cell contact between T cells and B cells is important for the suppressive function of CD9$^+$ B cells on T cells.

1. Pretreat each well of specific plates with transwell with 5 μg/mL anti-CD3e and anti-CD28 antibody in a final volume of 200 μL (*see* **Note 11**). Incubate the plate overnight at 4 °C.
2. The day after, wash each well twice with 200 μL D-PBS before seeding cells (*see* **Note 12**).
3. Seed 1 × 10^5 VPD450-stained CD4$^+$CD25$^-$ T cells in each well of both the receiver plate and the insert. The insert well is also loaded with different numbers of autologous CD19$^+$CD9$^+$ B cells or CD19$^+$CD9$^-$ B cells.
4. Culture the cells for 72 h and then analyze T-cell proliferation by following the dilution of the VPD450 dye by flow cytometry.

3.5 In Vivo Activity of CD9$^+$ B Cells

The protocol outlined in this section allows the evaluation of the in vivo immune suppressive activity of CD9$^+$ B cells through the CHS assay. As FACS sorting takes a long time to obtain the desirable cell number and is not good for cell viability, we developed a method for immunomagnetic cell enrichment of CD9$^+$ B cells. CD9$^+$ and CD9$^-$ B cells are enriched with FITC-microbeads from CD90.2$^-$ cells (which themselves are enriched with CD90.2-microbeads) and then stained with anti-CD9 antibody conjugated to FITC. CD19 KO mice reconstituted with either CD9$^+$ or CD9$^-$ B cells are first immunized with oxazolone in acetone/olive oil by application on the animal's abdominal skin and subsequently challenged with oxazolone in acetone/olive oil by application to the animal's ears. CHS is mediated by T cells and is reflected by the thickness of the swelling of the ears. Therefore, the suppressive activity of $CD9^+$ B cells on T-cell-mediated immune response can be monitored through the ear thickness.

1. Enrich B cells from mouse splenocytes or peritoneal cavity cells by negative selection using CD90.2 microbeads and following the instructions of the kit. Culture the obtained $CD90.2^-$ cells with the anti-CD40 antibody for 48 h and LPS for the terminal 5 h (*see* **Note 9** and **12**).
2. Collect the cultured cells, wash and stain with the anti-CD9-FITC antibody as outlined in **steps 1–5** in Subheading 3.2. $CD9^+$ B cells are enriched using FITC-microbeads and following the instructions of the manufacturer. $CD9^-$ B cells represent the flow through fraction and are re-purified over the column to remove residual $CD9^+$ B cells, while $CD9^+$ cells are eluted from the column as a final step. Wash cells twice with D-PBS and finally resuspend both fractions in D-PBS at the final concentration of 2×10^7 B cells/mL (*see* **Note 13**).
3. Reconstitute CD19 KO mice by injecting intravenously 0.1 mL of 2×10^7 B cells/mL ($CD9^+$ B cells or $CD9^-$ B cells) prepared as in **step 2**. Use a 29-G needle for the injection. As a control, inject 0.1 mL/mouse of D-PBS. For each condition, prepare groups of five CD19 KO mice of the same age and sex (*see* **Note 14**).
4. Two days later, induce skin inflammation in mice. Shave the hind flank hair of the mice with an electric or manual shaver. Mice are painted with a pipette and sensitized by a uniform topical application of 25 μL of 100 mg/mL oxazolone in acetone/olive oil (4:1 v/v) for two consecutive days.
5. On day 5, challenge sensitized mice by application of 10 μL of a 10 mg/mL oxazolone solution to the right ear (5 μL on the dorsal side and 5 μL on the ventral side). As a control, an identical amount of acetone/olive oil (4:1) is administered to the left ear.
6. Using a constant force, calibrated digital thickness gauge, perform three measurements of the thickness of the central portion of each ear lobe before challenge and 24, 48, 72, and 96 h after challenge (*see* **Note 15**).
7. Ear thickness is an indicator of T-cell-mediated immune response (i.e., smaller ear thickness shows greater immune suppressive activity). Therefore, by comparing ear thickness in CD19 KO mice reconstituted with either $CD9^+$ or $CD9^-$ cells, it is possible to evaluate $CD9^+$ B-cells suppressive activity.

4 Notes

1. These reagents will be required if the operator opts for a retro-orbital injection, rather than an intravenous injection, for the reconstitution of B-cell-deficient mice.
2. The spleen should be mashed on the cell strainer without cutting it into smaller sections or digesting it with enzymes. Most of the cells prepared in this way are alive and grow well.
3. Vortex speed should be limited to the lowest rate at which the suspension can rise on the wall of the tube. A higher-than-necessary vortex rate may damage the cells.
4. When analyzing B10 cells obtained from the in vitro differentiation of B10pro cells, the LPI + M stimulus should be added during the last 5 h of the 48 h B-cell stimulation with anti-CD40 antibody.
5. From one spleen of an adult mouse, it should be possible to obtain 20–25 million CD19^{+} B cells using CD19 microbeads. After FACS, the number of obtained CD9^{+}IL10^{+} B cells, CD9^{+}IL10^{-} B cells, and CD9^{-}IL10^{-} B cells will be approximately 0.2%, 0.4%, and 0.4–50%, respectively, of the total sorted B cells. The number of CD9^{+} B cells and CD9^{-} B cells obtained is around 5% and 5–20%, respectively, of the total sorted B cells. When comparing the sorted subsets, it is better to set the yield of cell subsets with higher frequency comparable to the one with lowest frequency.
6. Although the dilution ratio suggested by manufacturer's instructions frequently works well, each lot of live/dead dye working solution and antibody staining solution must be titrated for optimal dilution prior to use in a critical experiment.
7. The cell surface staining mixture can include antibodies other than those directed against CD19 and CD9. More specifically, antibodies recognizing other Breg markers, such as CD1d and CD5, can be added.
8. Most of the facilities capable of providing RNA-seq services can also undertake rRNA depletion and rRNA-depleted total RNA quantification. It is recommended to choose such a service provider.
9. The incubation with anti-CD40 antibody and LPS is important to prime B10 cells. Differently from the stimulation protocol outlined in Subheading 3.1.4, PMA and ionomycin are not employed because such treatment would cause secretion of other cytokines, including proinflammatory cytokines, as well as IL-10 and force the B10 cells to transition into effector B10 cells, which does not reflect the physiological condition.

10. A coarser indicator of the suppressive effect of $CD9^+$ B cells on T-cell proliferation is through the evaluation of the final ratio of T cells and B cells in the coculture.
11. In the transwell assay, the transwell plate is coated with an anti-CD28 antibody in addition to the anti-CD3e antibody. This because, differently from the normal T/B cell coculture, in the transwell assay T and B cells are physically separated (the receiver plate contains no B cells) and therefore the support to T-cell proliferation provided by B-cell molecules such as CD80 (which binds CD28) is missing.
12. The date of the experiment of B-cell enrichment should be properly scheduled in order to match the injection times of **step 3** in the same section.
13. After enrichment with FITC-microbeads, a total of five million $CD9^+$ B cells and 20 million $CD9^-$ B cells should be obtained starting from 100 million $CD90.2^-$ cells.
14. As an alternative to intravenous injection via the animal's tail vein, cells can be retro-orbitally injected as described in detail by Yardeni et al. [11]. Consult your Institution's Animal Care and Use Committee guidelines to determine if retro-orbital injection is permitted.
15. The reading of the gauge may keep changing as the thickness of the swelled ear is easy to deform under compression. Waiting an extended period of time to obtain a stable number is not advised as it would not accurately reflect the real ear thickness. It is recommended to record the number at a fixed time point post release of the gauge knob for all ears.

Acknowledgments

This work is supported by Guangzhou Basic and Applied Basic Research Foundation (202002030127) to JS; the Fundamental Research Funds for the Central Universities (20ykzd08) to JS; Natural Science Foundation of Guangdong Province (2018A030313563) to JS; Program for Guangdong Introducing Innovative and Entrepreneurial Teams (2016ZT06S252) to JS; Guangdong Financial Fund for High-Caliber Hospital Construction to JS; NIAID (1R01AI099195 and R01AI134988) to U.B.

References

1. Zou F, Wang X, Han X et al (2018) Expression and function of Tetraspanins and their interacting Partners in B Cells. Front Immunol 9:1606
2. Rosser EC, Mauri C (2015) Regulatory B cells: origin, phenotype, and function. Immunity 42 (4):607–612
3. Kalampokis I, Yoshizaki A, Tedder TF (2013) IL-10-producing regulatory B cells (B10 cells) in autoimmune disease. Arthritis Res Ther 15: S1
4. Blair PA, Norena LY, Flores-Borja F et al (2010) CD19(+)CD24(hi)CD38(hi) B cells

exhibit regulatory capacity in healthy individuals but are functionally impaired in systemic lupus erythematosus patients. Immunity 32 (1):129–140

5. van de Veen W, Stanic B, Yaman G et al (2013) IgG4 production is confined to human IL-10-producing regulatory B cells that suppress antigen-specific immune responses. J Allergy Clin Immunol 131(4):1204–1212
6. Sun J, Wang J, Pefanis E et al (2015) Transcriptomics identify CD9 as a marker of murine IL-10-competent regulatory B cells. Cell Rep 13(6):1110–1117
7. Yanaba K, Bouaziz JD, Haas KM et al (2008) A regulatory B cell subset with a unique CD1dhiCD5+ phenotype controls T cell-dependent inflammatory responses. Immunity 28(5):639–650
8. Lindner S, Dahlke K, Sontheimer K et al (2013) Interleukin 21-induced granzyme B-expressing B cells infiltrate tumors and regulate T cells. Cancer Res 73(8):2468–2479
9. Matsushita T, Tedder TF (2011) Identifying regulatory B cells (B10 cells) that produce IL-10 in mice. Methods Mol Biol 677:99–111
10. Kramer A, Green J, Pollard J et al (2014) Causal analysis approaches in ingenuity pathway analysis. Bioinformatics 30(4):523–530
11. Yardeni T, Eckhaus M, Morris HD et al (2011) Retro-orbital injections in mice. Lab Anim 40 (5):155–160

Chapter 18

il-10 Gene *Locus* DNA Methylation in Regulatory B Cells

Silvia Tonon, Eleonora Martinis, Carlo E. M. Pucillo, and Francesca Mion

Abstract

Epigenetic studies are becoming increasingly common in the immunology field thanks to the support of cutting edge technology and to their potential of providing a large amount of data at the single cell level. Moreover, epigenetic modifications were shown to play a role in autoimmune/inflammatory disorders, paving the way for the possibility of using the results of epigenetic studies for therapeutic purposes. In recent years, epigenetic marks such as DNA methylation, histone modifications and nucleosome positioning were shown to regulate B cell fate and function during an immune response, but very little has been done in the context of one of the most recently discovered B cell subsets, that is regulatory B cells. Although no consensus has yet been found on the identity of these immunosuppressive B cells, the role of the IL-10 cytokine is consolidated, both in the murine and human setting. In this chapter we will focus on the analysis of the methylation profile of a gene of interest and we will specifically describe cloning and pyrosequencing bisulphite sequencing PCR (BSP). Given the specific context, we will provide tips and tricks for the analysis of the *il-10* gene *locus*. Nonetheless, the methods presented are valid for the study of any gene of interest.

Key words IL-10, B cells, Methylation, Pyrosequencing, Bisulphite cloning sequencing

1 Introduction

B-cell lymphopoiesis is a complex process starting in the bone marrow where hematopoietic stem cells differentiate into multipotent progenitors and common lymphoid progenitors. Further differentiation steps lead to the formation of the early precursors for immature naïve B cells, which leave the bone marrow and reach the peripheral immune system where they complete their maturation [1–3]. During this developmental and maturation process, B cells undergo extensive changes in their epigenome. DNA methylation/demethylation, histone modification, and noncoding RNAs are the most studied epigenetic modifications, and it has been highlighted how abnormalities in these complex regulatory processes may contribute to the onset of autoimmune diseases [4].

DNA methylation is a mechanism involving the transfer of a methyl group onto the C5 position of the cytosine nucleobase, leading to the formation of 5-methylcytosine (5mC) [5]. DNA

Francesca Mion and Silvia Tonon (eds.), *Regulatory B Cells: Methods and Protocols*, Methods in Molecular Biology, vol. 2270, https://doi.org/10.1007/978-1-0716-1237-8_18, © Springer Science+Business Media, LLC, part of Springer Nature 2021

methylation occurs predominantly on cytosines followed by guanine residues (CpG methylation), but it has also been found at cytosines followed by adenine, thymine, or by another cytosine (non-CpG methylation) [6]. This epigenetic modification is catalyzed by the family of DNA methyltransferases (DNMTs), which transfer a methyl group from *S*-adenyl methionine to the cytosine [5]. Among the different family members, Dnmt3a and Dnmt3b can establish a new methylation pattern to unmodified DNA and are thus known as de novo DNMTs. Differently, Dnmt1 functions during DNA replication to copy the DNA methylation pattern from the parental DNA strand onto the newly synthesized daughter strand [5]. The reverse process, that is the replacement of 5mC with cytosine, takes place via either passive or active DNA demethylation. Passive demethylation is due to the absence of maintenance of methylation profiles during replication, which results in a consequent dilution of 5mC. Active demethylation entails instead the modification of the cytosine nucleobase via deamination and/or oxidation, followed by DNA repair-mediated replacement [6]. Depending on the genomic region, DNA methylation can have different effects on gene activity. It can regulate tissue-specific gene expression by recruiting proteins involved in gene repression or by inhibiting the binding of transcription factors to DNA, and it also takes part to the formation of chromatin by interacting with various other epigenetic mechanisms, such as histone modification, nucleosome positioning, and noncoding RNAs [7].

Concerning early B-cell differentiation, *mb-1* is an example of a gene whose expression is regulated by DNA methylation. The *mb-1* gene encodes the Igα subunit of the pre-BCR in pre-B cells and of the BCR in immature naïve B cells. It is methylated at CpG dinucleotides in hematopoietic stem cells, but it is gradually demethylated during B-cell commitment. The transcription factors EBF and E2A contribute to CpG demethylation and nucleosomal remodeling of the *mb-1* promoter, an event necessary for its transcriptional activation by Pax5 [8]. Another example of a B-cell-specific gene epigenetically regulated during early B-cell development is *Cd19*, which encodes a cell surface protein that participates in signal transduction mechanisms via the pre-BCR and BCR. Chromatin remodeling at the upstream enhancer sequences of *Cd19* occurs in multipotent progenitors and leads to the recruitment of E2A first, and, later, of EBF and Pax5 [9]. However, except for B-cell lineage genes (e.g., *cd19*, *pax5*, *ebf*) exhibiting an active epigenetic status, immature naïve B cells display an overall DNA hypermethylation, an enrichment of repressive histone posttranslational modifications (e.g., H3K9me3 and H3K27me3) and low levels of overall histone acetylation [4].

Moving to the mature B-cell compartment, the differentiation of naïve B cells to germinal center B cells and then to plasma cells or memory B cells is associated with changes in the DNA methylome. Upon B-cell activation, DNA demethylation occurs and promotes histone modifications such as H3K4me3, H3K9ac, H3K14ac, and H4K8ac on the V(D)J region, thereby leading to an open chromatin status. Thus, these epigenetic marks increase V(D)J region chromatin accessibility to the somatic hypermutation (SHR) machinery that includes AID enzyme (encoded by *AICDA* in humans and *Aicda* in mice) whose expression is, in turn, regulated by epigenetic modifications. Indeed, in naïve B cells, *Aicda* is silenced by DNA hypermethylation and by low levels of histone H3 acetylation after B-cell activation, the gene is demethylated and the *locus* becomes enriched in H3K4me3 and H3K9ac/K14ac. However, after class-switch recombination and SHM, *Aicda* gene is downregulated again as a result of its DNA remethylation [10]. Similarly, in memory B cells, characterized by a high expression of DNMT3a, a distinctive DNA methylation pattern reflects a differentiated gene expression profile, as compared to naïve B cells. These differentially expressed genes could probably be involved in the different function exerted by memory B cells in regard to their ability to induce a more rapid and robust activation response than that of their naïve counterpart [10].

Given the relevance of epigenetic modifications and, more specifically, of DNA methylation, on the B-cell differentiative process, we recently undertook a study aimed at understanding if DNA methylation could be involved in the expansion and/or differentiation of IL-10-producing regulatory B cells, the most widely studied regulatory B-cell subset [11]. Nowadays, it is well known that, among all its functions, the B cell can also suppress a variety of pathological immune responses through a series of mechanisms ranging from the release of cytokines (IL-10, IL-35, TGF-β) to cell–cell interactions [12]. If on the one hand, the B-cell regulatory function is well established, and on the other, an agreement has not yet been found on their phenotypic identity, let alone on the existence of a specific molecular marker. We searched the answer to this unsolved question at an epigenetic level and what we found was that the development of IL-10-producing B cells goes hand in hand with the methylation status of the *il-10* gene *locus* [13]. We demonstrated that murine B cells immediately prone and developmentally committed to IL-10 production (IL-10$^+$ B cells) are characterized by a demethylated region located 4.5 kb from the transcription starting site (TSS) of the *il-10* gene *locus* (murine conserved noncoding sequence, mCNS-4.5) and by a partially demethylated region located 9 kb upstream the TSS (mCNS-9). This signature allows to distinguish these cells from those that require a persistent stimulation to exert an IL-10-mediated regulatory function (IL-10$^-$ B cells), which do not demethylate mCNS-

4.5 and undergo partial demethylation on mCNS-9. In the human setting, IL-10$^+$ B cells isolated from the peripheral blood of healthy donors show demethylation only at hCNS-12.5 (hCNS, human conserve noncoding sequence), which is conserved with mCNS-9, but not at hCNS-6, conserved with mCNS-4.5 [13]. The pathogenesis of different B-cell-related malignancies is often linked to changes in DNA methylation, and we identified similarities in the *il-10* gene *locus* methylation profile between human IL-10$^+$ B cells and malignant B cells of chronic lymphocytic leukemia (CLL) and mantle cell lymphoma (MCL), which have been reported exploiting IL-10 synthesis to maintain an immunosuppressive environment permissive for clone expansion [13–15].

In this chapter, we present and outline two methods which can be employed when undertaking the study of the methylation profile of a specific gene *locus* of a cell subset of interest. Specifically, bisulphite cloning sequencing and pyrosequencing will be described. Although kept as general as possible, the protocols presented in this chapter refer to the *il-10* gene *locus*, in order to provide an important tool for the study of regulatory B cells.

2 Materials

2.1 General Equipment

1. Thermal cycler.
2. Spectrophotometer (e.g., Nanodrop).
3. PyroMark Q96 ID (Qiagen, or equivalent machines).
4. Bacterial shaker incubator.
5. Electrophoresis chamber.

2.2 General Kits and Reagents

1. Kit for DNA conversion with bisulfite (*see* **Note 1**).
2. DNA polymerase specific for uracil-containing templates (*see* **Note 2**).
3. 2% agarose gel.
4. TAE 1× buffer: 40 mM Tris, 20 mM acetic acid and 1 mM EDTA.

2.3 Reagents for Bisulfite Cloning Sequencing and Pyrosequencing

1. Kit for gel-purification of PCR products.
2. Primers for bisulfite cloning sequencing (primers for the *il-10* gene *locus* are listed in Table 1).
3. Primers for pyrosequencing (primers for the *il-10* gene *locus* are listed in Table 2).
4. Cloning kit for sequencing (*see* **Note 3**) and competent bacteria.
5. Sterile glass plating beads (4 mm).

Table 1
List of primers used for cloning BSP

Target	Chromosomic localization	N° CpG	Forward primer	Reverse primer
mCNS -9	chr1:131010441–131,010,839	11	AGTGTAAAGATTATAGGAAGGTT	CTACCCAACTCTAAAAATAC
mCNS – 4.5	chr1:131015283–131,015,667	6	TAGAGATGTTATTGGTGTTT	CCACTTATACACAATATAAC
mCNS -0.5	chr1:131019234–131,019,658	7	GTAGAGGAGGTATTAGAATTTTT	ACTTCTACATTACAACTATTTTT
mCNS +1.1	chr1:131021587–131,021,799	6	AGATTAGATAGGAGATTAGGTAAA	AAAAAAACCATAACTAAAACCCC
hCNS -12.5	chr1:206784418–206,784,795	10	AAGTTTTTTTGAAAGAGATG	AACCTCTTCTAACTCATAACTT
hCNS – 6	chr1:206777989–206,778,360	7	GGTGGTTAAGGTTTAAATAT	CTATATTCCTCTAAACTTTC
hCNS -0.5	chr1:206772534–206,772,918	6	TGGGTATTTATTTTAGGTTG	AAAAAAACCTCTTCATTCAT

Table 2
List of primers used for pyrosequencing BSP

Target		Amplification primers	Sequencing primers
mCNS-9	Fragment 1	For: AGTGTAAAGATTATAGGAAGGTT Rev: Biotin-TCCTCAAAAACATAACCAAA	AGGAAGGTTTTATTAAGTTT TTTAAGAAAGTGTTAGTTTT TTATTTTTTTTTTATATTTG
	Fragment 2	For: GTTTTGTTATTTAATGAAGGTTT Rev; biotin-ACCTTTTTCCTAAAAACAAC	AAGGTTTTTTTGGTTT AAAGTATCGGGGGTTA
mCNS-4.5	Fragment 1	For: ATTTGGGGTAGTTATGGATATA Rev; biotin-CAATTTAACTTTTACTCAAAAACC	AGTTATGGATATAGTTAAA AGTTATGGATATAGTTAAA
	Fragment 2	For: AGTTATATAAAGGGGAATTTTAT Rev; biotin-AAAACCCAAATTAAAACTAACC	ATTTTATATTGGTTGTTTA GTAATATTTGTTTGGTT

6. LB agar plate with antibiotic (*see* **Note 3**).
7. LB medium.
8. 13 mL culture tubes with ventilation cap.
9. Plasmid DNA purification kit (starting material: 1–5 mL overnight bacteria culture volume).

3 Methods

Several methods allow the study of CpG methylation, but the gold standard are those techniques based on the treatment of DNA with bisulfite, a chemical compound that is able to convert unmethylated cytosine (C) into uracil (U) while leaving methylated C (^{me}C) untouched (*see* Fig. 1). Using specific primers, selected regions are amplified by PCR and sequenced. Importantly, after amplification, U will be turned into thymine (T), while each ^{me}C is amplified as C. The methylation status is determined by quantifying the percentage of C and T obtained in correspondence of CpG sites in the

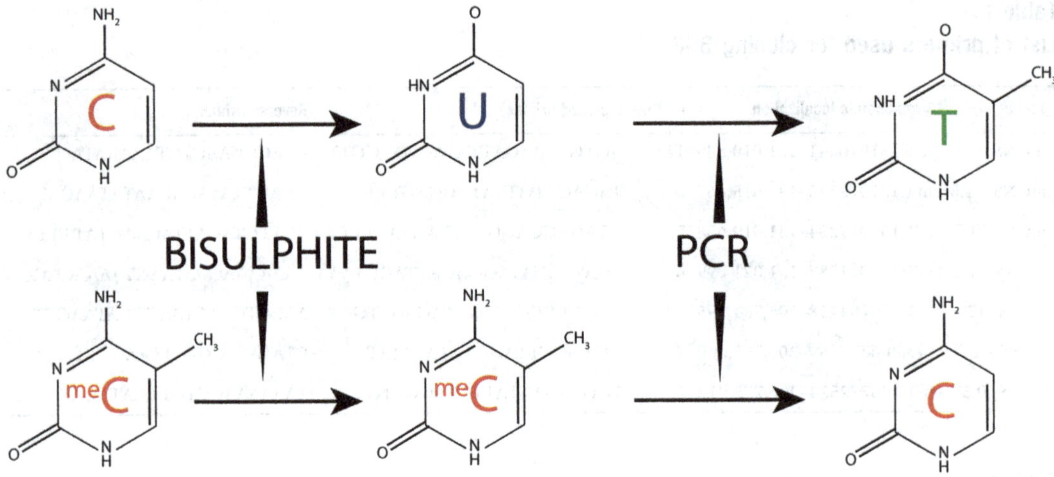

Fig. 1 DNA bisulfite conversion. Bisulfite converts into uracil only unmethylated cytosines. Then, the PCR step converts uracil into thymine and leaves cytosine unchanged

original genomic sequence. Hereafter we will describe two techniques that allow the study of specific regions across gene *loci*, reporting the example of the *il-10* gene *locus*: bisulphite cloning sequencing and pyrosequencing. Alternative methods for bisulfite-based methylation studies will only be briefly mentioned.

3.1 Preliminary Steps

Regardless of whether you want to use bisulphite cloning sequencing or pyrosequencing, the analysis of specific regions across the *il-10* gene *locus* involves a series of initial steps common to both procedures.

3.1.1 Bisulfite Conversion of DNA and Quantification

1. Purify the cells of interest by using a methodology that allows to obtain a very high grade of purity. Follow manufacturer's instruction of the chosen kit for DNA bisulfite conversion (*see* **Note 4**).
2. Quantify the converted DNA. Following conversion, the DNA is single-stranded and rich in uracil, and therefore should be quantified by using RNA settings on your spectrophotometer. Store samples at −20 °C.

3.1.2 Region of Interest (ROI) Identification

Here below we outline how to identify ROIs by taking advantage of the UCSC genome browser (https://genome-euro.ucsc.edu//cgi-bin/hgGateway) and VISTA (http://pipeline.lbl.gov/cgi-bin/gateway2?selector=vista).

1. On the UCSC main page, select the species, the assembly, and the chromosomic region (*see* Fig. 2a, red arrows). The user can also type the name of the gene.

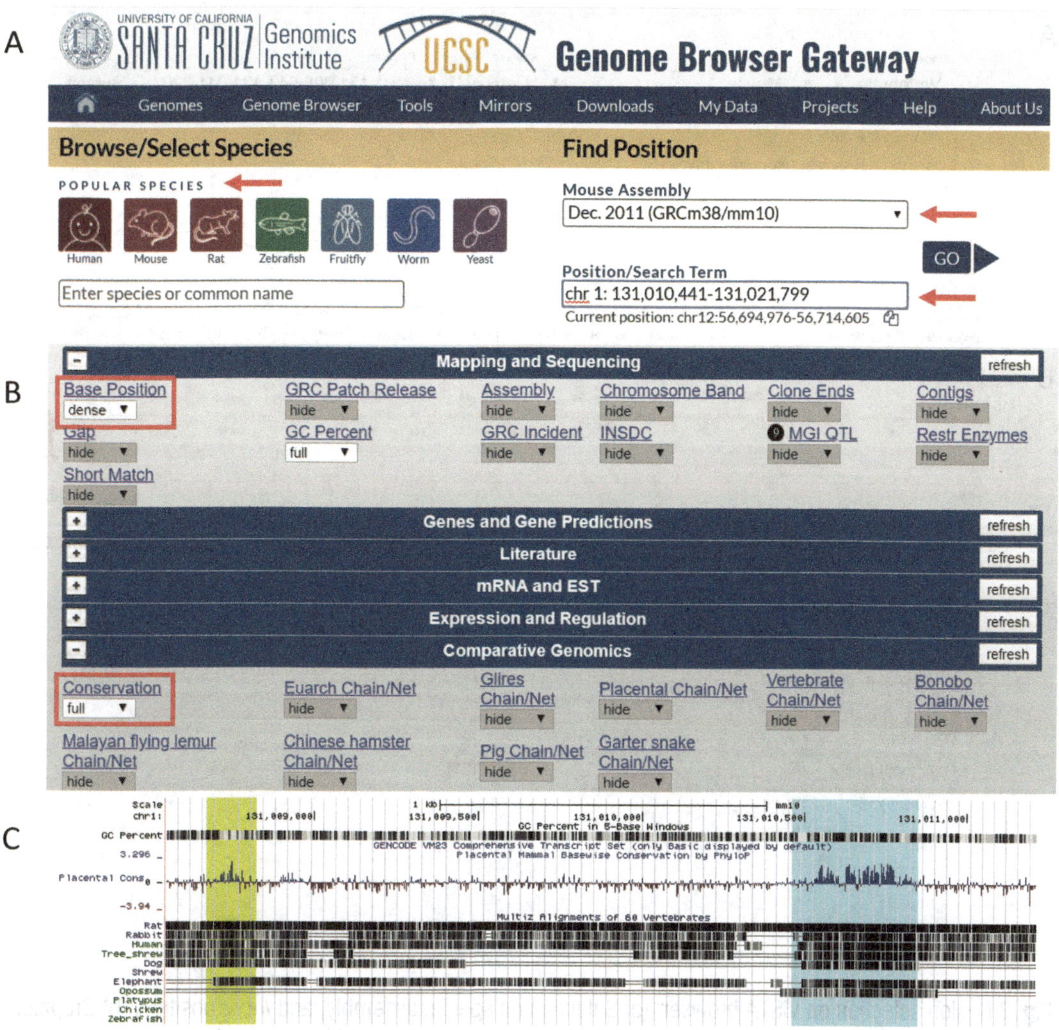

Fig. 2 Region selection on UCSC. (**a**) Selection on specie, assembly, and *locus* position. (**b**) Display of GC content and level of conservation. (**c**) Graphical display of conserved regions. To select regions, press on SHIFT + right click or ALT+ right click

2. Regions are selected on the basis of their level of conservation and their GC content. For this purpose, select "GC percent" and "conservation" among tracks (*see* Fig. 2b). As shown in Fig. 2c, the user can visually identify ROI and is guided in the interpretation of the result by a color scheme: the region highlighted in yellow is conserved (blue peak) but poor in GC content (light gray), while the region highlighted in light-blue has both characteristics (black in GC content bar and blue peak in conservation slots).
3. The selection process can also be integrated with data already present in literature or by taking advantage of VISTA. On the

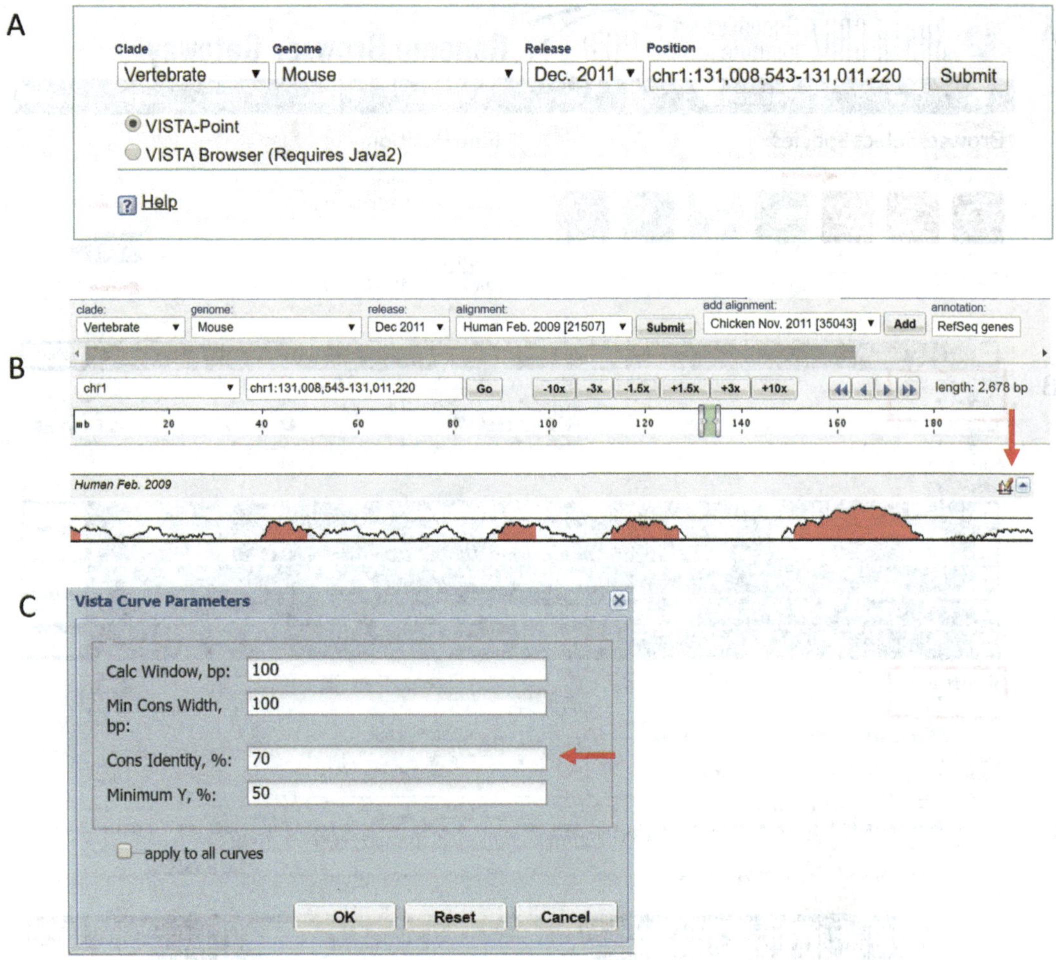

Fig. 3 Region selection on VISTA browser. (**a**) Selection on specie, assembly, and *locus* position. (**b**) Graphical display of conserved regions (pink). (**c**) Parameters of the curve. The panel is selected by clicking on the icon next to red arrow in panel (**b**)

main page, select the species, the assembly, and type the same chromosomic region analyzed in **step 2** (*see* Fig. 3a).

4. By default, mouse genome is aligned with human genome and regions that are >70% conserved are highlighted in pink (*see* Fig. 3b). The user can change the minimum level of conservation required by clicking on the pencil (*see* Fig. 3b, red arrow) and modifying "Cons Identity, %" (*see* Fig. 3c, red arrow).
5. Once ROIs are identified, the user can retrieve the native genomic DNA sequence on UCSC, zooming on the selected region (right click and "Zoom to Highlight"), going in the upper Menu and selecting, in series, "View," "DNA," "get DNA."

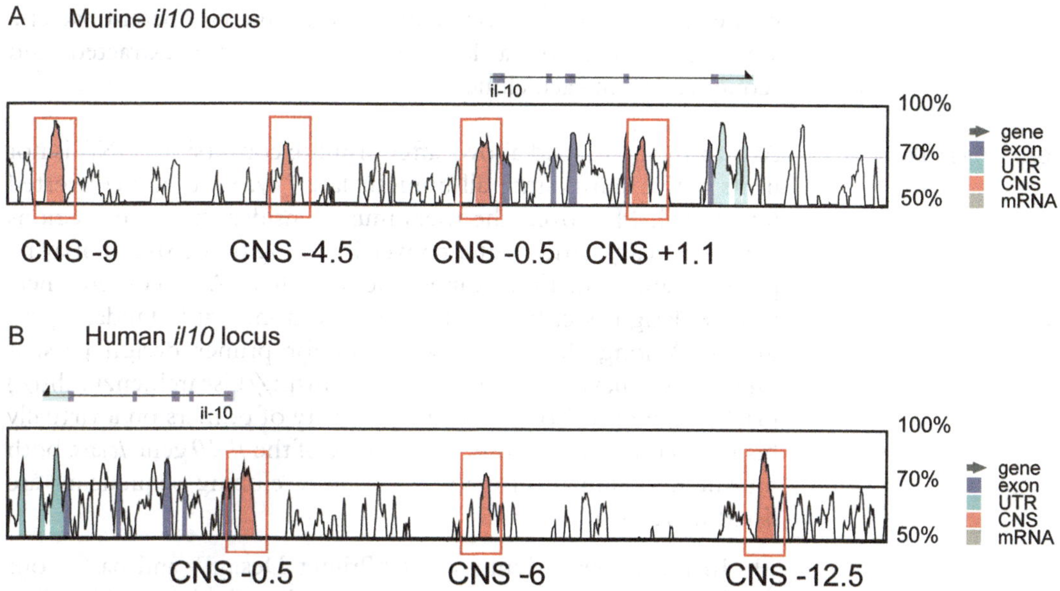

Fig. 4 *il-10* gene *locus* analysis. Representative figures for the murine (**a**) and human (**b**) *il-10* gene *locus* were generated taking advantage of the VISTA browser. Regions highlighted in pink have a high degree of conservation between mouse and human (>70%)

6. As an example, Fig. 4 shows the analysis of specific ROIs characterized by being conserved noncoding sequences (CNS), on the *il-10* gene *locus* for the murine (*see* Fig. 4a) and human (*see* Fig. 4b) setting. Murine regions were selected on GRCm38/mm10 assembly (chromosome 1: 131,010,441-131,021,799) and human regions on GRCh38/hg38 assembly (chr1: 206,784,453-206,772,920). In the murine setting, a total of four regions encompassing 30 CpGs were analyzed, while in the human context 22 CpG sites were selected among three fragments (chromosomic coordinates are listed in Table 1). In particular, mCNS-9 is evolutionary conserved with hCNS-12.5 and mCNS-4.5 with hCNS-6. In both species, the region near the TSS is conserved, while mCNS +1.1 was not analyzed in the human system because there were no conserved CpGs [13].

3.2 Cloning Bisulphite Sequencing PCR (Cloning BSP)

Direct Sanger sequencing of PCR products derived from bisulfite-converted DNA is fast but inefficient when analyzing regions with variable methylation. Since it is not a quantitative method, the peak highness will not correspond to the percentage of the nucleotide, resulting in the impossibility to quantify the grade of methylation. To overcome this problem, Sanger sequencing must be preceded by a vector-cloning step. This method allows to have a single-cell resolution since in each vector one single PCR product is present and sequenced. Briefly, selected regions are amplified with peculiar primers, amplicons are cloned into vectors, and competent bacteria are transformed. As a last step, plasmids are extracted and sequenced from each clone.

3.2.1 Primer Design

As already mentioned above, after bisulfite conversion, DNA is not in its native status since all unmethylated cytosines are converted into uracil. Moreover, the users must consider that some regions are particularly critical (after conversion, long polyT stretch may be present) and sometimes cannot be amplified. As a consequence, primer design is critical and cannot be done with standard programs. Among the several softwares for primer design present online, we have chosen BiSearch (http://bisearch.enzim.hu/) [16] that allows also to test the specificity of primers on a virtually bisulfite-converted genome. In the case of the *il-10* gene *locus*, both murine and human primers for bisulfite cloning sequencing are listed in Table 1.

1. In the general Menu, select "Primer Design" and paste your DNA-native sequence (selected as described in Subheading 3.1.2) in the appropriate slot (*see* Fig. 5a).
2. Select "Bisulfite." The software is set to draw the primers on the best strand from an efficiency point of view. In any case, if desired, the user can indicate to the software to design the primers on the sense or the antisense strand (*see* **Note 5**). At this point, primers can be searched.
3. Additionally, a number of other options are selectable to make the search more specific. The user can choose to force the design of primers at the level of specific parts of the regions of interest (*see* Fig. 5b) and set the maximum length of the PCR product (*see* **Note 6** and Fig. 5c). The user can also decide the minimum CpG number to be analyzed (*see* Fig. 5d) and select the genome on which the virtual PCR must be done to determine the specificity of primers for the ROI (*see* Fig. 5e). If possible, avoid the selection of primers containing CpG sites since this can lead to biased amplification of methylated/unmethylated strands.

3.2.2 PCR of Bisulfite-Converted DNA

1. For each PCR reaction, start with 10–20 ng of bisulfite-converted DNA and follow the manufacturer's instruction of the chosen DNA polymerase (*see* **Note 2**). Since the material is usually degraded, a minimum of 40 cycles should be included in the thermic protocol.
2. The PCR step is critical and must be optimized to obtain a single amplicon for each ROI. For this reason, checking the reaction on a 2% agarose gel is required each time.
3. If the amplicon is not unique, the user can choose to optimize the PCR reaction (e.g., adjusting annealing temperature or

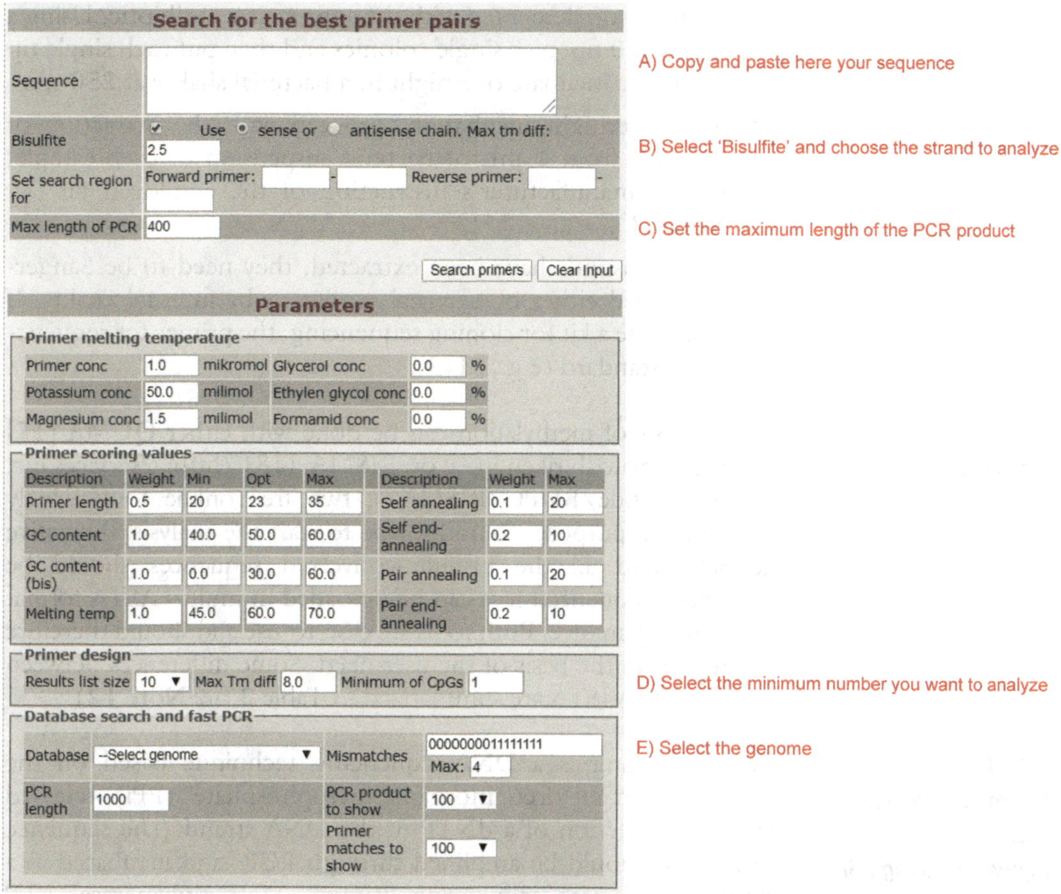

Fig. 5 Primer design with BiSearch. Shown is the webpage used for the generation of bisulfite-specific primers

primer concentration), or to gel purify the PCR product by using an appropriate kit.

3.2.3 Cloning, Plasmid Extraction, and Sequencing

1. Perform the cloning according to manufacturer's instruction of the chosen kit and proceed with the transformation of competent bacteria (*see* **Note 7**).
2. Plate different dilution of transformed bacteria on LB agar petri dishes containing the appropriate selection antibiotic. In order to obtain well spread single colonies, use sterile glass plating beads (8–10 per plate) and roll the plate for 1 or 2 minutes. Allow the suspension to dry, recover the beads and incubate overnight at 37 °C (*see* **Note 8**). Keep the remaining cell suspension at 4 °C (*see* **Note 9**). In order to have a good representation of the methylation percentage, 10–20 colonies should be picked, amplified, and sequenced.
3. The day after (*see* **Note 10**), prepare the desired quantity of tubes with ventilation cap (10–20), containing 2 mL of LB

medium supplemented with the appropriate antibiotic. Using a sterile p10 tip, pick single colonies and then put each single tip in a tube. Incubate overnight in a bacterial shaker at 250 rpm.

4. After overnight incubation, proceed with the extraction of plasmids from 1 mL of bacteria suspension of each sample. Follow manufacturer's instruction of the employed kit (*see* **Note 11**).
5. Once plasmids have been extracted, they need to be Sanger-sequenced either by external service or by internal facility. If you chose a kit for cloning sequencing, the primer for sequencing is standard (e.g., M13).

3.2.4 Analysis of Methylation

The analysis of methylation can be done with either QUMA [17] (http://quma.cdb.riken.jp/) or BISMA [18] (http://services.ibc.uni-stuttgart.de/BDPC/BISMA/), two free online tools widely used for this purpose. In both cases, to start the analysis, the native genomic and all the bisulfite-converted sequences should be uploaded. Sequenced files can be uploaded in multi-FASTA format or in one zip archive. Both tools are ease-to-use and should therefore be chosen on the basis of the user need. Some differences between QUMA and VISTA are summarized in Table 3 (*see* **Note 12**).

3.3 Pyrosequencing Bisulphite Sequencing PCR (pyrosequencing BSP)

Pyrosequencing is a DNA-sequencing technique based on the quantification of free inorganic pyrophosphate (PPi) released from the insertion of a dNTP in the DNA strand. The sequence of interest should be amplified through PCR, and incubated as a single strand with sequencing primers, DNA polymerase, ATP sulfurilase, luciferase, apyrase and the substrates luciferin and adenosine 5′ phosphosulfate. This is a sequencing-by-synthesis technique, so dNTPs are added to the reaction one at a time, sequentially. The DNA polymerase catalyzes the incorporation of a dNTP, and each time a dNTP is added a PPi is released. In the presence of adenosine 5′ phosphosulfate, the PPi is converted by

Table 3
Major characteristics of BISMA and QUMA analysis softwares

	BISMA	QUMA
Need of native genomic sequence	Yes	Yes
Sequenced regions upload	Multi-FASTA format/zip archive	Multi-FASTA format/zip archive
Statistical analysis between two samples	No	Yes
Exclusion of unconverted sequences	Yes	Yes
Alignment	Pairwise/multiple	Pairwise

ATP sulfurilase in ATP, and ATP acts as a substrate for the conversion of luciferin into oxyluciferin by luciferase. This last reaction generates visible light, proportional to the generated ATP, detected by a CCD camera and plotted on the pyrogram. Apyrase degrades unincorporated dNTPs and ATP, and the reaction starts again with a new dNTP.

3.3.1 Assay Design

Methylation is measured at each CpG site on a PCR amplicon. In this view, each CpG site should be considered as a C/T SNP. Each assay should not span more that 150–200 nucleotides. For example, in our analysis of the murine *il-10* gene *locus*, the assay was designed only on mCNS-9 and mCNS-4.5, and each region was divided into two different fragments [13]. For each region analyzed, a pair of amplification primers and one or more sequencing primers are necessary. Amplification and sequencing primers for the murine *il-10* gene *locus* are listed in Table 2. One of the amplification primers must be biotinylated at the 5′ to allow the isolation of single strand DNA during sequencing. Moreover, some important considerations must be kept in mind for primer design. First, avoid the selection of primers containing CpG sites since this can lead to biased amplification of methylated/unmethylated strands. Instead, for sequencing primers, it is reasonable to avoid CpG near the 3′ as this can lead to mispriming, preventing the synthesis of the sequencing filament, but it is equally important including amplification of Cs to verify bisulfite conversion. The design of amplification primers can be done with BiSearch as in Subheading 3.2.1, or by using specific softwares provided with the machine for pyrosequencing.

3.3.2 PCR

1. For each PCR reaction, start with 10–20 ng of bisulfite-converted DNA and follow manufacturer's instruction of the chosen DNA polymerase (*see* **Note 2**). Since the material is usually degraded, a minimum of 40 cycles should be included in the thermic protocol.
2. The PCR step is critical and must be optimized to obtain a single amplicon for each ROI. For this reason, checking the reaction on a 2% agarose gel is required each time. Avoid to gel purify the products and rather try to optimize the reaction (*see* **Note 13**).

3.3.3 Sequencing and Analysis

Briefly, biotinylated PCR products are immobilized and purified using Sepharose beads coated with streptavidin. Depending on the machine available, the procedures for amplicon isolation and the sequencing steps are different, for this reason we suggest to refer to manufacturer's instruction. As shown in Fig. 6, the software analysis modules of Qiagen Q96, Q48, and Q24 automatically provide the methylation percentage at each CpG site analyzed, together with a quality score for the sequencing (Pass, Check, Failed).

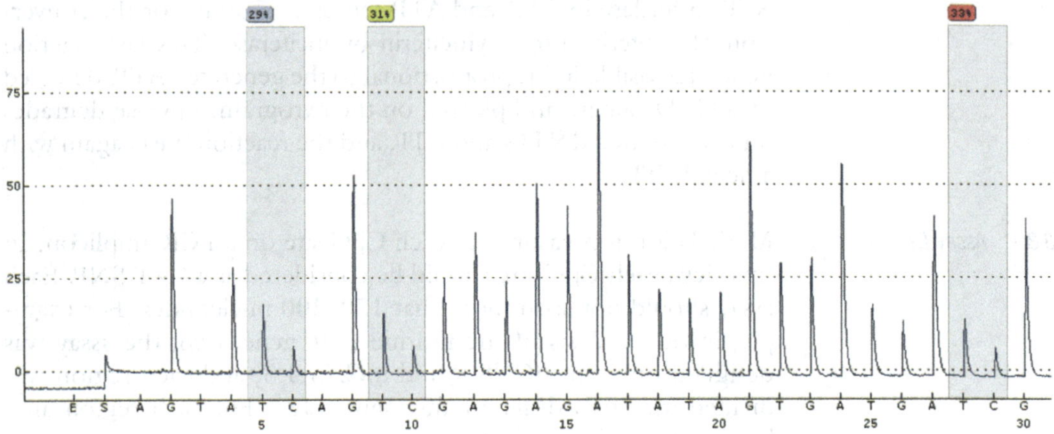

Sequence to analyze:
GGAC/TGGC/TGAGAAGGAAATATAGGTGAATAC/TGT

Position	1	2	3
Quality	Passed	Check	Failed
Meth (%)	29	31	33

Fig. 6 Example of a pyrogram. The pyrogram was generated with the Qiagen software analysis modules

3.4 Alternative Methods for Bisulfite-Based Methylation Studies

Cloning sequencing and pyrosequencing of PCR products derived from bisulfite-converted DNA allow the analysis of gene-specific methylation at a single base level, but these are not the only applicable techniques. Methylation-specific PCR (MSP) [19–21] is another technique that can be employed if the goal of the researcher is the analysis of gene-specific methylation. Depending on the detection system used, MSP can be qualitative or quantitative. In both cases, two sets of primers should be designed for a same region of interest, but with different sequences allowing the recognition of methylated or unmethylated DNA. In the case of qualitative MSP, primers should contain more CpG sites in their sequence, and PCR products are analyzed by gel electrophoresis. As shown in Fig. 7, if the DNA is fully methylated, the amplicon will be present only when the PCR is performed with the methylation primer set (M-primer), on the contrary if the DNA is completely unmethylated, the product will be present only when unmethylation primers (U-primer) are used. This technique is easy and cheap but difficult to interpret when the DNA presents intermediate methylation since the electrophoresis will reveal bands both for M-primers and U-primers. To avoid this problem, quantitative MSP should be employed as PCR products are detected by an intercalating dye or using TaqMan probes (MethyLight).

If a comprehensive analysis of the methylome is needed, employing NGS on bisulfite-converted DNA will be the right choice: whole-genome (WGBS) [22], reduced representation (RRBS) [23] or enhanced reduced representation (ERRBS) [24] bisulfite sequencing. After bisulfite conversion of genomic DNA,

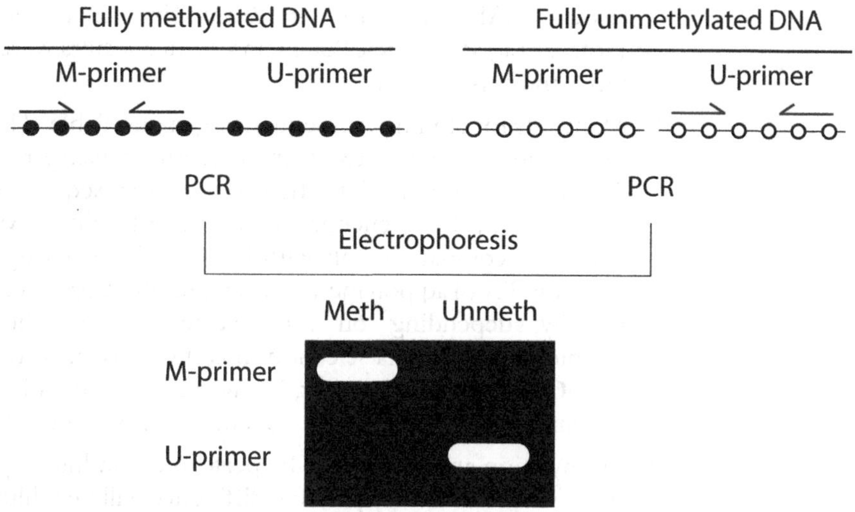

Fig. 7 Methylation-Specific PCR (MSP). Bisulfite-converted DNA is amplified by PCR both with the methylation primer (M-primer) and unmethylation primer (U-primer) set. The specific binding of primers is assessed by verifying the presence of the corresponding band by gel electrophoresis

the library is prepared, samples are sequenced, and all reads are mapped to the reference genome. While for WGBS the library is prepared from the entire converted genome, RRBS and ERRBS use the restriction enzyme MspI (which cleaves between Cs in 5′-CCGG-3′ sequences, regardless of the methylation status) to enrich the library in fragments containing CpG regions of the genomic DNA. Compared to RRBS, ERRBS has some modifications in the library preparation protocol, which allow a higher coverage of CpG sites. The choice of the method depends on the cost per sample and the coverage needed: WGBS can cover all CpG sites in the genome but at a high cost, on the contrary RRBS and ERRBS are cheaper but provide lower coverage.

Collectively, we recommend to start the analysis from cloning/ pyrosequencing BSP if you already know which gene needs to be analyzed, e.g., *il10* for regulatory B cells, otherwise NSG methods are preferable. Once the methylation status of the sample is established, MSP-based methods can be used for screening.

4 Notes

1. For our experiments we chose the EpiTect Fast Bisulfite Conversion kit from Qiagen because it is rapid and particularly well suited for low number of cells. However, many other kits are available.
2. We started with using a polymerase engineered for uracil-rich template (Roche, KAPA HiFi HotStart Uracil+ ReadyMix Kit), but we then switched to a high-fidelity DNA polymerase

(Roche, KAPA HiFi HotStart ReadyMix PCR Kit or Qiagen, HotStarTaq Plus DNA Polymerase) since results were comparable and it is cheaper.

3. Many kits for cloning and sequencing are available. The experiments published in [13] were performed using the pCR4-TOPO TA cloning kit (Invitrogen) for sequencing with TOP10 One Shot chemically competent cells (Invitrogen). This kit is compatible only with PCR products having an overhanging 3′A (Taq polymerase-amplified PCR products). Additionally, depending on the selected vector, the correct antibiotic for bacteria selection must be chosen. In the case of the pCR4-TOPO TA vector, LB agar plates containing 50 μg/mL ampicillin or 50 μg/mL kanamycin should be used.
4. Methylation analysis should be performed on highly pure cells because otherwise any possible difference will be "diluted" and lost. For example, in all the experiments published in [13], we bisulfite-converted the DNA from 100.000 IL-10^{+} and 100.000 IL-10^{-} splenic B cells obtained after an enrichment step through IL-10 secretion assay followed by FACS-sorting, a methodology that allows to have cells with a purity >95%.
5. Keep in mind that, after bisulfite conversion, DNA is not complementary anymore, so you should decide which strand to analyze. In our experiments, we analyzed the sense strand for the murine setting and the antisense strand in the human context since these are the strands on which the coding sequence of the gene is located.
6. It is recommended not exceeding 400–500 bp as bisulfite-converted DNA is highly degraded.
7. Competent bacteria are usually included in the kit for cloning. Alternatively, also homemade competent bacteria can be used considering that the efficiency of transformation could be lower.
8. Work under a bacteria-dedicated hood or near a Bunsen burner. Put the dishes in the incubator inverted.
9. The day after, check colonies: if they are not well spread or in insufficient number, then repeat the plating.
10. We suggest to perform the colony collection step late in the afternoon.
11. The extraction of each plasmid is relatively cheap but time-consuming. Alternatively, you can take advantage of services that allow to sequence the plasmids directly from single colonies transferred and expanded in a 96-well agar plate.
12. BISMA does not provide the statistical analysis between two samples. For this reason, we suggest the non-parametric Mann-Whitney test to compare the methylation percentage at each CpG site.

13. If primer dimers are present, try to prevent them from forming using different ratio of the forward and reverse primers, using a large excess of the non-biotinylated oligo.

References

1. Kulis M, Merkel A, Heath S et al (2015) Whole-genome fingerprint of the DNA methylome during human B cell differentiation. Nat Genet 47:746–756
2. Vale AM, Kearney JF, Nobrega A, et al (2015) Development and Function of B Cell Subsets, In: Molecular Biology of B Cells: Second Edition, pp. 99–119
3. Barneda-Zahonero B, Roman-Gonzalez L, Collazo O et al (2012) Epigenetic regulation of B lymphocyte differentiation, transdifferentiation, and reprogramming. Comp Funct Genomics 2012:1–10
4. Wu H, Deng Y, Feng Y et al (2018) Epigenetic regulation in B-cell maturation and its dysregulation in autoimmunity. Cell Mol Immunol 15:676–684
5. Moore LD, Le T, Fan G (2013) DNA methylation and its basic function. 38:28–38
6. Jang HS, Shin WJ, Lee JE et al (2017) CpG and non-CpG methylation in epigenetic gene regulation and brain function. Genes (Basel) 8:1–20
7. Jin B, Li Y, Robertson KD (2011) DNA methylation: superior or subordinate in the epigenetic hierarchy? Genes Cancer 2:607–617
8. Maier H, Ostraat R, Gao H et al (2004) Early B cell factor cooperates with Runx1 and mediates epigenetic changes associated with mb-1 transcription. Nat Immunol 10:1069–1077
9. Walter K, Bonifer C, Tagoh H (2008) Stem cell – specific epigenetic priming and B cell – specific transcriptional activation at the mouse Cd19 locus. Blood 112:1673–1682
10. Zan H, Casali P (2015) Epigenetics of peripheral B-cell differentiation and the antibody response. Front Immunol 6:1–20
11. Mauri C, Menon M, Mauri C et al (2017) Human regulatory B cells in health and disease : therapeutic potential. J Clin Invest 127:772–779
12. Rosser EC, Mauri C (2015) Regulatory B cells: origin, phenotype, and function. Immunity 42:607–612
13. Tonon S, Mion F, Dong J et al (2019) IL-10-producing B cells are characterized by a specific methylation signature. Eur J Immunol 49:1213–1225
14. Visser HPJ, Tewis M, Willemze R et al (2000) Mantle cell lymphoma proliferates upon IL-10 in the CD40 system. Leukemia 14:1483–1489
15. Alhakeem SS, McKenna MK, Oben KZ et al (2018) Chronic lymphocytic leukemia–derived IL-10 suppresses antitumor immunity. J Immunol 200:4180–4189
16. Arányi T, Váradi A, Simon I et al (2006) The BiSearch web server. BMC Bioinformatics 7:431
17. Kumaki Y, Oda M, Okano M (2008) QUMA: quantification tool for methylation analysis. Nucleic Acids Res 36:W170–W175
18. Rohde C, Zhang Y, Reinhardt R et al (2010) BISMA - fast and accurate bisulfite sequencing data analysis of individual clones from unique and repetitive sequences. BMC Bioinformatics 11:1–12
19. Herman JG, Graff JR, Myöhänen S et al (1996) Methylation-specific PCR: a novel PCR assay for methylation status of CpG islands. Proc Natl Acad Sci U S A 93:9821–9826
20. Eads CA, Danenberg KD, Kawakami K et al (2000) MethyLight: a high-throughput assay to measure DNA methylation. Nucleic Acids Res 28:e32–e00
21. Lo PK, Watanabe H, Cheng PC et al (2009) MethySYBR, a novel quantitative PCR assay for the dual analysis of DNA methylation and CpG methylation density. J Mol Diagnostics 11:400–414
22. Lister R, Pelizzola M, Dowen RH et al (2009) Human DNA methylomes at base resolution show widespread epigenomic differences. Nature 462:315–322
23. Meissner A, Gnirke A, Bell GW et al (2005) Reduced representation bisulfite sequencing for comparative high-resolution DNA methylation analysis. Nucleic Acids Res 33:5868–5877
24. Akalin A, Garrett-Bakelman FE, Kormaksson M et al (2012) Base-pair resolution DNA methylation sequencing reveals profoundly divergent epigenetic landscapes in acute myeloid leukemia. PLoS Genet 8:e1002781

Chapter 19

B-Cell Commitment to IL-10 Production: The VertX *Il10*^{egfp} Mouse

Akihiko Oka, Bo Liu, Jeremy W. Herzog, and R. Balfour Sartor

Abstract

Although the inflammatory cytokine IL-10 is pivotal in regulatory B-cell function, detecting IL-10-producing B cells by intracellular IL-10 staining requires multiple steps and tedious preparation. In contrast, the *Il10*-eGFP reporter mouse model (VertX), generated in 2009, allows easier and quicker detection of IL-10-producing B cells with the possibility of sorting viable cells without membrane permeabilization and ex vivo activation. Even though detecting IL-10^{+} cells is simpler, several nuances are important. For example, methanol-containing buffers delete GFP signal, while long-term fixation can maintain GFP intensity but decreases other intracellular signals (FOXP3, etc.). Here, we provide optimized and improved protocols for GFP detection in intestinal B cells and isolation techniques of lamina propria, spleen, mesenteric lymph node, peritoneum, and blood cells from VertX mice.

Key words Regulatory B cell, Interleukin-10, GFP, Mucosal immunology, Flow cytometry, Microbiota, Gnotobiotic mice

1 Introduction

B lymphocytes are able to both drive and inhibit inflammation. They contribute to maintain homeostasis by producing immunoglobulins and cytokines and through antigen presentation [1, 2]. Interleukin (IL)-10 is a key anti-inflammatory cytokine produced by lymphocytes, macrophages, dendritic cells, and epithelial cells [3]. Multiple studies suggest that IL-10-producing B cells play a pivotal role in maintaining mucosal homeostasis [1–4]. Dysfunctional or decreased IL-10-producing regulatory B cells have been observed in several immune-related diseases in human and rodent models [1, 5–9]. Resident microbiota and certain helminths can induce IL-10-producing B cells and attenuate inflammation [1, 2, 4, 10, 11]. Despite the critical protective role of IL-10-producing B cells, their dynamics and functional analyses remain elusive although these are cells being studied with emerging interest [8, 10, 11].

Francesca Mion and Silvia Tonon (eds.), *Regulatory B Cells: Methods and Protocols*, Methods in Molecular Biology, vol. 2270, https://doi.org/10.1007/978-1-0716-1237-8_19, © Springer Science+Business Media, LLC, part of Springer Nature 2021

Several techniques including flow cytometry, immunohistochemistry, quantitative PCR, and western blotting have been used to detect intracellular IL-10. Although flow cytometry is cell-specific and quite sensitive, it requires exacting and prolonged in vitro preparation (6–8 hours in general) before proceeding with the staining of the intracellular cytokine: (1) pharmacological cell stimulation with phorbol myristate acetate, ionomycin and lipopolysaccharide or other activators, (2) protein-transport-blocking with brefeldin A or monensin, (3) cell surface marker staining, and (4) cell fixation followed by the permeabilization of the cell membrane. These multiple steps may potentially change physiologic cytokine levels and transcriptional profiles, and decrease cell recovery. Cytokine reporter mice, characterized by the insertion of a reporter gene (green fluorescent protein [GFP] or other markers) into the target cytokine gene-promoter locus, constitute an improved tool to follow cytokine production since you avoid cell membrane permeabilization and skip long-term preparation. Moreover, by using cytokine reporter mice, the cytokine-producing cells are studied in their "intact" or native state. About 10 years ago, Dr. Karp and coworkers created the *Il10*-eGFP reporter mouse (VertX) with intact production of IL-10 [3], which is now commercially available from the Jackson Laboratory [12]. Further, germ-free (GF) VertX mice are available from the National Gnotobiotic Rodent Resource Center at the University of North Carolina at Chapel Hill (UNC-CH) [13].

This chapter describes the following methods with some critical notes for GFP detection: (1) cell isolation from spleen, mesenteric lymph node (MLN), intestinal lamina propria (LP), peritoneum, and peripheral blood mononuclear cells of VertX mice, (2) surface and intracellular staining for flow cytometry and flow sorting of GFP (IL-10)$^+$ B cells, and (3) representative functional analyses using VertX mice.

2 Materials

2.1 Mice

1. Specific pathogen-free (SPF) *Il10*-eGFP reporter (VertX, $Il10^{egfp}$) mice: provided by UNC-CH, and were originally obtained from Dr. Karp [3]. This strain is commercially available from the Jackson Laboratory (B6(Cg)-$Il10^{tm1.1Karp}$/J) [12]. The genetic background is C57BL/6 J.
2. GF VertX mice: provided by the National Gnotobiotic Rodent Resource Center at UNC-CH [13] where the GF strain was established by embryo transfer. The genetic background is C57BL/6 J.
3. SPF VertX;PI3Kδ^{D910A} mice: the phosphoinositide 3-kinase catalytic subunit p110δ (PI3Kδ) plays a critical role in IL-10

production by B cells [10, 11]. PI3Kp110δ$^{D910A/D910A}$ mutant (PI3Kδ^{D910A}) mice on the C57BL/6 J background, which have a loss-of-function (catalytically inactive) point mutation in a gene encoding the PI3K catalytic subunit p110δ, were previously obtained from Dr. Vanhaesebroeck [14]. VertX;PI3Kδ^{D910A} mice on a C57BL/6 J background were generated by crossing PI3Kδ^{D910A} with VertX mice at UNC-CH.

4. SPF C57BL/6 J mice: bred at UNC-CH, and were originally obtained from the Jackson Laboratory [15].

2.2 Equipment

1. Refrigerated centrifuge, unfixed angle centrifuge.
2. Autoclave.
3. CO_2 incubator.
4. Multi-position magnetic stirrer and stirrer bar.
5. Devices for immunomagnetic separation (magnet and stand, columns, 30-μm pre-separation filters).
6. Automated cell counter.
7. Instruments for organ harvest: forceps, scissors, paper, petri dish, and quad dish.
8. 50 mL glass beaker (or 50 mL polypropylene autoclavable beaker).
9. 15 mL and 50 mL conical tubes and 1.5 mL microcentrifuge tubes.
10. Flow cytometry: an analyzer with up to four laser wavelengths for laser excitation (e.g., BD LSR II cell analyzer), a cell sorter (e.g., FACSAria III cell sorter with FACSDiva software, version 8, BD), and a flow cytometry data analysis tool (FlowJo analysis, version 10, FlowJo).
11. 96-deep-well 1-mL plate.
12. Microplate shaker.
13. Vortex.
14. 20-G needle with cap, sterile.
15. Animal lancet, 4 mm point length, sterile.
16. 1 mL and 10 mL syringe, sterile.
17. 70-μm and 100-μm cell strainers.

2.3 Buffers and Reagents for Cell Isolation from Different Tissues

1. 10× Phosphate-buffered saline (PBS): 80 g NaCl, 2 g KCl, 17.8 g $Na_2HPO_4{\cdot}2H_2O$, 2.4 g KH_2PO_4, adjust final volume to 1000 mL with distilled water, sterilize by autoclaving, pH 6.8 (*see* **Note 1**).
2. Hank's balanced salt solution (HBSS): 8 g NaCl, 400 mg KCl, 140 mg $CaCl_2$, 100 mg $MgSO_4{\cdot}7H_2O$, 100 mg $MgCl_2{\cdot}6H_2O$,

60 mg $Na_2HPO_2 \cdot 2H_2O$, 60 mg KH_2PO_4, 1 g D-Glucose, 350 mg $NaHCO_3$, adjust final volume to 1000 mL, sterilize by autoclaving, pH 7.4.

3. Harvest buffer: 50 μg/mL gentamycin in 1× PBS.
4. Wash medium: 2.5% heat-inactivated fetal bovine serum (HI-FBS) and 100 U/mL penicillin-streptomycin in HBSS.
5. Red blood cell lysing buffer: 150 mM ammonium chloride, 10 mM potassium bicarbonate, and 0.1 mM EDTA (*see* **Note 2**).
6. Epithelial removal medium: 1 mM DL-dithiothreitol, 1 mM EDTA, 2.5% HI-FBS, and 100 U/mL penicillin-streptomycin in HBSS.
7. Digestion medium: 0.5 mg/mL collagenase Type IV, 2.5% HI-FBS and 100 U/mL penicillin-streptomycin in HBSS.
8. 100% Percoll (prepare 100 mL): 90% of Percoll (90 mL) + 10% of 10× PBS (10 mL).
9. 40% Percoll in HBSS (prepare 100 mL): 40% of 100% Percoll (40 mL) + 60% of HBSS (60 mL) (*see* **Note 3**).
10. 70% Percoll in HBSS (prepare 100 mL) = 70% of 100% Percoll (70 mL) + 30% of HBSS (30 mL) (*see* **Note 3**).
11. Heparin (stock 173 USP units/mg).
12. Anti-CD19 magnetic beads (*see* **Note 4**).
13. Modified MACS buffer: 10% HI-FBS in 1× PBS.

2.4 Reagents for the Identification of GFP⁺ B Cells by Flow Cytometry

1. Antibodies/reagents for cell staining (*see* Table 1). Every antibody/reagent needs to be titrated starting from manufacturer's instructions.
2. Compensation bead kit.
3. Fixation buffer: 4% paraformaldehyde and 0.01% Tween 20 in 1× PBS.
4. Phorbol 12-myristate 13-acetate (PMA, stock 1 mg/mL).
5. Ionomycin (stock 1 mg/mL).
6. GolgiStop (0.26% protein transport inhibitor monensin, BD).
7. Complete culture medium: 10% HI-FBS, 100 U/mL penicillin/streptomycin, 1 mM sodium pyruvate and 50 μM 2-mercaptoethanol in RPMI1640.
8. Permeabilization buffer: 0.1% Triton X-100, 0.5% bovine serum albumin (BSA) and 2 mM EDTA in 1× PBS.
9. CpG-ODN 1826 (stock 500 μM) (*see* **Note 5**).

Table 1
Antibodies/reagents for surface staining

Antibody/reagent	Clone	Fluorochrome	Isotype
Fc blocker (anti-CD16/CD32)	2.4G2	–	–
LIVE/DEAD fixable near-IR dead cell stain kit	–	APC-Cy7	–
CD45	30-F11	Pacific Orange	Rat IgG2b κ
B220 (CD45R)	RA3-6B2	Pacific blue	Rat IgG2a κ
CD19	6D5	BV605	Rat IgG2a κ

3 Methods

To date, several IL-10 reporter strains have been published (*see* Fig. 1) [3, 16–21] and nicely summarized by Bouabe [22]. The VertX strain was generated by inserting an internal ribosome entry site (IRES)-eGFP cassette along with polyadenylation sequence of bovine growth hormone (BGHpA) at the end of the last exon of the IL-10 gene [3, 22] (*see* Fig. 1). In contrast to some other reporter strains, such as *Il10*^{eYFP}, the IRES sequence enables the intact transcription of IL-10 along with eGFP under the control of the endogenous *Il10* promoter. *Il10* translation remains cap-dependent, whereas the translation of eGFP is driven by IRES [3, 22]. Furthermore, VertX strain has an advantage of stability of eGFP reporter mRNA because of the exchange of an endogenous mRNA-destabilizing 3′ untranslated region (3′UTR) for an exogenous mRNA-stabilizing polyadenylation sequence (BGHpA). In addition, BGHpA has higher mRNA and protein expression level than other polyadenylation sequences, such as simian vacuolating virus 40 (SV40pA) used in the other reporter strains [22]. Therefore, in VertX mice, functionally intact IL-10 protein can be secreted rapidly, whereas the GFP reporter protein remains intracellular longer [3, 22]. VertX mice indeed show higher reporter sensitivity compared to other reporter strains: many types of cells including B cells express eGFP reporter in VertX mice, whereas in some other reporter strains, only $CD4^+$ T cells express the reporter in the steady state [3, 22]. In this section, we describe cell isolation and GFP detection methods suitable for VertX mice.

3.1 Isolation of Cells from Several Tissues

The following protocols describe the procedures employed to isolate the total cell population from different organs. Regardless of the tissue under analysis, the subsequent purification of wild-type and of GFP^+ B lymphocytes from the total pool of cells is performed by positive selection using anti-CD19 magnetic beads and following manufacturer's instructions (*see* **Note 4**). Table 2 shows yields of both total and B cells obtained through these isolation protocols.

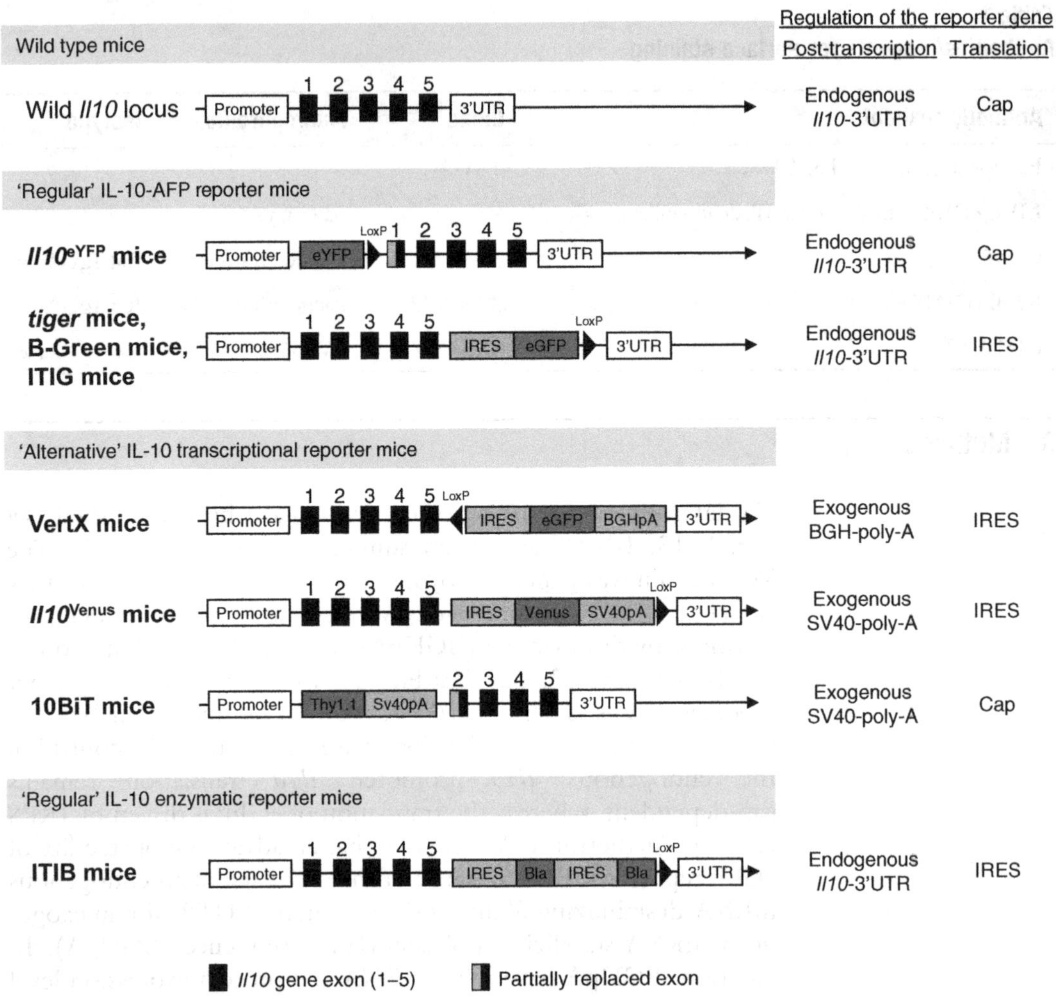

Fig. 1 *Il10* reporter allele in the *Il10* locus of reporter mice. 3′UTR: 3′ untranslated region. eYFP: enhanced yellow fluorescent protein. IRES: internal ribosome entry site. eGFP: enhanced green fluorescent protein. BGHpA: bovine growth hormone polyadenylation sequence. SV40pA: simian vacuolating virus 40 polyadenylation sequence. Thy1.1: Thymus cell antigen 1.1 (CD90.1). Bla: β-lactamase (reporter enzyme). References: *Il10*^{eYFP} mice [16], *tiger* mice [17], B-Green mice [20], ITIG mice [21], VertX mice [3], *Il10*^{Venus} mice [19], 10BiT mice [18], and ITIB mice [21]. Figure is adapted and modified from [22]

3.1.1 Isolation of Spleen and Mesenteric Lymph Node Cells

1. Harvest spleen and mesenteric lymph nodes (MLN) without fat tissue and place in cold harvest buffer.
2. Smash the spleen and MLN by a needle cap (or rubber plunger head) on 70-μm cell strainer and wash the strainer with 5 mL of cold wash media (*see* Fig. 2). Centrifuge at 450 × *g* for 5 min at 4 °C and discard supernatant.
3. For splenocytes (for MLN cells, go to **step 4**), resuspend pellet in red blood cell lysing buffer (5 mL/spleen) and incubate for 3–5 min at 18–22 °C. Add 10 mL of wash medium and filter

Table 2
Yield of cell isolation

($\times 10^6$ cells/mouse, mean $\pm$ SD)	MLN		Spleen		cLP		Peritoneum	PBMC
Mice	Total	$CD19^+$	Total	$CD19^+$	Total	$CD19^+$	Total	Total
GF VertX	12 ± 4.1	1.9 ± 0.4	73 ± 33	21 ± 5.9	2.7 ± 1.4	0.4 ± 0.2	N/A	N/A
SPF-colonized exGF VertX	45 ± 8.4	5.0 ± 1.5	184 ± 49	35 ± 7.2	5.3 ± 4.8	1.0 ± 0.2	N/A	N/A
SPF-raised VertX	16 ± 4.4	2.6 ± 0.5	86 ± 21	24 ± 8.6	4.1 ± 2.2	0.5 ± 0.3	6.5 ± 0.5	1.0 ± 0.5

GF: germ-free, SPF: specific pathogen-free, exGF: germ-free mice colonized for 2 weeks, MLN: mesenteric lymph node, cLP: colonic lamina propria, PBMC: peripheral blood mononuclear cell, N/A: not available, N = 3–37 mice/group, 8–14 weeks old

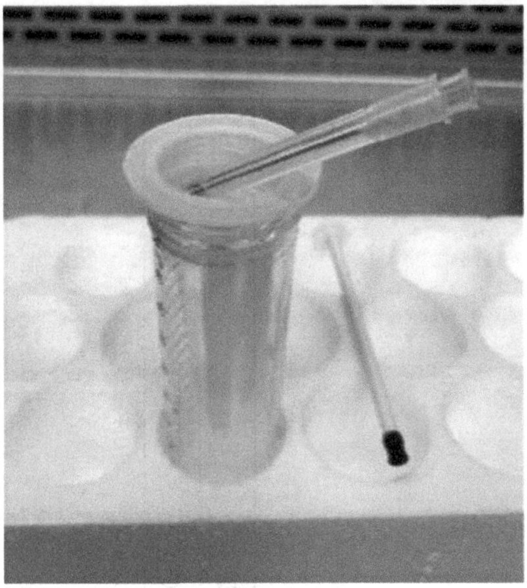

Fig. 2 Isolation of spleen and mesenteric lymph node cells. In order to obtain a single-cell population, spleens or mesenteric lymph nodes are smashed on a cell strainer by the needle cap (or rubber plunger head)

through a 70-μm cell strainer. Centrifuge at 450 × *g* for 5 min at 4 °C and discard supernatant. If the cell pellet looks still red, repeat **step 3**.

4. Resuspend cells in complete culture medium and count cells.

3.1.2 Isolation of Intestinal Lamina propria Mononuclear Cells

This protocol is suitable for colonic lamina propria. For small intestine, duodenum, and stomach, increase EDTA final concentration in epithelial removal medium from 1 mM to at least 3 mM.

1. To prepare the tissue, harvest colon without fat tissue and place in cold harvest buffer (*see* **Note 6**). Cut intestine longitudinally to remove luminal contents and wash in cold harvest buffer (*see* Fig. 3a). Remove mucus by rolling intestine on paper towel (*see* **Note** 7).
2. To remove the epithelial layer, cut intestine into 10 mm pieces and incubate in 20 mL of pre-warmed (37 °C) epithelial removal medium for 20 min at 37 °C with 250 rpm stir in 50 mL beaker (*see* Fig. 3b). Discard supernatant by aspiration with pipet (or pouring) and wash the intestine with pre-warmed (37 °C) wash medium to remove DL-dithiothreitol and EDTA (*see* **Note 8**).
3. To digest the lamina propria, incubate intestine in 20 mL of pre-warmed (37 °C) digestion medium for 30 min at 37 °C with 350 rpm stir in 50 mL beaker (*see* **Note 9**). Filter supernatant (containing lamina propria cells) and digested intestine

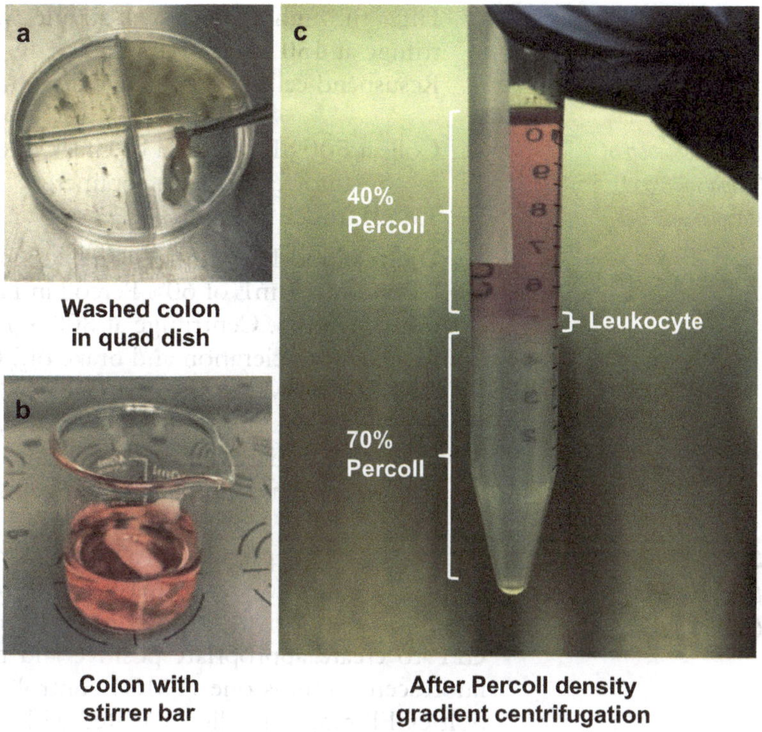

Fig. 3 Lamina propria cell isolation. (**a**) The colon is washed in a quad dish. (**b**) Incubation of colon pieces in beaker with stirrer bar. (**c**) Result of the Percoll density gradient centrifugation

through a 100-μm cell strainer with pre-warmed (37 °C) wash medium. Centrifuge at 450 × g for 10 min at 18–22 °C and discard the supernatant.

4. Resuspend the pellet in 5 mL of 40% Percoll in 15 mL conical tube. Carefully add 5 mL of 70% Percoll under the 40% Percoll layer with a 5 mL pipet (or dropper) without disrupting the 40/70% interface. Centrifuge at 800 × *g* for 20 min at 18–22 °C with slow acceleration and brake off. At the end of the centrifugation, collect the white layer (leukocyte layer) in the 40/70% interface with a 1000-μL tip (or dropper) (*see* Fig. 3c) (*see* **Note 10**). Resuspend in 50 mL of cold HBSS and centrifuge at 450 × *g* for 10 min at 4 °C and discard the supernatant. Resuspend cells in complete culture medium and count cells.

3.1.3 Isolation of Peritoneal Cells

1. Inject 10 mL of RPMI medium into the peritoneal cavity by 10 mL syringe with a 20-G needle. Tilt the mouse vertically and horizontally and collect the injected RPMI medium by a 10-mL syringe with a 20-G needle.

2. Filter through a 70-μm cell strainer with wash medium. Centrifuge at 450 × *g* for 10 min at 4 °C and discard supernatant. Resuspend cells in complete culture medium and count cells.

3.1.4 Isolation of Peripheral Blood Mononuclear Cells

1. Collect 500 μL of blood by cheek puncture with animal lancet or postmortem cardiac puncture into a heparin-coated 1.5 mL tube.
2. Dilute blood 1:1 with HBSS and then put 1 mL of the diluted blood onto 1 mL of 60% Percoll in HBSS for density gradient centrifugation. Centrifuge at 800 × *g* for 10 min at 18–22 °C with slow acceleration and brake off. Collect the white mononuclear cell layer at the interface of plasma/Percoll and resuspend in 15 mL of cold HBSS. Centrifuge at 450 × *g* for 10 min at 4 °C and discard the supernatant. Resuspend cells in complete culture medium and count cells.

3.2 Identification of GFP+ B Cells by Flow Cytometry

Because the GFP+ population is frequently small in VertX mice with dim GFP signal that can be masked with auto-fluorescence, precise negative and positive controls are required. A negative control for GFP to create appropriate positive and negative gates requires a fluorescence-minus-one (FMO) control, which is represented by non-eGFP reporter cells incubated with the same antibodies used to stain the experimental samples (*see* Fig. 4a) [23]. Importantly, some fixation and permeabilization buffers, especially the ones containing methanol, dampen GFP intensity (*see* Fig. 4b) [24], while the buffers described in this protocol do not.

3.2.1 Staining of Surface Markers for Flow Cytometry

1. Prepare samples by resuspending 1 × 10^6 cells in 45 μL of 1× PBS in a 96-well plate (*see* **Note 11**). The FMO control (non-eGFP reporter cells from C57BL/6 J mice) should be included as well as samples in the experimental plan (*see* **Note 12**).
2. For cell surface staining, incubate cells for 5 min at 4 °C with Fc blocker diluted according to manufacturer's instructions. Add 50 μL of titrated antibodies diluted in 1× PBS (*see* Table 1) and incubate at 4 °C for 20 min. After staining, add 100 μL of 1× PBS, centrifuge at 350 × *g* at 4 °C for 5 min and flick off supernatant.
3. To fix the samples, resuspend cells in 50 μL of pre-warmed (37 °C) fixation buffer and incubate at 37 °C for 5 min (*see* **Note 13**). Add 150 μL of 1× PBS, centrifuge at 350 × *g* for 5 min and flick off supernatant.
4. Resuspend cells in 200 μL of 1× PBS and keep at 4 °C before flow cytometry analysis. Representative results using this protocol are shown in Fig. 4.

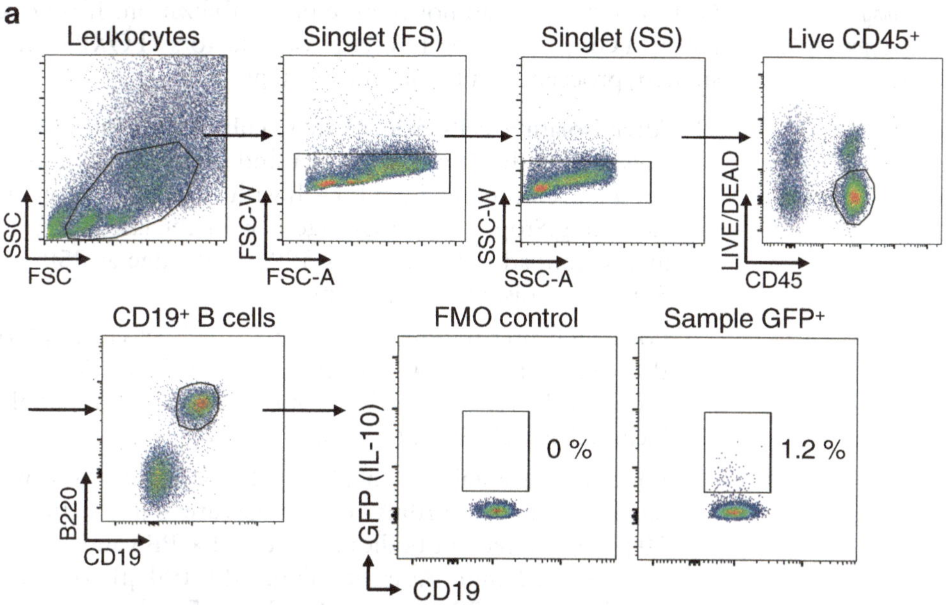

	<u>FMO control</u> Non-GFP-reporter cells (from C57BL6/J)	<u>Sample</u> GFP-reporter cells (from VertX)
LIVE/DEAD (APC-Cy7)	+	+
CD45 (Pacific Orange)	+	+
B220 (Pacific Blue)	+	+
CD19 (BV605)	+	+
GFP	–	+

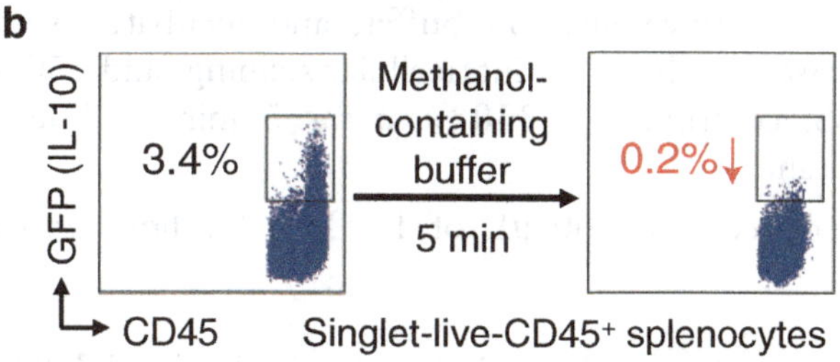

Fig. 4 GFP (IL-10) gating strategy. (**a**) Colonic lamina propria cells isolated from VertX mice were stained (LIVE/DEAD and anti-CD45, -B220 and -CD19 antibodies) and analyzed by flow cytometry. For the fluorescent-minus-one (FMO) control, non-eGFP reporter cells from the colonic lamina propria of C57BL6/J mice were stained by all antibodies and used to set the GFP-positive gate. (**b**) Splenocytes isolated from VertX mice were cultured with 500 nM CpG-ODN in complete culture medium for 24 h. The cultured splenocytes were stained with the LIVE/DEAD dye and anti-CD45 antibody and analyzed by flow cytometry. The flow dot plot shows singlet-live-CD45$^+$ splenocytes before exposure to methanol-containing buffer (left panel) and after incubation with methanol-containing buffer for 5 min (right panel). A reduction of GFP (IL-10) signal was observed when using a methanol-containing buffer

3.2.2 Staining Intracellular Cytokines for Flow Cytometry

GFP reporter cells do not require permeabilization. If other cytokines (TGF-β1 etc.) or transcriptional factors (FOXP3 etc.) are stained, proceed with the following steps.

1. After isolating cells from tissues, culture cells at 1–5 × 10^6 cells/mL with 50 ng/mL PMA and 1 μg/mL ionomycin in complete culture medium for 4 h with vortexing every 30 min. Add GolgiStop (1 μL/mL) together for the last 3 h. After 4 h incubation, add 10 mL of 1× PBS, centrifuge at 350 × *g* for 5 min, and discard supernatant.
2. For sample preparation, resuspend 1 × 10^6 cells in 45 μL of 1× PBS buffer in a 96-well plate (*see* **Note 11**). FMO control (non-eGFP reporter cells from C57BL/6 J) should be included as well as samples (*see* **Note 12**).
3. For cell surface staining, incubate cells for 5 min at 4 °C with Fc blocker diluted according to manufacturer's instructions. Add 50 μL of titrated antibodies diluted in 1× PBS and incubate at 4 °C for 20 min. After staining, add 100 μL of 1× PBS, centrifuge at 350 × *g* at 4 °C for 5 min, and flick off supernatant.
4. To fix cells, resuspend cells in 50 μL of pre-warmed (37 °C) fixation buffer and incubate at 37 °C for 5 min (*see* **Note 13**). Add 150 μL of 1× PBS, centrifuge at 350 × *g* for 5 min, and flick off supernatant.
5. For the permeabilization step, incubate 1 × 10^6 cells in 50 μL of permeabilization buffer at room temperature for 45 min with shaking at 360 rpm. Add 150 μL of 1× PBS, centrifuge at 350 × *g* for 5 min, and flick off supernatant.
6. For intracellular staining, add 100 μL of titrated antibodies diluted in permeabilization buffer, and incubate overnight (or at least for 2 h). After intracellular staining, add 150 μL of 1× PBS, centrifuge at 350 × *g* for 5 min, and flick off supernatant.
7. Resuspend cells in 200 μL of 1× PBS for flow cytometry analysis.

3.2.3 Special Compensation Controls for Flow Cytometry

For flow cytometry compensation, we use the bead kit which provides clearly separated positive and negative signals in contrast to actual cells. However, GFP and LIVE/DEAD dye compensations need actual cells. Although GFP can be detected by the FITC channel, GFP and FITC have different emission spectra. Therefore, we need GFP-expressing cells instead of FITC-antibody-stained cells. In order to obtain strong GFP signal, it is better to re-stimulate cells ex vivo with CpG-ODN because GFP expression in VertX mice is not so bright (dim) in a steady state. Similarly, as the LIVE/DEAD dye works for compromised membranes of apoptotic/necrotic cells (*see* **Note 14**), it is better to boil control cells to have strong dead signals.

1. For the GFP-positive control, culture overnight (or at least for 5 h) 1×10^6 cells from VertX with 500 nM CpG-ODN in complete culture medium in a 37 °C and 5% CO_2 incubator. Wash with 1× PBS and centrifuge at 350 × *g* for 5 min. Resuspend cells in 200 μL of 1× PBS for flow cytometry analysis (*see* **Note 15**).
2. For the LIVE/DEAD staining positive control, boil 1×10^6 non-eGFP reporter cells in hot water for 10 sec and stain with LIVE/DEAD staining dye in 1× PBS for 20 min. Wash with 1× PBS and centrifuge at 350 × *g* for 5 min. Resuspend cells in 200 μL of 1× PBS for flow cytometry analysis (*see* **Notes 14** and **16**).

3.3 Functional Analysis of GFP+ B Cell In Vivo and In Vitro

Here below, two representative methods that require the employment of VertX mice are described.

3.3.1 GFP+ B Cells in exGF VertX Mice

1. Collect fresh feces from specific pathogen-free (SPF) C57BL/6 J mice and pool together three feces in 3 mL of 1× PBS. Homogenize feces and inoculate to germ-free (GF) VertX mice by swabbing orally and rectally (conventionalization).
2. By 2 weeks after conventionalization, detect GFP+ B cells in the lamina propria. Isolate cells as in Subheading 3.1.2 and proceed with cell surface staining as in Subheading 3.2.1. Cells can be then sorted or simply analyzed by flow cytometry. Figure 5a shows the results of GFP (IL-10) induction in lamina propria B cells by resident microbiota colonization.
3. For the flow-sorting of GFP+ B cells, create GFP-positive and -negative gates based on the FMO control (*see* Subheading 3.2). According to the sequential assay (culture, RNA sequencing, quantitative PCR, etc.), sort cells directly into medium, TRIzol or RNAlater, etc. (when required by the case, add RNase inhibitor) [25] with a four-way-purity mode. Figure 5b shows the results of post-sorting.

3.3.2 Comparison of GFP Expression between Wild-Type and Gene-Modified B Cells

Several genes are involved in IL-10 signaling. If a certain gene is modified in GFP reporter mice, you can assess whether GFP expression remains unchanged or is either reduced or increased in gene-modified respect to wild-type mice. This allows to uncover a possible role for the modified gene in IL-10 signaling. For example, PI3Kδ signaling positively regulates IL-10 production [10, 11].

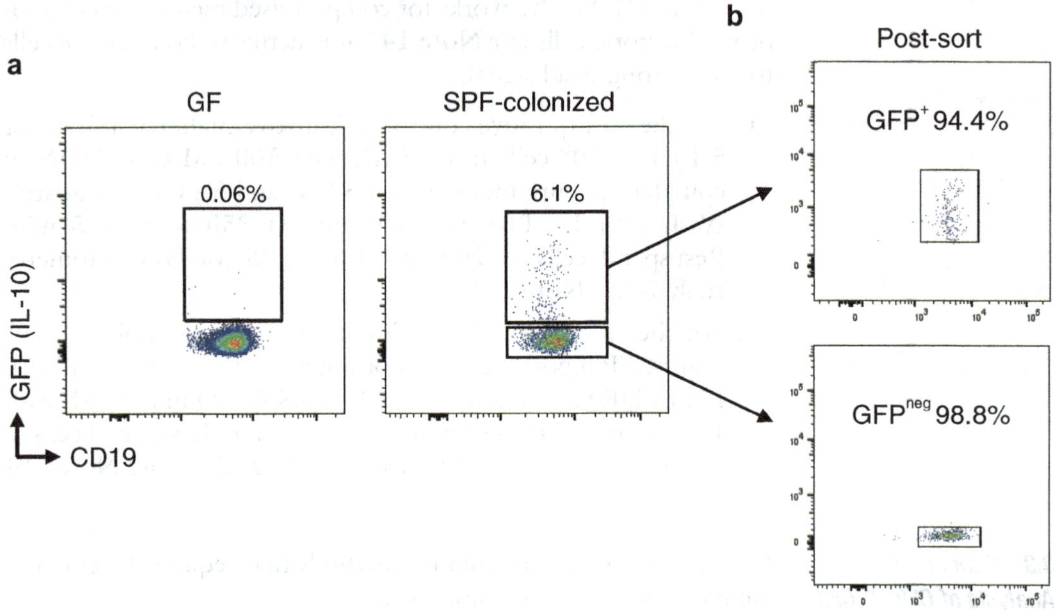

Fig. 5 GFP$^+$CD19$^+$ cells induced by specific pathogen-free (SPF) gut microbiota colonization in germ-free (GF) mice. Two weeks after colonization, colonic lamina propria cells isolated from non-eGFP reporter (C57BL6/J, as a fluorescent-minus-one [FMO] control) and VertX mice were stained (LIVE/DEAD dye and anti-CD45, -B220 and -CD19 antibodies) and flow-sorted in the four-way-purity mode. GFP gates were set based on the FMO control. (**a**) Colonic lamina propria GFP$^+$CD19$^+$ cells in GF and SPF-colonized GF VertX mice. (**b**) Post-sort analysis showing the purity of flow-sorted cells

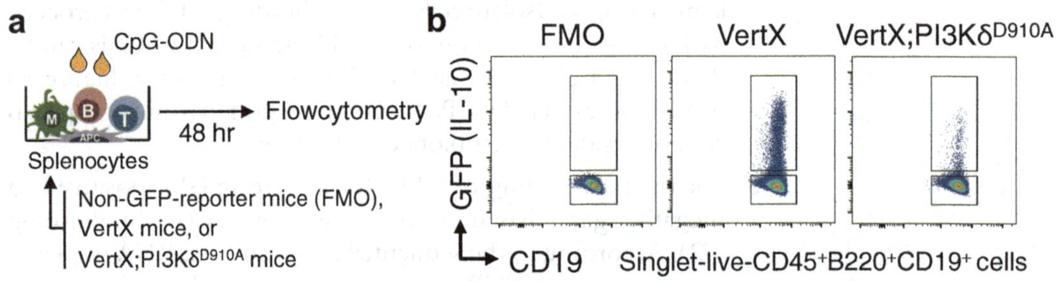

Fig. 6 GFP (IL-10) detection by flow cytometry. (**a**) Unfractionated splenocytes isolated from non-eGFP reporter (C57BL6/J, as a fluorescent-minus-one [FMO] control), VertX, and VertX;PI3Kδ^{D910A} mice were cultured with 500 nM CpG-ODN in complete medium for 48 h. The cultured cells were stained (LIVE/DEAD dye and anti-CD45, -B220 and -CD19 antibodies) and analyzed by flow cytometry. GFP gates were set based on the FMO control. (**b**) Flow dot plots showing singlet-live-CD45$^+$B220$^+$CD19$^+$ B cells and GFP-positive (upper) and -negative (lower) gates

1. Isolate total splenocytes (or MLN cells) from VertX and VertX; PI3Kδ^{D910A} mice. After counting cells, culture viable cells at 1×10^6 cells/mL in complete culture medium with 500 nM CpG-ODN. Incubate in a 37 °C 5% CO_2 incubator for 48 h (*see* Fig. 6a).

2. At the end of the 48-h stimulation, collect the cells and stain with antibodies directed against the surface markers CD45, B220, and CD19 as described in Subheading 3.2.1.
3. Run flow cytometry and compare GFP (IL-10) expression in B cells from VertX and VertX;PI3Kδ^{D910A} mice. Figure 6b shows reduced GFP (IL-10) production by PI3Kδ^{D910A} mutation compared to PI3Kδ wild type.

4 Notes

1. The pH of the 10× stock will be 6.8. When diluted to 1× PBS, the pH should change to 7.4 which is the normal pH for 1× PBS. If necessary, adjust pH using hydrochloric acid or sodium hydroxide.
2. The red blood cell lysing buffer can be homemade or purchased from different suppliers.
3. To see interface clearly, HBSS for 40% Percoll is phenol-red (+), while HBSS for 70% Percoll is phenol-red-free.
4. We routinely use CD19 microbeads from Miltenyi Biotec. The protocol for B cells isolation is according to the manufacturer's instruction, except for MACS buffer. Indeed, a modified MACS buffer was used (*see* Subheading 2.3).
5. CpG ODN1826 sequence: 5′- TCCATGACGTTCCT GACGTT-3′ [26].
6. Fat (adipose) tissue can reduce isolation yield and also potentially lead to contamination by immune cells present within the fat, such as macrophages, regulatory T cells, and natural killer T cells [27].
7. Mucus can reduce isolation yield due to clogging of the cell strainer.
8. The supernatant contains epithelial layer cells, which can be used for other assays [28].
9. To increase yield or shorten isolation time, additional collagenase, DNase I (40 μg/mL), or dispase (0.5–1 mg/mL) can be used [28–30]. Of note, these agents potentially disrupt lymphocyte surface markers likely due to contamination by proteases present in the enzyme preparations [31, 32]. Additional serum and trypsin inhibitor in digestion medium or overnight culture in complete culture medium after digestion may rescue this problem. Repeating short digestion rounds may help.
10. Do not take much Percoll with white layer cells since it reduces the efficacy of sequential centrifugation. If there is no pellet after centrifugation, add more HBSS to the cell suspension to dilute Percoll and centrifuge again.

11. Do not add FBS or BSA to the staining buffer when using LIVE/DEAD staining kit. The dyes in the kit react with proteins (FBS or BSA), resulting in no LIVE/DEAD signal. Use 1× PBS for staining buffer according to the manufacturer's manual.
12. For an optimal FMO control, use the same type of cells that means the same genetic background (C57BL6/J), same tissue, and same isolation process.
13. Do not incubate longer than 5 min. Long-term fixation significantly reduces intracellular fluorescence signals [33].
14. Another option is a compensation bead kit for LIVE/DEAD staining, the ArC Amine reactive compensation bead kit (Invitrogen), which does not require actual cells.
15. As a GFP compensation control, another option instead of using freshly isolated cells is to defreeze GFP^+ cells stored in RPMI1640 supplemented with 10% dimethyl sulfoxide and 10% HI-FBS. Wash thawed GFP^+ cells with 1× PBS and resuspend 1×10^6 cells in 200 μL of 1× PBS for flow cytometry analysis.
16. Do not permeabilize LIVE/DEAD stained cells. Permeabilization can reduce the intensity of the LIVE/DEAD dye.

Acknowledgments

We thank Dr. C.L. Karp for providing VertX mice and Dr. B. Vanhaesebroeck for providing $PI3K\delta^{D910A}$ mice. The authors are supported by grants from National Institute of Health (P01DK094779; P30DK034987; P40OD010995) and Crohn's & Colitis Foundation Research Fellowship Award (407007) and Gnotobiotic Facility. The UNC Flow Cytometry Core Facility is supported in part by P30CA016086 Cancer Center Core Support Grant to the UNC Lineberger Comprehensive Cancer Center. The flow cytometry research reported in this publication was supported in part by the North Carolina Biotech Center Institutional Support Grant 2012-IDG-1006.

References

1. Mizoguchi A, Mizoguchi E, Smith RN et al (1997) Suppressive role of B cells in chronic colitis of T cell receptor α mutant mice. J Exp Med 186:1749–1756
2. Tedder TF (2015) B10 cells: a functionally defined regulatory B cell subset. J Immunol 194:1395–1401
3. Madan R, Demircik F, Surianarayanan S et al (2009) Nonredundant roles for B cell-derived IL-10 in immune counter-regulation. J Immunol 183:2312–2320
4. Mishima Y, Liu B, Hansen JJ, Sartor RB (2015) Resident bacteria-stimulated IL-10-secreting B cells ameliorate T cell-mediated colitis by inducing Tr-1 cells that require IL-27-signaling. Cell Mol Gastroenterol Hepatol 1:295–310

5. Oka A, Ishihara S, Mishima Y et al (2014) Role of regulatory B cells in chronic intestinal inflammation: association with pathogenesis of Crohn's disease. Inflamm Bowel Dis 20:315–328
6. Mizoguchi A, Bhan AK (2006) A case for regulatory B cells. J Immunol 176:705–710
7. Wei B, Velazquez P, Turovskaya O et al (2005) Mesenteric B cells centrally inhibit $CD4^+$ T cell colitis through interaction with regulatory T cell subsets. Proc Natl Acad Sci U S A 102:2010–2015
8. Mauri C, Menon M (2017) Human regulatory B cells in health and disease: therapeutic potential. J Clin Invest 127:772–779
9. Mishima Y, Ishihara S, Aziz MM et al (2010) Decreased production of interleukin-10 and transforming growth factor-β in toll-like receptor-activated intestinal B cells in SAMP1/Yit mice. Immunology 131:473–487
10. Mishima Y, Oka A, Liu B et al (2019) Microbiota maintain colonic homeostasis by activating TLR2/MyD88/PI3K signaling in IL-10-producing regulatory B cells. J Clin Invest 130:3702–3716
11. Oka A, Mishima Y, Liu B et al (2019) Phosphoinositide 3-kinase P110δ-signaling is critical for microbiota-activated IL-10 production by B cells that regulate intestinal inflammation. Cells 8:1121. https://doi.org/10.3390/cells8101121
12. The Jackson Laboratory (2020) Mouse strain datasheet, B6(Cg)-Il10tm1.1Karp/J, Stock No:014530, Vert-X (or VertX). https://www.jax.org/strain/014530. Accessed 2 Feb 2020
13. The National Gnotobiotic Rodent Resource Center, University of North Carolina at Chapel Hill (2020). Price list Gnotobiotic mice. https://www.med.unc.edu/ngrrc/price-list/. Accessed 2 Feb 2020
14. Okkenhaug K, Bilancio A, Farjot G et al (2002) Impaired B and T cell antigen receptor signaling in p110delta PI 3-kinase mutant mice. Science 297:1031–1034
15. The Jackson Laboratory (2020) Mouse strain datasheet, C57BL/6J, Stock No:000664, Black 6. https://www.jax.org/strain/000664. Accessed 2 Feb 2020
16. Calado DP, Paixão T, Holmberg D, Haury M (2006) Stochastic monoallelic expression of IL-10 in T cells. J Immunol 177:5358–5364
17. Kamanaka M, Kim ST, Wan YY et al (2006) Expression of Interleukin-10 in intestinal lymphocytes detected by an Interleukin-10 reporter Knockin tiger mouse. Immunity 25:941–952
18. Maynard CL, Harrington LE, Janowski KM et al (2007) Regulatory T cells expressing interleukin 10 develop from $Foxp3^+$ and $Foxp3^-$ precursor cells in the absence of interleukin 10. Nat Immunol 8:931–941
19. Atarashi K, Tanoue T, Shima T et al (2011) Induction of colonic regulatory T cells by indigenous Clostridium species. Science 331:337–341
20. Neves P, Lampropoulou V, Calderon-Gomez E et al (2010) Signaling via the MyD88 adaptor protein in B cells suppresses protective immunity during Salmonella typhimurium infection. Immunity 33:777–790
21. Bouabe H, Liu Y, Moser M et al (2011) Novel highly sensitive IL-10–β-lactamase reporter mouse reveals cells of the innate immune system as a substantial source of IL-10 in vivo. J Immunol 187:3165–3176
22. Bouabe H (2012) Cytokine reporter mice: the special case of IL-10. Scand J Immunol 75:553–567
23. Roederer M (2002) Compensation in Flow Cytometry. Curr Protoc Cytom 22:Unit 1.14.1–Unit 1.1420
24. Schwarz MK, Scherbarth A, Sprengel R et al (2015) Fluorescent-protein stabilization and high-resolution imaging of cleared, intact mouse brains. PLoS One 10:e0124650. https://doi.org/10.1371/journal.pone.0124650
25. Tighe S, Held MA (2010) Isolation of total RNA from transgenic mouse melanoma subsets using fluorescence-activated cell sorting. Methods Mol Biol 632:27–44
26. Ballas ZK, Krieg AM, Warren T et al (2001) Divergent therapeutic and immunologic effects of Oligodeoxynucleotides with distinct CpG motifs. J Immunol 167:4878–4886
27. Lynch L, Michelet X, Zhang S et al (2015) Regulatory iNKT cells lack expression of the transcription factor PLZF and control the homeostasis of T(reg) cells and macrophages in adipose tissue. Nat Immunol 16:85–95
28. Weigmann B, Tubbe I, Seidel D et al (2007) Isolation and subsequent analysis of murine lamina propria mononuclear cells from colonic tissue. Nat Protoc 2:2307–2311
29. Sefik E, Geva-Zatorsky N, Oh S et al (2015) Individual intestinal symbionts induce a distinct population of $ROR\gamma^+$ regulatory T cells. Science 349:993–997
30. Ivanov II, McKenzie BS, Zhou L et al (2006) The orphan nuclear receptor RORγt directs the differentiation program of Proinflammatory $IL\text{-}17^+$ T helper cells. Cell 126:1121–1133

31. Mulder WMC, Koenen H, van de Muysenberg AJC et al (1994) Reduced expression of distinct T-cell CD molecules by collagenase/DNase treatment. Cancer Immunol Immunother 38:253–258
32. Abuzakouk M, Feighery C, O'Farrelly C (1996) Collagenase and Dispase enzymes disrupt lymphocyte surface molecules. J Immunol Methods 194:211–216
33. Grupillo M, Lakomy R, Geng X et al (2011) An improved intracellular staining protocol for efficient detection of nuclear proteins in YFP-expressing cells. BioTechniques 51:417–420

Part IV

Study of Regulatory B Cells in Pathological Settings

Chapter 20

Regulatory B Cells in Experimental Mouse Models of Arthritis

Diana E. Matei, Claudia Mauri, and Elizabeth C. Rosser

Abstract

Regulatory B cells (Breg) have been shown to have a role in the suppression of a wide variety of immune responses, yet they are deficient or defective in autoimmune diseases such as rheumatoid arthritis. For the study of autoimmune inflammation, experimental models of arthritis have acted as a valuable tool in understanding the development of Bregs and their role in maintaining immune homeostasis. In this chapter, we will focus on the study of transitional-2 marginal zone precursor (T2-MZP) Bregs in the context of two experimental arthritis models: antigen-induced arthritis (AIA) and collagen-induced arthritis (CIA). We will specifically focus on how to induce arthritis, as well as on methods for the isolation and functional study of Bregs both in vitro and in vivo.

Key words Arthritis, Regulatory B cells, Inflammation, IL-10, Autoimmunity, T2-MZP B cells

1 Introduction

Our group and others have shown that regulatory B cells (Breg) develop in response to inflammatory cues with the main aim of preventing the excessive damage caused by unrestrained inflammation. Experimental models of arthritis have been used as a model of inflammation to elucidate many intricacies of Breg development and function. For instance, by using the collagen-induced arthritis (CIA) model, previous work by this laboratory has revealed the importance of anti-CD40 stimulation in inducing IL-10 production and supporting the suppressive function of Bregs. CIA has also been pivotal in allowing us to identify splenic transitional-2-marginal zone precursor B cells (T2-MZP) as a candidate cell for a Breg phenotype [1, 2]. Moreover, by using the antigen-induced arthritis (AIA) model, we have also identified that the lack of arthritogenic inflammation, observed when mice are treated with gut microbiota-depleting antibiotics, leads to a significant reduction in the number of functional Bregs [3]. The use of the AIA model has also previously revealed that Bregs have the ability to

Francesca Mion and Silvia Tonon (eds.), *Regulatory B Cells: Methods and Protocols*, Methods in Molecular Biology, vol. 2270, https://doi.org/10.1007/978-1-0716-1237-8_20,

support regulatory T-cell (Treg) differentiation at the expense of pro-inflammatory CD4$^+$ and CD8$^+$ T-cell differentiation [4]. Although the suppressive function of Bregs is now well established, their phenotype has still not been fully elucidated, and it has been a hope in the field that a transcription factor specific for Bregs, similar to Foxp3 for Tregs, will eventually be found. Recent work from our group has shown, with the use of the AIA model, that the aryl hydrocarbon receptor (AhR) is highly expressed in IL-10$^+$CD19$^+$CD21^{hi}CD24^{hi} Bregs, and that this transcription factor skews their differentiation from pro-inflammatory B cells into regulatory B cells, finding supported by the exacerbated arthritis developed by B-cell-specific AhR-deficient mice [5].

These two models of arthritis are induced models, each with their own advantages and limitations. CIA is the most commonly used model of arthritis and is induced using an autoantigen, type II collagen, emulsified in complete Freund's adjuvant (CFA) to break immunological tolerance [1, 2, 6, 7]. This leads to the development of a polyarthritis, characterized by a monophasic inflammatory reaction of affected joints, including synovial hyperplasia and cartilage degradation. Though widely used, there are limitations associated with CIA, including problems for the inexperienced researcher setting up the model, as well as the fact that the housing conditions of experimental animals greatly affect the incidence and severity of arthritis. Furthermore, CIA is only successfully established in certain genetically susceptible mouse strains, such as the DBA/1, as there is a strong link between MHC class II haplotype and disease induction in this model [8].

Conversely, AIA is induced using a two-phase protocol that is based on firstly priming the immune system to methylated bovine serum albumin (mBSA) emulsified with CFA, followed 1 week later by an intra-articular injection of mBSA, which induces joint inflammation. The resulting mono-arthritic disease is defined by intense synovitis and pannus formation in the injected joint, although it does hold the disadvantage of an acute phase model where joint disease abates from day 3, therefore not fully representing human rheumatoid arthritis and its chronicity [4, 9, 10]. However, this model holds many advantages for the researcher, including 100% incidence in the C57BL/6 background which allows for the use of many available transgenic mice, a rapid disease course and, as arthritis is induced in the larger knee joint rather than the smaller joints of the paw, the ability to dissect out the inflamed synovia allowing direct analysis of cellular infiltrates by flow cytometry.

Here, we describe how to efficiently induce CIA and AIA, and how to assess the severity of arthritis. Furthermore, we show how CIA and AIA can be used as models of inflammation to assess the suppressive function of Bregs. Assessment of suppression by Bregs remains the gold standard for their identification, due to the heterogeneity of identified Breg phenotypes, such as the B10 cells with

$CD5^+CD1d^{hi}$ phenotype, the transitional-2 marginal zone precursor (T2-MZP) Bregs with $CD19^+CD21^{hi}CD24^{hi}CD23^+$ phenotype, the Tim-1^+ Bregs, and so on [11]. However, as we and others have identified T2-MZPs as B cells with the ability to suppress arthritis and other chronic inflammatory conditions, we will focus on how to assess the suppressive capacity of T2-MZPs both in vivo, using an adoptive transfer technique, and in vitro, using a standard suppression assay approach [1, 4, 12].

2 Materials

Prepare all solution in a sterile hood. Prepare and store all reagents at 4 °C (unless otherwise indicated). All solutions (apart from adjuvants) used for both antigen- and collagen-induced arthritis are endotoxin-free.

2.1 Antigen-Induced Arthritis

1. 8- to 12-week-old female or male mice (*see* **Note 1**).
2. Methylated Bovine Serum Albumin (mBSA): dissolve 80 mg of mBSA in 2 mL of sterile water by agitating overnight at 4 °C. Store at 4 °C for up to 6 months.
3. Complete Freund's adjuvant (CFA): in a fume hood, while wearing a facemask for safety, finely powder *M. tuberculosis* with a pestle and mortar. Resuspend powdered bacteria in incomplete Freund's adjuvant (IFA) before transferring into a sterile container. Final concentration should be 3 mg of *M. tuberculosis* per mL of IFA.
4. Needles: 25G × 5/8″ Needles (0.5 × 16 mm), 1 mL syringes, 29G × 1/2″ Insulin syringes (0.33 × 12 mm).
5. Gaseous Isoflurane: dial vaporizer to OFF and fill with isoflurane. Turn on O_2 flow rate to 1 L/min and set vaporizer to 3% (*see* **Note 2**).
6. Caliper (mechanical external measuring gage).

2.2 Collagen-Induced Arthritis

1. Bovine type II collagen (*see* **Note 3**).
2. 10 mM acetic acid.
3. 8- to 12-week-old male DBA/1 (H-2^q) mice.
4. Complete Freund's adjuvant: *see* above Subheading 2.1, **step 3** with the following change: final concentration should be 4 mg of *M. tuberculosis* per mL of IFA.
5. Needles: 25G × 5/8″ (0.5 × 16 mm) needles and 1 mL syringes.
6. Gaseous Isoflurane: *see* above Subheading 2.1, **step 5**.
7. Caliper (mechanical external measuring gage).

2.3 Adoptive transfer of T2-MZPs

1. Spleens from mice in remission from arthritis (*see* **Note 4**).
2. 5 mL syringes.
3. 70 μm cell strainers.
4. 15 mL and 50 mL tubes.
5. Polypropylene tubes for cell staining.
6. Red Blood Cell lysis buffer.
7. Recovery medium: 1% penicillin-streptomycin in RPMI-1640 medium.
8. Supplemented RPMI-1640: 10% fetal calf serum (FCS), 1% penicillin-streptomycin, and 50 μM 2-mercaptoethanol in RPMI-1640 medium.
9. Magnetic activated cell sorting (MACS) Buffer: 0.5% FCS, 2 mM ethylenediaminetetraacetic acid (EDTA) in 1× PBS.
10. Kit and associated equipment for immunomagnetic isolation of B cells (*see* **Note 5**).
11. Fluorochrome-conjugated anti-mouse CD19 (1D3), CD21 (7G6), CD23 (B3B4), and CD24 (M1/69) antibodies.
12. 4′,6-Diamidino-2-phenylindole (DAPI): stock solution 1 mg/mL.
13. Hanks' Balanced Saline Solution.
14. 29G × 1/2″ Insulin syringes (0.33 × 12 mm).
15. Cell sorter.

2.4 In Vitro Suppression Assay

1. Spleens from mice in remission from arthritis.
2. 5 mL syringes.
3. 70 μm cell strainers.
4. 15 mL and 50 mL tubes.
5. Supplemented RPMI-1640: 10% FCS, 1% penicillin-streptomycin, 50 μM 2-mercaptoethanol in RPMI-1640 medium.
6. MACS Buffer: 0.5% FCS, 2 mM EDTA in 1× PBS.
7. Kit and associated equipment for immunomagnetic isolation of B cells.
8. Fluorochrome conjugated anti-mouse CD19 (1D3), CD21 (7G6), CD23 (B3B4), CD24 (M1/69), CD4 (RM4–5), and CD25 (PC61.5) antibodies as well as fluorochrome-conjugated mAbs against mouse cytokines of interest (e.g., IL-10, TNFα, IL-17, IFNγ).
9. Fluorochrome-conjugated anti-mouse Foxp3 and anti-mouse Ki67 antibodies.
10. 4′,6-Diamidino-2-phenylindole (DAPI): stock solution 1 mg/mL.

11. Anti-CD3 (145-2C11) antibody, cell culture grade.
12. Phorbol 12-myristate 13-acetate (PMA): dilute in the appropriate medium at the final concentration of 50 ng/mL.
13. Ionomycin: dilute in the appropriate medium at the final concentration of 250 ng/mL.
14. Brefeldin A: dilute in the appropriate medium at the final concentration of 5 μg/mL.
15. Fixation and permeabilization buffers for intranuclear staining of transcription factors.
16. Fixation and permeabilization buffers for intracellular staining of cytokines.
17. Fluorescence-activated cell sorting (FACS) buffer: 0.05% FCS, 2 mM EDTA, and 0.001% sodium azide in 1× PBS.

3 Methods

Arthritis induction protocols are for 10 mice. Scale up volumes accordingly. All cell suspensions and associated buffers should be kept ice cold for cell isolation and collagen extraction.

3.1 Induction of Antigen-Induced Arthritis

1. Add 100 μL of the 40 mg/mL mBSA stock solution, 900 μL of PBS, and 1 mL of CFA in a sterile container. Using a 1-mL syringe, mix solution vigorously until mBSA is fully emulsified in CFA (*see* **Note 6**).
2. Place mice in induction chamber and anaesthetize using gaseous isoflurane. Move mice from induction chamber to individual nose cone face-down, and, using clippers, shave the area at the base of the back/pelvis proximal to the tail.
3. Draw up 100 μL of mBSA/CFA mixture into a 1-mL syringe with a 25G needle attached, being careful to exclude air bubbles.
4. Inject the full 100 μL of mBSA/CFA mixture into the subcutaneous fat at the base of the back at one or multiple sites, entering the skin just to the side of the spinal column. Transfer the mouse to a fresh cage to recover from the anesthesia. Immunize remaining animals using a fresh needle per cage or more frequently if needle becomes blunted.
5. Allow mice to rest for 7 days checking injection site daily (*see* **Note 7**).
6. After 7 days, dilute 100 μL of the 40 mg/mL mBSA stock solution in 100 μL of PBS in a 1.5-mL tube. Mix solution by pipetting up and down. Prepare a 1.5-mL tube containing PBS alone as a control.

7. Measure size of both knees from each mouse using calipers. Then place mice in induction chamber and anaesthetize using gaseous isoflurane. Move animals from induction chamber to individual nose cone face-up and, using clippers, shave the area around the knee joints.
8. Place 10 μL of mBSA/PBS mixture into a 29G insulin syringe and inject under the intra-articular ligament of the left knee. The needle should only be inserted slightly beyond the bevel. If the needle is in the joint, the knee should balloon slightly upon injection of mBSA/PBS. The right knee should receive an intra-articular injection of 10 μL of PBS as a control. Transfer mouse to a fresh cage to recover from anesthesia. Immunize remaining animals.
9. On each subsequent day post-intra-articular injection assess disease severity by assessing walking score and knee swelling. The walking score is graded as follows: 4, no walking; 3, walking on three legs; 2, limping on the inflamed leg; 1, limping on the inflamed leg only after pressure on the knee; and 0, normal walking. Knee swelling is measured using calipers and calculated as the percentage increase in knee size as compared with day 0 (pre-injection), or as a percentage difference between mBSA and PBS injected knees (*see* **Note 8**).
10. Following remission from arthritis, knee joints can be removed and fixed in formalin (10% v/v) for later analysis by histology.
11. When ready, joints are decalcified in EDTA (5% w/v), pH 7.3. Joints are placed in at least 15 volumes of EDTA for 2 weeks at 4 °C with occasional agitation. Depending on success of decalcification, EDTA solution can be replaced daily. Joints are rinsed, embedded in paraffin, then sectioned and stained with hematoxylin and eosin. The severity of joint inflammation is graded as follows: Normal, no damage; Mild, minimal synovitis, cartilage loss, and bone erosion limited to discrete foci; Moderate, synovitis, and erosion present but normal, intact joint architecture; Severe, synovitis, extensive erosion and joint architecture disrupted.

3.2 Induction of Collagen-Induced Arthritis

1. This protocol has been adapted from a previously published protocol [6].
2. Dissolve type II collagen in 10 mM acetic acid according to the manufacturer's instructions overnight at 4 °C, with vigorous mixture, to a final concentration of 4 mg/mL. Dissolved collagen can be stored at −80 °C until needed. Solution must be fully defrosted (on ice) before use.
3. Add 0.5 mL of dissolved type II collagen and 0.5 mL of CFA to a sterile container (or adjust volumes according to number of mice in a 1:1 mix). Using a 1-mL syringe, mix solution

together vigorously until collagen is fully emulsified in CFA. Emulsion should be thick enough to stay in container when upturned. Keep solution on ice.

4. Place mice in induction chamber and anaesthetize using gaseous isoflurane. Move mice from induction chamber to individual nose cone face-down, and, using clippers, shave the area at the base of the back/pelvis proximal to the tail. Draw up 50 μL of collagen/CFA emulsion into a 1-mL syringe with a 25G needle attached, being careful to exclude air bubbles.
5. Inject emulsion intra-dermally in the skin of the tail (inject at multiple sites if needed, in order to inject the total 50 μL). Immunize remaining animals using a fresh needle per cage or as needle becomes blunted.
6. Check mice for arthritis development every day 2 weeks post-immunization (*see* **Note 9**). Visible clinical arthritis usually develops around day 30.
7. Following arthritis onset, the clinical severity of arthritis is determined by measuring swelling of affected paws with calipers or by using the following scoring system. Arthritis is graded as follows: 3, ankylosis; 2, pronounced swelling; 1, slight swelling and/or erythema; 0, normal. Each limb is graded individually, thus there is a maximum score of 12 per mouse. The percentage incidence of arthritis among the experimental cohort can also be recorded.
8. Following remission from arthritis, affected paws can be removed and fixed in formalin (10% v/v) for later analysis by histology.
9. When ready, joints are then prepared and assessed for damage to articular structures (*see* Subheading 3.1, **step 11**). Alternatively, the proportion of eroded joints (defined as cartilage or bone with demarcated defects or filled with inflammatory tissue) can be determined.

3.3 Adoptive Transfer of T2-MZPs (In Vivo Suppression Assay)

As mentioned above, due to the heterogeneity of the known Breg phenotypes, the assessment of their suppressive function is the gold standard in their identification. Here we describe how to determine the suppressive capacity of transitional-2 marginal zone precursor (T2-MZP) Bregs with a $CD19^{+}CD21^{hi}CD24^{hi}CD23^{+}$ phenotype in vivo. The T2-MZP Breg population is expanded and activated in mice in remission from arthritis, which is why we use this particular time point in disease to isolate them.

3.3.1 Purification of T2-MZP B Cells

1. Dissect spleens from mice in remission from arthritis, put in tubes containing ice-cold recovery medium, and place directly on ice (*see* **Note 10**).

2. In a sterile hood, mash spleens through a 70-μm cell strainer (maximum 3 per strainer) into a 50-mL tube using the flat end of the plunger from a 5-mL syringe. Wash through filter with 15 mL of supplemented RPMI. Centrifuge for 10 min, 4 °C, 500 × *g*.
3. Discard supernatant and resuspend in 1 mL/spleen of red cell lysis buffer, leave for 2 min (*see* **Note 11**). Following incubation with red lysis buffer, fill tube to the top with supplemented RPMI. Centrifuge for 10 min, 4 °C, 500 × *g*.
4. Resuspend cells in 10 mL of MACS buffer per spleen and count. Centrifuge for 10 min, 4 °C, 500 × *g*.
5. Negatively isolate resting B cells using immunomagnetic separation technology. Follow the instructions of the employed kit and, at the end, count isolated cells. Centrifuge for 10 min, 4 °C, 500 × *g*.
6. Resuspend cells at 50×10^6 per mL in 1× PBS and stain with suggested antibody clones against CD19, CD21, CD23, and CD24 at a dilution of 1 in 125. Other clones will have to be optimized. Concurrently, prepare single stain controls for the compensation of the flow cytometer. Stain on ice for 20 min.
7. In the meantime, prepare collection tubes using polypropylene FACS tubes. Add 1–2 mL of a 1:1 mixture of FACS and MACS buffer to each 5 mL collection tube.
8. Following staining, wash cells twice in MACS buffer and resuspend at $30–50 \times 10^6$ cells per mL or appropriate concentration for cell sorter.
9. Transfer sample into filter-topped polypropylene FACS tubes, filtering through the lids to remove clumps in order to prevent blockage in the cell sorter.
10. Add DAPI at a final concentration between 0.05 and 0.1 μg/mL to the sample and to the single stained control. The staining with this fluorescent dye allows to differentiate between live and dead cells during sorting.
11. Take samples to cell sorter and sort T2-MZPs (*see* Fig. 1). Begin by excluding cellular debris and doublets using the forward and side scatter gating, followed by dead-cell exclusion using DAPI, and then selecting $CD19^+$ B cells. Within the B-cell gate, CD21 and CD24 expression allows exclusion of follicular B cells. Within the $CD21^{hi}CD24^{hi}$ T2 and MZ (marginal zone B cells) gate, CD23 will allow for the final sorting of T2-MZP Bregs as MZ B cells do not express this marker.

3.3.2 Adoptive Transfer of T2-MZP B Cells

1. While T2-MZPs are being sorted, immunize recipient mice with the intra-articular injection for AIA induction, or with the CII/CFA injection for CIA (*see* Subheadings 3.1 and 3.2).

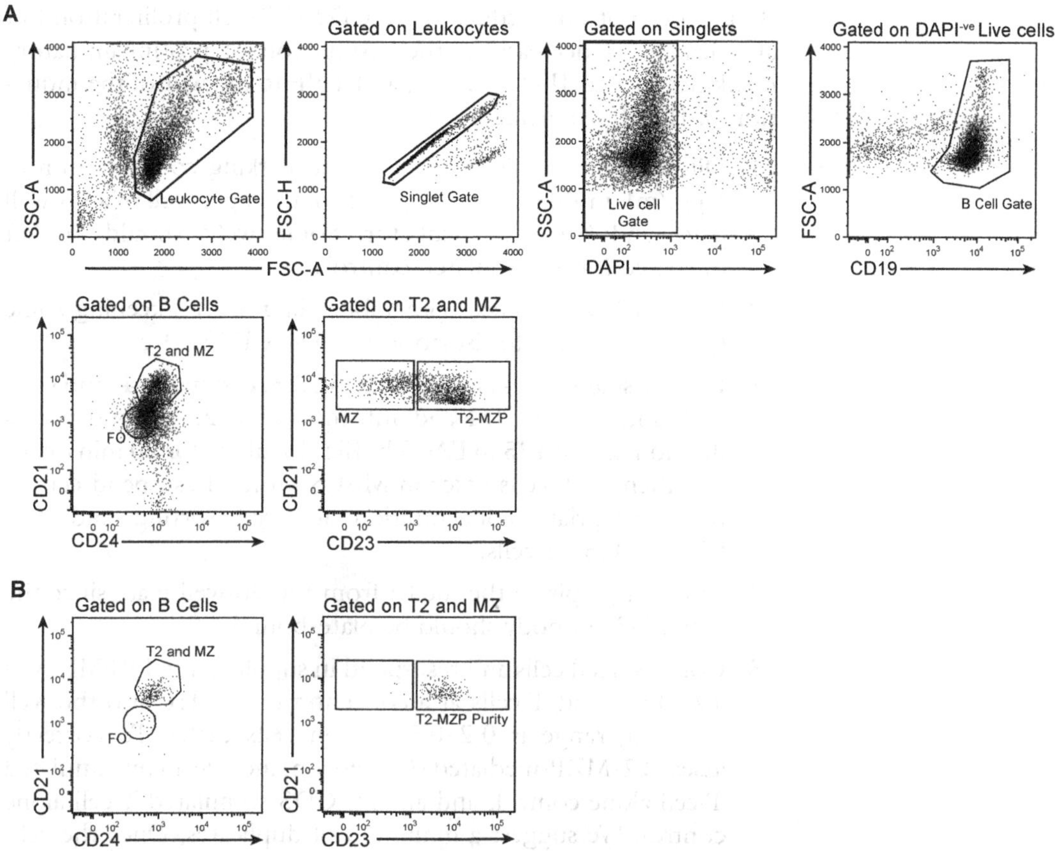

Fig. 1 Gating strategy and purity plots for T2-MZP isolation. Isolated B cells from mice in remission from arthritis were stained with antibodies against CD19, CD21, CD23, and CD24 for FACS. (**a**) Representative flow cytometry plots showing gating strategy for purification of T2-MZP B cells. (**b**) Representative flow cytometry plots showing purity of isolated T2-MZP B cells post-sort

2. After samples have been sorted, wash cells twice in Hanks' saline solution and count cells (*see* **Note 12**).
3. Resuspend T2-MZPs in Hanks' saline solution at appropriate concentration (*see* **Note 13**).
4. Heat recipient mice for 15 min in a heating chamber and inject T2-MZPs intravenously into a tail vein using an insulin needle (use PBS injection as control). Be careful to not aspirate the cells multiple times as this will damage cellular membranes and possibly lead to cell lysis.
5. Assess arthritis daily on subsequent days.

3.4 In Vitro Suppression Assay

The suppressive capacity of T2-MZP Bregs with a $CD19^{+}CD21^{hi}CD24^{hi}CD23^{+}$ phenotype can also be assessed in vitro, by evaluating their ability to suppress $CD4^{+}CD25^{-}$ T-cell proliferation, as well as to induce $CD4^{+}CD25^{+}Foxp3^{+}$ regulatory T cells differentiation. The suppressive effect of T2-MZP

Bregs does not only reduce CD4$^+$CD25$^-$ T-cell proliferation but also lead to a decrease in the production of pro-inflammatory cytokines such as IL-17, IFN-γ, and TNF-α, in favor of the induction of IL-10-producing Tregs.

1. Dilute the anti-CD3 antibody to a working concentration of 1 μg/mL in PBS. Add 200 μL of solution per well of a 96-well plate and place in incubator. Some wells should be left uncoated for unstimulated controls.
2. Purify T2-MZP B cells (*see* Subheading 3.3.1), keeping some splenocytes aside for isolation of CD4$^+$CD25$^-$ T cells.
3. Prepare splenocytes (*see* Subheading 3.3.1, **steps 1–4**) and stain with anti-mouse CD4 and anti-mouse CD25 antibodies at a dilution of 1 in 125 in FACS buffer. Incubate for 20 min on ice and then wash cells twice in MACS buffer. Resuspend cells at the appropriate concentration for cell sorting and sort CD4$^+$CD25$^-$ T cells.
4. After 2 h, aspirate the media from the 96-well plate since the anti-CD3 antibody should be plate-bound.
5. Count sorted cells and resuspend in supplemented RPMI. Add T2-MZPs and T cells at a concentration of 1:1 into the well (working range is 0.2–0.5 million cells each). To correctly assess T2-MZP-mediated suppression, include an unstimulated T-cell alone control, and an anti-CD3-stimulated T-cell alone control. We suggest a minimum of duplicates. Once the cells have been seeded, put the plate in the incubator for 48 h.
6. To determine the suppression of effector T-cell proliferation by T2-MZP B cells, collect cells and stain for Ki67 expression. Firstly, wash and stain samples with appropriate cell surface markers to allow for B-cell and T-cell discrimination, as per manufacturer's instructions or as described above in the pre-sort staining steps. After surface staining, wash, fix, and permeabilize the cells with an appropriate intranuclear fixation and permeabilization buffer set, according to kit instructions. Wash cells using an appropriate permeabilization wash buffer, add the anti-Ki67 antibody and incubate for 30 min at room temperature in the dark. Wash the cells in the same permeabilization buffer and finally resuspend in FACS buffer (*see* **Note 14**). A similar protocol can be used to analyze the expression of intranuclear Foxp3, in order to determine expansion of Tregs following contact with Bregs.
7. Lastly, to determine the effect of Breg suppression on the function of T cells, during the last 5 h of the 48 h co-culture, cells can be stimulated with 50 ng/mL PMA and 250 ng/mL ionomycin in the presence of 5 μg/mL Brefeldin A, and then stained intracellularly for the expression of cytokines such as IL-17, IFN-γ, TNF-α, and IL-10 (*see* **Note 15**).

4 Notes

1. Incidence of AIA is 100% regardless of mouse strain and sex. However, severity of disease does vary between strains. C57BL/6 and BALB/C mice are susceptible, whereas CBA mice are thought to be relatively resistant.
2. The anesthetic protocol used will depend on the equipment provided by the animal facility. However, we recommend the use of isoflurane as it is less toxic for animals than alternatives and has a faster recovery time. Alternatives include gaseous halothane, or a mixture of xylazine-HCL (5–10 mg/Kg)/ketamine-HCL (50–100 mg/Kg) can be used as an injectable anesthetic. Subcutaneous injections can be performed on un-anesthetized mice; however, for intra-articular injections mice must be fully asleep.
3. We strongly recommend using bovine type II collagen from Chondrex, as we have no experience using other suppliers.
4. The appropriate number of spleens must be calculated depending on strain and type of arthritis. Naïve spleens, or B cells from other organs, can be used; however, the protocol must be adjusted accordingly.
5. As the purposes of this step is only to enrich for B cells in order to make the cell sort run faster than if B cells were sorted directly from splenocytes, several different B-cell enrichment kits can be used, and, as 100% purity is not necessary, reagents can be diluted further than recommended. However, we would recommend using kits that negatively select for B cells.
6. Thorough emulsification is required for proper induction of arthritis, we recommend a minimum of 100 strokes with syringe, vortexing alone is not sufficient.
7. A rare side effect of injecting mice with CFA is the formation of an ulcer around the injection site (this is more likely to happen in genetically modified mice such as *Rag2*$^{-/-}$ or μMT animals). If this occurs, mice must be checked daily to make sure the wound is dry and healing properly. If not, mice must be sacrificed for humane reasons.
8. In order to keep consistent results, we suggest that the same researcher holds the calipers for every measurement, and that a colleague is employed to hold mice while measurement is taken thus allowing proper extension of the knee joint. Comparison of arthritic knee swelling to swelling of a PBS control injected knee adjusts disease scores to account for injection site inflammation so that only antigen-specific swelling is measured.
9. We usually find it is not necessary, but some researchers find that a booster injection is necessary to induce CIA. Booster

injections are carried out by emulsifying collagen 1:1 in incomplete Freund's adjuvant, and 100 μL is injected into mice on day 21 following the first injection.

10. In order to detect T-cell suppression, we recommend using donor animals which have the same type of experimental arthritis as recipient mice. The number of spleens dissected will depend on the following considerations: we calculate that approximately 0.8×10^6 T2-MZPs can be isolated from one C57BL/6 mouse in remission from AIA and 1.2×10^6 T2-MZPs can be isolated from one DBA mouse in remission from CIA. Furthermore, in order to see significant suppression in AIA, you need to transfer between 1.5 and 2×10^6 T2-MZPs per mouse, whereas, in CIA you only need to transfer between 4 and 10×10^5 T2-MZPs per mouse. Thus, the number of spleens dissected must be adjusted depending on the strain, type of arthritis, and number of recipients.
11. We do not recommend lysing more than five spleens together; if more spleens than this are lysed together, we find that cell viability is affected.
12. Do not forget to evaluate cell purities before processing isolated T2-MZPs further. Moreover, if surplus cells have been isolated, we recommend culturing cells with antigen (mBSA or collagen) and/or anti-CD40 (both 10 μg/mL) for 72 h to assess IL-10 production by ELISA. IL-10 data can be successfully paired with suppression assay data. Cells can also be put in Trizol™, or another appropriate extraction buffer, for assessment of gene transcription by RT-PCR.
13. When injecting intended numbers of cells in 100 μL volumes, we recommend drawing up 120 μL into the syringe to avoid losing cells in the dead space of the needle and syringe barrel (roughly equivalent to 20 μL).
14. Anti-Ki-67 antibodies from different sources might suggest specific staining protocols. Please follow specific manufacturer's instructions if different from our description. It is also advisable to titrate antibodies according to manufacturer's instructions in order to determine their working concentration, especially for transcription factor-specific antibodies.
15. We also recommend taking supernatants for assessment of cytokine levels by ELISA.

Acknowledgments

This work is funded by a Versus Arthritis program grant (21140) awarded to Claudia Mauri. Diana Matei is funded by a Versus Arthritis PhD studentship (21257) to C.M. Elizabeth Rosser is funded by a Versus Arthritis UK Foundation fellowship (21141).

References

1. Evans JG, Chavez-Rueda KA, Eddaoudi A, Meyer-Bahlburg A, Rawlings DJ, Ehrenstein MR, Mauri C (2007) Novel suppressive function of transitional 2 B cells in experimental arthritis. J Immunol 178(12):7868–7878. https://doi.org/10.4049/jimmunol.178.12.7868
2. Mauri C, Gray D, Mushtaq N, Londei M (2003) Prevention of arthritis by interleukin 10-producing B cells. J Exp Med 197 (4):489–501. https://doi.org/10.1084/jem.20021293
3. Rosser EC, Oleinika K, Tonon S, Doyle R, Bosma A, Carter NA, Harris KA, Jones SA, Klein N, Mauri C (2014) Regulatory B cells are induced by gut microbiota-driven interleukin-1beta and interleukin-6 production. Nat Med 20(11):1334–1339. https://doi.org/10.1038/nm.3680
4. Carter NA, Vasconcellos R, Rosser EC, Tulone C, Munoz-Suano A, Kamanaka M, Ehrenstein MR, Flavell RA, Mauri C (2011) Mice lacking endogenous IL-10-producing regulatory B cells develop exacerbated disease and present with an increased frequency of Th1/Th17 but a decrease in regulatory T cells. J Immunol 186(10):5569–5579. https://doi.org/10.4049/jimmunol.1100284
5. Piper CJM, Rosser EC, Oleinika K, Nistala K, Krausgruber T, Rendeiro AF, Banos A, Drozdov I, Villa M, Thomson S, Xanthou G, Bock C, Stockinger B, Mauri C (2019) Aryl hydrocarbon receptor contributes to the transcriptional program of IL-10-producing regulatory B cells. Cell Rep 29(7):1878–1892. e1877. https://doi.org/10.1016/j.celrep.2019.10.018
6. Brand DD, Latham KA, Rosloniec EF (2007) Collagen-induced arthritis. Nat Protoc 2 (5):1269–1275. https://doi.org/10.1038/nprot.2007.173
7. Carter NA, Rosser EC, Mauri C (2012) Interleukin-10 produced by B cells is crucial for the suppression of Th17/Th1 responses, induction of T regulatory type 1 cells and reduction of collagen-induced arthritis. Arthritis Res Ther 14(1):R32. https://doi.org/10.1186/ar3736
8. Grotsch B, Bozec A, Schett G (2019) In vivo models of rheumatoid arthritis. Methods Mol Biol 1914:269–280. https://doi.org/10.1007/978-1-4939-8997-3_14
9. Brackertz D, Mitchell GF, Mackay IR (1977) Antigen-induced arthritis in mice. I Induction of arthritis in various strains of mice. Arthritis Rheum 20(3):841–850. https://doi.org/10.1002/art.1780200314
10. Vasconcellos R, Carter NA, Rosser EC, Mauri C (2011) IL-12p35 subunit contributes to autoimmunity by limiting IL-27-driven regulatory responses. J Immunol 187 (6):3402–3412. https://doi.org/10.4049/jimmunol.1100224
11. Rosser EC, Mauri C (2015) Regulatory B cells: origin, phenotype, and function. Immunity 42 (4):607–612. https://doi.org/10.1016/j.immuni.2015.04.005
12. Blair PA, Chavez-Rueda KA, Evans JG, Shlomchik MJ, Eddaoudi A, Isenberg DA, Ehrenstein MR, Mauri C (2009) Selective targeting of B cells with agonistic anti-CD40 is an efficacious strategy for the generation of induced regulatory T2-like B cells and for the suppression of lupus in MRL/lpr mice. J Immunol 182 (6):3492–3502. https://doi.org/10.4049/jimmunol.0803052

Chapter 21

Regulatory and IgE⁺ B Cells in Allergic Asthma

John Paul Oliveria, Rita Agayby, and Gail M. Gauvreau

Abstract

Allergic asthma is triggered by inhalation of environmental allergens resulting in bronchial constriction and inflammation, which leads to clinical symptoms such as wheezing, coughing, and difficulty breathing. Asthmatic airway inflammation is initiated by inflammatory mediators released by granulocytic cells. However, the immunoglobulin E (IgE) antibody is necessary for the initiation of the allergic cascade, and IgE is produced and released exclusively by memory B cells and plasma cells. Acute allergen exposure has also been shown to increase IgE levels in the airways of patients diagnosed with allergic asthma; however, more studies are needed to understand local airway inflammation. Additionally, regulatory B cells (B_{regs}) have been shown to modulate IgE-mediated inflammatory processes in allergic asthma pathogenesis, particularly in mouse models of allergic airway disease. However, the levels and function of these IgE^+ B cells and B_{regs} remain to be elucidated in human models of asthma. The overall objective for this chapter is to provide detailed methodological, and insightful technological advances to study the biology of B cells in allergic asthma pathogenesis. Specifically, we will describe how to investigate the frequency and function of IgE^+ B cells and B_{regs} in allergic asthma, and the kinetics of these cells after allergen exposure in a human asthma model.

Key words Regulatory B cells, IgE^+ B cells, Allergic asthma, Inhaled allergen challenge, Airway inflammation, Sputum, Human immunology

1 Introduction

1.1 Allergic Asthma

Asthma is a chronic inflammatory disorder of the lower airways, with a high degree of variability in its severity, natural progression, response to treatment, and degree of bronchial hyperresponsiveness and airflow obstruction likely secondary to a complex integration of inflammatory mechanisms [1]. Allergic asthma, the predominant form of asthma in childhood, is the result of hyperactive responses to repeated exposure to common environmental allergens. These exposures, in turn, lead to the development of allergen-specific memory T- and B-cell responses and the resulting production of inflammatory mediators [1] that aid in the recruitment of allergic immune effector cells including T and B cells [2]. Activated $CD4^+$ T cells release type 2 cytokines which drive

Francesca Mion and Silvia Tonon (eds.), *Regulatory B Cells: Methods and Protocols*, Methods in Molecular Biology, vol. 2270, https://doi.org/10.1007/978-1-0716-1237-8_21, © Springer Science+Business Media, LLC, part of Springer Nature 2021

many of the inflammatory processes in allergic asthma. Specifically, IL-4 and IL-13 play pivotal roles in the synthesis of IgE by B cells, while IL-3 and IL-5 lead to differentiation and proliferation of eosinophils, mast cells, and basophils, all key effector cells contributing to asthmatic bronchial hyperresponsiveness [3, 4].

Bronchoprovocation with inhaled allergen in subjects with asthma has proven to be an effective model to study the intricate pathways associated with the development of allergic asthma [5, 6]. It is postulated that the development of allergic disease is a result of the initial allergen exposure priming the immune system and leading to a shift toward type 2 inflammation mediated by IgE-dependent pathways [1]. Allergen presentation by antigen-presenting cells (APCs) to naïve $CD4^+$ T cells is a pivotal event in the development of allergic responses [4]. Synthesis by B cells of antigen-specific IgE which binds to high-affinity IgE receptors (FcERI) on the surface of dendritic cells, granulocytic cells, such as mast cells and basophils, and becomes cross-linked by allergen, initiates cell activation and release of their inflammatory mediators, particularly histamine, leukotrienes, and the type 2 cytokines IL-4, IL-5, and IL-13. This leads to the influx of $CD4^+$ T cells and eosinophils into the airways [6], and thereby perpetuating type 2 inflammation. Thus, allergic asthmatics have been found to have higher levels of lymphocytes, eosinophils, basophils, and mast cells in their airways [6]. Eosinophilia is widely recognized as a hallmark of asthma, and fluctuation of these cells in blood and airways can be used to determine disease severity and treatment efficacy [6, 7]. Additionally, asthmatics also have higher levels of airway epithelial desquamation, goblet cell hyperplasia, and thicker basement membranes [4]. Ultimately, asthma has a broad presentation clinically with many different phenotypes, and cellularly with several different endotypes, and therefore, current management strategies must take these factors into consideration. Anti-IgE therapy has been used for several decades for treatment of asthmatic patients with high circulating IgE levels and has insofar proven to be clinically effective in the management of allergic asthma [8]. However, with the recognition of in situ IgE synthesis in asthma [9, 10], targeting local sources in the allergic tissue may be a more practical approach for treatment of allergic asthma. Thus, development of novel targets to regulate IgE synthesis for treatment of asthma and other allergic diseases is ongoing [11–13].

1.2 B Cells

Several diseases have B cells at the core of their pathogenesis, including, but not limited to, autoimmune disorders (multiple sclerosis [14, 15], systemic lupus erythematosus [16]), cancer (leukemia [17, 18]), and allergy (rhinitis [19], asthma [20–24]). B cells derive from the differentiation of hematopoietic stem cells. Most of their maturation occurs in the bone marrow, where they differentiate into functional effector or regulatory B cells [25–29].

Thereafter, they are released into peripheral compartments of the body (peripheral blood, secondary lymphoid organs, lymph nodes, and local tissues) [30]. B-cell surface markers allow for their characterization at different stages of development. These markers primarily include CD19, CD20, CD27, CD38, and CD138 [25–27, 31].

1.3 IgE$^+$ B Cells

IgM, IgD, IgG, IgE, and IgA form the five isotypes of immunoglobulins produced by B cells, whose expression and function depend on the heavy chain constant region of the B-cell receptor (BCR) [26, 32]. At the initial phases of development, B cells express IgM. Once the B cell encounters an antigen and is co-stimulated with CD40L, it becomes activated. This activation triggers isotype switching, a process facilitated by the activation-induced cytidine deaminase (AID) enzyme through which heavy chain genes are rearranged [32]. The mechanism of class switching involves deamination of residues of gene segments upstream of the heavy chain genes, called switch regions. This deamination produces double-stranded breaks secondary to a break in two switch regions [32]. As a result, certain portions of the heavy chain genes are excised, leaving behind the gene encoding the heavy chain of interest to be expressed [33]. Mu (μ), delta (δ), gamma (γ), epsilon (ε), and alpha (α) encode the heavy chains for IgM, IgD, IgE, and IgA, respectively [26, 32].

To reiterate, the pathogenesis of allergic asthma is driven by binding of IgE to FcεRI and the subsequent activation and degranulation of mast cells and basophils as a result of cross-linking by a specific antigen [34]. In effect, Van de Pol et al. have demonstrated increases in the levels of total serum and allergen-specific IgE following a single inhalation of house dust mite extract by allergic asthmatics [35]. In the airways, Wilson et al. have shown that allergen-specific IgE levels in bronchoalveolar lavage (BAL) were significantly increased following allergen challenge relative to saline challenge. Similarly, Oliveria et al. have shown that sputum supernatant total IgE is higher in allergic asthmatics compared to controls, and further increased at 7 hours post-allergen challenge [9, 10, 36]. It can therefore be concluded that B cells, through their production of IgE, play a key role in the local airway inflammation characteristic to allergic asthma.

1.3.1 IgE$^+$ B-Cell Kinetics and Compartmental Distribution

There are very few human studies evaluating IgE$^+$ B cells; however, we have gained insight from studies of murine models. Memory B cells (MBCs) and plasma cells (PCs) were studied in a murine parasitic infection model by Nduati et al. [37]. Their results showed that although MBCs were detectable in the blood at all times, PCs were only detectable shortly after parasitic infections (primary and secondary) and were thus highly time-sensitive with respect to the challenge [37]. In this regard, it can be alluded that a short time frame is needed to mobilize B cells into the blood following an inflammatory event. Similarly, Luger et al. found that mice who were given mucosal allergen challenge with ovalbumin (OVA) induced the production of PCs in the lung, spleen, and bone marrow but only for a short period following the challenge [38]. However, in both Luger et al. and Nduati et al.'s studies, a small population of those PCs were found to be long-lived in the spleen and bone marrow. These PCs were found to produce OVA-specific IgE, IgA, and IgG_1 [38]. Likewise, Chvatchko et al. demonstrated that, following inhalation challenge, murine B cells in the lungs were triggered toward increased antigen-driven differentiation, and, more specifically, toward OVA-specific IgE and IgG_1 production [39]. Despite these studies, the kinetics of B cells through various bodily compartments, such as lungs, blood, lymphatics, bone marrow, at different time points following challenges, remains to be elucidated, even in murine models. A further understanding of the expansion of B cells in asthma remains to be discovered. Although IgE^+ B cells are very rare and difficult to enumerate, advances in flow cytometry have allowed for their measurement in humans [40]. Oliveria et al. have been able to detect IgE^+ B cells in peripheral blood, bone marrow, tonsil, and airways by flow cytometry [10] and conducted studies to compare B-cell subsets across disease states (healthy controls, allergic non-asthmatics, and asthmatics), to examine the kinetics of these cells in peripheral blood (systemic compartment), bone marrow (hemopoietic compartment), tonsils (lymphatic compartment), and locally in sputum (airways compartment) after bronchoprovocation with inhaled allergen [9, 10]. They demonstrated higher levels of B cells and IgE^+ B cells in the airways of allergic asthmatics compared to controls, but found no differences in blood levels of these cell types. Furthermore, sputum B cells were positively correlated with sputum eosinophils, and sputum supernatant IgE and BAFF [9]. In subjects with mild allergic asthma, levels of B cells and IgE^+ B cells were noted to be elevated in the airways 7- and 24-hours post-bronchoprovocation challenge [10]; however no changes were observed in peripheral blood, bone marrow, or tonsils. Now that the levels of IgE^+ B cells have been reported across disease states, and after allergic provocation of airways in a human in vivo model, there are questions about function, development, and memory of these rare B-cell subsets that need to be explored. Particularly, we still do not know much about the regulation of these IgE^+ B-cell responses. There are B-cell-specific roles that modulate inflammation through cytokine or antibody-mediated processes, and these need to be explored within the context of allergy.

1.4 Regulatory B Cells (B_{regs})

In the early 1970s, the first postulated suppressive function of B cells was demonstrated through the transfer of B-cell-depleted splenocytes into OVA-sensitized guinea pigs which resulted in a decreased ability to dampen the inflammatory response [41, 42]. The exact mechanism by which the inflammatory response is dampened had not been further investigated until recently, wherein, in 1996, Wolf et al. demonstrated that B-cell-deficient mice could not recover from experimental autoimmune encephalomyelitis (EAE) [43, 44], suggesting a subset of B cells is required for immunomodulation. Similar observations were made regarding the B-cell-dependent immunomodulation in mouse models of inflammatory bowel disease [45], autoimmune diseases [46], and allergy [4, 47]. Interestingly, models of colitis [45], EAE [48], and arthritis [49] have found IL-10 to be a primary immunomodulatory cytokine, supporting the role of IL-10-producing B cells in these diseases. However, regardless of the disease, there is no universally accepted regulatory B-cell (B_{reg}) phenotype in the literature. Furthermore, the study of B_{reg} subsets and their functional mechanisms, specifically in allergic asthma, is still in its infancy and plenty of questions remain unanswered.

1.4.1 Development of B_{regs}

Significant attention was brought to the origin and function of B and T cells following the discovery of distinct lymphocyte subpopulations as unique aspects of the adaptive immune response over 40 years ago [50]. Cells expressing surface immunoglobulin receptors specific to antigenic epitopes are characterized as B (*bursal*) lymphocytes [50] and were demonstrated, in the early 1960s and 1970s, to be primarily responsible for the basic functions of antibody production and humoral immune responses [43]. However, several years later, as studies on B cells continued, complexities in their development, differentiation, maturation, and responses were observed. Of note was the role of B cells as antigen-presenting cells whereby they present peptides to T cells via MHC molecules on their surfaces [50]. Additionally, it was demonstrated that B cells have the ability to secrete a diverse array of cytokines that influence immune cell function and inflammatory processes [50]. B cells were found to have the ability to mount a robust secondary response with higher affinity to antigens through the process of somatic hypermutation within germinal centers [50]. The discovery of long-lived plasma cells and memory B cells provided crucial advancement in the understanding of the role of B cells in adaptive memory [51, 52]. B cells were found to have duality in their role in allergy and inflammation, wherein they possess the ability to class switch to IgE isotype in type 2 inflammatory environments and the further induction of the inflammatory cascade by IgE. Nevertheless, the recent discovery of regulatory B cells shed a different light [2]. Since the study of regulatory B cells is relatively novel in literature, the development and ontogeny of these cells remain to be elusive and future research is required.

1.4.2 Functions of B_{regs}

A paradigm shift was created upon the discovery of a tolerogenic role for B cells which consequently also shifted our understanding of B-cell function and role in diseases. Stimulation by TLR ligands, such as CpG and LPS, CD40:CD40L axis, and BCR agonists, activate B cells toward a regulatory phenotype [43]. The B_{regs} ability to produce IL-10, either constitutively or in response to stimulation, is often the definition of "activated" in the literature, though this definition can vary. The immunomodulatory function of B_{regs} has primarily been studied, in both mice [53] and humans [54], through its ability to modulate T-cell function in favor of a regulatory phenotype. Additionally, B_{regs} have also been shown to play an indirect immunomodulatory role in suppressing inflammatory processes through their ability to induce regulatory phenotypes in a variety of other immune cell subsets (e.g., DCs, T cells, and mast cells) [55]. Through their ability to produce anti-inflammatory cytokines (e.g., IL-10, TGF-β, and IL-35), B_{regs} indirectly aid in the suppression of Th1 and Th17 differentiation of $CD4^+$ T cells [55]. B_{regs} also play a crucial role in the maintenance of T_{reg} populations [24, 56]. When analyzing both the T_{reg} and B_{reg} regulatory functions, they have many distinct similarities and differences. Similar to the thymus-derived T_{regs}, the expression of genes responsible for the suppressive phenotype of B_{regs}, a distinct lineage of B cells, is influenced by specific factors [43]. However, the development and ontogeny of these cells remain unclear [43]. Like T_{regs}, B_{regs} possess regulatory capabilities through their ability to secrete anti-inflammatory cytokines that provide direct exhaustion and deletion of effector cells [57–60]. However, it is still unclear by which mechanism regulatory B cells elicit this function, and further research is required. Nevertheless, through their IgG_4 isotype, a type of blocking antibody that competes with the binding of IgE to allergen, B_{regs} have the unique ability to suppress the humoral immune response [61]. Despite the vast and continually growing knowledge of the role of B cells in immunity that we have gained in the literature, more remains to be elucidated and the persistence of scientific endeavors is crucial to providing clarity into the suppressive nature of B_{regs}.

1.4.3 IL-10 Production by B_{regs}

IL-10, produced primarily by clonally expanded Trl (regulatory T cells) and professional antigen-presenting cells, and at times also by mast cells, monocytes, and NK cells, is an important anti-inflammatory cytokine [62, 63]. IL-10 possesses anti-inflammatory properties through its ability to suppress naïve T-cell activation by blocking co-stimulatory signaling through CD2, CD28, and inducible T-cell co-stimulation (ICOS) in a rapid signal transduction cascade [62, 64, 65]. Specifically, CD28 tyrosine phosphorylation is inhibited which prevents the binding of phosphatidylinositol 3-kinase p85 [65, 66]. As a result, the entire

CD28 signaling pathway is inhibited, and thus, T-cell co-stimulatory pathways [65, 66]. Furthermore, IL-10 hinders the type 1 immune response by inducing expression of the suppressor of the cytokine signaling 3 (SOCS3) gene and the resulting inhibition of IFN-ϒ-induced phosphorylation of STAT1 [67]. IL-10 has the capacity to suppress total and allergen-specific IgE antibodies, and skew the humoral response from the IgE isotype to the non-inflammatory isotypes, IgG_4 and IgA, and hence plays a critical role in allergy and immune tolerance [68–70].

In summary, the ability to suppress activation of effector cells, production of inflammatory cytokines, and hence inflammation in general, characterizes IL-10 as an inflammatory cytokine [71]. In fact, evidences in allergic asthma demonstrating the capacity of regulatory T cells to suppress inflammation through secretion of IL-10 have been reported [72, 73]. The term regulatory B cell was coined in the early 2000s following the discovery of a subset of B cells with the capacity to produce IL-10 [74]. Currently, the terms regulatory B cells or B_{regs} and B10 cells are acceptable nomenclatures for IL-10-producing B cells. However, the phenotype of B_{regs} creates controversies in its studies due to its wide variability [75, 76]. Nevertheless, the commonly accepted attribute of B_{regs} is their ability to produce IL-10. In Iwata et al.'s study, B_{regs}, identified with the $CD19^+CD24^+CD27^+$ phenotype, were studied in both mice and humans and were found to be competent in the production of cytoplasmic IL-10 [76]. However, there is no clear knowledge of the pathways leading to the manifestation of these B cells. Additionally, B_{regs} were found to produce antigen-specific antibodies, specifically IgG_4, as was demonstrated in the study of Maseda et al., thus indicating that B_{regs} have the dual role of producing IL-10 as well as antigen-specific antibodies [61, 77, 78].

James et al. and van de Veen et al. demonstrated that IgG_4, produced by B cells following the induction of IL-10, can act as a blocking antibody for IgE-specific antigens. By doing so, the downstream IgE-mediated allergic cascade is inhibited. In fact, in James et al.'s study, grass pollen allergens were neutralized by IgG_4 antibodies, which subsequently resulted in reduced IgE-mediated events [77]. Similarly, in van de Veen et al.'s study, inflammatory immune responses induced by bee venom were dampened through IL-10-producing B_{regs} and their production of IgG_4 antibodies [61].

In summary, IL-10 induces B_{regs} to produce IgG_4 and together, these anti-inflammatory mediators suppress $CD4^+$ T-cell proliferation, IgE, and the allergic cascade [61, 77]. In a study of cow's milk allergy, Noh et al. found that B_{regs} produced IL-10 when stimulated with allergen. However, this same stimulation also increased apoptosis in the regulatory B-cell subpopulation [79–81]. Although numerous and phenotypically diverse regulatory B-cell subpopulations exist, they are all defined by their ability to produce IL-10 and their resulting significant roles in many autoimmune diseases, allergies, cancers, and infectious diseases. The phenotype and function of B_{regs} involved in such pathways, particularly with regard to allergic asthma, remain to be discovered.

1.4.4 Role of B_{regs} in Allergic Disease

Allergic diseases have complex and vastly heterogenous pathogenesis. Type 2 inflammatory responses to a specific allergen mediated by ways of sensitization and development of B- and T-cell responses are the means by which allergic diseases are established [2]. Hence, the focus of novel therapies are to shift the type 2 inflammatory response toward a healthy tolerogenic state [47, 82–84], which can be accomplished through various immunomodulatory approaches [2]. The in vivo induction of tolerance to the regimented and controlled administration of increasing allergen concentrations, called allergen immunotherapy (AIT), is a potentially curative therapy for allergic disease and represents a clinical model for tolerance induction [2].

Two mechanisms describe the role of B_{regs} in the allergic response: the cell-mediated and the humoral suppressive responses. The cell-mediated suppressive response is carried through the release of anti-inflammatory mediators (e.g., IL-10 and TGF-β). The humoral suppressive response is classified by the B cells' ability to isotype switch and produce IgG4 blocking antibodies.

The earliest discoveries of the role of B_{regs} in allergies occurred in guinea pigs through ovalbumin (OVA)-induced skin hypersensitivity reactions [41]. Similarly, a study in 1998, examined the frequency of IL-10$^+$ B cells in patients with bee venom allergy receiving immunotherapy and is the human study to first note evidence for B_{regs} [68]. Compared to IL-10$^-$ B cells, transcription analysis identified IL-10$^+$ B cells as being CD19$^+$CD73$^-$CD25$^+$CD71$^+$ [61].

These IL-10$^+$ B cells were appropriately named B_{regs} given that they are similar to Trl cells with regard to their ability to suppress antigen-specific T-cell proliferation via the IL-10-mediated response [61]. Those with bee venom allergy undergoing immunotherapy in the aforementioned study were found to have a two- to fivefold increase in the Brl CD19$^+$CD73$^-$CD25$^+$CD71$^+$IL-10$^+$ B-cell subset, specific for the major bee venom phospholipase A2 (PLA) approximately 4 months post-therapy [61]. In conclusion, following high-dose allergen exposure, we assist to an expansion of B_{reg} populations and thus to the maintenance of a tolerogenic response to specific allergens [61]. Moreover, B_{regs} have the ability to increase IgG_4 production relative to serum IgE levels, thus demonstrating humoral effects in allergic disease. B_{regs} are central to the humoral effects in allergic disease [61]. In fact, in the aforementioned study, IL-10 played an integral role in the B cells' ability to differentiate into the IgG_4-producing plasma cells and resulted in a 100-fold decrease in the IgE/IgG_4 ratio [61]. Hence, there is sufficient evidence to support the notion that B_{regs} play an integral part of the modulation of allergic disease, both through their ability to suppress effector T cells and skew the humoral response through the IgG_4 isotype. This has expanded our understanding of allergic disease and shows promise in the development of future therapies.

Through limited studies in allergic airway inflammation, we have gained tremendous insight into the mechanistic role played by B_{regs} [85]. Murine models of house dust mite (HDM) airway hyperresponsiveness have demonstrated that $CD9^+$ B cells were crucial to the production of suppressive mediators [86]. B1 cells, plasma cells, and marginal zone B cells are shown to express the adhesion molecule CD9 [86]. The adoptive transfer of $CD9^+$ B cells results in the suppression of Th2- and Th17-mediated inflammatory responses through IL-10-mediated mechanisms [86]. Additionally, FasL expression was upregulated on $CD5^+$ B1 cells following stimulation with cockroach allergen and mediated the apoptosis of effector $CD4^+$ T cells and thus controlled allergen-induced airway inflammation [23]. Furthermore, human trials have shown that the suppression of AHR-mediated inflammation is highly regulated by $IL\text{-}10^+$ B_{regs}. Specifically, IL-10 secretion resulted in the reversal of allergic airway inflammation through $CD19^+CD1d^{hi}CD5^+CD21^{hi}CD23^+IgD^+IgM^{hi}$ B_{regs} and positive expression of CD1d [87]. B_{regs} also recruit T_{regs} to the lungs, further suppressing airway inflammation [24, 85].

Further emphasizing the importance of B_{regs}, Amu et al., Sing et al., and Lundy et al. found that B_{reg}-deficient mice had higher levels of serum IgE, type 2 cytokines (IL-4 and IL-5), and eosinophilia [23, 24, 85]. They also found that adoptive transfer of B_{regs} into mice with allergic airway disease reversed the inflammatory phenotype [23, 24, 85].

In summary, B_{regs} produce IL-10 resulting in the production of IgG_4 and the recruitment of T_{regs} into the lungs, thus suppressing the allergic cascade and airway inflammation [23, 24, 85]. However, research regarding the role of B_{regs} in the pathogenesis and pathobiology of allergic asthma is limited and remains to be further elucidated.

1.4.5 Phenotypes of B_{regs}

Despite our partial understanding of the role of B_{regs} in various disease states, we still do not have a defined characterization of the B_{reg} phenotype. Moreover, the exact mechanism of their inception within specific disease contexts has not yet been elucidated. Currently two hypotheses have been considered: one states that B_{regs} are specific to a distinct B-cell lineage, whereas the other states that

B_{regs} are derived from a certain immunological microenvironment inducing B cells to take on this specific phenotype and function. In this light, a primary aim of future research in this field will be characterizing these phenotypes and highlighting those with the most suppressive functions to further understand their role in diseases. In a B_{reg} phenotype study by Oliveria et al., these phenotypes were evaluated, particularly FoxP3$^+$ B_{regs} were found to be lower in level in allergic asthmatics compared to controls. Furthermore, FoxP3$^+$ B_{regs} were evaluated in bone marrow, blood, and sputum, and it was demonstrated that at 7 hours post-challenge, FoxP3$^+$ B_{regs} increased in the blood, and at 24 hours post-challenge they decreased in the bone marrow and increased in the airways [88]. All together, these findings suggest that B_{regs} are trafficking to the airways after allergic stimulation. Oliveria et al. also conducted in vitro studies evaluating the role of IL-4 stimulation of B cells and found that IL-4 stimulation increases the levels of FoxP3$^+$IL-10$^+$ B cells after 72 hours of culture [88]. Thus, the allergic cascade has a role in the propagation of regulatory B cells and may be transiently increasing their functions to mitigate inflammatory mechanisms, but more comprehensive studies need to be done to confirm these conclusions. Particularly, for allergic diseases, we would benefit from gaining knowledge regarding B_{reg} trafficking and compartmentalization in the early and late phase of the allergic response. Among the investigated phenotypes, CD1d$^+$CD5$^+$ B_{regs}, CD5$^+$FoxP3$^+$ B_{regs}, and CD24$^+$CD38$^+$ B_{regs} have shown promise in reversing allergic airway inflammation, particularly in human and murine models.

CD1d$^+$CD5$^+$ B_{regs}

CD1d$^+$CD5$^+$ B_{regs} represent a splenic B-cell subset which exerts immunomodulatory effects through the production of IL-10 and plays a crucial role in the suppression of the acute phase reaction in contact hypersensitivity [46, 89, 90]. Moreover, it has been demonstrated that, in mice, CD19$^+$IL-10$^+$CD1d^{hi}CD5$^+$ CD21$^+$CD23$^+$ B_{regs} suppress allergic airway inflammation through the secretion of IL-10 and expression of CD1d [87]. Furthermore, murine and human models of autoimmune disease have demonstrated the involvement of B_{regs} in their pathogenesis, particularly systemic lupus erythematosus (SLE) and rheumatoid arthritis. In fact, defective CD1d expression resulted in altered B_{reg} stimulation and as a result, impaired invariant natural killer T cell (iNKT) number and function [91]. Normally, natural killer T (NKT) cells are activated through activation of their surface-membrane T-cell receptors (TCRs) secondary to CD1d expression. Overall, the expression of CD1d is a specific marker of B_{reg} that is implicated in both allergic and non-allergic diseases secondary to its unique suppressive pathways [92–94].

$CD5^+FoxP3^+$ B_{regs} The expression of FoxP3, an important transcription factor in T_{reg} development, was first identified in $CD19^+CD5^+$ B cells by Noh et al. in 2010 [75]. In human PBMCs, $CD5^+$ B-expressing FoxP3 made up 8.5 ± 3.5% of the $CD19^+$ B-cell pool and showed a significantly elevated apoptotic frequency of 63.44% [75]. These cells have been extensively studied in food allergy. In one study, subjects allergic to cow's milk protein (e.g., casein) presented decreased $CD5^+FoxP3^+$ B_{reg} upon allergen stimulation compared to milk-tolerant controls who actually showed an increase in this cell population [81]. Conversely, both allergic and tolerant individuals demonstrated an increase in $CD4^+FoxP3^+$ T_{reg}, suggesting that B_{regs} play a much broader role in food allergy beyond merely T_{reg}-mediated suppression [81]. More remains to be discovered regarding the role of $CD5^+FoxP3^+$ B_{regs} in the pathogenesis of allergic asthma.

$CD24^+CD38^+$ Bregs $CD24^+CD38^+$ regulatory B cells constitute a subset of transitional B cells localized primarily in the peripheral tissues [46, 55, 76, 95]. Following stimulation with CD40, these cells produce the highest levels of IL-10 among all other B_{regs} in peripheral blood ($CD24^+CD27^+$ B_{regs}, $CD1d^+$ B_{regs}) [46]. Additionally, they are the only subset currently demonstrated to directly suppress Th1 differentiation of $CD4^+$ cells which is speculated to be partially dependent on cellular contact between CD80–86 on B cells and CD28 on T cells, and they have the capacity to induce the differentiation of $CD4^+$ T cells into T_{regs} or Trl cells [95]. According to studies by Blair et al., $CD24^+CD38^+$ B_{regs} from SLE patients were defective in number and showed impaired IL-10 production following CD40 stimulation [95]. These patients were also unable to suppress Th1 responses secondary to defective STAT3 phosphorylation [95]. Although SLE could be the result of genetic predispositions, the above findings lead to the hypothesis that the observed B_{reg} dysfunction is the result of overstimulation secondary to the chronic inflammatory environment leading to B_{reg} exhaustion and loss of function [74]. $CD24^+CD38^+$ B_{regs} also contribute to immune dysfunction in HIV infection where they hinder viral clearance [96]. This subtype of B_{reg} plays an integral role in the establishment of graft tolerance through suppression of effector T cells and thus prevents the development of chronic graft versus host disease [97, 98]. To conclude, B_{regs} have a vast role in various disease processes, and our understanding of their function will potentially give rise to novel therapies and the possibility of creating transplantation tolerance. Nevertheless, their role in allergic disease is still not well understood.

$CD24^{+}CD27^{+}$ B_{regs}

$CD24^{+}CD27^{+}$ B_{regs} comprise a subset of memory B cells and represent the majority of IL-10-producing B10 cells [46, 55]. The production of TNF-α by circulating monocytes is regulated by these $CD24^{+}CD27^{+}$ B_{regs} [76]. It was found that individuals with allergic asthma have a significantly reduced number of $CD24^{+}CD27^{+}$ B_{regs} in addition to their defective production of IL-10 upon LPS stimulation relative to healthy patients [29]. As a result, the induction of T_{regs} in response to the Der p1 allergen was weaker, and this could potentially be responsible for the propagation of allergic asthma and hence warrants further research in $CD24^{+}CD27^{+}$ B_{regs} [29].

Other B_{regs} Phenotypes

There is no standard definition of the phenotypic characterization of B_{regs}, and as a result, certain established B_{reg} subtypes do not conform to the definition of IL-10-mediated suppression. A subset of plasmablasts identified as $CD27^{hi}CD38^{hi}$ is known as being IL-10-rich and is postulated to have a role in the anti-inflammatory humoral response [99]. Another unique B_{reg} subset, characterized by the $CD25^{hi}CD71^{hi}CD73^{lo}$ phenotype, is postulated to have a role in the induction of allergen tolerance through the production of IgG4 antibodies and the suppression of antigen-specific $CD4^{+}$ T cells [61]. In addition to IL-10-enriched B_{regs}, granzyme B (GrB)-expressing B cells, characterized by the $CD19^{+}CD38^{+}CD1d^{+}$ $IgM^{+}CD147^{+}$ phenotype, have been described to exert a suppressive function [100, 101]. Another subtype of B_{regs} characterized by the $CD39^{+}CD73^{+}$ phenotype was shown to drive the microenvironment away from an AT-mediated pro-inflammatory environment, through interaction with adenosine [102]. Additionally, the $CD35^{+}TSP\text{-}1^{+}$ B_{regs} subset has been shown to suppress allergic inflammation in the intestine through their ability to downregulate dendritic cell co-stimulatory molecules via TGF-β production, thus resulting in T_{reg} differentiation [103].

1.5 Summary

To summarize, B-cell subsets play important roles in the promotion and regulation of allergic disease. Future studies are required to further characterize and define subsets of IgE and B_{reg} phenotypes, and in particular, their individual contributions to allergic disease. Given that these cells have been shown to modulate the inflammatory processes in allergic asthma, much remains to be understood in this field. We provide a comprehensive overview of IgE^{+} B cells and regulatory B cells in the studies outlined in this chapter, utilizing a human model of allergic airway inflammation, rare samples spanning the airway, hematopoietic, lymphatic and peripheral compartments, and relevant experimental strategies in the field of immunology (*see* Fig. 1) [9, 10, 88]. Further, the advent of novel technologies being able to study these cells more in depth will allow us to better understand their undiscovered roles in disease.

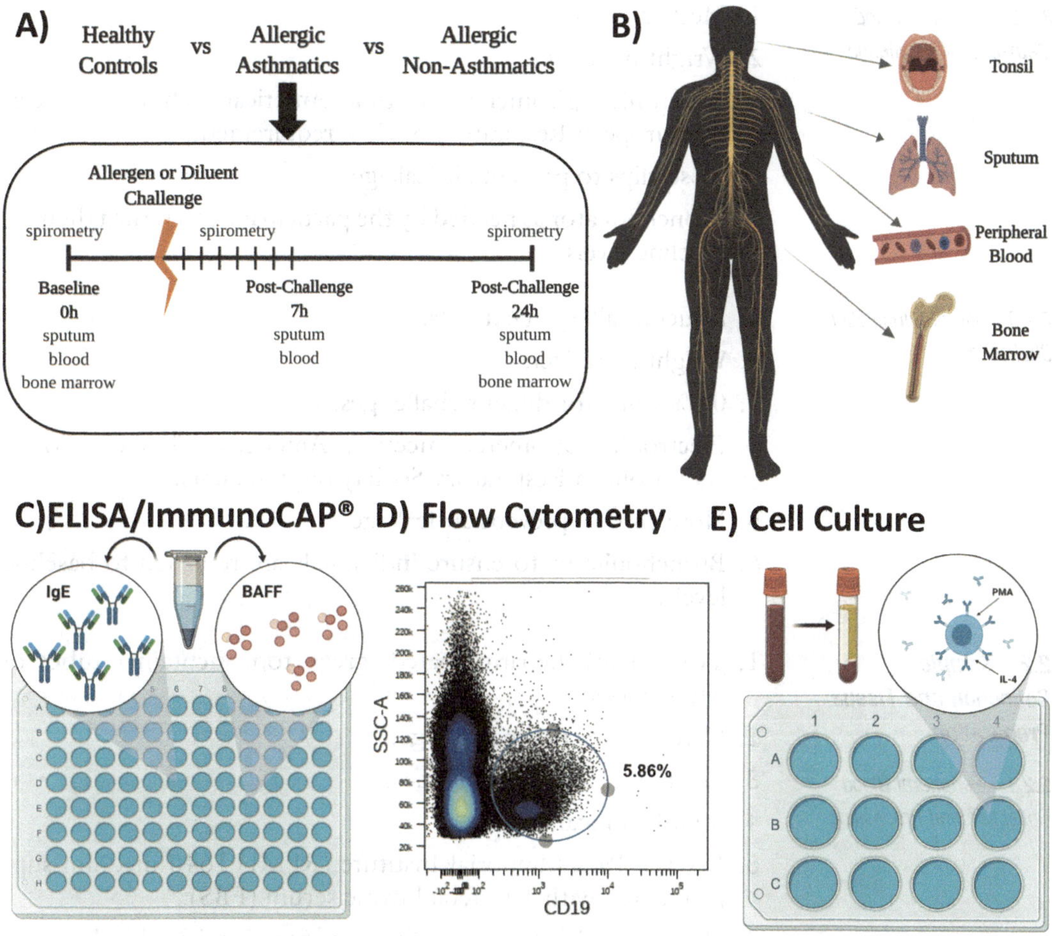

Fig. 1 Experimental workflow evaluating IgE+ B cells and regulatory B cells in allergic asthmatics. (**a**) Groups of individuals evaluated and experimental timeline for the human allergen inhalation challenge. (**b**) Specimens collected from human volunteers and evaluated for IgE+ B cells and regulatory B cells analysis. (**c**) ELISA and ImmunoCAP measurements for inflammatory mediators including BAFF, total IgE, and specific IgE. (**d**) Flow cytometry analysis of various sample cell suspensions at baseline between disease groups and pre- and post-allergen challenge. (**e**) Cell culture techniques employed to stimulate B cells and evaluate their regulatory capacity

2 Materials

2.1 Selection of Participants with Mild Allergic Asthma

2.1.1 Skin Prick Test

1. Histamine (positive control).
2. Diluting solution: 0.9% saline (negative control).
3. Allergen extracts resuspended in diluting solution.
4. Lancet to perform a small abrasion on the skin with the allergen extracts.
5. Pen and ruler to measure the wheal diameters.
6. Alcohol swabs to wipe allergen extract from skin.
7. Anti-histamines as needed by the participants.

2.1.2 Spirometry and Methacholine Challenge Test

1. Methacholine.
2. Wright nebulizer.
3. Electronic spirometer meeting American Thoracic Society/European Respiratory Society requirements.
4. Nose clips to prevent air leakage.
5. Bronchodilator as needed by the participants, to return them to baseline levels.

2.1.3 Allergen Inhalation Challenge

1. Aqueous allergen extracts.
2. Wright nebulizer.
3. 0.9% saline for diluent challenges.
4. Electronic spirometer meeting American Thoracic Society/European Respiratory Society requirements.
5. Nose clips to prevent air leakage.
6. Bronchodilator to ensure individuals are returned to baseline levels.

2.2 Sample Collection and Tissue Preparation

2.2.1 Peripheral Blood Collection and Processing

1. Two 10 mL heparin-coated, green top, vacutainer tubes of whole blood.
2. Cryovials for plasma storage.
3. Frosted, glass slides for smear.
4. 50 mL conical tubes.
5. Roswell Park Memorial Institute (RPMI) 1640 medium supplemented with 10% fetal bovine serum (FBS).
6. Density gradient medium for centrifugation-based isolation of peripheral blood mononuclear cells.
7. Ammonium chloride-based red cell lysing reagent.
8. Sterile disposable 10 mL and 20 mL pipettes.
9. Centrifuge.
10. $CD19^+$ isolation kit to isolate and purify B cells (*see* **Note 1**).

2.2.2 Bone Marrow Aspiration and Processing

1. Bone marrow aspiration needle.
2. Local anesthetic such as lidocaine.
3. 10 mL syringe.
4. 1 mL liquid heparin in syringe.
5. Cryovials for plasma storage.
6. Frosted, glass slides for smear.
7. 50 mL conical tubes.
8. RPMI 1640 medium supplemented with 10% FBS.

9. Density gradient medium for centrifugation-based isolation of peripheral blood mononuclear cells.
10. Ammonium chloride-based red cell lysing reagent.
11. Sterile disposable 10 mL and 20 mL pipettes.
12. Centrifuge.
13. Kit, device (magnet, column, etc.) and solutions for immunomagnetic separation of human CD138+ cells (*see* **Note 2**).
14. 100 μm sterile filter.

2.2.3 Tonsil biopsy Processing and Cell Isolation

1. Sterile, through-cut forceps.
2. Local anesthetic such as lidocaine.
3. 10 mL conical tubes.
4. Phosphate buffered saline (PBS): 8.00 g sodium chloride, 0.20 g potassium chloride, 1.44 g sodium phosphate, 0.24 g potassium phosphate, 1000 mL distilled water, pH adjusted to 7.4.
5. Petri dish.
6. RPMI 1640 medium supplemented with 10% FBS.
7. Disposable scalpel.
8. Sterile squeeze bulb pipettes.
9. 0.1% collagenase solution: 1 mL of 1% collagenase type I in 9 mL PBS.
10. 37 °C incubator with shaker.
11. 100 μm sterile filter.
12. Centrifuge.

2.2.4 Sputum Induction and Processing

1. 3%, 4%, and 5% saline.
2. Nebulizer (jet or ultrasonic) with output 0.2–1.0 mL/min.
3. Sterile cups with screw-on caps for sputum expectorant.
4. Petri dish.
5. Sterile forceps.
6. 10 mL and 50 mL conical tubes.
7. PBS.
8. 0.2% sputolysin reagent: a concentrate of dithiothreitol (DTT) in phosphate buffer.
9. Cryovials for sputum supernatant storage.
10. Trypan blue live/dead cell stainer.
11. Hemocytometer.
12. 50 μm nylon mesh cloth.

13. Frosted, glass slides for sputum cytospins.
14. Cytospin centrifuge.
15. Diff-Quik™ stain with hematoxylin and eosin (Microptic).

2.3 Circulating Protein Measurements

1. Squeeze bottle for wash buffer.
2. Paper towels and kim wipes.
3. Multi-channel pipettes.
4. Ice box and ice.
5. Human BAFF ELISA kit. Many different suppliers provide ELISA kits of sufficient quality to be used for BAFF detection. We used the BAFF ELISA kit from R&D Systems.
6. Total human IgE ELISA kit. Many different suppliers provide ELISA kits of sufficient quality to be used for BAFF detection. We used the total IgE ELISA kit from Abcam.
7. ELISA plate reader.
8. Phadia® 250 platform by ImmunoCAP® (ThermoFisher Scientific).

2.4 Flow Cytometry Staining

1. Trypan blue live/dead cell stainer.
2. Hemocytometer.
3. Round-bottom, 5 mL, polystyrene tubes with filter caps.
4. Cell staining medium (CSM): 0.5% bovine serum albumin (BSA), 0.1% sodium azide, 5 mM ethylenediaminetetraacetic acid (EDTA) in PBS.
5. Human FcR block reagent. (*see* **Note 3**).
6. Fluorochrome-conjugated antibodies for flow cytometry staining of surface (*see* Table 1) and intracellular (*see* Table 2) molecules of IgE^+ B cells and B_{regs}.
7. Homemade or commercially distributed fixation and permeabilization buffers.
8. Centrifuge.
9. Table top vortex.
10. Compensation beads.
11. Flow cytometer and flow cytometry data analysis software.

2.5 B-Cell Isolation, Culture, and Stimulation

2.5.1 B-Cell Isolation

1. Four 10 mL heparin-coated, green top, vacutainer tubes of whole blood.
2. $CD19^+$ isolation kit to isolate and purify B cells (*see* **Note 4**).
3. 50 mL conical tubes.
4. PBS.
5. Magnetic separation system.

Table 1
Surface antibodies used to characterize IgE^{+} B cells and B_{regs} subsets

Target	Clone	Fluorophore
CD4	RPA-T4	APC-H7
CD8	RPA-T8	FITC
CD5	UCHT2	Alexa Fluor 700
CD19	SJ25-C1	APC-Cy7
CD19	MOPC-21	PE-Cy7
CD1d	CD1d42	APC
CD24	ML5	PE-CF594
CD27	M-T271	PE-Cy7
CD27	M-T271	V450
CD38	HIT2	PE
CD38	HB7	V450
CD45	2D1	AmCyan
CD45	2D1	APC-H7
CD45	HI30	V450
CD138	MI15	FITC
CD138	MI15	PerCP-Cy5.5

Table 2
Intracellular antibodies used to characterize IgE^{+} B cells and B_{regs} subsets

Target	Clone	Fluorophore
FoxP3	PCH101	Alexa Fluor 488
IgE	MB10-5C4	APC
IgE	MB10-5C4	PE
IgG	IS11-3B2.2.3	APC
IgG	IS11-3B2.2.3	FITC
IL-10	JES3-9D7	PE

6. Sterile squeeze bulb pipette.
7. B-cell culture medium: RPMI medium supplemented with 10% FBS, 2.5% 4-(2-hydroxyethyl)-1-piperazine-ethane-sulfonic acid (HEPES), 0.5% Penicillin/Streptomycin, and 1% sodium pyruvate.

2.5.2 B-Cell Culture and Stimulation

1. Round-bottom, 96-well, individually packaged, sterile culture plates.
2. Trypan blue live/dead cell stainer.
3. Hemocytometer.
4. Purified human IL-4.
5. Phorbol 12-myristate 13-acetate (PMA).
6. Ionomycin.
7. 5% CO_2, 37 °C cell culture incubator.
8. Protein transport inhibitor cocktail made of monensin and brefeldin A.
9. Fluorochrome-conjugated antibodies for flow cytometry staining of surface (*see* Table 1) and intracellular (*see* Table 2) molecules of IgE^+ B cells and B_{regs}.

3 Methods

3.1 Selection of Participants with Mild Allergic Asthma

When recruited, study participants complete all allergic asthmatic testing aimed to confirm the allergic status (skin prick test) and airway hyperresponsiveness (methacholine challenge) (*see* Table 3). The results of the methacholine challenge and skin prick test confirm the eligibility for subjects with mild asthma to enter the study, while the results of the skin prick test titration are used to determine the allergen dose for inhalation, as previously described [104–110].

3.1.1 Determination of Allergic Status Using Skin Prick Testing

1. Prick the skin with a lancet containing a small amount of common aeroallergens. Additionally, histamine and saline are used as positive and negative controls, respectively.
2. Measure wheal size using a pen and ruler 10 min after skin prick. A wheal diameter > 2 mm is considered to be positive [104–106].

Table 3
Subject characterization using methacholine challenge and skin prick test resultss

	Methacholine challenge result	Skin prick test result
Allergic asthmatics	Positive	Positive
Allergic non-asthmatics	Negative	Positive
Healthy controls	Negative	Negative

3.1.2 Measurement of lung Function Using Spirometry

1. Subjects must perform spirometric maneuvers with full flow volume loop.
2. Determine the percent predicted forced expiratory volume in one second (FEV_1) using the third National Health and Nutrition Examination Survey (NHANES III) reference values. A FEV1 $\geq$ 70% of predicted [107] is considered to be normal lung function.
3. Subjects that develop asthmatic exacerbations or respiratory tract infections within 4 weeks of the study start date or are historically diagnosed by a physician with other underlying diseases other than asthma must be excluded. Spirometry must be performed following American Thoracic Society guidelines [108].

3.1.3 Airway Hyperresponsiveness Testing Using the Methacholine Challenge Test

1. The methacholine challenge test that determines airway responsiveness [109] should be conducted by a trained, experienced technician using the tidal breathing method from a Wright Nebulizer.
2. The methacholine provocative concentration causing at least a 20% fall in FEV_1 (PC_{20}) is calculated by linear interpolation.
3. The methacholine PC_{20} is required to be $\leq$16 mg/mL [107] for a subject to have airway hyperresponsiveness (*see* **Note 5**).

3.1.4 Inducing Symptomatic Allergic asthma Using the Inhaled Allergen Challenge

1. As detailed in [111], allergen challenge should be conducted by a trained, experienced technician with a physician at arms-length in the event of complications.
2. The allergen challenge is conducted with increasing concentrations of allergen inhaled by tidal breathing for 2 min each. FEV_1 is measured 10 min post-inhalation.
3. Allergen inhalation is stopped when the FEV_1 falls by at least 20%, then FEV_1 is measured regularly until 7 h post-challenge.
4. The early asthmatic response is the lowest fall in FEV_1 between 0 and 2 h, while the late asthmatic response is the lowest fall in FEV_1 between 3 and 7 h.
5. The diluent control challenge (negative control) consisted of three doses of the diluting solution instead of diluted allergen extract (*see* Fig. 1a).

3.2 Sample Collection and Tissue Preparation

All samples must be collected by trained physicians or technicians, ensuring excellent quality sampling, and stored in controlled conditions (*see* Fig. 1b). Our group is uniquely positioned where we have extensive experience employing the allergen inhalation challenge model, in addition to being able to obtain a wide array of human biological specimens (e.g., bone marrow, peripheral blood, sputum, and tonsil biopsies).

3.2.1 Collection of Venous Blood through Venipuncture

1. Peripheral blood must be collected into vacutainers containing heparin by an experienced, trained phlebotomist.
2. Perform total cell count using a hemocytometer. Prepare smears and stain with Diff-Quik™ for cell differentials.
3. Centrifuge 2 mL of the blood at 1000 × *g* for 10 min to collect plasma for measurement of total IgE levels.
4. Dilute the remaining blood in RPMI medium supplemented with 10% FBS at 1:1 and then layer on density gradient medium. Centrifuge at 800 × *g* for 20 min without break.
5. Collect the PBMC layer and store at 4 °C for flow cytometry staining (*see* **Note 6**).

3.2.2 Aspiration of Bone Marrow Sample from the Iliac Crest

1. Bone marrow must be aspirated from the iliac crest following local administration of lidocaine by a trained, experienced hematologist.
2. Collect 9 mL of bone marrow into a bone marrow aspiration syringe containing 1 mL of heparin.
3. The 10 mL of bone marrow is further diluted 1:1.5 with RPMI medium supplemented with 10% FBS and layered on top of 15 mL density gradient medium at room temperature. Centrifuge at 800 × *g* for 20 min without break (*see* **Note** 7).
4. The bone marrow mononuclear cell (BMMC) layer was collected and stored at 4 °C for flow cytometry staining of regulatory B cells (*see* **Note 8**).

3.2.3 Homogenization of Tonsil biopsy and Cell Isolation

1. Tonsil tissue must be collected from patients using a through-cut forceps technique following local administration of lidocaine by a trained, experience otolaryngologist (*see* **Note 9**).
2. Disrupt the biopsy mechanically with a disposable scalpel in a petri dish and then incubate the processed tissue in 0.1% collagenase for 2 h at 37 °C to further breakdown tissue collagen (*see* **Note 10**).
3. Wash cells with PBS, centrifuge at 500 × *g* for 10 min, and filter through a 100-μm filter. Cells can then be stained for flow cytometry analysis.

3.2.4 Induction of Sputum Samples

1. Induce sputum by inhalation of 3%, 4%, and 5% saline and select and process mucous plugs as previously described [112, 113] (*see* **Notes 11** and **12**).
2. Treat sputum with sputolysin reagent and filter through a nylon mesh. Pellet the cells by centrifugation and perform a total cell count.

3. Prepare two cytospins and stain with Diff-Quik for cell differentials. Store the remaining cells at 4 °C for flow cytometry staining.
4. Froze the fluid phase at −80 °C for measurements of total IgE, BAFF, and other inflammatory mediators.

3.3 Circulating IgE and BAFF Measurements

1. Use commercially available, sandwich, enzyme-linked immunosorbent assay (ELISA) kits to quantify total and allergen-specific IgE and BAFF in peripheral blood plasma and sputum fluid phase (*see* Fig. 1c and **Note 13**).
2. The lower limit of detection (LLOD) is 0.5 IU/mL for total IgE based on the Abcam kit, 0.1 IU/mL for allergen-specific IgE based on the ImmunoCAP® platform, and 2.68 pg/mL for BAFF based on the R&D Systems kit.
3. Quantify the absorbance using an appropriate plate reader (*see* **Note 14**).

3.4 Flow Cytometry Experiments

The ones presented here below are the first protocols to be developed to evaluate IgE$^+$ B cells and regulatory B cells (B_{regs}) in the sputum, as well as in other peripheral compartments, of allergic asthmatics using the allergen inhalation challenge model [9, 10, 88].

Classically, IgE$^+$ B cells have been difficult to detect in the blood due to cell rarity. However, methodological advances in flow cytometry with more lasers have allowed for B-cell subsets to be measured using greater than 10 fluorochrome-conjugated antibody panels. Recent papers have reported the measurement of IgE$^+$ B cells in the blood [40], nasal biopsies, and nasal lavage of patients with allergic rhinitis [114, 115]. However, with our methods we were able for the first time to consistently detect IgE$^+$ B cells in the blood, bone marrow, tonsil, and sputum of subjects.

We also evaluated different phenotypes of B_{regs} implicated in allergic disease [29, 81, 116] using flow cytometry. We observed a consistent decrease in the frequency of FoxP3-expressing B_{regs} in the bone marrow and an increase in the blood at 24 h post-allergen inhalation challenge. Although we were not able to measure different phenotypes of B_{regs} in the airways due to limited sample availability, we were the first to measure the numbers of CD19$^+$FoxP3$^+$ B cells in the sputum.

3.4.1 General Cell Staining Protocol for Flow Cytometry

1. Aliquot the isolated cells in cell staining tubes (*see* **Note 15**) and wash twice with CSM.
2. Incubate cells for 10 min with human FcR block reagent diluted in accordance to manufacturer's instructions to a final volume of 50 μl.

3. After 10 min, add the surface antibodies without washing. Depending on the specific sample (sputum, PBMC, BMMC, tonsil) being analyzed, incubate cells for 30 min at 4 °C with a different combination of antibodies directed against specific surface markers at a final volume of 200 μl (*see* Table 1 and Subheadings 3.4.2 and 3.4.3).
4. Following incubation, wash cells by 5 min centrifugation at 500 × *g* at 4 °C (*see* **Note 16**).
5. Proceed with the fixation/permeabilization step according to the manufacturer's instructions of the employed commercial kit (*see* **Note 17**).
6. Incubate cells with mouse and rat serum for 10 min (*see* **Note 18**).
7. After 10 min, add the intracellular antibodies without washing. Incubate cells with the antibodies directed against specific intracellular markers at a final volume of 200 μl for 30–60 min at room temperature (*see* Table 2 and Subheadings 3.4.2 and 3.4.3). Appropriate isotypes and fluorescence minus one (FMO) must be used as negative controls for fluorescent staining background and antibody specificity, respectively. Use compensation beads to adjust settings.
8. Following incubation, wash cells and acquire the samples using a flow cytometer capable of detecting up to 15 fluorochromes simultaneously.
9. Export the .fcs files from the flow cytometer and analyze them with a dedicated software (*see* Fig. 1d).

3.4.2 Gating Strategy to Identify the Rare Population of IgE⁺ B Cells

1. To identify IgE^+ B cells among total sputum cells, samples should be surface stained with antibodies to CD45 (APC-H7), CD19 (PE-Cy7), and intracellularly stained with antibodies to IgE (PE). As shown in Fig. 2a, place a gate around all the cells, excluding debris and doublets, in the forward scatter (FSC) and side scatter (SSC) plots. Plot SSC-A and CD45 and gate on the $SSC^{low}CD45^+$ lymphocyte population (*see* Fig. 2b). Then draw a gate around the $CD19^+$ B-cell population on the CD45 and CD19 plot (*see* **Note 19**). Plot $CD19^+$ B cells with IgE and analyze IgE^+ B cells in the airways (*see* **Note 20** and Fig. 2b). Figure 2 also shows a representative analysis of how the frequency of the CD19 population changes among the participants of the allergic asthma study (*see* Fig. 2c) and in the course of allergen challenge (*see* Fig. 2d).
2. To identify IgE^+ B cells among memory B cells (MBCs, $CD27^+CD38^-$), plasmablasts or pre-plasma cells (PPCs, $CD27^+CD38^+$) and plasma cells (PCs, $CD38^+CD138^+$) from peripheral blood and tonsil, samples should be surface stained

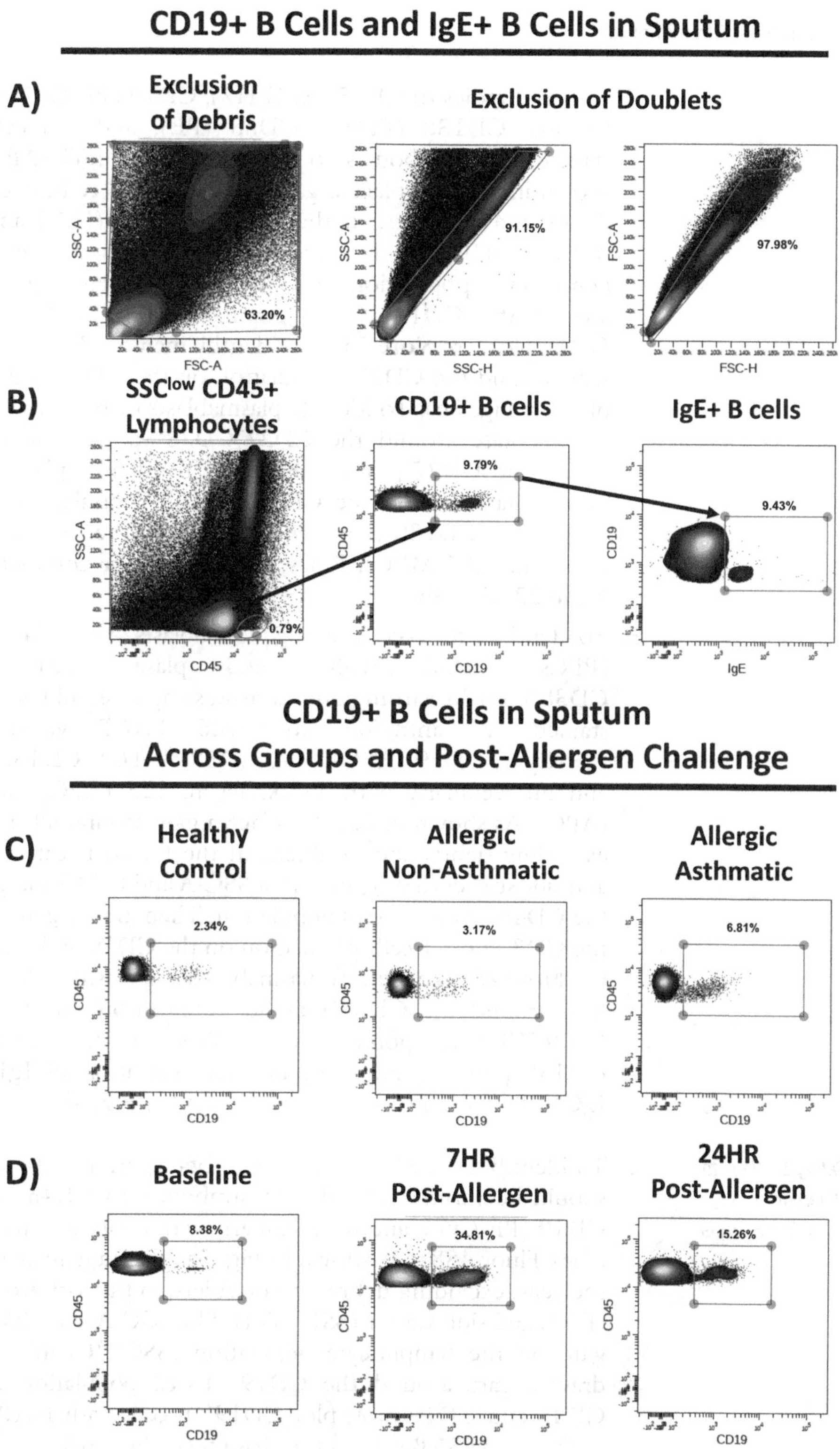

Fig. 2 Representative gating strategy for $CD19^+$ and IgE^+ B cells in sputum. (**a**) Exclusion of debris and isolation of single cells. (**b**) Identification of total lymphocytes, $CD19^+$ B cells, and IgE^+ B cells. (**c**) $CD19^+$ B-cell proportions as a percent of $CD45^+$ lymphocytes across groups (controls and allergic asthmatics). (**d**) $CD19^+$ B cell proportions as a percent of $CD45^+$ lymphocytes in allergic asthmatics pre- and post-allergen inhalation challenge

with antibodies to CD45 (APC-H7), CD19 (PE-Cy7), CD27 (V450), CD138 (FITC), CD38 (PE), and intracellularly stained with antibodies to IgE (APC) and IgG (APC). As shown in Fig. 3a, place a gate around all the cells, excluding debris and doublets, in the forward scatter (FSC) and side scatter (SSC) plots. Plot SSC-A and CD45 and gate on the lymphocyte population ($SSC^{low}CD45^{+}$). Then draw a gate around the $CD19^{+}$ B-cell population on the CD45 and CD19 plot (*see* **Note 21**). To identify memory B cells, draw a gate around the $CD27^{+}$ population on the CD19 and CD27 plot (*see* Fig. 3b). To identify plasmablasts or pre-plasma cells, draw a gate around the $CD27^{+}CD38^{+}$ population on the CD38 and CD27 plot (*see* Fig. 3c). To identify plasma cells, draw a gate around the $CD38^{+}CD138^{+}$ population on the CD38 and CD138 plot (*see* Fig. 3d). Further evaluation of IgE^{+} and IgG^{+} MBCs, PPCs, and PCs can be conducted (*see* **Note 22**, Fig. 3b-d).

3. To identify IgE^{+} B cells among plasmablasts or pre-plasma cells (PPCs, $CD38^{+}CD138^{-}$) and plasma cells (PCs, $CD38^{+}CD138^{+}$) from bone marrow, samples should be surface stained with antibodies to CD45 (PerCP-Cy5.5), CD3 (PE-Cy7), CD19 (APC-Cy7), CD38 (FITC), CD138 (PE), and intracellularly with antibodies to IgE (APC) and IgG (APC). As shown in Fig. 4a, place a gate around all the cells, excluding debris and doublets, in the forward scatter (FSC) and side scatter (SSC) plots. Plot SSC-A and CD45 and gate on the $CD45^{+}$ lymphocytes population. Then draw a gate around the $CD3^{-}$ non-T cells population on the CD19 and CD3 plot (*see* **Note 23**). To identify plasmablasts and plasma cells, draw a gate around the $CD38^{+}CD138^{-}$ population for PPCs and $CD38^{+}CD138^{+}$ population for PCs on the CD38 and CD138 plot (*see* Fig. 4a). Further evaluation of IgE^{+} and IgG^{+} PPCs and PCs can be conducted (*see* Fig. 4b-c).

3.4.3 Gating Strategy to Identify Different Regulatory B-Cell Subsets

1. To identify $FoxP3^{+}$ B cells among total sputum cells, samples should be surface stained with antibodies to CD45 (V450), CD19 (PE-Cy7), and intracellularly with antibodies to FoxP3 (Alex Fluor 488). As shown in Fig. 5a, place a gate around all the cells, excluding debris and doublets, in the forward scatter (FSC) and side scatter (SSC) plots. Plot SSC-A and CD45 and gate on the lymphocyte population ($SSC^{low}CD45^{+}$). Then draw a gate around the $CD19^{+}$ B-cell population on the CD45 and CD19 plot, plot $CD19^{+}$ B cells with FoxP3, and analyze $FoxP3^{+}$ B cells in the airways (*see* Fig. 5b).
2. To identify regulatory B cells among total B cells from peripheral blood and bone marrow, samples should be surface stained with antibodies to CD19 (PE-Cy7), CD1d (APC), CD5 (Alexa

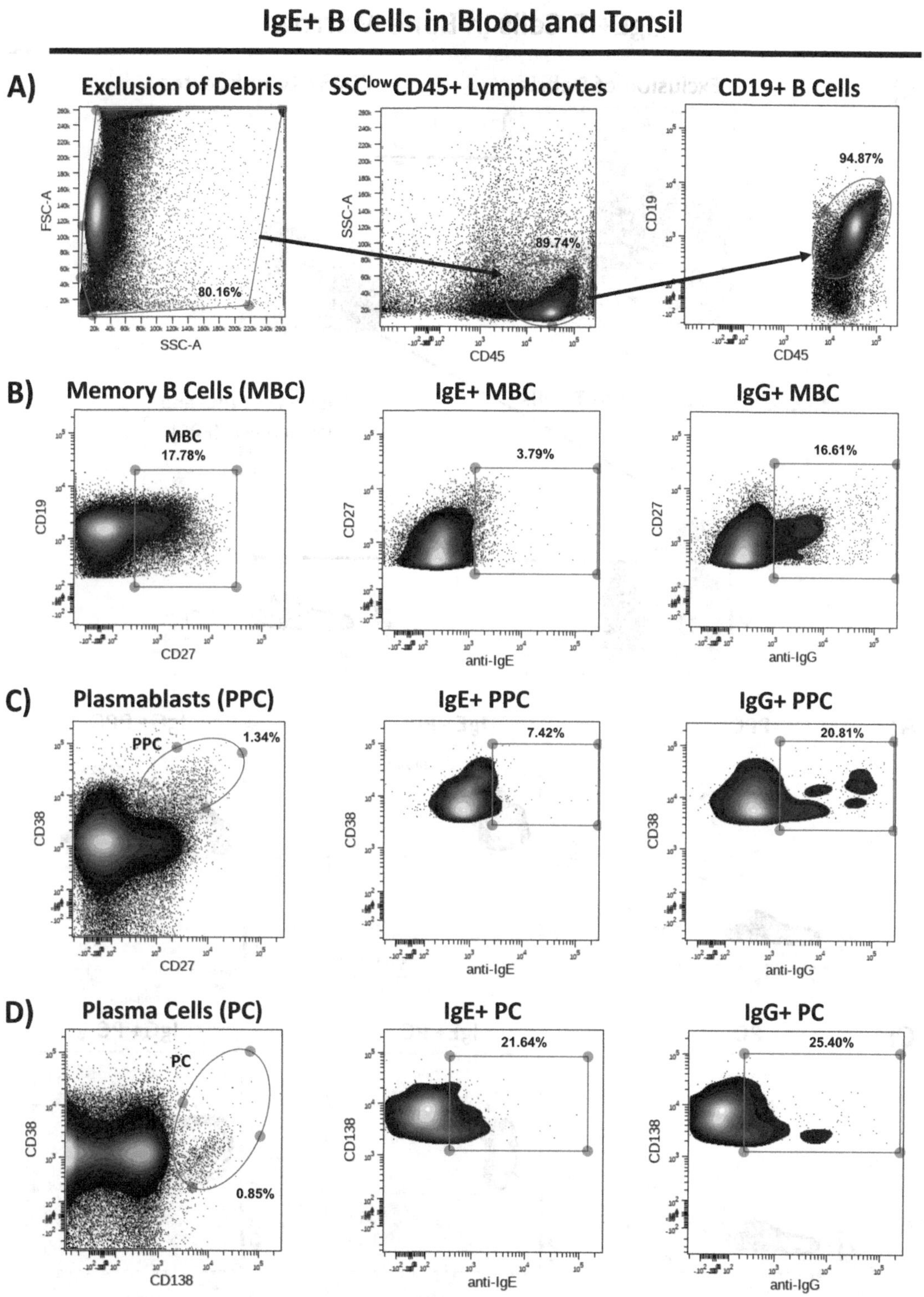

Fig. 3 Representative gating strategy for IgE$^+$ B cells in peripheral blood and tonsil. (**a**) Exclusion of debris and isolation of single cells and identification of CD19$^+$ B cells. (**b**) Identification of memory B cells and IgE$^+$ and IgG$^+$ memory B cells. (**c**) Identification of plasmablasts and IgE$^+$ and IgG$^+$ plasmablasts. (**d**) Identification of plasma cells and IgE$^+$ and IgG$^+$ plasma cells

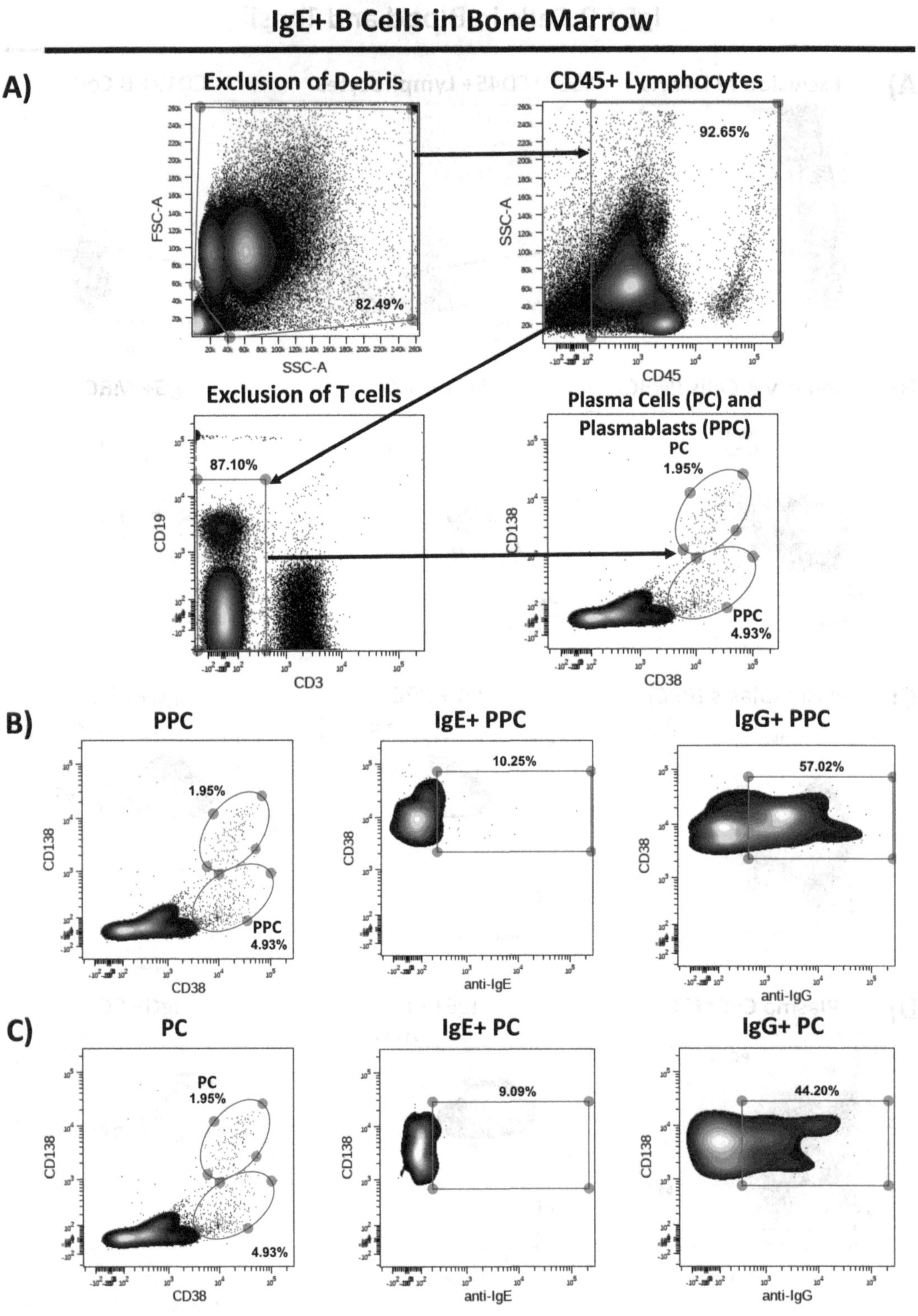

Fig. 4 Representative gating strategy for IgE$^+$ B cells in the bone marrow. (**a**) Exclusion of debris and isolation of single cells, identification of CD3$^-$ cells, and identification of plasmablasts and plasma cells. (**b**) Identification of plasmablasts and IgE$^+$ and IgG$^+$ plasmablasts. (**c**) Identification of plasma cells and IgE$^+$ and IgG$^+$ plasma cells

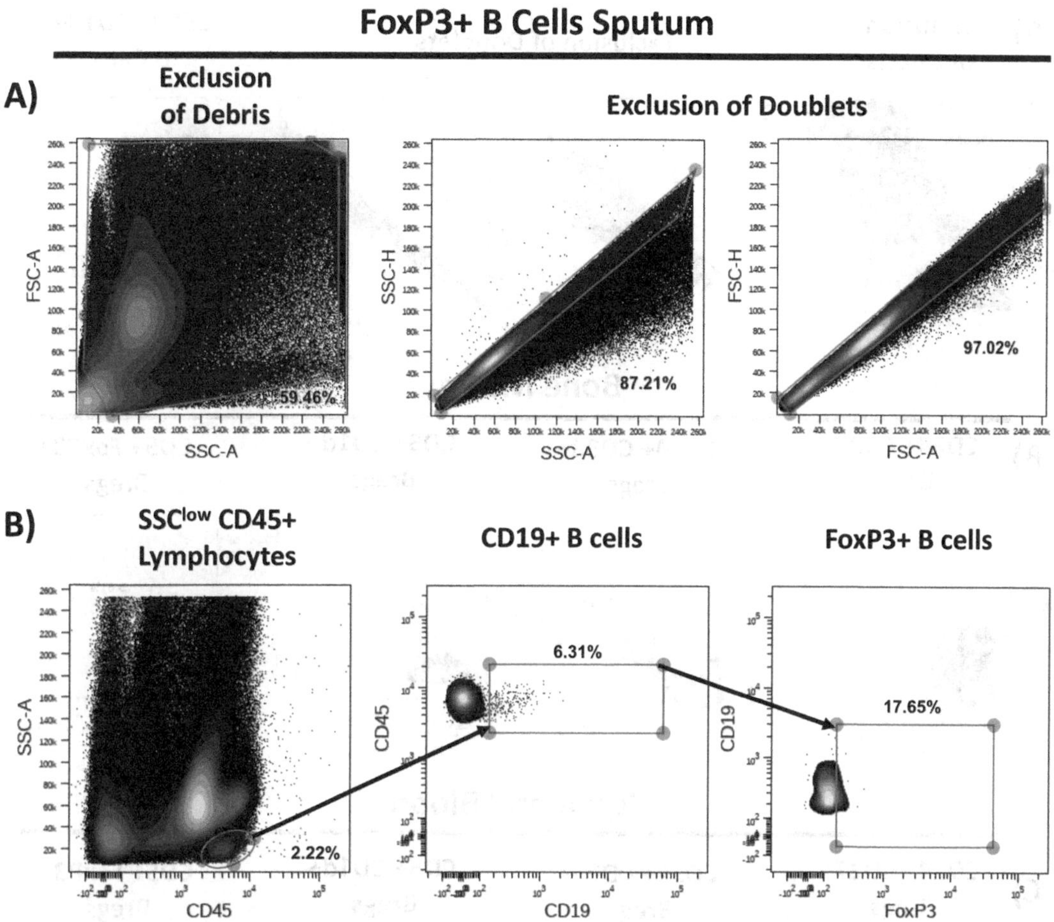

Fig. 5 Representative gating strategy for FoxP3+ B cells in sputum. (**a**) Exclusion of debris and isolation of single cells. (**b**) Identification of total lymphocytes, CD19+ B cells and FoxP3+ B cells

Fluor 700), CD24 (PE-CF594), CD27 (V450), CD38 (PE), and intracellularly with antibodies to IgE (APC), IL-10 (PE), and FoxP3 (Alexa Fluor 488). As shown in Fig. 6a, place a gate around all the cells, excluding debris and doublets, in the forward scatter (FSC) and side scatter (SSC) plots. Plot SSC-A and CD19 and gate on the B-cell population ($SSC^{low}CD19^{+}$). To identify the different regulatory B-cell subsets in peripheral blood and bone marrow, a combination of plots are used as seen in Fig. 6b-c. Briefly, plot CD24 and CD27 and gate on the $CD24^{+}CD27^{+}$ B_{reg} population. Second, plot CD24 and CD38 and gate on the $CD24^{+}CD38^{+}$ B_{reg} population. Third, plot CD1d and CD5 and gate on the $CD1d^{+}CD5^{+}$ B_{reg} population. Last, plot CD5 and FoxP3 and gate on the $CD5^{+}FoxP3^{+}$ B_{reg} population.

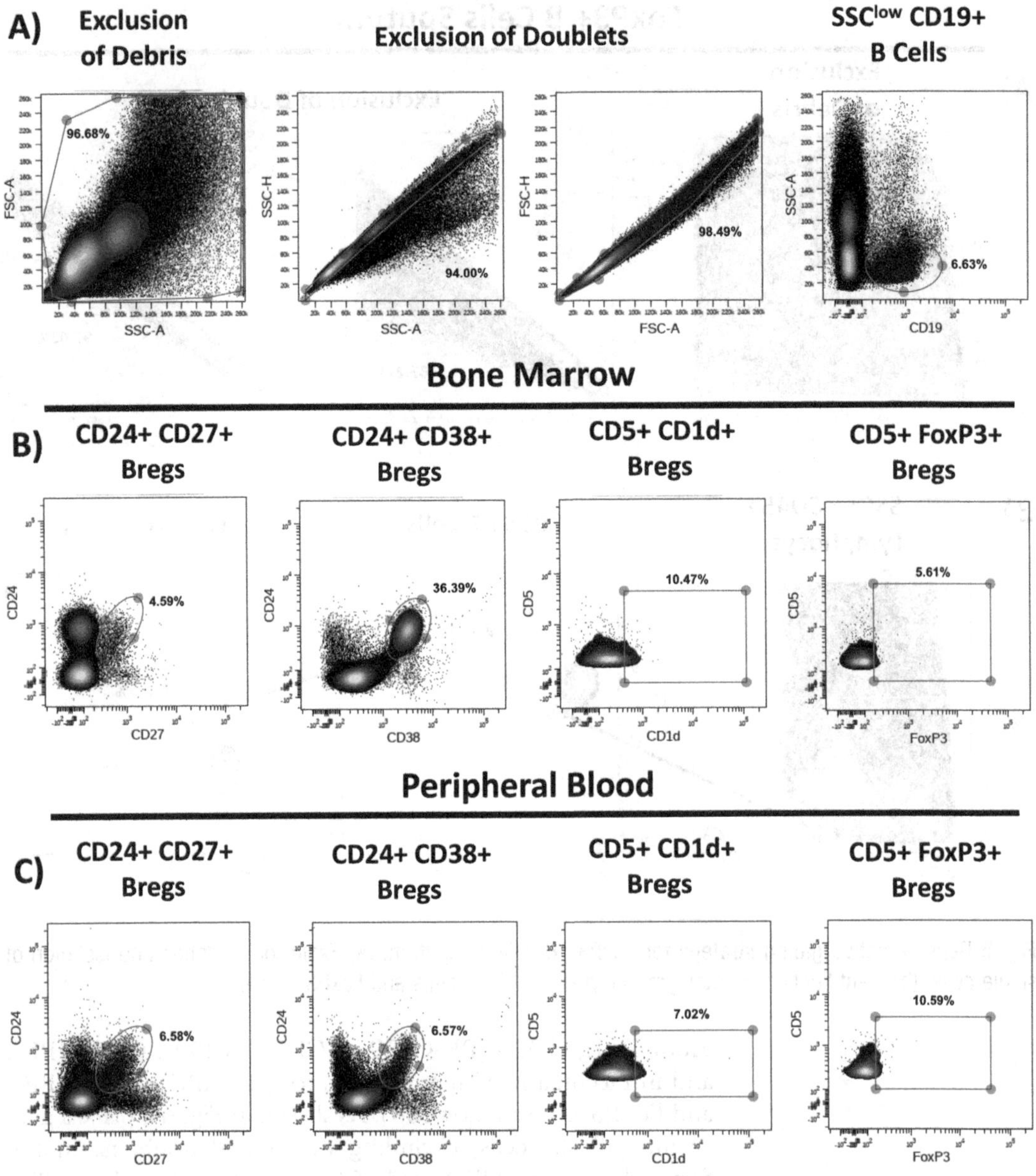

Fig. 6 Representative gating strategy for regulatory B cells in the bone marrow and peripheral blood. (**a**) Exclusion of debris and isolation of single cells. (**b**) B_{reg} populations in the bone marrow. (**c**) B_{reg} populations in peripheral blood

3.5 B_{regs} Functional Assay

The initiation of type 2 inflammation in allergic asthmatics includes the production of the IL-4 and IL-13 cytokines which are known to promote maturation of IgE-producing B cells [9, 10]. In a growing body of literature, B_{regs} have been proposed to suppress IgE-mediated allergic inflammation through the secretion of IL-10 [24, 61, 81, 117]. In murine models, a deficiency in B_{regs} has been associated with increased serum IgE, increased type-2-cytokines, and increased eosinophilia [24, 85]. In light of these considerations, when studying B_{regs} in the context of allergic asthma, it is very important to investigate the functional capacity of B_{regs} to express IL-10 in vitro. In this section we provide the protocols to assess how molecules produced during inflammation in allergic asthmatics, such as IL-4, affect the B-cell capacity to express FoxP3 and IL-10, which are both important markers for B_{regs} functions.

3.5.1 Isolation of Peripheral Blood CD19+ B Cells by Magnetic-Based Cell Separation

1. Collect the PBMC layer after density gradient centrifugation of peripheral blood (*see* Subheading 3.2.1).
2. Isolate human CD19+ B cells from whole blood by immunomagnetic separation (*see* **Note 4**). Follow the manufacturer's instructions of the employed kit.
3. At the end of the isolation process, wash and count purified cells. Before culturing, check the purity of isolated B cells by assessing the expression of the CD45, CD19, and CD20 markers by flow cytometry (*see* **Note 24**).
4. Suspend isolated cells at a concentration of 1×10^6 B cells/mL in B-cell culture medium (*see* **Note 25**).

3.5.2 B-Cell Stimulation with IL-4 to Determine Functional Expression of IL-10 and FoxP3

1. Plate isolated B cells in a round-bottom 96-well plate at a starting density of 2×10^5 cells in a final culture volume of 200 μl (*see* Fig. 1e).
2. Culture B cells in B-cell culture medium alone (negative control) or supplemented with either 15 ng/mL PMA and 0.5 μg/mL ionomycin (positive control) or with increasing concentrations (5 ng/mL, 25 ng/mL, and 50 ng/mL) of IL-4.
3. Incubate B cells in a humidified 37 °C, 5% CO_2 incubator for 72 h. Every 12 h, gently agitate the culture plate for approximately 3 sec (*see* **Note 26**).
4. Six hours before the end of culture, add to the culture suspension a protein transport inhibitor cocktail of 1 μmol/l brefeldin A and 1 μmol/l monensin to block cytokine secretion (*see* **Note 27**).
5. Collect cells and transfer to staining tubes. Proceed with cell surface (CD19, CD5, CD24, CD27) and intracellular (IL-10, FoxP3) staining as described in Subheading 3.4.1.
6. Analyze by flow cytometry the frequency of different B_{reg} subpopulations (*see* Subheading 3.4.3).

3.6 Next Generation Methods

The ones reported here below are not methodological protocols but rather the descriptions of two cutting edge techniques that allow to simultaneously study IgE+ B cells and regulatory B cells. Mass cytometry (CyTOF) and multiplexed imaging (IMC and MIBIscope) are next generation technologies still in their infancy of utility that can permit to quantify and characterize IgE$^+$ B cells and B_{regs} with much more resolution than what is already available in literature.

3.6.1 Mass Cytometry (CyTOF)

A big limitation when studying IgE$^+$ B cells and B_{regs} is the technological limitation in being able to quantify these cells. With the advancements in flow cytometry techniques and the availability of many new fluorochromes, it has been possible to adequately study IgE$^+$ B cell and B_{regs} subsets in separate flow cytometry experiments. However, the ability to simultaneously study IgE$^+$ B cells and B_{regs} within one experiment would be ideal since it would give us the ability to accurately compare the ratio of these cell types and heterogenous cell states; better examining the balance in cellular quantities between inflammation and regulation within the context of allergic asthma pathogenesis. Specifically, utilizing mass cytometry or cytometry by time-of-flight mass spectrometry (CyTOF), and specifically quantifying and characterizing IgE$^+$ B cells and B_{regs} would be beneficial to the better understanding of the proportions of these cell subpopulations [118] (*see* Fig. 7a). Mass cytometry is still a fairly underused, versatile technology used for the analysis of cells on a single-cell level [119–126]. Unlike flow cytometry, mass cytometry allows for simultaneous measurement of more intracellular and extracellular biomarkers, with greater precision [120, 122]. In flow cytometry, cells of interest are labeled with fluorochrome-conjugated antibodies, and the interactions of the cell with a laser lead to fluorescent emission of light at variable wavelengths, allowing for the detection and quantification of up to 20 cellular markers [122]. Mass cytometry involves the labeling of cells with metal-tagged antibodies for the detection and quantification of up to 50 cellular markers, which is almost double compared to flow cytometry [122]. The ability to simultaneously explore more cellular parameters allows for better understanding of complex cellular systems and signaling pathways that contribute to our current understanding of B-cell biology [127]. Glass et al. prepared the first B-cell atlas, evaluating the expression of 351 surface molecules on B cells using mass cytometry, as well as interrogate transcription, translation, metabolism, and signaling in B cells [127, 128]. They identified four specific markers (CD45RB, CD11c, CD73, CD95) that distinguished phenotypically and isotypically distinct B-cell subsets [127]. The next step would be to explore the intracellular environment of B cells, evaluating transcription factors, cytokine expression, and other inflammatory mediators, particularly within the context of regulatory B cells. One of the most practical approach to deeply learn B-cell biology is to continue employing next generation technologies like mass cytometry. Quantifying cells based on mass and charge allows us to circumvent fluorochrome light detection overlap and autofluorescence, which are large limitations of flow cytometry [122]. Lastly,

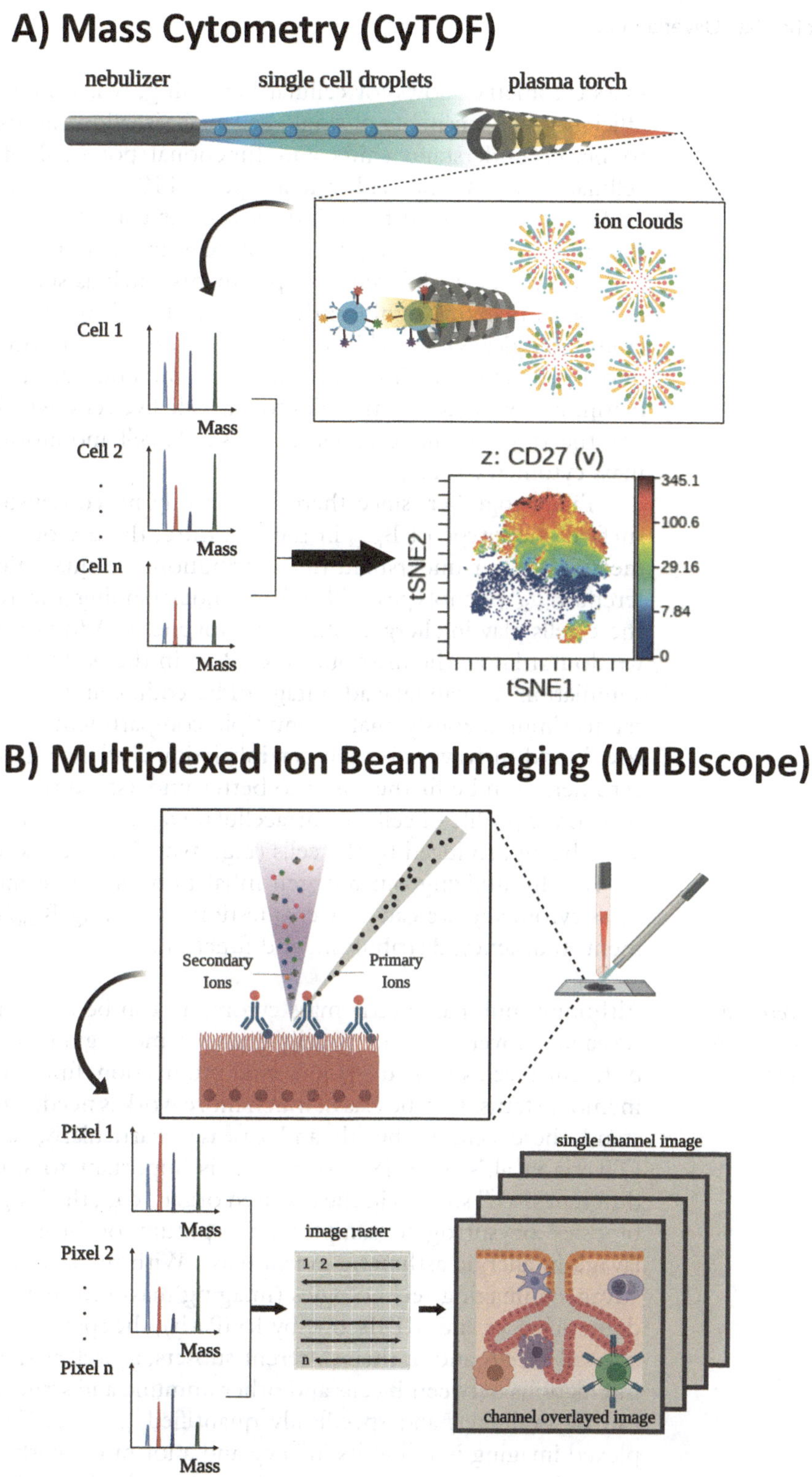

Fig. 7 Next generation technologies to evaluate IgE^{+} B cells and regulatory B cells. (**a**) Multiparameter cytometry using mass cytometry (CyTOF) technology with the ability to simultaneously measure more than 40 antigens simultaneously, on the cell surface or intracellularly. (**b**) Multidimensional imaging using multiplexed ion beam imaging (MIBIscope) technology with the ability to simultaneously measure more than 40 targets in tissues, simultaneously revealing spatial localization of structural, cellular, and subcellular features

mass cytometry allows for cellular barcoding, which improves the efficiency and sensitivity of single-cell analysis, allowing researchers to better understand shifts and functional potential of specific cellular subsets and sub-phenotypes [119, 122, 123, 129–132]. Capitalizing on the utility of cellular barcoding to increase the efficiency in the acquisition of cells from multiple patients and/or cells from different compartments, such as spleen, blood, and bone marrow, significantly increases the throughput of precious biological samples [119, 123]. Furthermore, Hartmann et al. developed and quality controlled a method using CD298 platinum-conjugated antibodies to barcode live cells, which broadens the downstream capabilities of single-cell monitoring using mass cytometry [132].

Taken together, since there is currently no consensus on the surface phenotype of B_{regs} in the literature, the use of mass cytometry to better understand the distribution and quantities of different B_{regs} phenotypes will aid in understanding the roles that these cells play in allergic asthma pathogenesis. Additionally, since we do not know the distribution of B_{regs} in the body after allergic stimulation, we can take advantage of barcoding and mass cytometry to simultaneously analyze multiple compartments (bone marrow, blood, airways) after allergen inhalation challenge. Lastly, mass cytometry can be further used to better understand the single-cell proteomic profile of cells by intracellular staining of different cytokines being produced by the cells (e.g., type 2 cytokines; IL-4 and IL-13). By utilizing our allergen inhalation challenge model and mass cytometry, we can answer questions regarding B_{regs} development, transiency, distribution, and function.

3.6.2 Multiplexed Ion Beam Imaging Time of Flight (MIBI-TOF)

Although multiparametric mass cytometry can be a useful tool in revealing novel states of B cells giving a more granular look on different B cell states (developmental progression, functional state, memory status, isotype class), much more work is needed to understand these cells in health and disease. Particularly, as seen in Oliveria et al.'s work [9, 10, 88], it is important to study these different B-cell subsets in the diseased organ (e.g., the lungs such as biopsies or surrogate samples like sputum or bronchoalveolar lavage in allergic asthmatic individuals). With the advent of more advanced imaging technologies (imaging mass cytometry by Fluidigm Sciences and MIBIscope by IonPath), the spatial localization of total B cells and of their different subsets, as well as the cell–cell interactions between B cells and other immune and structural cells, can be evaluated and specifically quantified (*see* Fig. 7b). Multiplexed imaging is still in its infancy and a lot more work is needed to: (i) learn more interesting biological mechanisms [133, 134], (ii) work with the high-dimensional data and develop more robust and innovative analytical pipelines [134, 135], and (iii) develop concurrent methodological approaches leveraging the imaging technology platforms to perform multi-omic-type experimental studies. Similar to how mass cytometry is the next generation technology for flow cytometry, imaging mass cytometry (IMC) and MIBIscope is the next generation technology for immunohistochemistry [129]. Multiplexed imaging yields rich spatial information that cannot be achieved by mass or flow cytometry [129, 134]. Imaging has always been able to provide spatial information, such as localization of cell surface or intracellular markers, points of cell contact and interaction, spatial heterogeneity of various cell populations. However, with multiplexed imaging and through the using of the full potential of greater than 40 antigens measured simultaneously, novel cell subsets, different cellular clusters/niches can be revealed, and spatial arrangement of immune cells can be uncovered [134, 136–138]. In the work by Zhao et al., authors determined that different B-cell subsets occupy different niches in lymphoid tissues, where marginal zone B cells and memory B cells are spatially located in different anatomical spaces within the gut lymphoid tissues [136]. This data shows that there is B-cell diversity and heterogeneity that is still widely unknown, even within healthy individuals, let alone various disease states. Much more work using high-dimensional imaging platforms to study B cells is needed, particularly in allergic diseases, since IgE produced by B cells plays an important role in disease pathogenesis [138].

4 Notes

1. To isolate CD19$^+$ B cells from whole blood, we use the RosetteSep™ CD19$^+$ B-cell enrichment kit (STEMCELL Technologies). This negative selection kit enriches the B-cell population through a two-step protocol: first non-B cells are bound to a tetramer-antibody cocktail, while the following centrifugation with the RosetteSep™ density gradient medium will enrich B cells in the visible layer, and pellet non-B cells and red blood cells.
2. We used the StraightFrom® Whole Blood CD138 MicroBeads (Miltenyi Biotec) since it allows the isolation of CD138$^+$ cells directly from blood or blood products without the need for density gradient centrifugation. The AutoMACS running buffer and AutoMACS rinsing solution were used accordingly.
3. The FcR block reagent is used to prevent unwanted binding of antibodies to human Fc receptor-expressing cells. In alternative to the FcR block reagent, both mouse and rat serum can be used during staining for flow cytometric analysis to inhibit non-specific binding of mouse and rat monoclonal antibodies, respectively. Although many different suppliers provide the FcR block reagent, we used the one from Miltenyi Biotec.

4. EasySep™ $CD19^+$ B-cell isolation kit (STEMCELL Technologies) is used to isolate and purify $CD19^+$ B cells by positive selection. This kit isolates $CD19^+$ B cells directly from whole blood and the isolation process is quick and efficient, yielding high purity of functional B cells. Compared to the RosetteSep $CD19^+$ B-cell enrichment kit, the EasySep $CD19^+$ B-cell isolation kit provides a final product with a much greater purity, and this is fundamental when cells must be put in culture for downstream experiments. Indeed, although good at depleting other cells, B-cell isolation through negative selection still has other cellular contaminations, which can be easily removed in silico (e.g., gating desired cells and/or gating out undesired cells) but are not suitable with cell culture.
5. To be considered to have airway hyperresponsiveness, the methacholine PC_{20} must be below 16 mg/mL. Methacholine is a smooth muscle agonist, and by inhaling concentrations of methacholine higher than 16 mg/mL, even healthy subjects with healthy airways can experience bronchoconstriction.
6. For the peripheral blood studies evaluating the kinetics of IgE^+ B cells [10], peripheral blood can be collected into heparin tubes and enriched for B cells using the RossetteSep™ isolation kit. B cells can then be stained for flow cytometry.
7. The suggested dilution is based on experience evidences that show that this dilution generates the optimal viscosity to perform an undisrupted layer on the density gradient.
8. Since the bone marrow is a reservoir for $CD138^+$ plasma cells, a $CD138^+$ isolation kit can be used to isolate and enrich plasma cells in the bone marrow studies evaluating the kinetics of IgE^+ B cells [10]. Incubate the mononuclear cell layer with anti-$CD138^+$ microbeads before proceeding with immunomagnetic separation. If using the magnetic-activated cell sorter (MACS) system from Miltenyi, then you can increase $CD138^+$ cell purity by passing the labeled cells through a LS column twice, and by slowly plunging the LS column each time. Isolated plasma cells can be stained for flow cytometry.
9. The physician should consistently collect 0.5 cm^3 pieces of tonsil tissue from willing donors. This will allow to yield enough cells in order to stain 2×10^6 cells per sample tube for flow cytometry analysis.
10. After mechanical disruption of the tissue, the petri dish must be thoroughly washed with PBS three times to ensure that all cells were collected before further chemical digestion. Place the petri dish above a black colored piece of paper to visualize any remnants of cells. Moreover, filter three times the digested tissue to ensure there is no clumping of cells or remnants of collagen milieu.

11. The collection of mucous plugs must be done by trained and experienced technicians. Indeed, this staff is trained to collect "milky white" mucous plugs rich in cells, and to make sure to not include excess saliva and other debris, which could contaminate the sample with buccal epithelial cells. Sputum mucous plug collection must be done above a black colored piece of paper to visualize no remnants of cells. The increasing salt concentrations gradually increase ciliary transport of sputum from the trachea and allow for the mucous plugs to be coughed up by the sputum donor.
12. Encouragement of the participant during expectoration of sputum and live demonstration by the technician was shown to result in optimal samples with adequate cell numbers for flow cytometry staining. Visualization of the expectoration process yields optimal samples.
13. All samples should be pre-aliquoted after collection and processing, and stored at −80 °C. This ensures no freeze–thaw of samples which helps to avoid any inaccurate results from unmeasurable protein degradation.
14. It is important to note whether the samples for protein measurements have been diluted or run neat. For example, our sputum supernatant values were multiplied by the sputum processing dilution factor of 8 in order to get the correct detected levels.
15. To consistently obtain reliable bone marrow and peripheral blood B-cell measurements, the quantity of cells stained per sample tube should be 2×10^6 cells. This needs to be consistent throughout the duration of the study. If there are not enough cells (a very rare situation), use 1×10^6 cells per sample tube. To consistently obtain reliable sputum B-cell measurements, 5×10^5 cells per sample tube is required.
16. Perform centrifugation at a speed of $500 \times g$ before fixation and permeabilization, and drop down in speed of $300 \times g$ after fixation and permeabilization to ensure cells remain intact.
17. The addition of fixation and permeabilization solution should be done at a slow, dropwise fashion while the cell suspension is maintained under slow vortexing to avoid any clumping of cells.
18. The use of mouse and rat serum is useful to decrease the background signal of intracellular antibodies in flow cytometry.
19. In addition, selected $CD19^+$ B cells can be analyzed for CD27 and CD138 expression to isolate memory B cells (MBCs) and plasma cells (PCs). IgE^+ MBCs and PCs can also be enumerated in the airways.

20. IgG+ B cells, MBCs, and PCs can also be enumerated in the airways.
21. By using the RosetteSep™ CD19+ B-cell enrichment kit, the CD19+ B-cell population was above 90% of the total CD45 parent gate.
22. This gating strategy can be used for cells isolated from tissue (e.g., tonsil) and peripheral blood.
23. Since a CD138+ isolation kit was used to isolate CD138+ cells, a CD3 in silico depletion was needed to remove any T cells from the analysis, as a subset of T cells also express CD138.
24. By using the EasySep™ CD19+ B-cell isolation kit, the purity was consistently above 98.5%.
25. Resuspend the isolated B cells in B-cell culture medium to ensure they remain "happy" after magnetic isolation and let them rest for 2 h at 37 °C before beginning culture protocols.
26. Since it is known that B cells suffer during culture, a trypan blue viability count was performed before and 72 h after the start of culture to count viable and death cells. B-cell viabilities were above 99.3% and 82.1%, respectively.
27. Every 2 h during the 6 h protein transport inhibition period, gently agitate the culture plate for approximately 3 sec.

Acknowledgments

Our thanks to Ms. Vanessa Luk for editorial support. J.P.O. was supported by a Canadian Institutes of Health Research Postdoctoral Fellowship.

References

1. Lotvall J, Akdis CA, Barcharier LB, Bjermer L, Casale TB, Custovic A, Lemanske RF Jr, Wardlaw AJ, Wenzel SE, Greenberger PA (2015) Asthma endotypes: a new approach to classification of disease entities within the asthma syndrome. J Allergy Clin Immunol 127(2):355–360. https://doi.org/10.1016/j.jaci.2010.11.037
2. Akdis CA, Akdis M (2015) Mechanisms of allergen-specific immunotherapy and immune tolerance to allergens. World Allergy Organization Journal 8(1):17–17. https://doi.org/10.1186/s40413-015-0063-2
3. Wills-Karp M (1999) Immunologic basis of antigen-induced airway hyperresponsiveness. Annu Rev Immunol 17(1):255–281. https://doi.org/10.1146/annurev.immunol.17.1.255
4. Wills-Karp M (2004) Interleukin-13 in asthma pathogenesis. Immunol Rev 202 (1):175–190. https://doi.org/10.1111/j.0105-2896.2004.00215.x
5. Gauvreau GM, Evans MY (2007) Allergen inhalation challenge: a human model of asthma exacerbation. Contrib Microbiol 14:21–32. https://doi.org/10.1159/0000107052
6. Smith SG, Gauvreau GM (2007) IL-13 is a novel therapeutic target in allergic asthma. Expert Reviews in Clinical Immunology 3:671–675
7. Nair P, O'Byrne PM (2016) Measuring eosinophils to make treatment decisions in asthma. Chest 150(3):485–487. https://doi.org/10.1016/j.chest.2016.07.009

8. Holgate S, Casale T, Wenzel S, Bousquet J, Deniz Y, Reisner C (2005) The anti-inflammatory effects of omalizumab confirm the central role of IgE in allergic inflammation. J Allergy Clin Immunol 115 (3):459–465. https://doi.org/10.1016/j.jaci.2004.11.053
9. Oliveria JP, Salter BM, Phan S, Obminski CD, Munoz CE, Smith SG, Scime T, Watson RM, Sehmi R, Gauvreau GM (2017) Asthmatic subjects with allergy have elevated levels of IgE+ B cells in the airways. J Allergy Clin Immunol 140(2):590–593.e9. https://doi.org/10.1016/j.jaci.2016.12.981
10. Oliveria JP, Salter BM, MacLean J, Kotwal S, Smith A, Harris JM, Scheerens H, Sehmi R, Gauvreau GM (2017) Increased IgE+ B cells in sputum, but not blood, bone marrow, or tonsils, after inhaled allergen challenge in subjects with asthma. Am J Respir Crit Care Med 196(1):107–109. https://doi.org/10.1164/rccm.201611-2274LE
11. Gauvreau GM, Arm JP, Boulet LP, Leigh R, Cockcroft DW, Davis BE, Mayers I, FitzGerald JM, Dahlen B, Killian KJ, Laviolette M, Carlsten C, Lazarinis N, Watson RM, Milot J, Swystun V, Bowen M, Hui L, Lantz AS, Meiser K, Maahs S, Lowe PJ, Skerjanec A, Drollmann A, O'Byrne PM (2016) Efficacy and safety of multiple doses of QGE031 (ligelizumab) versus omalizumab and placebo in inhibiting allergen-induced early asthmatic responses. J Allergy Clin Immunol 138 (4):1051–1059. https://doi.org/10.1016/j.jaci.2016.02.027
12. Gauvreau GM, Harris JM, Boulet L-P, Scheerens H, Fitzgerald JM, Putnam WS, Cockcroft DW, Davis BE, Leigh R, Zheng Y, Dahlén B, Wang Y, Maciuca R, Mayers I, Liao XC, Wu LC, Matthews JG, O'Byrne PM (2014) Targeting membrane-expressed IgE B cell receptor with an antibody to the M1 prime epitope reduces IgE production. Sci Transl Med 6(243):243ra85. https://doi.org/10.1126/scitranslmed.3008961
13. Maurer M, Giménez-Arnau AM, Sussman G, Metz M, Baker DR, Bauer A, Bernstein JA, Brehler R, Chu C-Y, Chung W-H, Danilycheva I, Grattan C, Hébert J, Katelaris C, Makris M, Meshkova R, Savic S, Sinclair R, Sitz K, Staubach P, Wedi B, Löffler J, Barve A, Kobayashi K, Hua E, Severin T, Janocha R (2019) Ligelizumab for chronic spontaneous Urticaria. N Engl J Med 381(14):1321–1332. https://doi.org/10.1056/NEJMoa1900408
14. Monson NL (2008) The natural history of B cells. Curr Opin Neurol 21(Suppl 1):S3–S8. https://doi.org/10.1097/01.wco.0000313358.53553.c7
15. Matsushita T, Yanaba K (2008) Regulatory B cells inhibit EAE initiation in mice while other B cells promote disease progression. J Clin Investig 118(10):3420–3430. https://doi.org/10.1172/JCI36030
16. Watanabe R, Ishiura N, Nakashima H, Kuwano Y, Okochi H, Tamaki K, Sato S, Tedder TF, Fujimoto M (2010) Regulatory B cells (B10 cells) have a suppressive role in murine lupus: CD19 and B10 cell deficiency exacerbates systemic autoimmunity. J Immunol 184(9):4801–4809. https://doi.org/10.4049/jimmunol.0902385
17. Jurlander J, Lai CF, Tan J, Chou CC, Geisler CH, Schriber J, Blumenson LE, Narula SK, Baumann H, Ma C (1997) Characterization of interleukin-10 receptor expression on B-cell chronic lymphocytic leukemia cells. Blood 89(11):4146–4152
18. Balkwill F, Montfort A, Capasso M (2013) B regulatory cells in cancer. Trends Immunol 34 (4):169–173. https://doi.org/10.1016/j.it.2012.10.007
19. Hulse KE, Norton JE, Suh L, Zhong Q, Mahdavinia M, Simon P, Kern RC, Conley DB, Chandra RK, Tan BK, Peters AT, Grammer LC, Harris KE, Carter RG, Kato A, Schleimer RP (2013) Chronic rhinosinusitis with nasal polyps is characterized by B-cell inflammation and EBV-induced protein 2 expression. Journal of Allergy and Clinical Immunology 131(4):1075–1083.e1077. https://doi.org/10.1016/j.jaci.2013.01.043
20. Dullaers M, De Bruyne R, Ramadani F, Gould HJ, Gevaert P, Lambrecht BN (2012) The who, where, and when of IgE in allergic airway disease. J Allergy Clin Immunol 129 (3):635–645. https://doi.org/10.1016/j.jaci.2011.10.029
21. Oettgen HC, Geha RS (2001) IgE regulation and roles in asthma pathogenesis. J Allergy Clin Immunol 107(3):429–440. https://doi.org/10.1067/mai.2001.113759
22. Gould HJ, Sutton BJ (2008) IgE in allergy and asthma today. Nat Rev Immunol 8 (3):205–217. https://doi.org/10.1038/nri2273
23. Lundy SK, aa B, Martens TF, Lukacs NW (2005) Deficiency of regulatory B cells increases allergic airway inflammation. Inflamm Res 54(12):514–521. https://doi.org/10.1007/s00011-005-1387-0
24. Amu S, Saunders SP, Kronenberg M, Mangan NE, Atzberger A, Fallon PG (2010)

Regulatory B cells prevent and reverse allergic airway inflammation via FoxP3-positive T regulatory cells in a murine model. Journal of Allergy and Clinical Immunology 125 (5):1114–1124.e1118. https://doi.org/10.1016/j.jaci.2010.01.018

25. Kato A, Hulse KE, Tan BK, Schleimer RP (2013) B-lymphocyte lineage cells and the respiratory system. J Allergy Clin Immunol 131(4):933–957. https://doi.org/10.1016/j.jaci.2013.02.023
26. Pieper K, Grimbacher B, Eibel H (2013) B-cell biology and development. J Allergy Clin Immunol 131(Fig 1):959–971. https://doi.org/10.1016/j.jaci.2013.01.046
27. Hagman J, Lukin K (2006) Transcription factors drive B cell development. Curr Opin Immunol 18(2):127–134. https://doi.org/10.1016/j.coi.2006.01.007
28. Vadasz Z, Toubi E (2014) The many faces of B regulatory cells. Isr Med Assoc J 16 (10):631–633
29. van der Vlugt LEPM, Mlejnek E, Ozir-Fazalalikhan A, Janssen Bonas M, Dijksman TR, Labuda La, Schot R, Guigas B, Möller GM, Hiemstra PS, Yazdanbakhsh M, Smits HH (2014) CD24(hi)CD27(+) B cells from patients with allergic asthma have impaired regulatory activity in response to lipopolysaccharide. Clin Exp Allergy 44 (4):517–528. https://doi.org/10.1111/cea.12238
30. Perez-Andres M, Paiva B, Nieto WG, Caraux A, Schmitz A, Almeida J, Vogt RF, Marti GE, Rawstron AC, Van Zelm MC, JJM VD, Johnsen HE, Klein B, Orfao A (2010) Human peripheral blood B-cell compartments: a crossroad in B-cell traffic. Cytometry Part B, Clinical Cytometry 78(Suppl 1):S47–S60. https://doi.org/10.1002/cyto.b.20547
31. Samitas K, Lötvall J, Bossios A (2010) B cells: from early development to regulating allergic diseases. Arch Immunol Ther Exp 58 (3):209–225. https://doi.org/10.1007/s00005-010-0073-2
32. Stavnezer J, Guikema JEJ, Schrader CE (2008) Mechanism and regulation of class switch recombination. Annu Rev Immunol 26:261–292. https://doi.org/10.1146/annurev.immunol.26.021607.090248
33. Hussaarts L, van der Vlugt LEPM, Yazdanbakhsh M, Smits HH (2011) Regulatory B-cell induction by helminths: implications for allergic disease. J Allergy Clin Immunol 128(4):733–739. https://doi.org/10.1016/j.jaci.2011.05.012
34. Galli SJ, Tsai M (2012) IgE and mast cells in allergic disease. Nat Med 18(5):693–704. https://doi.org/10.1038/nm.2755
35. Pol MAVD, Lutter R, Ree RVV, Zee JSVD, Van De Pol MA, Van Ree R, van der Zee JS (2012) Increase in allergen-specific IgE and ex vivo Th2 responses after a single bronchial challenge with house dust mite in allergic asthmatics. Allergy: European. J Allergy Clin Immunol 67(8):67–73. https://doi.org/10.1111/j.1398-9995.2011.02722.x
36. Wilson DR, Merrett TG, Varga EM, Smurthwaite L, Gould HJ, Kemp M, Hooper J, Till SJ, Durham SR (2002) Increases in allergen-specific IgE in BAL after segmental allergen challenge in atopic asthmatics. Am J Respir Crit Care Med 165 (1):22–26. https://doi.org/10.1164/ajrccm.165.1.2010112
37. Nduati EW, Ng DHL, Ndungu FM, Gardner P, Urban BC, Langhorne J (2010) Distinct kinetics of memory B-cell and plasma-cell responses in peripheral blood following a blood-stage Plasmodium chabaudi infection in mice. PLoS One 5(11): e15007–e15007.
38. Luger EO, Fokuhl V, Wegmann M, Abram M, Tillack K, Achatz G, Manz RA, Worm M, Radbruch A, Renz H (2009) Induction of long-lived allergen-specific plasma cells by mucosal allergen challenge. Journal of Allergy and Clinical Immunology 124 (4):819–826.e814.
39. Chvatchko Y, Kosco-Vilbois MH, Herren S, Lefort J, Bonnefoy JY (1996) Germinal center formation and local immunoglobulin E (IgE) production in the lung after an airway antigenic challenge. J Exp Med 184 (6):2353–2360. https://doi.org/10.1084/jem.184.6.2353
40. Wong KJ, Timbrell V, Xi Y, Upham JW, Collins AM, Davies JM (2015) IgE+ B cells are scarce, but allergen-specific B cells with a memory phenotype circulate in patients with allergic rhinitis. Allergy 70(4):420–428. https://doi.org/10.1111/all.12563
41. Katz SI, Parker D, Turk JL (1974) B-cell suppression of delayed hypersensitivity reactions. Nature 251(5475):550–551. https://doi.org/10.1038/251550a0
42. Neta R, Salvin SB (1974) Specific suppression of delayed hypersensitivity: the possible presence of a suppressor B cell in the regulation of delayed hypersensitivity. J Immunol 113 (6):1716–1725

43. Mauri C, Menon M (2015) The expanding family of regulatory B cells. Int Immunol 27 (10):479–486. https://doi.org/10.1093/intimm/dxv038
44. Wolf SD, Dittel BN, Hardardottir F, Janeway CA (1996) Experimental autoimmune encephalomyelitis induction in genetically B cell–deficient mice. J Exp Med 184 (6):2271–2278. https://doi.org/10.1084/jem.184.6.2271
45. Mizoguchi A, Mizoguchi E, Takedatsu H, Blumberg RS, Bhan AK (2002) Chronic intestinal inflammatory condition generates IL-10-producing regulatory B cell subset characterized by CD1d upregulation. Immunity 16(2):219–230. https://doi.org/10.1016/s1074-7613(02)00274-1
46. Miyagaki T, Fujimoto M, Sato S (2015) Regulatory B cells in human inflammatory and autoimmune diseases: from mouse models to clinical research. Int Immunol 27 (10):495–504. https://doi.org/10.1093/intimm/dxv026
47. Gauvreau GM, Hessel EM, Boulet L-P, Coffman RL, O'Byrne PM (2006) Immunostimulatory sequences regulate interferon-inducible genes but not allergic airway responses. Am J Respir Crit Care Med 174(1):15–20. https://doi.org/10.1164/rccm.200601-057OC
48. Fillatreau S, Sweenie CH, McGeachy MJ, Gray D, Anderton SM (2002) B cells regulate autoimmunity by provision of IL-10. Nat Immunol 3(10):944–950. https://doi.org/10.1038/ni833
49. Mauri C, Gray D, Mushtaq N, Londei M (2003) Prevention of arthritis by interleukin 10–producing B cells. J Exp Med 197 (4):489–501. https://doi.org/10.1084/jem.20021293
50. LeBien TW, Tedder TF (2008) B lymphocytes: how they develop and function. Blood 112(5):1570–1580. https://doi.org/10.1182/blood-2008-02-078071
51. Fagraeus A (1948) The plasma cellular reaction and its relation to the formation of antibodies in vitro. J Immunol 58(1):1–13
52. Jacob J, Kelsoe G, Rajewsky K, Weiss U (1991) Intraclonal generation of antibody mutants in germinal centres. Nature 354 (6352):389–392. https://doi.org/10.1038/354389a0
53. Carter NA, Vasconcellos R, Rosser EC, Tulone C, Muñoz-Suano A, Kamanaka M, Ehrenstein MR, Flavell RA, Mauri C (2011) Mice lacking endogenous IL-10–producing regulatory B cells develop exacerbated disease and present with an increased frequency of Th1/Th17 but a decrease in regulatory T cells. J Immunol 186(10):5569–5579.
54. Flores-Borja F, Bosma A, Ng D, Reddy V, Ehrenstein MR, Isenberg DA, Mauri C (2013) CD19+ CD24hiCD38hi B cells maintain regulatory T cells while limiting TH1 and TH17 differentiation. Science Translational Medicine 5 (173):173ra23
55. Rosser EC, Mauri C (2015) Regulatory B cells: origin, phenotype, and function. Immunity 42(4):607–612. https://doi.org/10.1016/j.immuni.2015.04.005
56. Zhang Y, Eliav Y, S-u S, Schreiber TH, Podack ER, Tadmor T, Rosenblatt JD (2013) B lymphocyte inhibition of antitumor response depends on expansion of Treg but is independent of B-cell IL-10 secretion. Cancer Immunol Immunother 62 (1):87–99. https://doi.org/10.1111/j.1398-9995.2011.02610.x
57. Moldaver D, Larché M (2011) Immunotherapy with peptides. Allergy 66(6):784–791
58. Larché M (2006) Peptide immunotherapy. Immunol Allergy Clin N Am 26 (2):321–332. https://doi.org/10.1016/j.iac.2006.02.005
59. Ca A, Akdis M (2011) Mechanisms of allergen-specific immunotherapy. J Allergy Clin Immunol 127(1):18–27.; quiz 28-19. https://doi.org/10.1016/j.jaci.2010.11.030
60. Akdis M, Ca A (2014) Mechanisms of allergen-specific immunotherapy: multiple suppressor factors at work in immune tolerance to allergens. J Allergy Clin Immunol 133 (3):621–631. https://doi.org/10.1016/j.jaci.2013.12.1088
61. van de Veen W, Stanic B, Yaman G, Wawrzyniak M, Söllner S, Akdis DG, Rückert B, Akdis CA, Akdis M (2013) IgG4 production is confined to human IL-10-producing regulatory B cells that suppress antigen-specific immune responses. J Allergy Clin Immunol 131(4):1204–1212. https://doi.org/10.1016/j.jaci.2013.01.014
62. Couper KN, Blount DG, Riley EM (2008) IL-10: the master regulator of immunity to infection. J Immunol 180(9):5771–5777. https://doi.org/10.4049/jimmunol.180.9.5771
63. van de Veen W, Stanic B, Wirz OF, Jansen K, Globinska A, Akdis M (2016) Role of regulatory B cells in immune tolerance to allergens and beyond. J Allergy Clin Immunol 138 (3):654–665. https://doi.org/10.1016/j.jaci.2016.07.006

64. Banchereau J, Pascual V, O'garra A (2012) From IL-2 to IL-37: the expanding spectrum of anti-inflammatory cytokines. Nat Immunol 13(10):925–931. https://doi.org/10.1038/ni.2406
65. Taylor A, Akdis M, Joss A, Akkoç T, Wenig R, Colonna M, Daigle I, Flory E, Blaser K, Akdis CA (2007) IL-10 inhibits CD28 and ICOS costimulations of T cells via src homology 2 domain—containing protein tyrosine phosphatase 1. Journal of Allergy and Clinical Immunology 120 (1):76–83.
66. Taylor A, Verhagen J, Blaser K, Akdis M, Akdis CA (2006) Mechanisms of immune suppression by interleukin-10 and transforming growth factor-β: the role of T regulatory cells. Immunology 117(4):433–442. https://doi.org/10.1111/j.1365-2567.2006.02321.x
67. Ito S, Ansari P, Sakatsume M, Dickensheets H, Vazquez N, Donnelly RP, Larner AC, Finbloom DS (1999) Interleukin-10 inhibits expression of both interferon alpha–and interferon gamma-induced genes by suppressing tyrosine phosphorylation of STAT1. Blood 93 (5):1456–1463. https://doi.org/10.1182/blood.V93.5.1456
68. Akdis CA, Blesken T, Akdis M, Wüthrich B, Blaser K (1998) Role of interleukin 10 in specific immunotherapy. J Clin Invest 102 (1):98–106. https://doi.org/10.1172/JCI2250
69. Meiler F, Klunker S, Zimmermann M, Akdis CA, Akdis M (2008) Distinct regulation of IgE, IgG4 and IgA by T regulatory cells and toll-like receptors. Allergy 63 (11):1455–1463. https://doi.org/10.1111/j.1398-9995.2008.01774.x
70. Cox L, Nelson H, Lockey R, Calabria C, Chacko T, Finegold I, Nelson M, Weber R, Bernstein DI, Blessing-Moore J, Khan DA, Lang DM, Nicklas RA, Oppenheimer J, Portnoy JM, Randolph C, Schuller DE, Spector SL, Tilles S, Wallace D (2011) Allergen immunotherapy: a practice parameter third update. J Allergy Clin Immunol 127 (1 Suppl):S1–55. https://doi.org/10.1016/j.jaci.2010.09.034
71. Moore KW, de Waal Malefyt E, Coffman RL, O'Garra A (2001) Interleukin-10 and the Interleukin-10 receptor. Annu Rev Immunol 19:683–765. https://doi.org/10.1146/annurev.immunol.19.1.683
72. Thorburn AN, Hansbro PM (2010) Harnessing regulatory T cells to suppress asthma: from potential to therapy. Am J Respir Cell Mol Biol 43(5):511–519. https://doi.org/10.1165/rcmb.2009-0342TR
73. Chu K-H, Chiang B-L (2012) Regulatory T cells induced by mucosal B cells alleviate allergic airway hypersensitivity. Am J Respir Cell Mol Biol 46(5):651–659. https://doi.org/10.1165/rcmb.2011-0246OC
74. Mauri C, Bosma A (2012) Immune regulatory function of B cells. Annu Rev Immunol 30:221–241. https://doi.org/10.1146/annurev-immunol-020711-074934
75. Noh J, Choi WS, Noh G, Lee JH (2010) Presence of Foxp3-expressing CD19(+)CD5(+) B cells in human peripheral blood mononuclear cells: human CD19(+)CD5(+)Foxp3(+) regulatory B cell (Breg). Immune Network 10(6):247–249. https://doi.org/10.4110/in.2010.10.6.247
76. Iwata Y, Matsushita T, Horikawa M, Dilillo DJ, Yanaba K, Venturi GM, Szabolcs PM, Bernstein SH, Magro CM, Williams AD, Hall RP, St Clair EW, Tedder TF (2011) Characterization of a rare IL-10-competent B-cell subset in humans that parallels mouse regulatory B10 cells. Blood 117(2):530–541. https://doi.org/10.1182/blood-2010-07-294249
77. James LK, Bowen H, Calvert RA, Dodev TS, Shamji MH, Beavil AJ, McDonnell JM, Durham SR, Gould HJ (2012) Allergen specificity of IgG(4)-expressing B cells in patients with grass pollen allergy undergoing immunotherapy. Journal of Allergy and Clinical Immunology 130 (3):663–670.e663. https://doi.org/10.1016/j.jaci.2012.04.006
78. Maseda D, Smith SH, DiLillo DJ, Bryant JM, Candando KM, Weaver CT, Tedder TF (2012) Regulatory B10 cells differentiate into antibody-secreting cells after transient IL-10 production in vivo. J Immunol 188 (3):1036–1048. https://doi.org/10.4049/jimmunol.1102500
79. Noh J, Noh G, Lee SJ, Lee JH, Kim A, Kim HS, Choi WS (2012) Tolerogenic effects of interferon-gamma with induction of allergen-specific interleukin-10-producing regulatory B cell (Br1) changes in non-IgE-mediated food allergy. Cell Immunol 273(2):140–149. https://doi.org/10.1016/j.cellimm.2011.12.006
80. Noh J, Lee JH, Noh G, Bang SY, Kim HS, Choi WS, Cho S, Lee SS (2010) Characterisation of allergen-specific responses of IL-10-producing regulatory B cells (Br1) in cow Milk allergy. Cell Immunol 264(2):143–149. https://doi.org/10.1016/j.cellimm.2010.05.013

81. Noh J, Noh G, Kim HS, Kim AR, Choi WS, Ra K, Choi WS (2012) Allergen-specific responses of CD19(+)CD5(+)Foxp3(+) regulatory B cells (Bregs) and CD4(+)Foxp3(+) regulatory T cell (Tregs) in immune tolerance of cow milk allergy of late eczematous reactions. Cell Immunol 274(1–2):109–114. https://doi.org/10.1016/j.cellimm.2012.01.005

82. Leaker BR, Singh D, Lindgren S, Almqvist G, Eriksson L, Young B, O'Connor B (2019) Effects of the toll-like receptor 7 (TLR7) agonist, AZD8848, on allergen-induced responses in patients with mild asthma: a double-blind, randomised, parallel-group study. Respir Res 20(1):288–288. https://doi.org/10.1186/s12931-019-1252-2

83. Ma L, Xiao X, Ma Y, Wu H, Qiu S, Li J, Yang P, Liu Z (2017) Effect of activation of toll-like receptor 7 in the inhibition of allergic asthma on a mouse model. J Trans Res 9 (5):2143–2152

84. Campbell JD, Sa K, Kozy HM, Ja L, Sweetwood R, Chu M, Cunningham CR, Salamon H, Lloyd CM, Coffman RL, Hessel EM (2014) A limited CpG-containing oligodeoxynucleotide therapy regimen induces sustained suppression of allergic airway inflammation in mice. Thorax 1:565. https://doi.org/10.1136/thoraxjnl-2013-204605

85. Singh A, Carson WF, Secor ER, La G, Ra F, Clark RB, Thrall RS, Schramm CM (2008) Regulatory role of B cells in a murine model of allergic airway disease. J Immunol 180 (11):7318–7326. https://doi.org/10.4049/jimmunol.180.11.7318

86. Braza F, Chesne J, Durand M, Dirou S, Brosseau C, Mahay G, Cheminant M-A, Magnan A, Brouard S (2015) A regulatory CD 9+ B-cell subset inhibits HDM-induced allergic airway inflammation. Allergy 70 (11):1421–1431. https://doi.org/10.1111/all.12697

87. Noh G, Lee JH (2011) Regulatory B cells and allergic diseases. Allergy, Asthma Immunol Res 3(3):168–177. https://doi.org/10.4168/aair.2011.3.3.168

88. Oliveria JP, El-Gammal AI, Yee M, Obminski CD, Scime TX, Watson RM, Howie K, O'Byrne PM, Sehmi R, Gauvreau GM (2018) Changes in regulatory B-cell levels in bone marrow, blood, and sputum of patients with asthma following inhaled allergen challenge. J Allergy Clin Immunol 141(4):1495. https://doi.org/10.1016/j.jaci.2017.11.013

89. Yanaba K, Bouaziz J-DD, Haas KM, Poe JC, Fujimoto M, Tedder TF (2008) A regulatory B cell subset with a unique CD1dhiCD5+ phenotype controls T cell-dependent inflammatory responses. Immunity 28(5):639–650. https://doi.org/10.1016/j.immuni.2008.03.017

90. Watanabe R, Fujimoto M, Ishiura N, Kuwano Y, Nakashima H, Yazawa N, Okochi H, Sato S, Tedder TF, Tamaki K (2007) CD19 expression in B cells is important for suppression of contact hypersensitivity. Am J Pathol 171(2):560–570. https://doi.org/10.2353/ajpath.2007.061279

91. Bosma A, Abdel-Gadir A, Isenberg DA, Jury EC, Mauri C (2012) Lipid-antigen presentation by CD1d+ B cells is essential for the maintenance of invariant natural killer T cells. Immunity 36(3):477–490. https://doi.org/10.1016/j.immuni.2012.02.008

92. Liu F, Ji J, Li X, Li X, Xu J, Yue H, Zhao S, Fan H, Hou Y (2017) Decreased CD1d level is associated with CD86 over-expression in B cells from systemic lupus erythematosus. Acta Biochim Biophys Sin 49(4):328–337. https://doi.org/10.1093/abbs/gmx011

93. Chaudhry MS, Karadimitris A (2014) Role and regulation of CD1d in Normal and pathological B cells. J Immunol 193 (10):4761–4768. https://doi.org/10.4049/jimmunol.1401805

94. Brutkiewicz RR (2006) CD1d ligands: the good, the bad, and the ugly. J Immunol 177 (2):769–775. https://doi.org/10.4049/jimmunol.177.2.769

95. Pa B, Noreña LY, Flores-Borja F, Rawlings DJ, Da I, Ehrenstein MR, Mauri C (2010) CD19+CD24hiCD38hi B cells exhibit regulatory capacity in healthy individuals but are functionally impaired in systemic lupus erythematosus patients. Immunity 32 (1):129–140. https://doi.org/10.1016/j.immuni.2009.11.009

96. Siewe B, Stapleton JT, Martinson J, Keshavarzian A, Kazmi N, Demarais PM, French AL, Landay A (2013) Regulatory B cell frequency correlates with markers of HIV disease progression and attenuates anti-HIV CD8+ T cell function in vitro. J Leukoc Biol 93(5):811–818. https://doi.org/10.1189/jlb.0912436

97. Nouël A, Simon Q, Jamin C, Pers J-O, Hillion S (2014) Regulatory B cells: an exciting target for future therapeutics in transplantation. Front Immunol 5:11. https://doi.org/10.3389/fimmu.2014.00011

98. Khoder A, Sarvaria A, Alsuliman A, Chew C, Sekine T, Cooper N, Mielke S, De Lavallade H, Muftuoglu M, Curbelo IF (2014) Regulatory B cells are enriched within

the IgM memory and transitional subsets in healthy donors but are deficient in chronic GVHD. Blood 124 (13):2034–2045.

99. Masson a d, Bouaziz JD, Le Buanec H, Robin M, O'Meara a PN, Rybojad M, Hau E, Monfort JB, Branchtein M, Michonneau D, Dessirier V, Sicre de Fontbrune F, Bergeron a IR, Dhedin N, Bengoufa D, Peffault de Latour R, Xhaard a BM, Bensussan a SG (2015) CD24hiCD27+ and plasmablast-like regulatory B cells in human chronic graft-versus-host disease. Blood 125:1830. https://doi.org/10.1182/blood-2014-09-599159

100. Ray A, Wang L, Dittel BN (2015) IL-10-independent regulatory B-cell subsets and mechanisms of action. Int Immunol 27 (10):531–536. https://doi.org/10.1093/intimm/dxv033

101. Lindner S, Dahlke K, Sontheimer K, Hagn M, Kaltenmeier C, Barth TF, Beyer T, Reister F, Fabricius D, Lotfi R (2013) Interleukin 21–induced granzyme B–expressing B cells infiltrate tumors and regulate T cells. Cancer Res 73(8):2468–2479. https://doi.org/10.1158/0008-5472.CAN-12-3450

102. Saze Z, Schuler PJ, Hong C-S, Cheng D, Jackson EK, Whiteside TL (2013) Adenosine production by human B cells and B cell–mediated suppression of activated T cells. Blood 122(1):9–18. https://doi.org/10.1182/blood-2013-02-482406

103. Zhang H-P, Wu Y, Liu J, Jiang J, Geng X-R, Yang G, Mo L, Liu Z-Q, Liu Z-G, Yang P-C (2013) TSP1-producing B cells show immune regulatory property and suppress allergy-related mucosal inflammation. Sci Rep 3:3345. https://doi.org/10.1038/srep03345

104. Pepys J (1975) New tests to assess lung function. inhalation challenge tests in asthma. The New England Journal of Medicine 293 (15):758–759. https://doi.org/10.1056/NEJM197510092931507

105. Hendrick DJ, Davies RJ, D'Souza MF, Pepys J (1975) An analysis of skin prick test reactions in 656 asthmatic patients. Thorax 30 (1):2–8. https://doi.org/10.1136/thx.30.1.2

106. Clarke CW, Mitchell J, Nunn AJ, Pepys J (1982) Reproducibility of prick skin tests to five allergens. Clin Allergy 12(1):1–8. https://doi.org/10.1111/j.1365-2222.1982.tb03120.x

107. Bousquet J, Clark TJH, Hurd S, Khaltaev N, Lenfant C, O'Byrne P, Sheffer A (2007) GINA guidelines on asthma and beyond. Allergy 62(2):102–112. https://doi.org/10.1111/j.1398-9995.2006.01305.x

108. Miller MR, Hankinson J, Brusasco V, Burgos F, Casaburi R, Coates A, Crapo R, Enright P, van der Grinten CPM, Gustafsson P, Jensen R, Johnson DC, MacIntyre N, McKay R, Navajas D, Pedersen OF, Pellegrino R, Viegi G, Wanger J (2005) Standardisation of spirometry. Eur Respir J 26 (2):319–338. https://doi.org/10.1183/09031936.05.00034805

109. Cockcroft DW, Killian DN, Mellon JJ, Hargreave FE (1977) Bronchial reactivity to inhaled histamine: a method and clinical survey. Clin Allergy 7(3):235–243. https://doi.org/10.1111/j.1365.2222.1977.tb01448

110. O'Byrne PM, Dolovich J, Hargreave FE (1987) Late asthmatic responses. Am Rev Respir Dis 136(3):740–751. https://doi.org/10.1164/ajrccm/136.3.740

111. Diamant Z, Gauvreau GM, Cockcroft DW, Boulet LPP, Sterk PJ, de Jongh FHC, Dahlén B, O'Byrne PM (2013) Inhaled allergen bronchoprovocation tests. The Journal of Allergy and Clinical Immunology 132 (5):1045–1055.e1046. https://doi.org/10.1016/j.jaci.2013.08.023

112. Pizzichini E, Pizzichini MM, Efthimiadis A, Evans S, Morris MM, Squillace D, Gleich GJ, Dolovich J, Hargreave FE (1996) Indices of airway inflammation in induced sputum: reproducibility and validity of cell and fluid-phase measurements. Am J Respir Crit Care Med 154(2 Pt 1):308–317. https://doi.org/10.1164/ajrccm.154.2.8756799

113. Sohani ZN, Strinich TX, Watson B, Smith SG, Torek A, Howie KJ, Gauvreau GM (2011) Reproducibility of sputum differential cell counts is not affected by squamous epithelial cells. J Asthma 48(9):952–956. https://doi.org/10.3109/02770903.2011.617477

114. Kleinjan A, Vinke JG, Severijnen LWFM, Fokkens WJ (2000) Local production and detection of (specific) IgE in nasal B-cells and plasma cells of allergic rhinitis patients. Eur Respir J 15(3):491–497. https://doi.org/10.1034/j.1399-3003.2000.15.11.x

115. Zürcher AW, Derer T, Lang AB, Stadler BM (1996) Culture and IgE synthesis of nasal B cells. Int Arch Allergy Immunol 111 (1):77–82. doi:https://doi.org/10.1159/000237349

116. Kamekura R, Shigehara K, Miyajima S, Jitsukawa S, Kawata K, Yamashita K, Nagaya T, Kumagai A, Sato A, Matsumiya H, Ogasawara N, Seki N, Takano K, Kokai Y, Takahashi H, Himi T,

Ichimiya S (2015) Alteration of circulating type 2 follicular helper T cells and regulatory B cells underlies the comorbid association of allergic rhinitis with bronchial asthma. Clin Immunol 158(2):204–211. https://doi.org/10.1016/j.clim.2015.02.016

117. Natarajan P, Singh a MNJT, Secor ER, La G, Thrall RS, Schramm CM (2012) Regulatory B cells from hilar lymph nodes of tolerant mice in a murine model of allergic airway disease are CD5+, express TGF-β, and co-localize with CD4+Foxp3+ T cells. Mucosal Immunol 5(6):691–701. https://doi.org/10.1038/mi.2012.42

118. Hoh RA, Joshi SA, Liu Y, Wang C, Roskin KM, Lee J-Y, Pham T, Looney TJ, Jackson KJL, Dixit VP, King J, Lyu S-C, Jenks J, Hamilton RG, Nadeau KC, Boyd SD (2016) Single B-cell deconvolution of peanut-specific antibody responses in allergic patients. J Allergy Clin Immunol 137(1):157–167. https://doi.org/10.1016/j.jaci.2015.05.029

119. Yao Y, Liu R, Shin MS, Trentalange M, Allore H, Nassar A, Kang I, Pober JS, Montgomery RR (2014) CyTOF supports efficient detection of immune cell subsets from small samples. J Immunol Methods 415:1–5. https://doi.org/10.1016/j.jim.2014.10.010

120. Proserpio V, Mahata B (2016) Single-cell technologies to study the immune system. Immunology 147(2):133–140. https://doi.org/10.1111/imm.12553

121. Bendall SC, Simonds EF, Qiu P, Amir E-aD, Krutzik PO, Finck R, Bruggner RV, Melamed R, Trejo A, Ornatsky OI, Balderas RS, Plevritis SK, Sachs K, Pe D, Tanner SD, Nolan GP (2011) Single-cell mass cytometry of differential immune and drug responses across a human hematopoietic continuum. Science 332(6030):687–696. https://doi.org/10.1126/science.1198704

122. Bendall SC, Nolan GP, Roederer M, Chattopadhyay PK (2012) A deep profiler's guide to cytometry. Trends Immunol 33(7):323–332. https://doi.org/10.1016/j.it.2012.02.010

123. Bodenmiller B, Zunder ER, Finck R, Chen TJ, Savig ES, Bruggner RV, Simonds EF, Bendall SC, Sachs K, Krutzik PO, Nolan GP (2012) Multiplexed mass cytometry profiling of cellular states perturbed by small-molecule regulators. Nat Biotechnol 30(9):858–867. https://doi.org/10.1038/nbt.2317

124. Qiu P, Simonds EF, Bendall SC, Gibbs KD, Bruggner RV, Linderman MD, Sachs K, Nolan GP, Plevritis SK (2011) Extracting a cellular hierarchy from high-dimensional cytometry data with SPADE. Nat Biotechnol 29(10):886–891. https://doi.org/10.1038/nbt.1991

125. Gaudilliere B, Fragiadakis GK, Bruggner RV, Nicolau M, Finck R, Tingle M, Silva J, Ganio EA, Yeh CG, Maloney WJ, Huddleston JI, Goodman SB, Davis MM, Bendall SC, Fantl WJ, Angst MS, Nolan GP (2014) Clinical recovery from surgery correlates with single-cell immune signatures. Science Translational Medicine 6 (255):255ra131-255ra131.

126. Bendall SC, Nolan GP (2012) From single cells to deep phenotypes in cancer. Nat Biotechnol 30(7):639–647. https://doi.org/10.1038/nbt.2283

127. Glass DR, Tsai AG, Oliveria JP, Hartmann FJ, Kimmey SC, Calderon AA, Borges L, Glass MC, Wagar LE, Davis MM, Bendall SC (2020) An integrated multi-omic single-cell atlas of human B cell identity. Immunity 53 (1): 217-232.e5. https://doi.org/10.1016/j.immuni.2020.06.013

128. Kimmey SC, Borges L, Baskar R, Bendall SC (2019) Parallel analysis of tri-molecular biosynthesis with cell identity and function in single cells. Nat Commun 10 (1):1185–1185. https://doi.org/10.1038/s41467-019-09128-7

129. Hartmann FJ, Bendall SC (2019) Immune monitoring using mass cytometry and related high-dimensional imaging approaches. Nat Rev Rheumatol 16:87. https://doi.org/10.1038/s41584-019-0338-z

130. Hartmann FJ, Babdor J, Gherardini PF, Amir EAD, Jones K, Sahaf B, Marquez DM, Krutzik P, O'Donnell E, Sigal N, Maecker HT, Meyer E, Spitzer MH, Bendall SC (2019) Comprehensive Immune Monitoring of Clinical Trials to Advance Human Immunotherapy. Cell reports 28 (3):819–831.e814.

131. Hartmann FJ, Simonds EF, Vivanco N, Bruce T, Borges L, Nolan GP, Spitzer MH, Bendall SC (2019) Scalable Conjugation and Characterization of Immunoglobulins with Stable Mass Isotope Reporters for Single-Cell Mass Cytometry Analysis. Methods in molecular biology (Clifton, NJ) 1989:55–81.

132. Hartmann FJ, Simonds EF, Bendall SC (2018) A universal live cell barcoding-platform for multiplexed human single cell analysis. Sci Rep 8(1):10770–10770. https://doi.org/10.1038/s41598-018-28791-2

133. Angelo M, Bendall SC, Finck R, Hale MB, Hitzman C, Borowsky AD, Levenson RM, Lowe JB, Liu SD, Zhao S, Natkunam Y, Nolan GP (2014) Multiplexed ion beam

imaging of human breast tumors. Nat Med 20 (4):436–442. https://doi.org/10.1038/nm.3488

134. Keren L, Bosse M, Marquez D, Angoshtari R, Jain S, Varma S, Yang S-R, Kurian A, Van Valen D, West R, Bendall SC, Angelo M (2018) A Structured Tumor-Immune Microenvironment in Triple Negative Breast Cancer Revealed by Multiplexed Ion Beam Imaging. Cell 174 (6):1373–1387.e1319.

135. Keren L, Bosse M, Thompson S, Risom T, Vijayaragavan K, McCaffrey E, Marquez D, Angoshtari R, Greenwald NF, Fienberg H, Wang J, Kambham N, Kirkwood D, Nolan G, Montine TJ, Galli SJ, West R, Bendall SC, Angelo M (2019) MIBI-TOF: A multiplexed imaging platform relates cellular phenotypes and tissue structure. Sci Adv 5 (10):eaax5851-eaax5851.

136. Zhao Y, Uduman M, Siu JHY, Tull TJ, Sanderson JD, Y-CB W, Zhou JQ, Petrov N, Ellis R, Todd K, Chavele K-M, Guesdon W, Vossenkamper A, Jassem W, D'Cruz DP, Fear DJ, John S, Scheel-Toellner D, Hopkins C, Moreno E, Woodman NL, Ciccarelli F, Heck S, Kleinstein SH, Bemark M, Spencer J (2018) Spatiotemporal segregation of human marginal zone and memory B cell populations in lymphoid tissue. Nat Commun 9 (1):3857–3857. https://doi.org/10.1038/s41467-018-06089-1

137. Kwak K, Quizon N, Sohn H, Saniee A, Manzella-Lapeira J, Holla P, Brzostowski J, Lu J, Xie H, Xu C, Spillane KM, Tolar P, Pierce SK (2018) Intrinsic properties of human germinal center B cells set antigen affinity thresholds. Sci Immunol 3 (29): eaau6598-eaau6598.

138. Oliveria JP (2020) Multiomic approaches to study B cells: sequencing, cytometry, imaging, and beyond. J Allergy Clin Immunol 146 (2): 456-457 https://doi.org/10.1016/j.jaci.2020.03.012

Chapter 22

Regulatory B Cells in Type 1 Diabetes

Joanne Boldison, Larissa Camargo Da Rosa, and F. Susan Wong

Abstract

Type 1 diabetes is an organ-specific autoimmune disease characterized by immune-mediated beta cell destruction in pancreatic islets, which results in deficient insulin production. B cells have a dual role in type 1 diabetes pathogenesis. A pathogenic role for B cells has been widely described and is supported by the observation of a delay in the loss of C-peptide following B-cell depletion by Rituximab, in the first year after diagnosis. However, it is now clear that B cells, under certain conditions, can delay and prevent the onset of type 1 diabetes as demonstrated in mouse models. In this chapter, we describe the methods required to study the phenotype and function of regulatory B cells in the context of diabetes.

Key words Type 1 diabetes, B cells, Dendritic cells, Regulation, NOD mouse

1 Introduction

Type 1 diabetes (T1D) is an organ-specific autoimmune disease characterized by immune-mediated beta cell destruction in pancreatic islets, which results in deficient insulin production. Although T cells directly damage insulin-producing beta cells, B cells play a key role in this multifactorial process (fully reviewed in [1]). B-cell involvement in disease pathogenesis was demonstrated by the use of the anti-CD20 antibody Rituximab in clinical trials, where beta-cell function was preserved in the first year [2]. However, in T1D, a dual role for B cells is evident. Individuals with T1D have reduced regulatory B cells in peripheral blood, compared to healthy subjects [3, 4]. Regulatory B cells mitigate autoimmunity via the production of anti-inflammatory cytokines such as IL-10, which can modulate pathogenic T cells [5]. Furthermore, B cells can influence the differentiation of dendritic cells (DCs) [6–8], which are key cells in the initiation of disease [9].

Non-obese diabetic (NOD) mice develop spontaneous T1D and parallel pathological outcomes, similar to humans. Regulatory B cells can also prevent the onset of disease in the NOD mouse model [10–12]. In NOD mouse colonies worldwide,

Francesca Mion and Silvia Tonon (eds.), *Regulatory B Cells: Methods and Protocols*, Methods in Molecular Biology, vol. 2270, https://doi.org/10.1007/978-1-0716-1237-8_22,

approximately 20% of NOD mice remain normoglycemic and "protected" from diabetes, despite their genetic predisposition [13]. B cells and, more specifically, anergic CD40$^+$IL-10-producing B cells are found in the pancreatic islets of long-term normoglycemic mice (protected) [3], may confer this protection. Recently, we have reported that B cells from NOD mice, which have developed diabetes, have lost the capacity to produce IL-10, whereas B cells from naturally protected NOD animals have an increased frequency of IL-10-producing B cells [14]. Furthermore, we demonstrated that B-cell regulation of mature bone-marrow-derived dendritic cells (BM-DCs) is compromised in mice that have developed diabetes [14]. Here we describe useful and detailed protocols for the study of the phenotype and function of regulatory B cells in T1D, using the NOD mouse model.

2 Materials

2.1 Mice

We suggest housing mice in specific pathogen-free ventilated cabinet for housing of rodents in open cages (scantainers). The particular strains of mice described below are used to provide a specific example of an antigen-specific test system (*see* **Note 1**). Depending on the chosen antigen, other strains of mice would be required.

1. Wild-type (WT) NOD mice.
2. NOD.PI2^{tg} mice (commercially available from Jackson laboratory, strain 005739) to provide bone-marrow-derived dendritic cells (NOD.PI2^{tg} BM-DCs) expressing insulin peptides endogenously, and thus, not requiring exogenous antigen.
3. G9C$\alpha^{-/-}$NOD mice (commercially available from Jackson laboratory, strains 032569 [A22Calpha], crossed with 032568 [B2Calpha]), a T-cell receptor (TCR) transgenic mouse, to provide responding CD8$^+$ T cells that respond to an insulin peptide, the particular antigen used in our system.

2.2 Equipment

1. Shaking water bath.
2. Dissecting microscope.
3. 40 μm cell strainer.
4. 1 mL and 5 mL syringe.
5. Sterile tweezers.
6. 25 gauge (G) and 30 G needle.
7. Petri dish.
8. 15 mL tubes.
9. Glass Dounce homogeniser (similar to a glass pestle and mortar), sterilized by autoclave or alcohol.

10. 24-well and 6-well plates.
11. 5 mL polypropylene tubes for flow cytometry analysis (FACS tubes).

2.3 Reagents for Tissue Preparation

All reagents and materials should be used sterile or sterilized prior to use either by autoclave or alcohol. Tissues should be prepared in a suitable sterile environment. Surgical equipment (scissors, forceps, clamps) is required to excise murine tissues.

1. RMPI complete medium: RPMI 1640 supplemented with 5% fetal bovine serum (FBS), 2 mM L-glutamine, 100 U/mL Penicillin, 100 μg/mL Streptomycin, and 50 μM β-2-mercaptoethanol.
2. Deionized water.
3. 10× sterile phosphate buffered saline (PBS): 1.37 M NaCl; 27 mM KCl; 100 mM Na_2HPO_4; 18 mM KH_2PO_4.
4. IMDM complete medium: IMDM supplemented with 5% fetal bovine serum (FBS), 2 mM L-glutamine, 100 U/mL Penicillin, 100 μg/mL Streptomycin, and 50 μM β-2-mercaptoethanol.
5. Hanks' Balanced Salt Solution with Ca^{2+} and Mg^{2+} (HBSS):1.26 mM $CaCl_2$; 0.49 mM $MgCl_2$-6H20; 0.40 mM $MgSO_4$-7H20; 5.33 mM KCl; 0.44 mM KH_2PO_4; 4.16 mM $NaHCO_3$; 137.93 mM NaCl; 0.33 mM Na_2HPO_4, 5.55 mM D-Glucose.
6. Collagenase solution: dissolve collagenase P in HBSS at the final concentration of 1.1 mg/mL. Keep cold (*see* **Note 2**).
7. Histopaque-1077 and Histopaque-1119. Prepare 10 mL per pancreas in a ratio of 5 mL Histopaque-1077: 6 mL Histopaque-1119.
8. Trypsin.

2.4 Reagents for Cell Culture and Flow cytometry Analysis

1. Reagents for immunomagnetic isolation of B cells and of $CD8^+$ T cells (*see* **Note 3**).
2. 1.5 ng/mL Granulocyte Macrophage Colony Stimulating Factor (GM-CSF).
3. 5 μg/mL lipopolysaccharide (LPS) from *Escherichia coli* 026: B6.
4. 5 μg/mL anti-CD40 antibody (clone FGK45).
5. Phorbol 12-mistrate 13 acetate (PMA)/Ionomycin/Monensin cocktail (PIM): 50 ng/mL PMA, 500 ng/mL ionomycin, and 3 μg/mL monensin.
6. FACS buffer: 0.5% bovine serum albumin (BSA) and 0.1% sodium azide in 1× PBS. Store at 4 °C.

Table 1
Antibodies used for cell surface and intracellular staining

Target cell type	Antibody	Fluorochrome	Clone
B cell	CD19	AF700	6D5
	CD24	BV650	M1/69
	CD38	PeCy7	90
	CD21	PECF594	7G6
	CD23	PE	B3B4
	CD1d	BV510	1B1
	CD5	FITC	53–7.3
	CD44	PerCPCy5.5	IM7
	CD138	BV711	281–2
	IL-10	APC	Jes5-16e3
	TGFβ	BV421	TW7-16B4
Dendritic cell	CD11c	PeCy7	N418
	CD11b	APC or BV421	M1/70
	MHC I	PE	SF1–1.1
	MHC II	FITC	10–3-6
	CD80	BV650	16-10A1
	CD86	AF700	PO3
	PD-L1	APC	10F-962
	CD45RB	PerCPCy5.5	C363–16.7
CD8 T cell	CD8	PE CF594	53–6.7
	CD44	PerCPCy5.5	IM7

7. Fixation/Permeabilization solution and permeabilization buffer (*see* **Note 4**).
8. Fc block reagent: anti-mouse CD16/32 antibody. Use 1 μg per test.
9. Fluorescence-conjugated antibodies (*see* Table 1). Each antibody should be appropriately titrated before starting experiments as the exact quantity used will vary per batch.
10. Compensation beads.
11. Carboxyfluorescein succinimidyl ester (CFSE) cell proliferation dye. Dilute the stock concentration according to manufacturer's instructions.
12. G9 insulin B15–23 peptide (optional).

3 Methods

3.1 Tissue Preparation

Regardless of the organ of interest, sacrifice mice according to approved methods and national laws of respective institutes.

3.1.1 Isolation of Cells from the Spleen

1. Depending on the experimental requirement, isolate the spleen from WT or G9C$\alpha^{-/-}$NOD mice (*see* **Note 1**) and collect it in a 15-mL tube containing 5 mL of RPMI complete medium.
2. Under the hood, homogenize the tissue with a glass homogenizer and centrifuge the cell suspension at 400 × *g* for 5 min. Decant the supernatant.
3. Lyse the erythrocytes by hypo-osmotic shock: flick to resuspend the cell pellet, add 900 μL of water and immediately add 100 μL of 10× PBS, then add 5 mL of RMPI complete medium.
4. Centrifuge at 400 × *g* for 5 min and decant the supernatant. Resuspend cells in 10 mL of RPMI complete medium and filter the cell suspension with a 40-μm cell strainer.
5. Count cells. Cells can now be used for either B cell or CD8$^+$ T cell (*see* Subheading 3.3.2) isolation or for flow cytometric analysis.

3.1.2 Isolation of Cells from the Bone Marrow

1. Collect hind legs (tibia and femur) from either WT NOD or NOD.PI2^{tg} mice (*see* **Note 1**) and remove the foot from the leg. Using scissors and forceps, remove all fur and as much muscle as possible. Refer to [15] for a detailed description of how to perform this step. Place the bones into a tube and add 15–30 mL of RPMI complete medium.
2. Under the hood, transfer the tibias and femurs from the tube to a petri dish and cut the ends off each bone with scissors or a scalpel. Fill a 5-mL syringe with RPMI complete medium and fit a 25-G needle. Insert the needle into the bone and gently flush to expel all bone marrow into a petri dish. Bones should be white when all bone marrow is removed.
3. Collect all bone marrow suspension using a syringe without the needle and expel cells through the needle into a clean 50-mL tube. This step will ensure cell dissociation. Wash petri dish with RPMI complete medium to collect all the cells and centrifuge cells at 600 × *g* for 10 min.
4. Wash cells in a suitable volume of RPMI complete medium and spin again, then resuspend cells in fresh RPMI complete medium and count. If needed, cells can be passed through a 40-μm cell strainer.
5. Cells are now ready for B-cell analysis by flow cytometry. Alternatively, cells can be seeded and undergo the protocol for bone-marrow-derived dendritic cell differentiation (*see* Subheading 3.3.1.1).

3.1.3 Isolation of Cells from Pancreatic Lymph Nodes

1. Excise WT NOD pancreatic lymph nodes which are located deep in the abdomen, under the stomach, by the pancreas. Make a vertical incision in the midline, exposing all the organs of the abdominal cavity of the mouse. Locate the spleen, the pancreas, and the stomach on the left side. Lift the stomach, and the pancreatic lymph nodes will be found beneath, attached to the pancreas at the caudal end. Remove the lymph nodes and place them in a petri dish with 1 mL of RPMI complete medium.
2. Dissociate lymph nodes using a 30-G needle to release lymphocytes. Briefly, hold the lymph node with sterile tweezers and use a needle attached to a 1-mL syringe to tease apart the lymph nodes, this will release the required lymphocytes into the RMPI complete medium.
3. Transfer the cell suspension to a FACS tube, rinsing the petri dish with fresh RPMI complete medium in order to collect all cells.
4. Filter cells with a 40-μm cell strainer.
5. Cells are now ready for analysis by flow cytometry.

3.1.4 Isolation of Cells from WT NOD Pancreatic Islets

To ensure good viability and a sufficient number of pancreatic islets, the pancreas should be inflated, via the common bile duct, with a collagenase solution before being excised and digested. It is recommended prior to inflation and isolation of pancreatic islets to see references [16, 17], as inflations can require technical skill.

1. Before beginning the inflation protocol, prepare the collagenase solution as described in Subheading 2.3. Bring Histopaque to room temperature and heat the shaking water bath to 37 °C.
2. Once euthanized the mouse, expose the thoracic cavity and remove rib cage, taking care not to puncture the heart or liver.
3. Locate gall bladder and common bile duct. Rotate duodenum to locate entry of the common bile duct at the ampulla and clamp securely.
4. Insert a needle into common bile duct starting at gall bladder. Gently infuse the collagenase solution, ensuring entry into and inflation of the pancreas. Fully inflate the pancreas with collagenase solution.
5. Remove clamps. Gently remove pancreas from bowels, taking care not to tear the tissue to prevent leakage of the collagenase solution.
6. Place the pancreas in a conical tube with 2 mL of collagenase solution and put on ice.

7. To digest the pancreas, place the tube with the inflated pancreas in the shaking water bath at 37 °C for 8 min. After 8 min, give tube a firm shake by hand to disperse tissue, tilt tube, and check progress of digestion. If larger clumps remain, then repeat shaking incubation, checking at 2 min intervals.
8. When fully digested, add 5 mL of HBSS and spin at 300 × *g* for 3 min at 4 °C.
9. Discard supernatant, wash again in 5 mL HBSS and spin at 300 × *g* for 3 min at 4 °C.
10. After washing, discard supernatant, remove all liquid and resuspend well in 10 mL of Histopaque solution (*see* Subheading 2.3).
11. Spin at 300 × *g* for 20 min at room temperature. Islets will be in the supernatant.
12. Collect supernatant in 20 mL of HBSS. Spin at 450 × *g* for 10 min at 4 °C. At this point, islets will be in the pellet. Resuspend in complete IMDM medium.
13. Under a dissecting microscope, hand-pick islets into a tube containing complete IMDM medium. After hand-picking, centrifuge islets at 400 × *g* for 5 min.
14. To obtain a single cell suspension, resuspend islets in 500 μL of trypsin and place in the 37 °C water bath for 5 min, shaking tubes at intervals. The islets will disperse into single cells.
15. Add 5 mL of complete IMDM medium and spin at 400 × *g* for 5 min.
16. Resuspend in complete IMDM medium and culture overnight at 37 °C, 5% CO_2 (*see* **Note 5**).

3.2 Phenotypical Characterization of Regulatory B Cells

Characterization of IL-10-expressing B cells can be performed in NOD mice that are at various stages of diabetes development, for example, prediabetic or diabetic animals (*see* Fig. 1). It is also possible to compare B cells from a diabetes-prone NOD strain to other nondiabetes-prone mice, such as the BALB/C strain. Overall, various comparisons can be made, depending on the scientific question (i.e., female versus male NOD mice). However, when comparing IL-10-expressing B cells from pancreatic islets, only the diabetes-prone NOD strain can be used, due to lack of pancreatic immune cell infiltrate in other nondiabetes-prone mice.

Although great effort has been devoted to phenotypically characterize regulatory B cells, to date the production of IL-10 remains the hallmark of this functional subset. As reported in Table 2, several B-cell populations have been described to exert regulatory functions, and each of this subset is characterized by the expression of specific surface markers. Here below we describe the protocols to detect either intracellular IL-10 (*see* Subheading 3.2.3) or surface

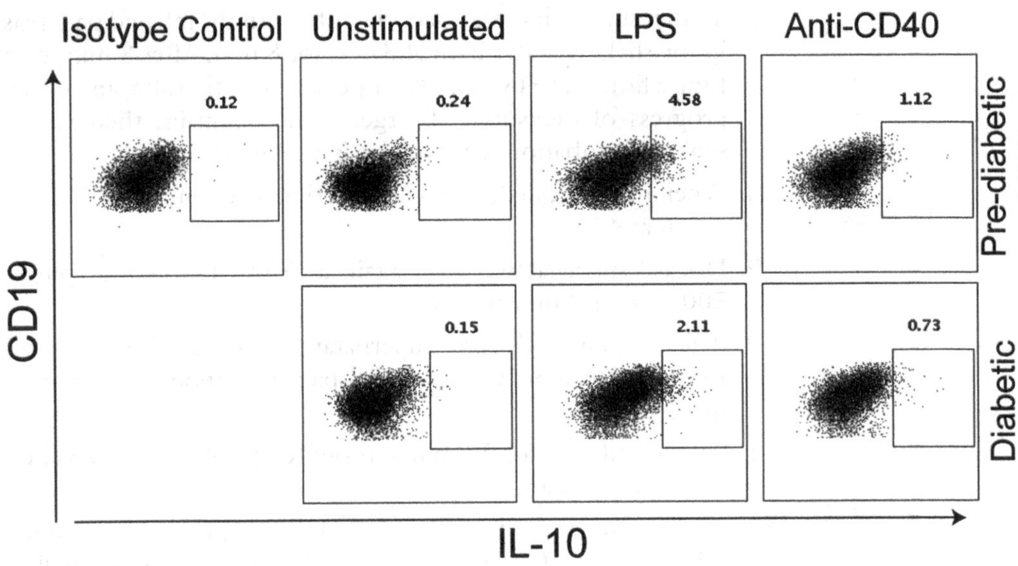

Fig. 1 Analysis of IL-10-expressing B cells in prediabetic and diabetic WT NOD mice. IL-10$^+$CD19$^+$ B cells were analyzed among prediabetic and diabetic WT NOD mouse splenocytes, either unstimulated or stimulated with LPS or anti-CD40 antibody for 24 h. IL-10$^+$ B cells were analyzed by flow cytometry and were gated on singlets, live, CD19$^+$ cells

Table 2
Subsets of mouse regulatory B cells

Regulatory cytokine	B cell subset	Surface Marker	Reference
IL-10	Regulatory B10 cells	CD5$^+$CD1d^{hi}CD43$^-$, Tim-1$^+$	[21, 22]
IL-10	Regulatory marginal zone (MZ) B cells	CD19$^+$CD21^{hi}CD23^{lo}	[23]
IL-10	Transitional (T2-MZP) regulatory B cells	CD19$^+$CD21^{hi}CD23^{hi}CD24^{hi}	[24, 25]
IL-10	Regulatory plasmablasts/ plasma cells	CD138$^+$, CD44^{hi}	[26, 27]
IL-10	Tim-1$^+$ regulatory B cells	CD19$^+$Tim-1$^+$	[28, 29]
TGFβ	TGF-β producing B cells	Tim-1$^+$, CCR6^{hi}, CXCR3^{hi}	[10, 30, 31]
IL-35 and IL-10	Regulatory plasmablasts	IgM$^+$CD138^{hi}TACI$^+$CXCR4$^+$CD1d^{int}Tim-1^{int}	[32]
IL-35	CD5$^+$CD1d^{hi}FcγRIII B cells	CD5$^+$CD1d^{hi}FcγRIII, TACI, IgM	[33]
IL-35	IL-35-producing Breg cells	Ebi3$^+$p35$^+$	[34]

markers associated with regulatory B cells (*see* Subheading 3.2.2) in WT NOD mice. While intracellular IL-10 staining requires an in vitro stimulation step with PMA and ionomycin (*see* Subheading 3.2.1, **step 3**), if only cell surface analysis is needed then no cell stimulation is necessary and B cells from WT NOD splenocytes, pancreatic lymph nodes, or pancreatic islets can be assessed immediately after isolation.

3.2.1 Cell Stimulation

The following protocol can be performed either on the totality of cells isolated by a specific organ (*see* Subheading 3.1) or on only purified B cells obtained using immunomagnetic separation protocols. Indeed, if the aim of the experiment is detecting B-cell IL-10 production in the supernatant, immunomagnetic separation should be performed to obtain a pure B-cell population. On the contrary, in the case of tissues such as pancreatic lymph nodes and pancreatic islets, where often only few B cells are present, a flow cytometric analysis on the totality of isolated cells is more appropriate (*see* **Note 6**).

1. Culture cells in a 24-well plate, seeded at 1×10^6/well in 2 mL of IMDM complete medium. When using pancreatic islets, more than one NOD mouse (depending on the age of the mouse) is recommended if performing stimulation with different agents. Pool together the collected pancreatic islets and divide the cells equally for each stimulation (*see* **Note 7**).
2. Add either 5 μg/mL LPS or 5 μg/mL anti-CD40 antibody. As a negative control, also prepare an unstimulated well (*see* **Note 8**). Culture for 24 h at 37 °C, 5% CO_2.
3. If cells will be intracellularly stained to test IL-10 production, then add PIM to cells during the last 3 h of culture. If the aim is to detect cytokine production by ELISA, then supernatant should be removed prior to the addition of the PIM cocktail.
4. Harvest wells in FACS tubes for cell surface and intracellular staining.

3.2.2 Cell Staining for the Detection of Surface Markers on B Cells

1. Collect cells from Subheading 3.2.1, pellet by centrifugation at $400 \times g$ for 5 min at 4 °C and wash them with FACS buffer.
2. Resuspend cells in the residual volume, add 1 μg of FcBlock reagent and incubate for 5 min at 4 °C.
3. Add the appropriate amount of surface fluorochrome-conjugated antibodies (*see* Table 1) and incubate for 30 min in the dark at 4 °C.
4. Wash twice with 1 mL of FACS buffer. If the aim is to proceed with intracellular cytokine staining, then continue with the protocol described in Subheading 3.2.2. Otherwise, resuspend the cells in 200 μL of FACS buffer and analyze the sample immediately by flow cytometry.

3.2.3 Cell Staining for the Detection of IL-10-Expressing B Cells

1. Following extracellular staining, add 200 μL of Fixation/Permeabilization solution (*see* **Note 4**) and incubate in the dark for 20 min at 4 °C.
2. Wash cells twice with permeabilization buffer and then resuspend cells in the appropriate amount of fluorochrome-conjugated antibodies for intracellular markers (*see* Table 1), diluted in permeabilization buffer. Incubate for 30 min in the dark at 4 °C (*see* **Note 9**).
3. Wash cells twice in permeabilization buffer and resuspend in 200 μL of FACS buffer. Samples are ready to be analyzed on a flow cytometer.

3.3 Functional Characterization of Regulatory B Cells

The regulatory function of NOD B cells can be assessed either directly on bone-marrow-derived dendritic cells (BM-DCs, *see* Subheading 3.3.1) or on T cells (*see* Subheading 3.3.2). Figure 2 shows a scheme of the experimental design and set up to study this important aspect of regulatory B cells. Of note, when assessing bystander B-cell regulation of T cells, it is important to consider the ability of B cells to present the antigen (*see* **Note 10**). Evaluation of B-cell regulation on both BM-DC or T-cell functionality requires a T-cell transgenic mouse model (either $CD8^+$ or $CD4^+$ T cells that recognize a diabetogenic antigen). In the system described here, it is a $CD8^+$ TCR G9C$\alpha^{-/-}$ mouse model.

3.3.1 B-Cell Regulation of BM-DCs Function

In order to assess whether NOD B cells can regulate BM-DCs, several aspects can be addressed. First, one can assess whether there is a change in the phenotype and/or in the produced cytokines following coculture (*see* steps 2A and 3A of Fig. 2). Moreover, the functionality of DCs in regard to antigen presentation to T cells can also be investigated (*see* steps 2B-D and 3B-D of Fig. 2).

Set up of the B Cell–DC Coculture

1. First, differentiate bone-marrow-derived dendritic cells (BM-DCs) from either NOD or NOD.PI2^{tg} mice. Isolate the bone marrow as described in Subheading 3.1.2 and seed bone marrow cells at 5 × 10^6/well in a 6-well plate in 5 mL of RPMI complete medium supplemented with 1.5 ng/mL GM-CSF (this should be titrated for optimal DC survival and differentiation). After 6 days, BM-DCs are mature (*see* **Note 11**). Activate BM-DCs by culturing the cells overnight with 5 μg/mL LPS.
2. Using a cell scraper, harvest LPS-activated BM-DCs from the 6-well plate (BM-DCs are adherent cells and require scraping off of the bottom of the wells). Wash wells with RPMI complete medium and centrifuge cells at 400 × *g* at room temperature. Discard the supernatant and wash with RPMI complete medium. Resuspend in IMDM complete medium and count cells.

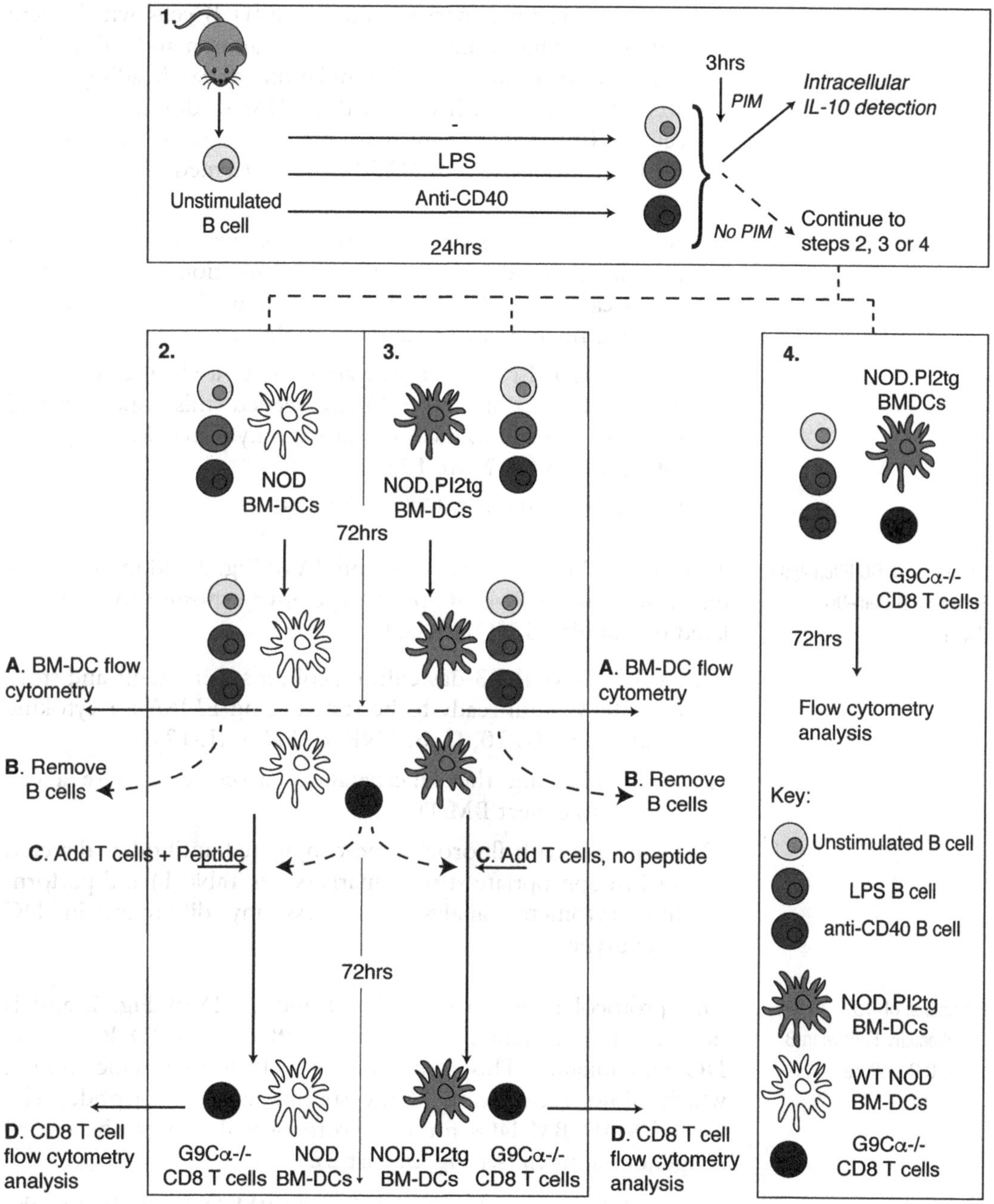

Fig. 2 Experimental setup and design for the functional characterization of regulatory B cells. **1.** Stimulation of B cells using LPS or anti-CD40 antibody and PMA/Ionomycin/Monensin (PIM) for the detection of intracellular IL-10 by flow cytometric analysis. If continuing to steps 2, 3, or 4, PIM should not be added. **2, 3.** Coculture between B cells and either wild-type NOD BM-DCs (**2**) or NOD.PI2tg BM-DCs (**3**) for 72 h. Following the 72 h incubation, the coculture can be used for monoclonal antibody staining and flow cytometric analysis of BM-DCs to detect the effect of B-cell regulation (**a**), or the assay can continue through the following steps. In this second case (BM-DC/T cell coculture), B cells are removed (**b**) and antigen-specific CD8 T^+ cells with peptide (WT NOD BM-DCs [**2**]) or without peptide (NOD.PI2tg BM-DCs [**3**]) are added (**c**). After a 72-h culture,

3. At the same time, harvest splenic NOD B cells which were purified through immunomagnetic separation and cultured in the presence or absence of stimulation (*see* Subheading 3.2.1, **steps 1–3**), and wash wells with IMDM medium. Centrifuge cells at 400 × *g* at room temperature and wash with IMDM medium. Resuspend in IMDM complete medium and count cells.
4. In a 24-well plate, seed 1.2×10^6 B cells/well. When preparing the plate, consider that each B-cell condition (unstimulated, LPS-treated, anti-CD40 antibody-treated) should be cultured either in the presence or absence of BM-DCs.
5. Add 4×10^5 BM-DCs to the appropriate wells. Prepare also a well in which only BM-DCs are seeded: this condition will serve as a control to measure the capacity of B cells to regulate DC function (*see* **Note 12**).
6. Culture for 3 days at 37 °C, 5% CO_2.

Evaluation of DC Phenotype Following B Cell–DC Coculture

This protocol refers to steps 2A and 3A of Fig. 2 and incorporates direct analysis on BM-DC phenotype after exposure to unstimulated or stimulated NOD B cells.

1. At the end of the 3-day culture, collect supernatants and store at −80 °C until ready to be tested using ELISA for cytokine production (IL-10, IL-6, TNF-α, IFN-γ, IL-12).
2. After collecting the supernatants, harvest cells. Use a cell scraper to collect BM-DCs.
3. Stain cells with fluorochrome-conjugated antibodies directed against appropriate surface markers (*see* Table 1) and perform flow cytometry analysis to assess any difference in DC phenotype.

Evaluation of DC Functionality Following B Cell-DC Coculture

This protocol refers to steps 2B-D and 3B-D of Fig. 2 and is designed to ascertain the tolerogenic effect of NOD B cells on DC functionality. This step requires a TCR transgenic mouse, which allows recognition of the specific antigenic peptide. The use of NOD BM-DCs for this protocol will require the use of exogenous antigen (*see* Fig. 2, part 2).

1. Carefully remove B cells, leaving the BM-DCs attached to the bottom of the wells, then wash wells with IMDM complete medium.

Fig. 2 (continued) $CD8^+$ T-cell staining and flow cytometry analysis are performed (**d**). **4**. Triple culture of B cells, BM-DCs (only NOD.PI2tg BM-DCs), and antigen-specific $G9C\alpha^{-/-}$ $CD8^+$ T cells for 72 h, followed by flow cytometric analysis

2. Prepare splenic $CD8^+$ T cells, using a $CD8^+$ T-cell isolation kit. In the system described here, $CD8^+$ T cells from the G9C$\alpha^{-/-}$ mouse are used. $CD8^+$ T cells are stimulated either exogenously with the G9 insulin B15–23 peptide or by intrinsic antigen-specific presentation using NOD.PI2^{tg} BM-DCs.
3. Seed 2×10^5 antigen-specific $CD8^+$ T cells in each well in IMDM complete medium. Include $CD8^+$ T cells in culture with BM-DCs that have not been exposed to B cells as a control.
4. Culture for a further 3 days at 37 °C, 5% CO_2 before harvesting for T-cell analysis (*see* **Note 13**).

3.3.2 B-Cell Regulation of Antigen-Specific $CD8^+$ T-Cell Function: B Cell–DC–$CD8^+$ T-Cell Cocultures

This protocol refers to step 4 in Fig. 2 and should be used to assess B-cell regulation of T cells. Here, the employed in vitro system is not based on the use of an exogenous antigen, but rather on a mouse model that allows intrinsic presentation of the antigen (in this case proinsulin) by BM-DCs to antigen-specific T cells.

1. Prepare NOD.PI2^{tg} BM-DCs and NOD B cells as in Subheading 3.3.1.1.
2. Prepare $CD8^+$ T cells from the spleen of a TCR transgenic mouse (in this case the G9C$\alpha^{-/-}$ mouse) through immunomagnetic separation. If the readout is different from a $CD8^+$ T-cell proliferation assay, then go directly to **step 3**. Conversely, label the $CD8^+$ T cells with CFSE. Resuspend cells at 2×10^6/mL in PBS and label them with CFSE for 15 min at 37 °C. Centrifuge the labeled cells at $400 \times g$ for 5 min and resuspend in warm complete IMDM medium and incubate for a further 30 min at 37 °C. Spin cells at $400 \times g$ for 5 min and resuspend in fresh complete IMDM medium and determine cell number.
3. In each experimental well of a 24-well plate, seed 1.2×10^6 B cells, 4×10^5 BM-DCs, and 2×10^5 $CD8^+$ T cells in order to have a 6:2:1 ratio (*see* **Note 12**). For control wells, seed BM-DCs only, BM-DCs with $CD8^+$ T cells, B cells only, $CD8^+$ T cells only.
4. Culture for 3 days at 37 °C, 5% CO_2 before harvesting for T-cell analysis (*see* **Note 13**).

4 Notes

1. The NOD/Caj (nonobese diabetic) is the main murine model used to study type 1 diabetes. These mice develop spontaneous type 1 diabetes with many parallels to human type 1 diabetes. Female mice are generally used as they have higher incidence of disease (NOD mice are fully reviewed in [1]). NOD.PI2^{tg} mice have a transgene that encodes expression of PI2 (proinsulin 2)

on the MHC class II promotor I-Eα [18] (NOD-Tg(H2-Ea-Ins2)1Wehi/WehiJ). These mice are used here as an example of a mouse that can supply DCs expressing MHC–peptide complexes without the need for addition of exogenous peptide or protein. G9C$\alpha^{-/-}$.NOD mice are genetically modified to express the T-cell receptor derived from the CD8 T-cell clone G9C8, responsive to amino acids 15–23 of the insulin B chain [19]. G9C$\alpha^{-/-}$.NOD mice are generated by crossing the A22Calpha (NOD.Cg-*Tcra*^{tm1Mjo} Tg(TcraG9C8)22Fsw/J) and the B2Calpha (NOD.Cg-*Tcra*^{tm1Mjo} Tg(TcrbG9C8)2Fsw/J) mice. These mice are used as an example of a T-cell receptor transgenic mouse, in which the majority of the CD8$^+$ T cells are antigen-specific.

2. Keep in mind that 6–7 mL of collagenase solution is needed per mouse.
3. Nowadays several suppliers provide reliable kits for immunomagnetic separation of different immune cell types.
4. Fixation/Permeabilization solutions can be bought as a kit from various suppliers. However, these solutions can also be individually homemade using separate components.
5. It is essential to rest pancreatic islets overnight as some cell surface markers can be cleaved due to collagenase digestion and therefore it may affect flow cytometric analysis.
6. Detecting IL-10 production from pancreatic lymph nodes can be difficult, owing to the sensitivity of B cells from this anatomical site to PMA and ionomycin. For this reason, when analyzing cells from pancreatic lymph nodes, it is recommended to limit stimulation time and to use lower concentrations of stimulants. Alternatively, do not assess IL-10 production but just phenotype regulatory B cells by analyzing surface marker expression.
7. Although differences can be found depending on the age and on the grade of insulitis of mice, B-cell numbers in pancreatic islets are low. Therefore, it can be useful to pool together pancreatic samples and, following this, splitting the pooled cells for the different culture conditions. This will ensure that there will be sufficient cells for the unstimulated, LPS, and anti-CD40 antibody stimulation conditions.
8. Regulatory B cells can be induced with either LPS or an anti-CD40 agonist, in combination with PMA/Ionomycin stimulation. The LPS and anti-CD40 antibody working concentrations, as well as the length of stimulation, should be titrated prior to use, to optimize IL-10 production and limit cell death. It should be noted that B-cell stimulation through

CD40 induces very little IL-10 secretion; on the contrary LPS can be used as B-cell stimulation agent when interested in detecting secreted IL-10 by ELISA since it is a strong inducer of IL-10 production and secretion [14, 20].

9. If using commercial rather than homemade solutions for cell fixation and permeabilization, the researcher can choose among different fixation and permeabilization kits that meet different needs. For example, if the Blimp1 transcription factor is used in addition to IL-10 for B-cell phenotyping, a nuclear fixation/permeabilization kit should be used.

10. If working with T-cell receptor transgenic $CD8^+$ or $CD4^+$ T cells, the use of NOD BM-DCs will require the addition of a specific peptide antigen. However, wild-type NOD BM-DCs will not allow the detection of bystander B-cell regulation in BM-DC-B cell-$CD8^+$ T-cell cultures (*see* Subheading 3.3.2) as the B cells within the culture will also be able to present the antigen. Thus, it will not be possible to assess the effects of sole dendritic cell antigen presentation, with bystander B-cell regulation. Another approach is to use whole antigen protein-pulsed (in this case the G9 insulin B15–23 peptide) BM-DCs which are obtained from WT NOD mice. More specifically, BM-DCs are fed with the antigenic protein for 24 h before being washed and cocultured with both T cells and B cells. However, it should be noted that the G9 insulin B15–23 peptide is a low affinity peptide, and pre-pulsing BM-DCs may not provide sufficiently robust stimulation of the T cell.

11. BM-DCs can be used for both the protocols described in Subheadings 3.3.1 and 3.3.2. The one provided in the Methods section is just a brief description of the steps required to differentiate BM-DCs. Refer to reference [15] for a full and detailed protocol.

12. All ratios for BM-DCs, B cells, and CD8 T cells should be titrated prior to set up. It is particularly important to ensure sufficient activation of $CD8^+$ T cells by BM-DCs to be able to detect and measure any suppression by B cells in the culture. Both WT NOD and antigen peptide expressing NOD.PI2^{tg} dendritic cells should be individually titrated, due to antigen presentation differences.

13. Several T-cell analyses can be performed. If the aim is assessing whether B cell primed DCs affect T-cell proliferation, then antigen-specific $CD8^+$ T cells should be labeled with a cell proliferation dye (i.e., CFSE) before being put in culture with BM-DCs. However, if the analysis involves evaluating the expression of surface activation markers, such as CD69, a shorter culture time would be more appropriate.

References

1. Pearson JA, Wong FS, Wen L (2016) The importance of the non obese diabetic (NOD) mouse model in autoimmune diabetes. J Autoimmun 66:76–88. https://doi.org/10.1016/j.jaut.2015.08.019
2. Pescovitz MD, Greenbaum CJ, Bundy B, Becker DJ, Gitelman SE, Goland R, Gottlieb PA, Marks JB, Moran A, Raskin P, Rodriguez H, Schatz DA, Wherrett DK, Wilson DM, Krischer JP, Skyler JS, Group TDTA-CS (2014) B-lymphocyte depletion with rituximab and β-cell function: two-year results. Diabetes Care 37(2):453–459. https://doi.org/10.2337/dc13-0626
3. Kleffel S, Vergani A, Tezza S, Ben Nasr M, Niewczas MA, Wong S, Bassi R, D'Addio F, Schatton T, Abdi R, Atkinson M, Sayegh MH, Wen L, Wasserfall CH, O'Connor KC, Fiorina P (2015) Interleukin-10+ regulatory B cells arise within antigen-experienced CD40+ B cells to maintain tolerance to islet autoantigens. Diabetes 64(1):158–171
4. Deng C, Xiang Y, Tan T, Ren Z, Cao C, Huang G, Wen L, Zhou Z (2016) Altered peripheral B-lymphocyte subsets in type 1 diabetes and latent autoimmune diabetes in adults. Diabetes Care 39(3):434–440. https://doi.org/10.2337/dc15-1765
5. Fillatreau S, Sweenie CH, McGeachy MJ, Gray D, Anderton SM (2002) B cells regulate autoimmunity by provision of IL-10. Nat Immunol 3(10):944–950. https://doi.org/10.1038/ni833
6. Morva A, Lemoine S, Achour A, Pers JO, Youinou P, Jamin C (2012) Maturation and function of human dendritic cells are regulated by B lymphocytes. Blood 119(1):106–114. https://doi.org/10.1182/blood-2011-06-360768
7. Maddur MS, Kaveri SV, Bayry J (2012) Regulation of human dendritic cells by B cells depends on the signals they receive. Blood 119(16):3863–3864. https://doi.org/10.1182/blood-2012-02-408948
8. Maddur MS, Sharma M, Hegde P, Stephen-Victor E, Pulendran B, Kaveri SV, Bayry J (2014) Human B cells induce dendritic cell maturation and favour Th2 polarization by inducing OX-40 ligand. Nat Commun 5:4092. https://doi.org/10.1038/ncomms5092
9. Ferris ST, Carrero JA, Unanue ER (2016) Antigen presentation events during the initiation of autoimmune diabetes in the NOD mouse. J Autoimmun 71:19–25. https://doi.org/10.1016/j.jaut.2016.03.007
10. Tian J, Zekzer D, Hanssen L, Lu Y, Olcott A, Kaufman DL (2001) Lipopolysaccharide-activated B cells down-regulate Th1 immunity and prevent autoimmune diabetes in nonobese diabetic mice. J Immunol 167(2):1081–1089
11. Xiao Z, Mohamood AS, Uddin S, Gutfreund R, Nakata C, Marshall A, Kimura H, Caturegli P, Womer KL, Huang Y, Jie C, Chakravarti S, Schneck JP, Yagita H, Hamad AR (2011) Inhibition of Fas ligand in NOD mice unmasks a protective role for IL-10 against insulitis development. Am J Pathol 179(2):725–732. https://doi.org/10.1016/j.ajpath.2011.04.016
12. Hussain S, Delovitch TL (2007) Intravenous transfusion of BCR-activated B cells protects NOD mice from type 1 diabetes in an IL-10-dependent manner. J Immunol 179(11):7225–7232
13. Anderson MS, Bluestone JA (2005) The NOD mouse: a model of immune dysregulation. Annu Rev Immunol 23:447–485. https://doi.org/10.1146/annurev.immunol.23.021704.115643
14. Boldison J, Da Rosa LC, Davies J, Wen L, Wong FS (2019) Dendritic cells license regulatory B cells to produce IL-10 and mediate suppression of antigen-specific CD8 T cells. Cell Mol Immunol 17:843. https://doi.org/10.1038/s41423-019-0324-z
15. Madaan A, Verma R, Singh AT, Jain SK, Jaggi M (2014) A stepwise procedure for isolation of murine bone marrow and generation of dendritic cells. J Biol Methods 1. https://doi.org/10.14440/jbm.2014.12
16. Carter JD, Dula SB, Corbin KL, Wu R, Nunemaker CS (2009) A practical guide to rodent islet isolation and assessment. Biol Proc 11:3–31. https://doi.org/10.1007/s12575-009-9021-0
17. Szot GL, Koudria P, Bluestone JA (2007) Murine pancreatic islet isolation. J Vis Exp 7:255. https://doi.org/10.3791/255
18. French MB, Allison J, Cram DS, Thomas HE, Dempsey-Collier M, Silva A, Georgiou HM, Kay TW, Harrison LC, Lew AM (1997) Transgenic expression of mouse proinsulin II prevents diabetes in nonobese diabetic mice. Diabetes 46(1):34–39. https://doi.org/10.2337/diab.46.1.34
19. Wong FS, Siew LK, Scott G, Thomas IJ, Chapman S, Viret C, Wen L (2009) Activation of insulin-reactive CD8 T-cells for development of autoimmune diabetes. Diabetes 58(5):1156–1164

20. Yanaba K, Bouaziz JD, Matsushita T, Tsubata T, Tedder TF (2009) The development and function of regulatory B cells expressing IL-10 (B10 cells) requires antigen receptor diversity and TLR signals. J Immunol 182(12):7459–7472. https://doi.org/10.4049/jimmunol.0900270
21. Yanaba K, Bouaziz JD, Haas KM, Poe JC, Fujimoto M, Tedder TF (2008) A regulatory B cell subset with a unique CD1dhiCD5+ phenotype controls T cell-dependent inflammatory responses. Immunity 28(5):639–650. https://doi.org/10.1016/j.immuni.2008.03.017
22. Iwata Y, Matsushita T, Horikawa M, Dilillo DJ, Yanaba K, Venturi GM, Szabolcs PM, Bernstein SH, Magro CM, Williams AD, Hall RP, St Clair EW, Tedder TF (2011) Characterization of a rare IL-10-competent B-cell subset in humans that parallels mouse regulatory B10 cells. Blood 117(2):530–541. https://doi.org/10.1182/blood-2010-07-294249
23. Gray M, Miles K, Salter D, Gray D, Savill J (2007) Apoptotic cells protect mice from autoimmune inflammation by the induction of regulatory B cells. Proc Natl Acad Sci U S A 104 (35):14080–14085. https://doi.org/10.1073/pnas.0700326104
24. Blair PA, Chavez-Rueda KA, Evans JG, Shlomchik MJ, Eddaoudi A, Isenberg DA, Ehrenstein MR, Mauri C (2009) Selective targeting of B cells with agonistic anti-CD40 is an efficacious strategy for the generation of induced regulatory T2-like B cells and for the suppression of lupus in MRL/lpr mice. J Immunol 182 (6):3492–3502. https://doi.org/10.4049/jimmunol.0803052
25. Evans JG, Chavez-Rueda KA, Eddaoudi A, Meyer-Bahlburg A, Rawlings DJ, Ehrenstein MR, Mauri C (2007) Novel suppressive function of transitional 2 B cells in experimental arthritis. J Immunol 178(12):7868–7878
26. Matsumoto M, Baba A, Yokota T, Nishikawa H, Ohkawa Y, Kayama H, Kallies A, Nutt SL, Sakaguchi S, Takeda K, Kurosaki T, Baba Y (2014) Interleukin-10-producing plasmablasts exert regulatory function in autoimmune inflammation. Immunity 41 (6):1040–1051. https://doi.org/10.1016/j.immuni.2014.10.016
27. Neves P, Lampropoulou V, Calderon-Gomez-E, Roch T, Stervbo U, Shen P, Kühl AA, Loddenkemper C, Haury M, Nedospasov SA, Kaufmann SH, Steinhoff U, Calado DP, Fillatreau S (2010) Signaling via the MyD88 adaptor protein in B cells suppresses protective immunity during Salmonella typhimurium infection. Immunity 33(5):777–790. https://doi.org/10.1016/j.immuni.2010.10.016
28. Ding Q, Yeung M, Camirand G, Zeng Q, Akiba H, Yagita H, Chalasani G, Sayegh MH, Najafian N, Rothstein DM (2011) Regulatory B cells are identified by expression of TIM-1 and can be induced through TIM-1 ligation to promote tolerance in mice. J Clin Invest 121 (9):3645–3656. https://doi.org/10.1172/JCI46274
29. Xiao S, Brooks CR, Sobel RA, Kuchroo VK (2015) Tim-1 is essential for induction and maintenance of IL-10 in regulatory B cells and their regulation of tissue inflammation. J Immunol 194(4):1602–1608
30. Parekh VV, Prasad DV, Banerjee PP, Joshi BN, Kumar A, Mishra GC (2003) B cells activated by lipopolysaccharide, but not by anti-Ig and anti-CD40 antibody, induce anergy in CD8+ T cells: role of TGF-beta 1. J Immunol 170 (12):5897–5911
31. Lee KM, Stott RT, Zhao G, SooHoo J, Xiong W, Lian MM, Fitzgerald L, Shi S, Akrawi E, Lei J, Deng S, Yeh H, Markmann JF, Kim JI (2014) TGF-beta-producing regulatory B cells induce regulatory T cells and promote transplantation tolerance. Eur J Immunol 44(6):1728–1736
32. Shen P, Roch T, Lampropoulou V, O'Connor RA, Stervbo U, Hilgenberg E, Ries S, Dang VD, Jaimes Y, Daridon C, Li R, Jouneau L, Boudinot P, Wilantri S, Sakwa I, Miyazaki Y, Leech MD, McPherson RC, Wirtz S, Neurath M, Hoehlig K, Meinl E, Grützkau A, Grün JR, Horn K, Kühl AA, Dörner T, Bar-Or A, Kaufmann SHE, Anderton SM, Fillatreau S (2014) IL-35-producing B cells are critical regulators of immunity during autoimmune and infectious diseases. Nature 507 (7492):366–370. https://doi.org/10.1038/nature12979
33. Zhang Y, Li J, Zhou N, Wu M, Xu J, Shen C, An X, Shen G, Yang M, Zhang C, Tao J (2017) The unknown aspect of BAFF: inducing IL-35 production by a CD5. J Invest Dermatol 137 (12):2532–2543. https://doi.org/10.1016/j.jid.2017.07.843
34. Wang RX, Yu CR, Dambuza IM, Mahdi RM, Dolinska MB, Sergeev YV, Wingfield PT, Kim SH, Egwuagu CE (2014) Interleukin-35 induces regulatory B cells that suppress autoimmune disease. Nat Med 20(6):633–641

Chapter 23

Analysis of Regulatory B Cells in Experimental Autoimmune Uveitis

Jin Kyeong Choi and Charles E. Egwuagu

Abstract

Regulatory B cells (Bregs) that produce IL-35 and IL-10 (i35-Bregs) regulate central nervous system (CNS) autoimmune diseases including uveitis. In the mouse model of uveitis, i35-Breg cells suppress intraocular inflammation by inducing expansion of IL-10-producing B cells (B10), IL-10-producing T cells (Tregs), and IL-35-producing T cells (iT_R35), suggesting that i35-Bregs orchestrate an immune-suppressive milieu that regulates immunity during autoimmune diseases. In this chapter, we discuss uveitis and therapeutic challenges that necessitate the development of cell-based therapies for the treatment of these potentially blinding diseases that cause 10% visual handicap. We then describe the methods we set up for ex vivo generation of i35-Breg cells employed in i35-Breg immunotherapy in uveitis and in other CNS autoimmune diseases.

Key words Regulatory B cells, i35-Breg, Uveitis, EAU, IL-35, IL-10, CNS autoimmune disease

1 Introduction

Uveitis is a general term that groups diverse intraocular inflammatory diseases such as birdshot retinochoroidopathy, Behcet's disease, and ocular sarcoidosis, and it accounts for 10% of severe visual handicaps in the United States [1, 2]. Similarly to other central nervous system (CNS) tissues, the neuroretina is an immune privileged tissue comprised of intricate and highly vulnerable physiology shielded by the blood-ocular barrier [3]. The endothelial and parenchymal basement membranes, pericytes, and perivascular space are barrier-forming constituents that limit paracellular and transcellular diffusion, while allowing import of nutrients and export of toxic metabolites out of the neuroretina [3]. Ocular immune privilege is maintained by retinal microglia and resident ocular parenchymal cells that constitutively secrete immunosuppressive and anti-inflammatory cytokines which inactivate immu-

Francesca Mion and Silvia Tonon (eds.), *Regulatory B Cells: Methods and Protocols*, Methods in Molecular Biology, vol. 2270, https://doi.org/10.1007/978-1-0716-1237-8_23,

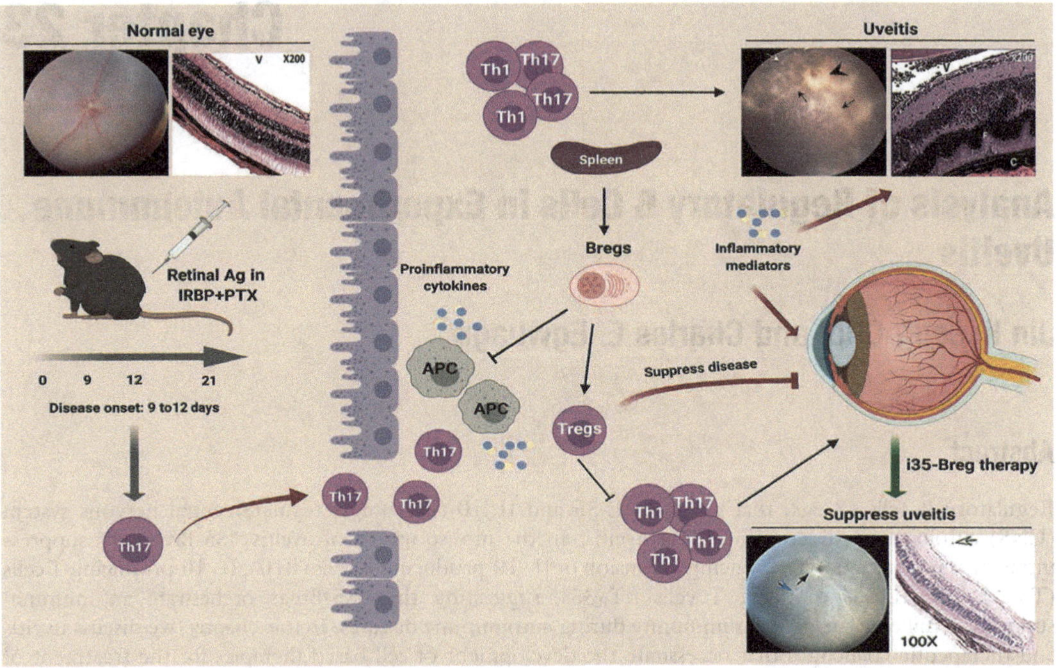

Fig. 1 Schematic representation of early events associated with loss of immune privilege of the eye, Th17/Th1-mediated pathology in the neuroretina and efficacy of Regulatory B-cell (Breg) immunotherapy in suppressing uveitis. Retinal fold (F); Choroiditis (C); Granuloma (G); Vitreous (V)

nological effector cells [4, 5]. However, during uveitis, lymphocytes bearing receptors specific to retinal proteins (uveitogenic T cells) breach the blood-ocular-barrier, attack and destroy photoreceptor cells. Thus, extravasation of inflammatory cells into the neuroretina plays an important role in the development of uveitis, and these cells are prime therapeutic targets (*see* Fig. 1). However, therapeutic intervention in uveitis presents formidable challenges, due to the need of striking a balance between controlling pathogenic immune responses on one hand and preventing generalized immunosuppression that would undermine the patients' vital immune surveillance functions and immunity.

Although steroids constitute an effective therapy for uveitis, serious adverse effects preclude their prolonged use. Immune modulation therapies that target inflammatory cells, cytokines, and cytokine receptors have been used in uveitis, and these include anti-IL-2R, anti-TNF-α, Etanercept (Enbrel®), and Infliximab (Remicade®) therapies. However, these biologics are mostly used as steroid-sparing agents that allow reduction of therapeutic dose of steroids. Although some of these biologics are used in uveitis, the therapeutic efficacy is a matter of some debate. Thus, there is considerable impetus to develop more effective biologics and cell-based therapies for uveitis. Experimental autoimmune uveitis

(EAU) shares essential immunopathogenic features of human uveitis, and this animal model provides a useful framework for evaluating therapies purported to suppress and ameliorate uveitis.

The cytokines belonging to the interleukin-12 (IL-12) family have profound effects on lymphocyte developmental decisions and have emerged as important biologics that regulate immunity [6]. The family is comprised of pro-inflammatory members (IL-12, IL-23, IL-39) implicated in several autoimmune diseases while two members (IL-27, IL-35) suppress CNS inflammation [7–10] and contribute to mechanisms that ameliorate uveitis in mice [11–13]. Regulatory B cells (Bregs) that secrete IL-35 (i35-Bregs) have recently been shown to suppress uveitis and encephalomyelitis [8, 14]. These studies suggest that the i35-Breg can produce both IL-10 and IL-35 in a time-dependent manner, although production of either cytokine is mutually exclusive [8, 14]. At early time points in culture, Bregs predominantly produce IL-10, but, at later time points, the majority of these cells produce IL-35. Thus, IL-10-producing Bregs and IL-35-producing Bregs are not distinct lineages but represent transitory states of the i35-Breg lineage. In this chapter, we describe the methods to generate and enrich Breg cells that exclusively produce IL-35 and the efficacy of autologous i35-Breg therapy in uveitis.

2 Materials

2.1 General Instrumentation

1. Tissue culture hood.
2. Incubator at 37 °C with 5% CO_2 atmosphere.
3. 0.2 μm syringe filters with 1 mL syringes.
4. Hamilton 1 mL glass syringes.
5. 16-Gauge blunt-end needles.
6. Alcohol swab and gauze.
7. 27-Gauge needles and 1 mL syringes.
8. 40- and 70-μm pore-size nylon cell strainers.
9. Refrigerated centrifuge and microcentrifuge for 96-well plates and conical tubes.
10. Plastic serological pipettes.
11. 15 mL and 50 mL polypropylene conical tubes.
12. 5 mL polystyrene round-bottom flow tubes.
13. 1.5–1.7 mL microcentrifuge tubes.
14. Photomicroscope.
15. Electroretinography console.
16. Ganzfeld dome.

17. Dissecting microscope.
18. Cell counting chamber or cell viability analyzer such as Vi-Cell XR cell viability analyzer (Beckman Coulter).
19. Cell sorter, flow cytometer, and software for analyzing flow cytometry data.

2.2 Tissue Dissection and Cell Culture Reagents

1. Incomplete culture medium: RPMI-1640.
2. Complete culture medium: 1% L-glutamine, 10% fetal bovine serum (FBS), 1% HEPES, 1% sodium pyruvate, 1% MEM nonessential amino acids, 1% penicillin/streptomycin, and 0.1% mercaptoethanol in RPMI-1640.
3. Red blood cell lysing buffer: 150 mM NH_4Cl, 10 mM $KHCO_3$, and 0.1 mM Na_2EDTA in distilled water.
4. Mouse restrainer with tail access.
5. Sterile scissors and forceps.
6. Sterile 100 mm Petri dishes.
7. Phosphate-buffered saline (PBS): 8 g NaCl, 0.2 g KCl, 1.44 g Na_2HPO_4, and 0.24 g KH_2PO_4 in 1 liter distilled water. Keep sterile.
8. Trypan blue solution.
9. 6-Well tissue culture plates.
10. Collagenase.
11. DNase.

2.3 Reagents for the Study of i35-Breg Cells

1. Fluorescence-activated cell sorting (FACS) buffer: 2% fetal calf serum (FCS), 2 mM EDTA, 0.1% sodium azide in PBS.
2. Cell sort collection buffer: 1 mL FBS in 15 mL conical tubes.
3. Magnetic-activated cell sorting (MACS) buffer: 0.5% bovine serum albumin (BSA) and 2 mM EDTA in PBS, pH 7.2.
4. Equipment for immunomagnetic separation (e.g., columns and magnets).
5. CD45R/B220 MicroBeads.
6. Cell stimulation reagents: LPS (*Escherichia coli* 0111: B4) and anti-mouse CD40 (clone FGK4.5/FGK45).
7. Phorbol 12-myristate 13-acetate (PMA).
8. Ionomycin.
9. Brefeldin A.
10. 4′,6-Diamidino-2-phenylindole (DAPI) viability dye for dead cell exclusion.
11. PE rat anti-mouse CD138 antibody, clone 281–2.

12. APC anti-human/mouse IL-12/IL-35 p35 antibody, clone 27537.
13. PerCP anti-mouse EBI3 antibody, clone 355022.
14. Dye for the discrimination of viable from nonviable cells in multicolor flow cytometric applications. Reconstitute the dye according to manufacturer's instructions.
15. Fixation and permeabilization solutions for intracellular staining.

2.4 Mice and Immunization Reagents

1. 6- to 8-week-old C57BL/6 J for CD45.2$^+$ recipient mice.
2. 6- to 8-week-old B6.SJL-*Ptprc*^{a} *Pepc*^{b}/BoyJ (CD45.1$^+$) for donor mice.
3. Interphotoreceptor retinoid-binding protein peptide ($IRBP_{651–670}$).
4. Complete Freund's adjuvant (CFA): Incomplete Freund's (IFA) supplemented with heat-killed *Mycobacterium tuberculosis* (strain H37Ra) at a final concentration of 2.5 mg/mL.
5. 1% mouse normal serum: restore the lyophilized normal mouse serum with sterile water in order to obtain a 1% solution. Filter through a 0.2-μm filter.
6. *Bordetella pertussis* toxin (PTX). Lyophilized powder in 50 μg vials.

2.5 Reagents for the Assessment of Uveitis

1. Ketamine.
2. Xylazine.
3. Midrin P: 0.5% tropicamide, 0.5% phenylephrine hydrochloride eye drops.
4. 4% glutaraldehyde.
5. 4% formaldehyde.
6. Alcohol.
7. Methacrylate.
8. Photomicroscope.
9. Gonioscopic prism solution.

3 Methods

3.1 Induction of EAU

EAU is a T-cell-mediated autoimmune disease that serves as a model of human intraocular inflammatory disease [11, 14]. EAU is induced in susceptible species by active immunization with ocular-specific proteins (or peptides derived from them) and is transferable to naive syngeneic animals by injection of in vitro-activated CD4$^+$ MHC class II-restricted T cell lines specific to retinal antigens. The mouse EAU model is commonly induced by immunization with $IRBP_{651–670}$, a 140-kDa retinal glycoprotein that functions in the transport of retinoids between the neuroretina and retinal pigment epithelium. For immunization, the $IRBP_{651–670}$ is emulsified in CFA (*see* **Note 1**).

1. Prepare CFA by pestle crushing in a porcelain mortar 100 mg of heat-killed *Mycobacterium tuberculosis* to a fine powder, and mix with 40 mL of IFA. Store indefinitely at 4 °C.
2. Dissolve the $IRBP_{651–670}$ peptide in PBS to a final concentration of 10 mg/mL (*see* **Note 2**).
3. Make an emulsion of the $IRBP_{651–670}$ peptide in CFA (1:1; v/v) by vortexing for 10 min at high speed, and sonicate 1 time with 30 sec bursts. After mixing peptide and CFA, ensure that the amount of emulsion is sufficient, bearing in mind that 300 μg peptide in 0.2 mL emulsion must be provided to each mouse. Emulsion for two additional mice should be prepared.
4. Spin-down the emulsion for 5 min at 300 × *g* to remove bubbles from the emulsion, and vortex briefly to mix. Well-made emulsion should appear as a very sticky cream.
5. Draw emulsion into a 1-mL Hamilton glass syringe using 16-Gauge blunt-end needles. Make sure that no air bubble is present in the syringe. Replace the 16-Gauge needle with a 23-Gauge needle to proceed with immunization.
6. Prepare a 10-μg/mL PTX stock solution by adding the filtered 1% mouse serum solution to the PTX vial (*see* **Note 3**).
7. Use 6- to 8-weeks-old female C57BL/6 J mice (*see* **Note 4**). Inject 100 μL of the $IRBP_{651–670}$ emulsion subcutaneously into the back of the mouse, and 50 μL to each thigh. After $IRBP_{651–670}$, immediately inject intraperitoneally 1 μg/mouse (100 μL) of PTX stock solution (*see* **Note 5**). Return the animal to the cage for daily evaluation of EAU development.

3.2 Assessment of Uveitis and Pathological Score

Initial signs of uveitis in C57BL/6 J mice are observed by day 13 post-immunization (p.i.), with full-blown uveitis occurring between day 16 and day 22 p.i.. Disease progression is monitored by fundoscopy, histology, optical coherence tomography (OCT), and electroretinography (ERG).

1. Fundoscopy: This is a noninvasive method routinely used to examine the retina of a dilated eye pupil under a binocular microscope. EAU severity is evaluated at various time points during the course of the disease. Briefly, following administration of systemic anesthesia (intraperitoneal injection of 1.4 mg/mouse ketamine and of 0.12 mg/mouse xylazine), the pupil is dilated by topical administration of 1% tropicamide ophthalmic solution. At least six images (two posterior central

retinal view, four peripheral retinal views) are taken from each eye by positioning the endoscope and viewing from superior, inferior, lateral, and medial fields, and each individual lesion is identified, mapped, and recorded (*see* **Note 6**).

2. Histology: This technique is generally used to assess and grade pathological lesions and involves enucleation of the eye. Eyes are fixed in 4% glutaraldehyde for 30 min and transferred to a 4% formaldehyde solution. Specimens are then dehydrated through graded alcohol series, embedded in methacrylate, and 4 μm serial transverse sections are cut and stained with hematoxylin and eosin. Photographs of representative sections are taken on a photomicroscope.
3. Optical coherence tomography: This noninvasive procedure allows visualization of internal microstructures of various eye structures in living animals. It allows the spatial localization and assessment of the extent of accumulation of inflammatory cells in vitreous and optic nerve head. Before OCT imaging is performed, each animal is anesthetized, and the pupils dilated. The anesthetized mouse is immobilized using adjustable holder that rotates easily allowing for horizontal or vertical scanning. Each scan is performed at least twice, with realignment each time. The dimension of the scan (in depth and transverse extent) is adjusted until the optimal signal intensity and contrast are achieved.
4. Electroretinogram: This technique measures changes in electrical potentials in response to light stimulation of the retina and is a well-established tool for identifying gross physiologic changes indicative of defects in cone and/or rod signaling functions and visual function defects. Before ERG recordings, mice are dark-adapted overnight, and experiments performed under dim red illumination. Mice are anesthetized with a single intraperitoneal injection of 1.4 mg/mouse ketamine and 0.12 mg/mouse xylazine and pupils dilated with Midrin P drops. ERGs are recorded using an electroretinography console that generates and controls the light stimulus. Dark-adapted ERG is recorded with a single flash delivered in a Ganzfeld dome with intensity of −4 to 1 log cd·s/m^2 delivered in 6 steps. Light-adapted ERG was obtained with a 20 cd/m^2 background, and light stimuli started at 0.3 to 100 cd·s/m^2 in six steps. Gonioscopic prism solution is used to provide good electrical contact and maintain corneal moisture. A reference electrode (gold wire) is placed in the mouth, and a ground electrode (subcutaneous stainless-steel needle) is positioned at the base of the tail. Signals are differentially amplified and digitized. Amplitudes of the major ERG components (a- and b-wave) are measured by automated methods.

3.3 Isolation of Regulatory or Inflammatory Cells from the Neuroretina

To characterize inflammatory cells that cross the blood–retina barrier during EAU, mice should be euthanized and perfused with PBS. Enucleated eyes are put in a Petri dish containing incomplete culture medium for immediate isolation of the retina under a dissecting microscope.

1. Cut the eye along the limbus of the eye, and then carefully remove lens and cornea.
2. Peel off the retina and remove the attached optic nerve.
3. Digest the freshly isolated retina with 1 mg/mL collagenase in incomplete culture medium containing 10 μg/mL DNase for 1 h at 37 °C. Cells are pipetted intermittently every 30 min. Digestion is quenched with 5–10 folds volume of 10% FBS in complete culture medium.
4. Wash the cells twice in complete culture medium and count cells using the trypan blue dye exclusion method and either a counting chamber or a cell viability analyzer.

3.4 Isolation of Splenocytes

Isolate cells from the spleen of unimmunized or EAU-bearing mice and sort primary B cells based on the positive expression of the CD19 or B220 markers.

1. Euthanize B6 CD45.1$^+$ mice via CO_2 asphyxiation and dissect the spleen from animals.
2. Place the spleen in a sterile Petri dish with 10–15 mL of complete culture medium.
3. Under a sterile tissue culture hood, gently rub the spleen between the frosted end of a glass slide or plunger (butt) of a disposable 1 mL syringe, to gradually break the tissue apart into a suspension. Repeat the mechanic disruption procedure until no large pieces of tissue remain in the buffer.
4. Use 10 mL plastic serological pipettes to recover the splenocyte suspension from the dish into a 50-mL conical tube. Pass the cell suspension several times through a 70-μm pore-size nylon cell strainer or filter. Make sure the cell suspension contains no visible fragments.
5. Centrifuge the cells in 50 mL conical tubes for 10 min at 300 × g, 4 °C.
6. Discard supernatant and resuspend cell pellet in 2 mL of red blood cell lysis buffer for 5 min.
7. Wash the pellet once in PBS by centrifuging 10 min at 300 × g, 4 °C.
8. Resuspend cells in 10 mL complete culture medium and determine the cell number.

3.5 Regulatory B-Cell Enrichment and Isolation

Bregs that produce IL-10 and/or IL-35 (i35-Breg) suppress CNS autoimmune diseases and are enriched in CD138$^+$ B cells. Although i35-Bregs can produce both IL-10 and IL-35, these cells are developmentally and functionally distinct from the CD5^{hi}CD1d^{hi} B10 subset that exclusively produce IL-10. Here we describe the method we use to generate and enrich i35-Bregs that exclusively produce IL-35 from CD138$^+$ cells (*see* Fig. 2a and **Note** 7).

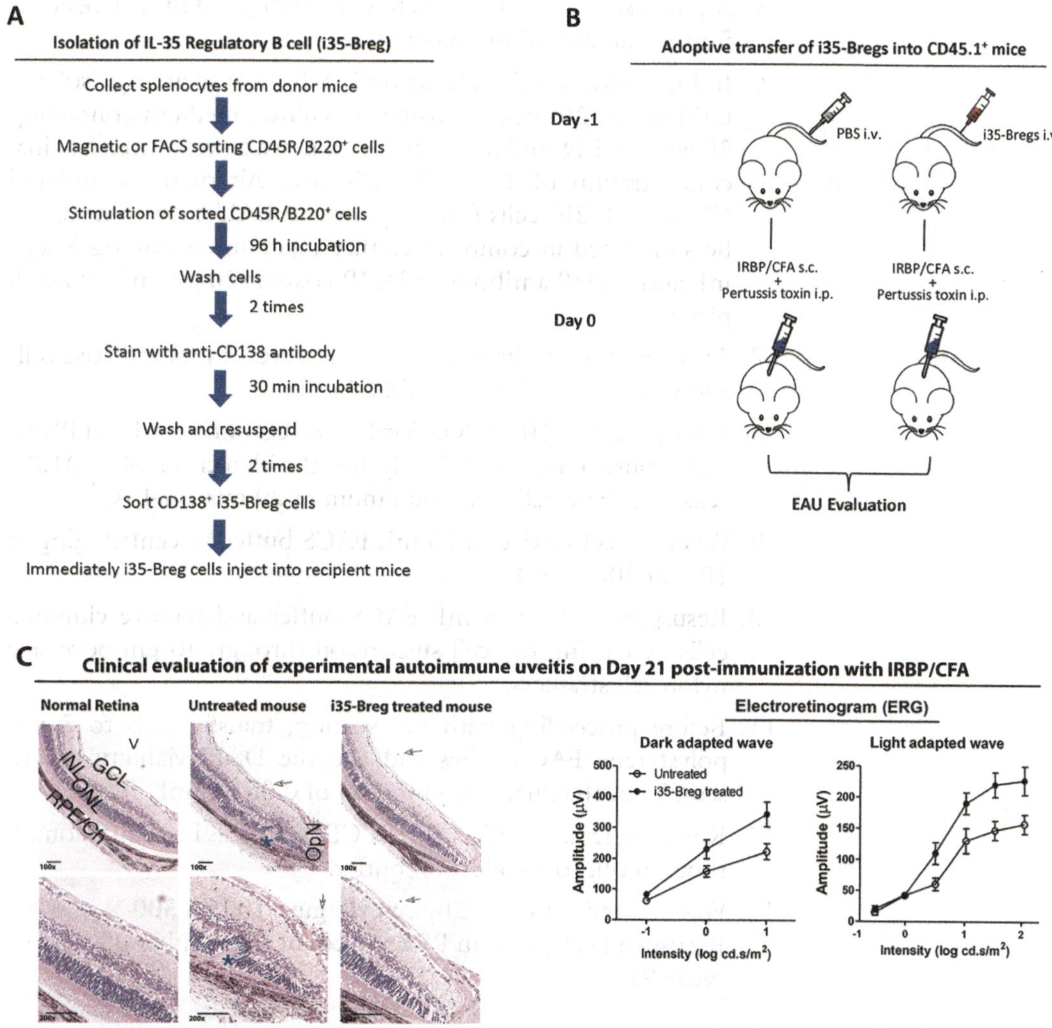

Fig. 2 Schematic and diagrammatic representations of procedures for (**a**) ex vivo generation of IL-35-producing Regulatory B cells (i35-Bregs) and (**b**) autologous transfer of the CD45.2$^+$ Breg cells to CD45.1$^+$ mice as treatment for experimental autoimmune uveitis (EAU)

3.5.1 Induction and Isolation of CD138⁺ Cells

1. Isolate splenocytes from healthy or EAU-bearing C57BL/6 J mice as described in Subheading 3.4.
2. Centrifuge the isolated spleen cell suspension at 300 × *g* for 10 min and resuspend the cell pellet in MACS buffer. Determine the cell number.
3. Isolate CD45R/B220⁺ cells by immunomagnetic separation, using the specific microbeads and columns according to manufacturer's instructions (*see* **Note 8**).
4. Wash the obtained cells once more in 10 mL PBS by centrifuging at 10 min 300 × *g*, 4 °C.
5. Aspirate supernatant completely and resuspend the cell pellet in fresh complete culture medium.
6. Induce plasma cell differentiation by resuspending isolated CD45R/B220⁺ cells in complete culture medium containing 25 μg/mL LPS and incubate for 96 h in a 6-well plate, at a final concentration of 1×10^6 cells/mL. Alternatively, isolated CD45R/B220⁺ cells from healthy and EAU-bearing mice can be stimulated in complete culture medium containing 5 μg/mL anti-CD40 antibody in IRBP-coated (20 μg/mL) 96-well plates.
7. At the end of the 96 h incubation, harvest the stimulated cells and wash twice with cold FACS buffer.
8. Resuspend 1×10^8 cells in 5 mL of FACS buffer and add PE rat anti-mouse CD138 antibody for the detection of CD138⁺ cells. Incubate cells for a minimum of 20 min on 4 °C.
9. Wash the cells twice in 10 mL FACS buffer by centrifuging at 10 min 300 × *g*, 4 °C.
10. Resuspend cells in 5 mL FACS buffer and remove clumped cells by passing the cell suspension through 40-μm pore-size nylon cell strainers.
11. Before proceeding with cell sorting, transfer cells to 5 mL polystyrene FACS tubes and add the DAPI viability dye to samples at the final concentration of 0.05 μg/mL.
12. Run samples and collect sorted CD138⁺ cells in 15 mL conical tubes in cell sort collection buffer.
13. Wash sorted cells twice by centrifuging 10 min 300 × *g*, 4 °C. Resuspend cell pellet in PBS and count the number of cells (*see* **Note 9**).

3.5.2 Detection of IL-35-Producing CD138⁺ Cells by Intracellular Cytokine Staining

Determine the percentage of IL-35-producing B cells among sorted CD138⁺ cells by intracellular cytokine staining using monoclonal Abs specific to p35 or Ebi3.

1. Plate sorted CD138⁺ cells at 1×10^6 cells/mL and add 50 ng/mL PMA, 500 ng/mL ionomycin, and 5 μg/mL Brefeldin A in complete culture medium. Incubate for 5 h.

2. After 5 h incubation, wash cells twice with cold PBS and stain the cells with a dye specific for the discrimination of viable from nonviable cells in multicolor flow cytometric applications for 20 min at 4 °C.
3. Wash the cells twice in FACS buffer by centrifuging at 10 min at 300 × *g*, 4 °C and add 200 μL/well intracellular fixation buffer for 30 min on 4 °C.
4. Permeabilize cells by washing twice with permeabilization buffer and centrifuge 10 min at 300 × *g*, 4 °C.
5. Add the anti-mouse p35 and Ebi3 antibodies diluted according to manufacturer's instructions in 100 μL permeabilization buffer. Incubate for 1 h at 4 °C.
6. Wash the cells twice and resuspend in 200 μL FACS buffer. Transfer cells to 5 mL polystyrene FACS tubes and acquire data on a flow cytometer. Analyze data using a software specific for the analysis of flow cytometry data, e.g., FlowJo. A representative intracellular staining analysis of i35-Breg cells is shown in Fig.3.

3.6 Adoptive transfer of IL-35-Producing B Cells in Recipient Uveitis Mice

To establish if i35-Bregs can directly suppress uveitis, it is necessary to induce EAU in C57BL/6 J mice ($CD45.2^+$), purify i35-Breg cells from the spleen of the donor $CD45.2^+$ mouse, and examine whether adoptive transfer of the i35-Breg cells would suppress EAU in a $CD45.1^+$-recipient congenic mouse. B6 CD45.1 (recipient) and B6 CD45.2 (donor) mice should be age-matched (*see* **Note 10**). The i35-Bregs are transferred to naïve $CD45.1^+$ mice (1×10^7 cells/mouse), and EAU is induced 24 h after cell transfer. Efficacy of the i35-Bregs treatment is evaluated starting from 10 days after adoptive transfer (*see* Fig. 2b).

1. The day before EAU induction, prepare i35-Bregs in fresh complete medium (*see* Subheading 3.5.1) and inject 10^7 cells in a < 200 μL volume per mouse by tail vein injection. For this procedure, the mouse should be placed under a heat lamp to promote peripheral vasodilation. Then the mouse should be mechanically restrained using a mouse restrainer with a tail access chamber. Finally, the tail should be swabbed with alcohol gauze and placed horizontally for cell injection through a 27-Gauge needle.
2. On day 0, induce EAU by immunization with $IRBP_{651-670}$ in CFA emulsion (*see* Subheading 3.1).
3. From day 10, start monitoring mice (*see* **Note 11**).
4. After 14 days post-immunization, examine the eyes using a microscope with coaxial illumination to assess disease severity.

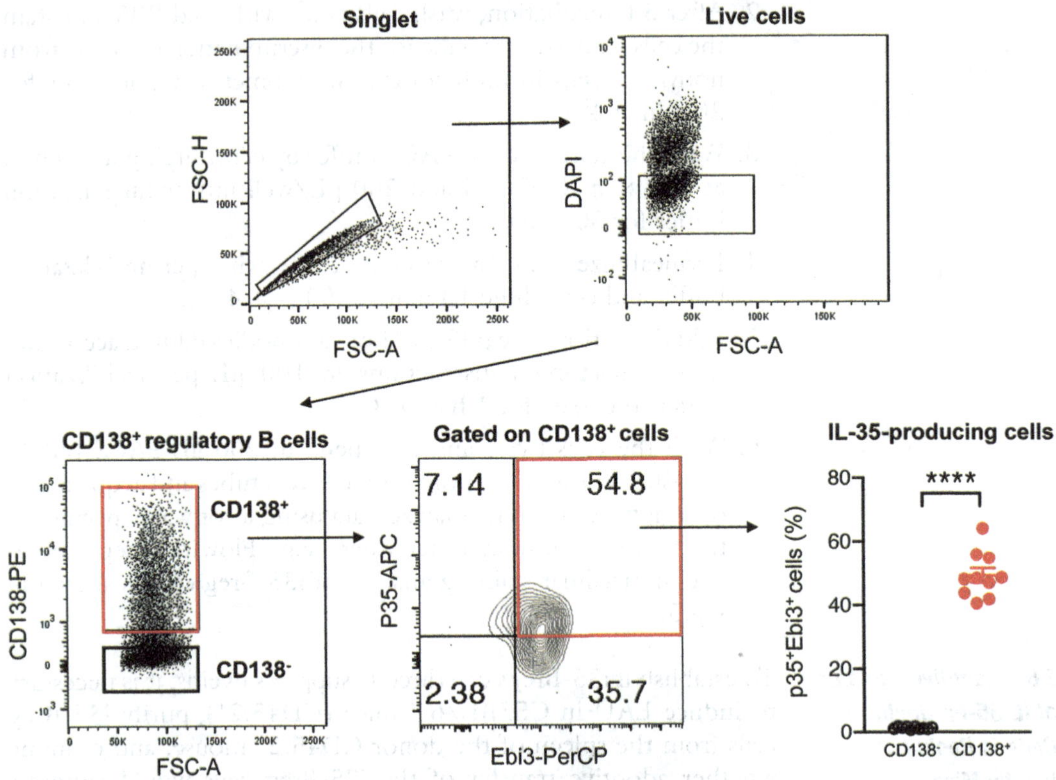

Fig. 3 Gating strategy for the analysis of IL-35-producing CD138$^+$ B cells. Live cells from LPS-stimulated B220/CD45R cells were stained with an anti-CD138 antibody and sorted by FACS. CD138$^+$ or CD138$^-$ cells were then subjected to intracellular cytokine staining analysis. The representative flow cytometry plot shows the percentage of IL-35-expressing CD138$^+$ B cells (p35$^+$ and Ebi3$^+$). Bar chart shows the mean percentage of IL-35 expressing CD138$^+$ or CD138$^-$ cells from 10 independent i35-Breg preparations. ****$p < 0.0001$

5. After 21 days post-immunization, use one of the eyes of every mouse for histological analysis. Use the other remaining eye to isolate the retina cells and to evaluate the inflammatory cell changes in the i35-Bregs treatment group using FACS analysis.

4 Notes

1. The emulsion of the $IRBP_{651–670}$ peptide in CFA must be mixed well and prepared just before using it as the suspended *Mycobacterium tuberculosis* easily settles at the bottom of the bottle.
2. If you purchase a large quantity of the $IRBP_{651–670}$ peptide (50 mg/vial), do not try to dissolve it all at once since it does not dissolve well. This makes it difficult to ascertain the true concentration of the peptide. Using the recommended dose is crucial to obtain reproducible results in the induction of EAU.

3. The PTX vial contains 50 μg of the powdered toxin. It is expedient to add 5 mL of 1% sterile normal mouse serum to the vial to make the 10 μg/mL PTX stock solution.
4. The C57BL/6 mouse strain must not be used in EAU studies since it presents the RD8 mutation in the Crb1 gene. The RD8 mutation is a single nucleotide deletion in the Crb1 gene, which results in a form of retinal degeneration having a distinct clinical appearance. The C57BL/6 J strain does not have the RD8 mutation and can therefore be employed [15].
5. To induce severe EAU in most susceptible mouse species, concurrent injection of *Bordetella pertussis* toxin is required.
6. To avoid a subjective bias in scoring Fundoscopy examinations, evaluation of the fundus photographs is conducted without knowledge of the mouse identity by a masked observer.
7. The use of p35 and/or Ebi3 reporter mouse strain would facilitate ex vivo production of i35-Breg cells. However, a IL-35 (p35/Ebi3) reporter mouse is not commercially available.
8. It is important to work fast and keep the cells cold (do not work at room temperature). This prevents capping of antibodies on the cell surface and non-specific cell labeling.
9. When working with normal mice, we generally obtain 70×10^6 cells from mouse spleen processing, then 25×10^6 CD45R/B220$^+$ cells after immunomagnetic separation, and we end up with 0.5×10^6 viable regulatory plasmacytes per mouse after FACS sorting. In EAU-bearing mice, the number of cells varies depending on disease severity.
10. CD45.1 and CD45.2 mice are widely used in adoptive transfer studies to track the donor and recipient cells. B cells expressing either CD45.1$^+$ or CD45.2$^+$ can be distinguished by FACS using mouse antibodies that recognize either CD45 haplotypes. We use these mice to track donor and recipient Breg cells in mouse tissues during EAU.
11. Depending on the experimental goal, the end point of the EAU study can vary and the mouse might be euthanized from 15 to 21 days after immunization.

References

1. Nussenblatt RB (1990) The natural history of uveitis. Int Ophthalmol 14(5–6):303–308
2. Nussenblatt RB (1991) Proctor lecture. Experimental autoimmune uveitis: mechanisms of disease and clinical therapeutic indications. Invest Ophthalmol Vis Sci 32(13):3131–3141
3. Wraith DC, Nicholson LB (2012) The adaptive immune system in diseases of the central nervous system. J Clin Invest 122(4):1172–1179
4. Streilein JW (2003) Ocular immune privilege: therapeutic opportunities from an experiment of nature. Nat Rev Immunol 3(11):879–889

5. Caspi RR (2010) A look at autoimmunity and inflammation in the eye. J Clin Invest 120 (9):3073–3083
6. Vignali DA, Kuchroo VK (2012) IL-12 family cytokines: immunological playmakers. Nat Immunol 13(8):722–728
7. Fitzgerald DC, Ciric B, Touil T, Harle H, Grammatikopolou J, Das Sarma J, Gran B, Zhang GX, Rostami A (2007) Suppressive effect of IL-27 on encephalitogenic Th17 cells and the effector phase of experimental autoimmune encephalomyelitis. J Immunol 179(5):3268–3275
8. Shen P, Roch T, Lampropoulou V, O'Connor RA, Stervbo U, Hilgenberg E, Ries S, Dang VD, Jaimes Y, Daridon C, Li R, Jouneau L, Boudinot P, Wilantri S, Sakwa I, Miyazaki Y, Leech MD, McPherson RC, Wirtz S, Neurath M, Hoehlig K, Meinl E, Grutzkau A, Grun JR, Horn K, Kuhl AA, Dorner T, Bar-Or A, Kaufmann SH, Anderton SM, Fillatreau S (2014) IL-35-producing B cells are critical regulators of immunity during autoimmune and infectious diseases. Nature 507 (7492):366–370
9. Zundler S, Neurath MF (2015) Interleukin-12: functional activities and implications for disease. Cytokine Growth Factor Rev 26 (5):559–568
10. Wang X, Wei Y, Xiao H, Liu X, Zhang Y, Han G, Chen G, Hou C, Ma N, Shen B, Li Y, Egwuagu CE, Wang R (2016) A novel IL-23p19/Ebi3 (IL-39) cytokine mediates inflammation in lupus-like mice. Eur J Immunol 46(6):1343–1350
11. Amadi-Obi A, Yu CR, Liu X, Mahdi RM, Clarke GL, Nussenblatt RB, Gery I, Lee YS, Egwuagu CE (2007) T(H)17 cells contribute to uveitis and scleritis and are expanded by IL-2 and inhibited by IL-27/STAT1. Nat Med 13 (6):711–718
12. Choi JK, Dambuza IM, He C, Yu CR, Uche AN, Mattapallil MJ, Caspi RR, Egwuagu CE (2017) IL-12p35 inhibits Neuroinflammation and ameliorates autoimmune encephalomyelitis. Front Immunol 8:1258
13. Dambuza IM, He C, Choi JK, Yu CR, Wang R, Mattapallil MJ, Wingfield PT, Caspi RR, Egwuagu CE (2017) IL-12p35 induces expansion of IL-10 and IL-35-expressing regulatory B cells and ameliorates autoimmune disease. Nat Commun 8(1):719
14. Wang RX, Yu CR, Dambuza IM, Mahdi RM, Dolinska MB, Sergeev YV, Wingfield PT, Kim SH, Egwuagu CE (2014) Interleukin-35 induces regulatory B cells that suppress autoimmune disease. Nat Med 20(6):633–641
15. Mattapallil MJ, Wawrousek EF, Chan CC, Zhao H, Roychoudhury J, Ferguson TA, Caspi RR (2012) The Rd8 mutation of the Crb1 gene is present in vendor lines of C57BL/6N mice and embryonic stem cells, and confounds ocular induced mutant phenotypes. Invest Ophthalmol Vis Sci 53 (6):2921–2927

Chapter 24

Purification and Immunophenotypic Characterization of Human $CD24^{hi}CD38^{hi}$ and $CD24^{hi}CD27^{+}$ Regulatory B Cells in Transplantation

Rowa Y. Alhabbab and Giovanna Lombardi

Abstract

Transplantation is still the treatment of choice for organ failure; however, allograft induces inflammatory immune responses that require immunosuppressive treatment. The role of regulatory B cells (Bregs) in downregulating inflammation has been reported to be significant in several diseases including transplant rejection. Many reports have analyzed different B-cell subpopulations, including Bregs, in tolerant, stable, and rejecting transplant recipients as well as the influence of immunosuppressant on the frequencies and functions of the different B-cell subsets. In this chapter, the key techniques required to investigate human Breg frequencies and functions in transplant patients are discussed.

Key words Human Bregs, $CD24^{hi}CD38^{hi}$ Bregs, $CD24^{hi}CD27^{+}$ Bregs, Breg frequency, Breg function, Transplantation

1 Introduction

Transplantation is currently the treatment of choice for end stage organ failure. Early studies have reported that graft survival can be prolonged in renal transplant patients by utilizing human anti-CD20-depleting antibodies to remove B cells [1]. In contrast, a study by Clatworthy et al. reported that 85% of kidney transplant recipients who have received B-cell depleting antibody treatment suffered from cellular rejection, whereas only 14% showed cellular rejection upon receiving anti-CD25 antibodies, which interfere with the binding of IL-2 to its receptor, inhibiting T-cell proliferation and survival [2]. Moreover, it was also suggested by the same study that the lack of B cells induced the production of several pro-inflammatory cytokines such as TNF-α that might stimulate antigen-presenting cells, and in turn activate T cells, suggesting that the treatment with anti-CD20 antibodies can deplete B cells with a

Francesca Mion and Silvia Tonon (eds.), *Regulatory B Cells: Methods and Protocols*, Methods in Molecular Biology, vol. 2270, https://doi.org/10.1007/978-1-0716-1237-8_24,

regulatory role during the response to allograft [2]. Subsequently, Newell and colleagues have reported that tolerant kidney transplant recipients, no longer receiving immunosuppressive drugs, expressed high levels of B-cell genes encoding the variable region segments of Ig light chains including RNA for IGKV4–1, IGLL21, and IGKV1D-13 [3]. This genetic profile was also associated with an increase in B-cell numbers, particularly in naïve, memory, and IL-10^{+} immature B cells, compared to stable recipients under immunosuppressive drugs. The authors have also suggested to use the presence of this "B-cell genetic signature" to select patients who would not require immunosuppressive treatment [3, 4]. Although a study by Chesneau et al. have also reported increased levels of total B cells in kidney tolerant patients compared to stable recipients on immunosuppressant, the regulatory capacity of the total B cells was IL-10 and TGF-β-independent and their function was mainly mediated by the action of granzyme-B inducing apoptosis of T cells [5]. In another study, it was proposed that the differences in the profiles of total B-cell frequencies and regulatory function between tolerant and non-tolerant renal transplant recipients were due to the effect of the immunosuppressive drugs on the B cells in non-tolerant patients [6]. Two human regulatory B-cell (Breg) subpopulations have been identified, the immature transitional $CD24^{hi}CD38^{hi}$ and the memory $CD24^{hi}CD27^{+}$ Bregs [7]. Both human Breg subpopulations have been reported by several groups for their essential anti-inflammatory role in many diseases [7]. In human transplant, as mentioned earlier and discussed later, most of the studies have correlated Breg frequencies among peripheral blood mononuclear cells (PBMCs) isolated from allograft receiving patients with graft survival, immunosuppressant therapy, and the level of serum anti-human leukocyte antigen (HLA) antibodies, with some studies reporting human Breg suppressive capacities and cytokines production in vitro. A study by Cherukuri et al. has analyzed the lymphocyte populations in two groups of renal transplant patients, one group receiving alemtuzumab induction plus tacrolimus monotherapy and the other receiving basiliximab induction and tacrolimus plus mycophenolate mofetil therapy. The authors have shown differences in the B-cell profile 25 months posttreatment, with an increase in several B-cell subsets including transitional $CD24^{hi}CD38^{hi}$ B cells in patients that received alemtuzumab therapy. Moreover, they have reported that patients with lower levels of B cells had worse graft function, and this was independent of their treatment regimen. They have also reported that with alemtuzumab treatment the patient's transitional $CD24^{hi}CD38^{hi}$ B-cell numbers were decreased as HLA-specific antibodies levels increased [8]. A subsequent study by the same group comparing the frequency of $CD24^{hi}CD38^{hi}$ B cells and IL-10/TNF-α ratio in healthy subjects, patients with stable renal transplant and rejecting patients reported no differences in transitional $CD24^{hi}CD38^{hi}$ B-cell frequencies, IL-10 expression as well as in IL-10/TNF-α ratio between healthy and stable patients. Nevertheless, rejecting patients showed low frequencies in their transitional $CD24^{hi}CD38^{hi}$ B cells as well as a significant reduction in their IL-10/TNF-α ratio compared to healthy and stable subjects [9]. These data collectively emphasize the crucial role that B cells, in particular transitional $CD24^{hi}CD38^{hi}$ Bregs, play in renal transplant survival. An additional study with renal transplant patients prior of receiving the allograft and on five subsequent occasions up to 1 year posttransplant reported a protective role provided by transitional $CD24^{hi}CD38^{hi}$ B cells against acute rejection episodes, while a lack of any association between the transitional $CD24^{hi}CD38^{hi}$ B-cell numbers and the production of donor-specific as well as donor non-specific antibodies was observed [10]. Moreover, Latorre et al. have found that stable renal transplant patients for up to 28 years showed an increase in transitional $CD24^{hi}CD38^{hi}$ B cell levels that positively correlated with graft survival independently of patient's treatment regimen [11]. Schlosser et al. have studied longitudinally up to 1 year B-cell subsets distribution in renal transplant patients who received ABO-compatible and ABO-incompatible organs. They reported a decrease in both activated B cells as well as in the plasmablast population in patients with no signs of rejection, whereas rejecting patients showed a significant increase in the same B-cell subsets. Moreover, they found that ABO-incompatible renal transplant recipients that suffered from acute rejections 1 year after depleting their B cells had an increase in their activated B cells and plasmablasts and a decrease in transitional $CD24^{hi}CD38^{hi}$ as well as in memory $CD24^{hi}CD27^{+}$ Bregs [12]. In agreement with the previous study, Svachova and colleagues found that in patients undergoing renal transplant rejection, transitional $CD24^{hi}CD38^{hi}$ B cells were absent [13]. In liver transplant patients, Zhou et al. observed a significant decrease in the $CD24^{hi}CD27^{+}$ memory B cells during allograft rejection, while a significant increase in the same population of B cells was found in patients that responded well to the anti-rejection drugs [14]. Collectively, these data outline the important role of B cells, particularly Bregs, in maintaining as well as inducing allograft tolerance. In the present chapter, we describe several techniques that can be applied to any cohort of patients, including transplant patients, and to healthy controls, focusing on human Breg phenotyping. We describe how to purify and coculture Bregs, and we include some methods to study the serum levels of anti-HLA antibodies as well as the anti-HLA cellular response from transplant patients.

2 Materials

2.1 General Equipment

1. 20 mL disposable plastic serological pipettes.
2. Pipette controller.
3. 50 mL conical sterile centrifuge tubes.
4. Temperature-controlled centrifuge.
5. Plastic sterile pipettes.
6. Sterile fluorescence-activated cell sorting (FACS) tubes with filters.
7. Sterile 96-well round-bottom plate.
8. 1.5 mL tubes or U-shape 96-well plate.
9. Time controlled shaker.
10. Vortex.
11. Flow cytometer (e.g., LSRFortessa) and related analysis software.
12. Cell sorter (e.g., BD FACSAria).
13. ELISPOT plate reader.

2.2 Buffers and Reagents

1. Density gradient medium for the isolation of mononuclear cells from peripheral blood (e.g., Lymphoprep and StemCell).
2. 1× sterile phosphate buffered saline (PBS).
3. FACS buffer: 0.5% fetal calf serum (FCS) and 2 mM EDTA in 1× PBS, on ice.
4. Trypan-blue.
5. Distilled water (dH_2O).

2.3 Antibodies and Reagents for Flow Cytometry

1. Dye for the discrimination of viable from nonviable cells in multicolor flow cytometric applications (e.g., Fixable Viability Stain 780, BD). Reconstitute and use the dye according to manufacturer's instructions.
2. Polystyrene microparticles for the optimization of fluorescence compensation settings in multicolor flow cytometric analyses (e.g., compbeads, BD). Purchase the beads according to the isotype of the antibodies used in the staining.
3. Fluorescent-conjugated human monoclonal antibodies (*see* Table 1).
4. 1× CellFix: dilute 10× concentrate CellFix (BD) 1:10 in dH_2O (*see* **Note 1**).
5. Fixation/permeabilization kit for intracellular staining.
6. Carboxyfluorescein succinimidyl ester (*CFSE*) for T-cell proliferation assay.
7. 4′,6-Diamidino-2-phenylindole (DAPI).

Table 1
List of antibodies required for phenotyping

Antibodies	Clone
Anti-human-CD19-BV650	HIB19
Anti-human-CD24-PE-CF594	ML5
Anti-human-CD38-BV421	HB-7
Anti-human-CD27-BV510	M-T271
Anti-human-CD138-Alexa700	MI15
Anti-human-IgD-FITC	lA6–2
Anti-human-IgM-APC	MHM-88
Anti-human-CD4-BUV395	RPA-T4
Anti-human-IFN-γ-FITC	B27
Anti-human-TNF-α-Alexa700	Mab11
Anti-human-IL-10-APC	JES3-19F1

2.4 Reagents for Cell Enrichment and Isolation

1. Human B cells isolation kit based on immunomagnetic separation (e.g., B Cell Isolation Kit II, human, Miltenyi).
2. Equipment for immunomagnetic separation (e.g., columns and magnets).
3. Human T cells isolation kit (e.g., RosetteSep human T-cell enrichment cocktail, Stemcell).
4. Human CD25 Microbeads II (Miltenyi).

2.5 Reagents for Cell Culture and Assay

1. Reagents for T-cell expansion and activation such as Human T activator CD3/CD28 Dynabeads (ThermoFisher). Alternative methods to activate human T cells can be used (*see* **Note 2**).
2. X-VIVO 15 medium: serum-free hematopoietic cell medium (*see* **Note 3**).
3. Phorbol myristate acetate (PMA) and ionomycin (*see* **Note 4**).
4. Brefeldin A Solution (1000×).

2.6 Reagents for Serum Anti-HLA Antibodies Detection

1. FlowPRA HLA Class I & II Screening kit (One Lambda Inc) which contains: HLA-Class I Screening Beads, HLA-Class II Screening Beads, 10× Wash Buffer, and 100× anti-Human IgG–FITC (*see* **Note 5**).
2. Fixing solution: dilute 1.35 mL of formaldehyde (37%) in 100 mL of PBS.

2.7 Enzyme-Linked Immunosorbent Spot (ELISPOT) Assay for the Detection of Anti-HLA Cellular Responses by IFN-γ

1. Human IFN-γ ELISPOT kit, which should contain anti-IFN-γ monoclonal coated plates, biotinylated detection monoclonal antibodies, streptavidin-alkaline phosphatase (ALP), 5-bromo-4-chloro-3-indolyl phosphate (BCIP)/nitro blue tetrazolium (NBT) plus substrate (*see* **Note 6**).
2. X-VIVO 15 medium containing 10% human AB serum.
3. 0.5% FCS in 1× PBS.
4. PBMCs isolated from patients that have received allograft.
5. Materials for recipient PBMCs activation (*see* **Note 7**).

3 Methods

3.1 Peripheral Blood Mononuclear Cells (PBMCs) Isolation

Whole blood components including red blood cells and plasma elements can block and slow the flow cytometry machine and can influence the results of coculture studies. For these reasons, for flow cytometry procedures, as well as for any culture or enrichment processes, it is preferable to work on purified PBMCs. Here below we describe the protocol for PBMCs isolation (*see* Fig. 1).

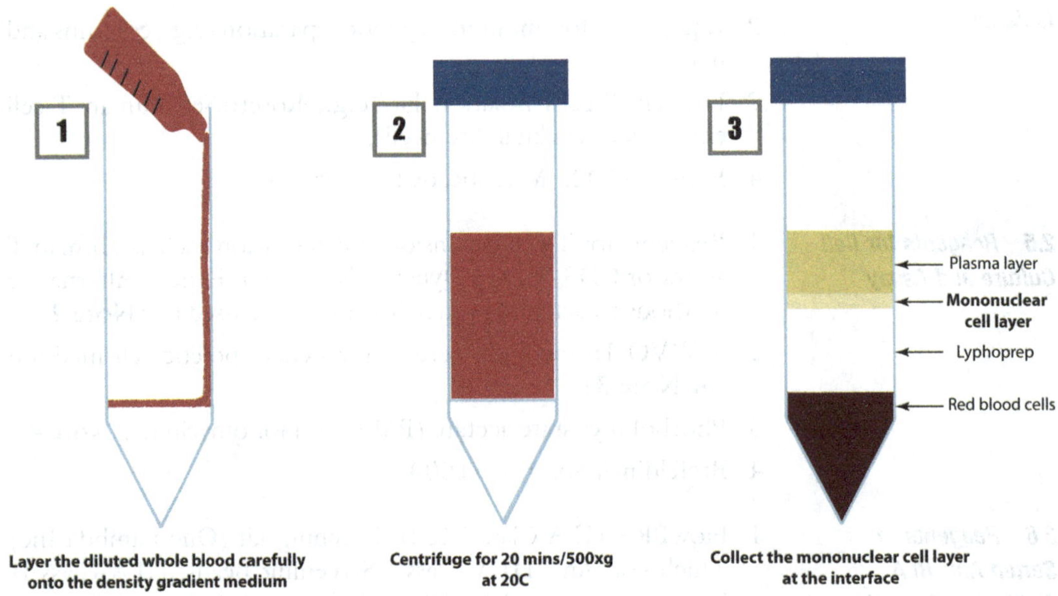

Fig. 1 Main steps of PBMC isolations from total blood. To isolate PBMCs from total blood, the diluted blood is layered over the density gradient medium, and, after centrifugation, the blood components are separated into plasma, mononuclear (PBMCs), and red blood cell layers

1. Dilute whole blood with sterile PBS at a ratio of 1:2.
2. Using disposable plastic serological pipettes, layer the diluted whole blood carefully onto the density gradient medium (e.g., Lymphoprep) in a sterile tube, following manufacturer's instructions.
3. Centrifuge the layered blood for 20 min/500 × *g* (low to no break) at 20°C.
4. Collect the mononuclear cell layer at the interface by sterile plastic pipettes and transfer it into new sterile tube.
5. Wash twice the transferred cell layer by adding sterile PBS to reach the top of the tube and centrifuging at 500 × *g* for 10 min at 4°C.
6. After washing, count the cells by using trypan-blue either manually by light microscope or by automated cell-counting machine.
7. Subsequently, use the isolated PBMCs for the different methods listed below including B cells phenotyping and enrichment.

3.2 B-Cell Subsets Phenotyping

1. Transfer 1–2 × 10^6 PBMCs per well into U-bottom-shaped 96-well plate, and centrifuge for 5 min at 200 × *g* at 4°C.
2. Add the cell viability dye. If using the Fixable Viability Stain 780, then mix 0.5 μL from the reconstituted dye in 1 mL PBS and transfer 200 μL into the well containing cells. Incubate in dark for 30 min at room temperature.
3. During incubation, prepare the appropriate anti-human antibody mix. For B-cell subsets phenotyping, add the fluorochrome-conjugated monoclonal antibodies to CD19, CD24, CD38, and CD27, optionally, and depending on the study antibodies to CD138, IgM, and IgD can be added (*see* Table 1). Dilute the antibodies in the mix as recommended by the manufacturer, which is usually 5 μL of each antibody per one million cells in a total of 100 μL FACS buffer. However, the antibodies concentration should be optimized to the minimum working dilution.
4. At the same time also prepare the compensation tubes by using the compensation beads. Follow manufacturer's instructions.
5. After incubation with the cell viability dye, wash the cells three times with PBS (200 × *g* for 5 min). Stain the cells by adding 100 μL of the prepared antibodies mix to the cell pellets.
6. Incubate for 20 min in the fridge at 4°C, then wash the cells twice with FACS buffer, and fix through 15 min incubation with 100 μL of 1× cellFix per well at 4°C.
7. After fixing, wash the cells twice and resuspend in 200 μL FACS buffer.
8. Acquire the cells by the flow cytometer and analyze the data using the appropriate software.

3.3 Isolation of B-Cell Subsets by FACS Sorting

Before sorting the B-cell subsets of interest (*see* Table 2) by FACS, it is advisable to isolate B cells from total PBMCs by immunomagnetic separation. Indeed, working on purified B cells allow to minimize the sorting time and to increase the purity of the isolated B-cell subsets by FACS. Wash the isolated PBMCs once by FACS buffer and, after discarding the supernatant, proceed to immunomagnetic separation following the instructions of the employed kit. Count the obtained cells by using trypan-blue and use the isolated B cells for B-cell subsets purification by FACS sorting.

1. Centrifuge the purified B cells for 5 min at 200 × *g* and discard the supernatant.
2. Stain the cell pellet, directly and without adding FACS buffer, with fluorochrome conjugated monoclonal antibodies (*see* Table 1) either to CD19, CD24, CD38 to study transitional Bregs, or to CD19, CD24, CD27 to study memory Bregs, in the concentrations recommended by the manufacturers or as optimized. Incubate the cells for 30 min at 4°C.
3. During incubation, prepare both the collection and the compensation tubes. For the collection tubes, add 300 μL of X-VIVO 15 medium into sterile FACS sorting tubes, and prepare the compensation beads as described by manufacturer's instructions.
4. At the end of incubation, wash the cells twice, once with FACS buffer and once with X-VIVO 15 medium. Subsequently, resuspend the cell pellet with 300 μL of X-VIVO 15 medium and keep everything on ice until the end of the sorting process (*see* **Note 8**).
5. Run samples on a cell sorter and collect populations of interest. If the initial staining contains antibodies for CD19, CD24, and CD38, then $CD19^{+}CD24^{hi}CD38^{hi}$ transitional Breg, $CD19^{+}CD24^{hi}CD38^{-}$ memory Breg, and $CD24^{int}CD38^{int}$

Table 2
B-cell subsets phenotyping

Phenotype	Population
$CD19^{+}CD24^{hi}CD27^{+}IgM^{hi}IgD^{hi}CD38^{-}$	Non-switched memory B cells
$CD19^{+}CD24^{hi}CD27^{+}CD38^{-}IgM^{-}IgD^{-}$	Switched memory B cells
$CD19^{+}CD24^{hi}CD38^{hi}CD27^{-}IgM^{hi}IgD^{hi}$	Transitional immature B cells
$CD19^{+}CD24^{inter}CD38^{inter}IgM^{+}IgD^{+}$	Naïve B cells
$CD19^{+}CD38^{hi}CD27^{hi}IgM^{lo}IgD^{-}CD24^{-}$	Plasmablast
$CD19^{+}CD38^{hi}CD27^{hi}IgM^{-}IgD^{-}CD24^{-}CD138^{+}$	Plasma cells
CD80, CD86, and CD69	B cells activation markers

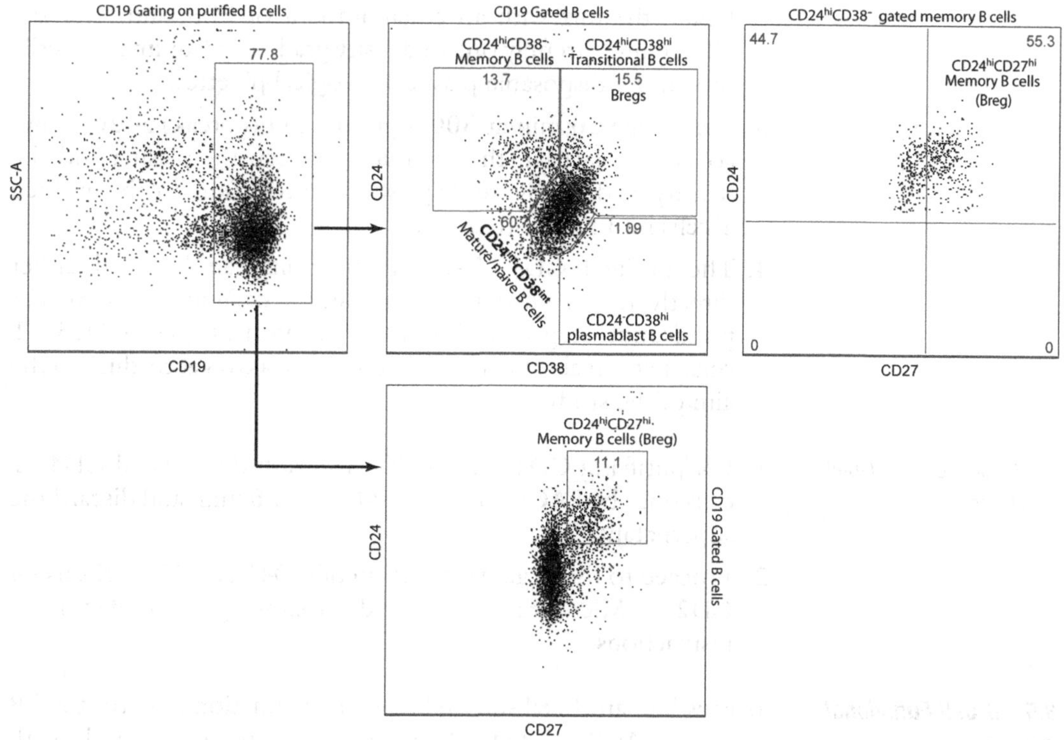

Fig. 2 Gating strategies for the identification of human CD24^{hi}CD38^{hi} and CD24^{hi}CD27^{+} regulatory B cells. Representative dot plots show the gating on CD19^{+} B cells as the initial step. Based on the fluorochrome-conjugated monoclonal antibodies used, the strategy follows in the gating of memory, transitional, mature, and plasmablast B cells and ends with the identification of CD27^{hi}CD24^{hi} memory B cells as represented at the top. Alternatively, CD19^{+} B cells can be directly analyzed for CD24 and CD27 expression, leading to the identification of CD24^{hi}CD27^{hi} memory B cells, as shown at the bottom

mature B cells can be isolated. If the initial staining contains antibodies for CD19, CD24, CD27, then CD19^{+}CD24^{hi}CD27^{hi} memory Breg and CD19^{+}CD24^{-}CD27^{-} non-Bregs can be collected (*see* Fig. 2).

3.4 CD4^{+}CD25^{-} T-Cell Enrichment

CD4 $^{+}$CD25^{-} T-cell enrichment requires a two-step procedure made of a first isolation of untouched CD4^{+} T cells and a subsequent purification of CD4^{+}CD25^{-} T cells by depleting CD4^{+}CD25^{+} T cells. Purified CD4^{+}CD25^{-} T cells are mainly used to study the effect of Bregs on regulatory T (Treg)-cell induction as well as Breg suppressive capacity on T cells' cytokines production and proliferation.

3.4.1 CD4^{+} T-Cell Enrichment

1. Add 50 μL of rosetteSep human T-cell enrichment cocktail to every 1 mL of whole blood and incubate for 20 min at room temperature on a rotator (*see* **Note 9**).

2. Dilute the mix with an equal amount of PBS, and layer the diluted mix carefully onto a density gradient medium in a sterile tube using disposable plastic serological pipettes.
3. Centrifuge 20 min at 500 × *g* (low to no break) at 20°C and collect the layer at the interface between the plasma and the density medium by sterile plastic pipettes. Transfer the purified T cells into a new sterile tube.
4. The purified $CD4^+$ T-cell populations can be used either directly for in vitro functional assays or undergo a further purification step that allows the isolation of $CD4^+CD25^-$ T cells that can also be used for functional assays according to the aim of the study.

3.4.2 $CD4^+CD25^-$ T-Cell Enrichment

1. For purifying $CD4^+CD25^-$ T cells, wash the isolated $CD4^+$ T cells once by FACS buffer at 200 × *g* for 5 min, and discard the supernatant.
2. Proceed to the negative selection of $CD4^+CD25^-$ T cells using CD25 Microbeads II and following manufacturer's instructions.

3.5 B-Cell Functional Assays

To asses human B-cell subsets' regulatory function in vitro, total B cells or FACS sorted B-cell subsets are cocultured with $CD4^+CD25^-$ effector T cells. After incubation, the suppression capacity of B cells is measured through evaluating T-cell proliferation by flow cytometry and cytokines production either by flow cytometry (intracellular) or ELISA (extracellular, in cell culture supernatant).

3.5.1 Suppression Assay: T-Cell Proliferation

One of the major challenges facing the field of transplantation is the management of immunosuppression, and, in this view, the study of the immunosuppressive properties of B cells acquires even greater relevance. One way to measure the regulatory function of B cells is by coculturing effector $CD4^+CD25^-$ T cells isolated from HLA-$A2^+$ individuals with total B cells or FACS-sorted B-cell subsets that are obtained from HLA-$A2^-$ individuals. Indeed, the HLA-A2 mismatch is an additional method to allow the two populations (T cells and B cells) to be distinguished when acquired by FACS to measure T cells' proliferation.

1. Stain the effector T cells with 2.5 μM CFSE by adding the CFSE solution to the cells, and incubate for 5 min in the dark at room temperature.
2. Wash the CFSE stained effector T cells twice with X-VIVO 15 medium, and then resuspend the cells in X-VIVO 15 medium at one million cells/mL.

3. Activate the CFSE stained effector T cells by adding the appropriate amount of anti-CD3/CD28 activator beads as recommended by the manufacturer. Keep some non-stimulated CFSE stained effector T cells without anti-CD3/CD28 activator beads to be used as a control.
4. Place the non-activated and the anti-CD3/CD28 beads activated effector T cells into a 96-well plate at 1–2 × 10^5 cells per well according to the number of cells obtained after purifying both the effector T cells and, most importantly, the Breg cells obtained after sorting (*see* **Note 10**).
5. Wash the total B cells or FACS-sorted B-cell subsets with X-VIVO 15 medium, and coculture them at 1:1 ratio with activated effector T cells. As a control, one well for both activated as well as non-activated effector T cells should be left without B cells. Incubate the cells for 5 days at 37°C with 5% CO_2.
6. After incubation, spin the cells at 200 × *g* for 5 min, discard the supernatant and wash twice with PBS.
7. Stain the cells with a cell viability dye and then with fluorochrome-conjugated monoclonal antibodies to CD19 and CD4 (*see* Table 1). Refer to Subheading 3.2 for the protocol of cell surface staining.
8. Acquire the cells by flow cytometry and analyze CFSE profile to assess the suppression of T-cell proliferation (*see* Fig. 3).

3.5.2 Suppression Assay: Cytokines Quantification by Intracellular Cytokine Staining

1. Set up the $CD4^+CD25^-$ T cells/B cells (total or FACS sorted) coculture as in Subheading 3.5.1 (do not stain the cells with CFSE). Incubate the cells for 3 days at 37°C with 5% CO_2.
2. Following the 3 days coculture, carefully collect 100 μL of the supernatants from each well without touching the cells at the

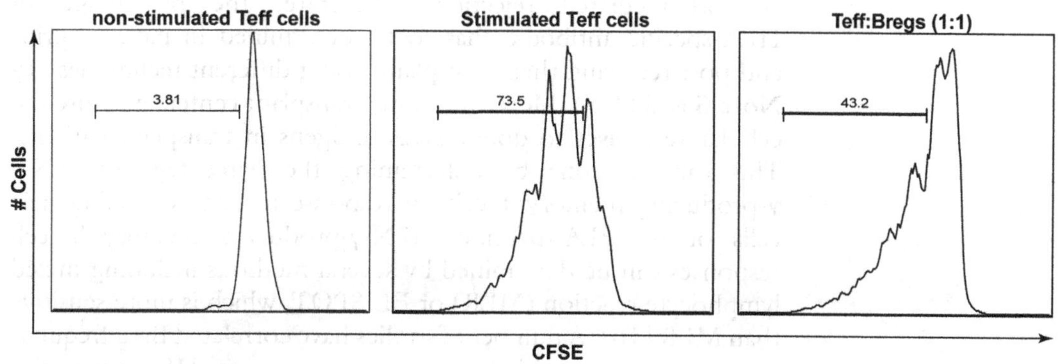

Fig. 3 $CD4^+CD25^-$ T-cell proliferation and suppression. Representative histograms showing non-stimulated and CD3/CD28 beads stimulated $CD4^+CD25^-$ T (Teff) cells, as well as the suppression of beads-activated Teff proliferation by Bregs upon coculturing at 1:1 ratio

bottom of the well (*see* **Note 11**). Top up the wells with 100 μL of new X-VIVO 15 medium and then add 50 ng/mL PMA, 250 ng/mL Ionomycin, and brefeldin A (1:1000) for 4–5 h at 37°C.

3. After the incubation, spin the cells at 200 × *g* for 5 min, discard the supernatant and wash twice with PBS.
4. Stain the cells with a cell viability dye and then with fluorochrome-conjugated monoclonal antibodies to CD19 and CD4 (*see* Table 1). Refer to Subheading 3.2 for the protocol of cell surface staining.
5. Following cell surface staining, fix the cells for 30 min in fridge with the intracellular fixative solution, then wash twice the cells with 1× permeabilization buffer at 200 × *g* for 5 min.
6. Incubate the cells with 1× permeabilization buffer for 30 min in the fridge. During incubation, prepare the mix of the fluorochrome conjugated monoclonal antibodies to IL-10, TNF-α, IL17, and IFN-γ (*see* Table 1) at the recommended concentrations by the providing company in a final volume of 100 μL of 1× permeabilization buffer per well.
7. Spin the cells and resuspend with the appropriate fluorochrome-conjugated monoclonal antibodies mix. Incubate for 20 min at 4°C.
8. Wash the cells twice with 1× permeabilization buffer, then one last wash with FACS buffer.
9. Resuspend the cells with 200 μL of FACS buffer and acquire by flow cytometry (*see* **Note 12**).

3.6 HLA-Related Testing

In the immunopathogenesis of allograft rejection, an important role is played by the immune response against human leukocyte antigens (HLA). For years, B cells have been known to be the cells producing the antibodies against donor HLA antigens, leading to antibody-mediated rejection. Therefore, the percentage of HLA-specific antibodies has to be determined in patients prior and post receiving their transplant, using different techniques (*see* **Note 5** and [15]). Moreover, some transplant centers measure the cellular responses to donor HLA antigens in transplant patients. This can be done by determining the percentage of IFN-γ-producing memory T cells in response to panels of allogeneic cells or to HLA peptides. IFN-γ-producing memory T cell responses can be determined by several methods including mixed lymphocyte reaction (MLR) or ELISPOT, which is more sensitive than MLR [16]. A number of studies have correlated Breg frequencies and function with the levels of serum anti-HLA antibodies or/and anti-HLA cellular responses in transplant patients. In this view, the following two sections discuss the methods for measuring the levels of anti-HLA antibodies in the serum and anti-HLA cellular response.

3.6.1 Detection of Serum Anti-HLA Antibodies

The FlowPRA kit is an assay used to detect anti-HLA antibodies in human sera using flow cytometry. We suggest using this kit since it is easy to follow. However, the user can replace it by another antigen-coated beads technology such as Luminex that is based on a similar principle (*see* **Note 5**). To preform FlowPRA beads test, follow the manufacturer's instructions and acquire the samples using flow cytometry.

3.6.2 Assessment of Anti-HLA Cellular Response

One of the assays that allows to assess the anti-HLA cellular responses is the dosage of IFN-γ by ELISPOT. Generally, IFN- γ ELISPOT is done in a 96-well plate coated with capture antibodies against IFN-γ, and then the cells of interest are added to the wells with or without the antigens. To measure the anti-donor responses by transplant patients the antigens are either donor PBMC or HLA peptides (*see* Table 3). After an incubation, IFN-γ is secreted by the recipient cells and captured by the coating specific antibodies. Subsequently, the cells are washed out, and anti-IFN-γ biotinylated detection antibodies are added to bind to the IFN-γ captured by the coating antibodies. Next, an enzyme conjugated to streptavidin is added, and then precipitated with precipitating substrate. After incubation and upon the emergence of coloured spots, each spot represents a single IFN-γ secreting cell that is counted by image-based reader. The final readout is represented as the number of cells producing IFN-γ per the number of the plated cells.

Table 3
Test suspensions for the ELISPOT plate

Responder cells	Activating antigens	Final volume per well
4–5 × 10^5 recipient PBMCs, isolated from patients that received the allograft.	20 μg/mL HLA-derived peptides. For HLA peptides design and synthesis, reader is referred to reference [17].	100 μL of X-VIVO 15 medium containing 10% human AB serum
3 × 10^5 recipient PBMCs, isolated from patients that received allograft.	(a) 3 × 10^5 CD3 depleted living donor PBMCs, (b) 3 × 10^5 CD2 depleted dead donor splenocytes, or (c) 3 × 10^5 bank splenocytes. (*see* **Note 7**)	100 μL of X-VIVO 15 medium containing 10% human AB serum.
Positive controls, 3 × 10^5 recipient PBMCs	(a) 10 μg/mL PPD, or/and (b 100 ng/mL anti-CD3 antibodies.	100 μL of X-VIVO 15 medium containing 10% human AB serum
Negative control, with or without 3 × 10^5 recipient PBMCs	No activating antigens	100 μL of X-VIVO 15 medium containing 10% human AB serum

1. Prepare the anti-IFN-γ ELISPOT plate under sterile conditions by washing the plate four times with 200 μL PBS per well, then incubate 200 μL X-VIVO 15 medium containing 10% human AB serum per well for 30 min at room temperature to prime the plate.
2. After preparing the ELISPOT plate, remove the X-VIVO 15 medium containing 10% human AB serum and add the test suspension under sterile conditions. The test suspension can differ depending on the way PBMCs are activated (*see* Table 3).
3. After adding the test suspension to the ELISPOT plate, incubate at 37°C with 5% CO_2 for 48 h.
4. After the incubation, remove the cells and wash the plate by adding 200 μL PBS per well. Dilute the detection antibody to 1 μg/mL with 0.5% FCS-PBS and transfer 100 μL per well.
5. Incubate for 2 h at room temperature, subsequently wash as described in **step 4**, then add 100 μL per well from the 1:1000 diluted streptavidin-ALP in 0.5% FCS-PBS.
6. Following 1 hour incubation at room temperature, wash the plate as described in **step 4**, and add 100 μL per well from the filtered ready to use substrate solution.
7. Wash the plate extensively with tap water upon the development of distinct spots to stop the color expansion and leave the plate to dry.
8. Count the spots by using ELISPOT reader.

4 Notes

1. If the cells will not be acquired on the same day (within a maximum of 5 days post-staining), it is useful to fix cells after immunofluorescence staining with monoclonal antibodies and prior to flow cytometric analysis. BD CellFIX™ can be used to fix human peripheral blood cell suspensions.
2. Human T activator CD3/CD28 Dynabeads is the most commonly used reagent to activate human T cells. Alternatively, in vitro T-cell activation can be performed by a step protocol. Prepare a 10-μg/mL solution of anti-CD3 (clone UCHT1) antibody in PBS and coat a 96-well plate overnight at 4 °C. After washing with PBS, add 1×10^5 T cells per well together with anti-CD28 (clone CD28.2) antibody at 5 μg/mL.
3. We have been using the X-VIVO 15 serum-free hematopoietic cell medium for culture and coculture experiments because it is modified to support CD3 T cells' proliferation, and it can also be supplemented with L-glutamine and gentamicin to prevent

the growth of gram-positive, gram-negative, and mycoplasma. However, X-VIVO 15 medium can be replaced with RPMI 1640 medium supplemented with 100 U/mL penicillin/streptomycin.

4. PMA and ionomycin can be replaced by the Cell Activation Cocktail (without Brefeldin A, BioLegend), a pre-mixed cocktail with optimized concentrations of PMA and ionomycin. It is ready to use, just follow the manufacturer's instructions. However, price wise buying PMA and ionomycin individually is much cheaper, and once optimized the same setting can be used all the time.
5. Anti-HLA antibodies can be detected with several methods including complement-dependent cytotoxicity (CDC), enzyme-linked immunosorbent assay, or by using antigen-coated beads technology (Luminex or FlowPRA). For many years, CDC has been used as the golden method to detect anti-HLA class I and II antibodies; however, this method has been replaced by the antigen-coated beads technology due to its high sensitivity. The results obtained from both the Luminex and FlowPRA methods are represented as panel reaction antibody (PRA), which indicates the percentage of cells or HLA-coated beads that provide positive reaction with patient serum. Both Luminex and FlowPRA have the same principle; therefore, any technique can be utilized based on the user preference. The major supplier company providing kits to detect anti-HLA class I and II is One Lambda, Thermo Fisher Scientific.
6. The positive control for this assay is constituted by anti-CD3 monoclonal antibody-stimulated PBMCs. The user can optionally decide to include one additional positive control such as purified protein derivative (PPD), which is known as a powerful PBMCs stimulator.
7. Recipient PBMCs can be activated in transplant by several methods. A method requires the usage of nonpolymorphic HLA-derived peptides (for peptide design refer to reference [17]). Instead, in the case of donor-specific ELISPOT, CD2-depleted splenocytes from dead donors and CD3-depleted living donor PBMCs are needed. CD2 and CD3 depletion can be made by using StemCell kits, following manufacturer's instructions. The test can also include splenocytes collected from different donors (bank) to investigate the recipient immune response to HLA class I and class II complete mismatch.
8. DAPI can be used to follow viable cells during FACS sorting by adding 1:1000 into the cells just before acquiring.

9. Through the rosetteSep human T-cell enrichment cocktail, T cells are isolated by negative selection. Unwanted cells are crosslinked to red blood cells that pellet during standard density gradient centrifugation, allowing T-cell isolation. Kits to isolate T cells are not limited to rosetteSep, but other companies such as Miltenyi provide several kits with the same quality.
10. Keep in mind that Bregs number after sorting are usually very low allowing to test the cells regulatory function only at a ratio of 1:1.
11. The collected supernatants can be stored at −80°C to be used in the future to measure the produced cytokines by the cocultured cells via several techniques such as ELISA.
12. Remember to prepare compensation tubes each time prior to acquiring cells by flow cytometry, as well as control wells including wells that contain only non-activated, wells containing only activated cells, and wells with activated cells for isotype staining.

References

1. Lefaucheur C, Nochy D, Andrade J, Verine J, Gautreau C, Charron D, Hill GS, Glotz D, Suberbielle-Boissel C (2009) Comparison of combination plasmapheresis/IVIg/anti-CD20 versus high-dose IVIg in the treatment of antibody-mediated rejection. Am J Transplant 9(5):1099–1107. https://doi.org/10.1111/j.1600-6143.2009.02591.x
2. Clatworthy MR, Watson CJ, Plotnek G, Bardsley V, Chaudhry AN, Bradley JA, Smith KG (2009) B-cell-depleting induction therapy and acute cellular rejection. N Engl J Med 360 (25):2683–2685. https://doi.org/10.1056/NEJMc0808481
3. Newell KA, Asare A, Kirk AD, Gisler TD, Bourcier K, Suthanthiran M, Burlingham WJ, Marks WH, Sanz I, Lechler RI, Hernandez-Fuentes MP, Turka LA, Seyfert-Margolis VL, Immune Tolerance Network STSG (2010) Identification of a B cell signature associated with renal transplant tolerance in humans. J Clin Invest 120(6):1836–1847. https://doi.org/10.1172/JCI39933
4. Sagoo P, Perucha E, Sawitzki B, Tomiuk S, Stephens DA, Miqueu P, Chapman S, Craciun L, Sergeant R, Brouard S, Rovis F, Jimenez E, Ballow A, Giral M, Rebollo-Mesa I, Le Moine A, Braudeau C, Hilton R, Gerstmayer B, Bourcier K, Sharif A, Krajewska M, Lord GM, Roberts I, Goldman M, Wood KJ, Newell K, Seyfert-Margolis V, Warrens AN, Janssen U, Volk HD, Soulillou JP, Hernandez-Fuentes MP, Lechler RI (2010) Development of a cross-platform biomarker signature to detect renal transplant tolerance in humans. J Clin Invest 120(6):1848–1861. https://doi.org/10.1172/JCI39922
5. Chesneau M, Michel L, Dugast E, Chenouard A, Baron D, Pallier A, Durand J, Braza F, Guerif P, Laplaud DA, Soulillou JP, Giral M, Degauque N, Chiffoleau E, Brouard S (2015) Tolerant kidney transplant patients produce B cells with regulatory properties. J Am Soc Nephrol 26(10):2588–2598. https://doi.org/10.1681/ASN.2014040404
6. Rebollo-Mesa I, Nova-Lamperti E, Mobillo P, Runglall M, Christakoudi S, Norris S, Smallcombe N, Kamra Y, Hilton R, Bhandari S, Baker R, Berglund D, Carr S, Game D, Griffin S, Kalra PA, Lewis R, Mark PB, Marks S, Macphee I, McKane W, Mohaupt MG, Pararajasingam R, Kon SP, Seron D, Sinha MD, Tucker B, Viklicky O, Lechler RI, Lord GM, Hernandez-Fuentes MP, Indices of Tolerance EUC (2016) Biomarkers of Tolerance in kidney transplantation: are we predicting Tolerance or response to immunosuppressive treatment? Am J Transplant 16(12):3443–3457. https://doi.org/10.1111/ajt.13932
7. Alhabbab RY, Nova-Lamperti E, Aravena O, Burton HM, Lechler RI, Dorling A, Lombardi G (2019) Regulatory B cells: development, phenotypes, functions, and role in

transplantation. Immunol Rev 292 (1):164–179. https://doi.org/10.1111/imr.12800
8. Cherukuri A, Salama AD, Carter C, Smalle N, McCurtin R, Hewitt EW, Hernandez-Fuentes-M, Clark B, Baker RJ (2012) An analysis of lymphocyte phenotype after steroid avoidance with either Alemtuzumab or Basiliximab induction in renal transplantation. Am J Transplant 12(4):919–931. https://doi.org/10.1111/j.1600-6143.2011.03891.x
9. Cherukuri A, Rothstein DM, Clark B, Carter CR, Davison A, Hernandez-Fuentes M, Hewitt E, Salama AD, Baker RJ (2014) Immunologic human renal allograft injury associates with an altered IL-10/TNF-alpha expression ratio in regulatory B cells. J Am Soc Nephrol 25(7):1575–1585. https://doi.org/10.1681/ASN.2013080837
10. Shabir S, Girdlestone J, Briggs D, Kaul B, Smith H, Daga S, Chand S, Jham S, Navarrete C, Harper L, Ball S, Borrows R (2015) Transitional B lymphocytes are associated with protection from kidney allograft rejection: a prospective study. Am J Transplant 15(5):1384–1391. https://doi.org/10.1111/ajt.13122
11. Latorre I, Esteve-Sole A, Redondo D, Giest S, Argilaguet J, Alvarez S, Peligero C, Forstmann I, Crespo M, Pascual J, Meyerhans A (2016) Calcineurin and mTOR inhibitors have opposing effects on regulatory T cells while reducing regulatory B cell populations in kidney transplant recipients. Transpl Immunol 35:1–6. https://doi.org/10.1016/j.trim.2016.01.004
12. Schlosser HA, Thelen M, Dieplinger G, von Bergwelt-Baildon A, Garcia-Marquez M, Reuter S, Shimabukuro-Vornhagen A, Wennhold K, Haustein N, Buchner D, Heiermann N, Kleinert R, Wahba R, Ditt V, Kurschat C, Cingoz T, Becker J, Stippel DL, von Bergwelt-Baildon M (2017) Prospective analyses of circulating B cell subsets in ABO-compatible and ABO-incompatible kidney transplant recipients. Am J Transplant 17 (2):542–550. https://doi.org/10.1111/ajt.14013
13. Svachova V, Sekerkova A, Hruba P, Tycova I, Rodova M, Cecrdlova E, Slatinska J, Honsova E, Striz I, Viklicky O (2016) Dynamic changes of B-cell compartments in kidney transplantation: lack of transitional B cells is associated with allograft rejection. Transpl Int 29(5):540–548. https://doi.org/10.1111/tri.12751
14. Zhou H, Zhan F, Zhang H, Gu J, Mu X, Gao J, Rao J, Ji G, Ni X, Lu L, Xia Y (2019) The proportion of CD19(+)CD24(hi)CD27(+) regulatory B cells predicts the occurrence of acute allograft rejection in liver transplantation. Ann Transl Med 7(18):465. https://doi.org/10.21037/atm.2019.08.05
15. Uffing A, Hidalgo LG, McMullan C, Perry J, Milford EL, Murakami N, Yeung MY, Guleria I, Wood IG, Akalin E, Azzi J, Chandraker AK, Riella LV (2019) Preformed donor-specific antibodies against HLA class II and graft outcomes in deceased-donor kidney transplantation. Transplant Direct 5(5):e446. https://doi.org/10.1097/TXD.0000000000000893
16. Zitzner JR, Tambur AR (2012) Role of ELISPOT assays in risk assessment pre- and post-kidney transplantation. Cell 1(2):100–110. https://doi.org/10.3390/cells1020100
17. Smith HJ, Hanvesakul R, Bentall A, Shabir S, Morgan MD, Briggs D, Cockwell P, Borrows R, Larche M, Ball S (2011) T lymphocyte responses to nonpolymorphic HLA-derived peptides are associated with chronic renal allograft dysfunction. Transplantation 91(3):279–286. https://doi.org/10.1097/TP.0b013e318203862d

INDEX

Francesca Mion and Silvia Tonon (eds.), *Regulatory B Cells: Methods and Protocols*, Methods in Molecular Biology, vol. 2270, https://doi.org/10.1007/978-1-0716-1237-8, © Springer Science+Business Media, LLC, part of Springer Nature 2021

Q

R

S

T

U

V

W

9781071612361